Acquired Speech and Language Disorders

Acquired Speech and Language Disorders: A Neuroanatomical and Functional Neurological Approach

Second Edition

Bruce E. Murdoch

Director
Centre for Neurogenic Communication Disorders Research
The University of Queensland

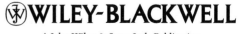

A John Wiley & Sons, Ltd., Publication

KH

Wiley-Blackwell is an imprint of John Wiley & Sons, formed by the merger of Wiley's global Scientific, Technical and Medical business with Blackwell Publishing.

Registered office
John Wiley & Sons Ltd, The Atrium, Southern Gate, Chichester, West Sussex, PO19 8SQ, United Kingdom

Editorial office
John Wiley & Sons Ltd, The Atrium, Southern Gate, Chichester, West Sussex, PO19 8SQ, United Kingdom

For details of our global editorial offices, for customer services and for information about how to apply for permission to reuse the copyright material in this book please see our website at www.wiley.com/wiley-blackwell.

Library of Congress Cataloging-in-Publication Data

Murdoch, B. E., 1950–
    Acquired speech and language disorders : a neuroanatomical and functional neurological approach / Bruce E. Murdoch. – 2nd ed.
        p. ; cm.
    Includes bibliographical references and index.
    ISBN 978-0-470-02567-3 (pbk. : alk. paper)   1. Language disorders.   2. Brain damage.
3. Neuroanatomy.   I. Title.
    [DNLM: 1. Language Disorders–physiopathology.   2. Speech Disorders–physiopathology.
3. Language Disorders–etiology.   4. Nervous System–anatomy & histology.   5. Nervous System Diseases–complications.   6. Speech Disorders–etiology. WL 340.2 M974a 2010]
    RC423.M738 2010
    616.85'5–dc22

A catalogue record for this book is available from the British Library.   2009014223

Set in 10/12 pt Sabon by Aptara®, Inc., New Delhi, India

1   2010

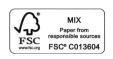

11/17/16

Contents

Neuroanatomical and neuropathological framework of speech and language

1

Introduction

Human communication in the form of speech-language behaviour is dependent upon processes which occur in the nervous system. Consequently, knowledge of the basic structure and function of the human nervous system is an essential pre-requisite to the understanding of the anatomical, physiological and pathological basis of human communication disorders. With this in mind, the materials presented in the present chapter are in-tended to provide the reader with an introductory knowledge of the anatomy of the human nervous system. Such knowledge is necessary prior to dis-cussion of the signs, symptoms and neurological mechanisms underlying the various acquired neu-rogenic speech-language disorders in later chap-ters. Where necessary, more detailed information regarding the anatomy of specific brain structures important for speech-language function is pro-vided in subsequent relevant chapters.

The nervous system is an extremely complex organization of structures which serves as the main regulative and integrative system of the body. It receives stimuli from the individual's in-ternal and external environments, interprets and integrates that information and selects and ini-tiates appropriate responses to it. Consider this process in the context of a spoken conversation between two persons. The words spoken by one partner in the conversation, in the form of sound waves, are detected by receptors in the inner ear of the second partner and conveyed to the cere-bral cortex of the brain via the auditory pathways where they are perceived and interpreted. Follow-ing integration with other sensory information, a response to the verbal input is formulated in the language centres of the brain and then passed to the motor areas of the brain (i.e. areas that con-trol muscular movement) for execution. Nerve impulses from the motor areas then pass to the muscles of the speech mechanism (e.g. tongue, lips, larynx, etc.) leading to the production of a verbal response by the second person.

Speech is produced by the contraction of the muscles of the speech mechanism, which include the muscles of the lips, jaw, tongue, palate, phar-ynx and larynx as well as the muscles of respi-ration. These muscle contractions, in turn, are controlled by nerve impulses which descend from the motor areas of the brain to the level of the brainstem and spinal cord and then pass out to the muscles of the speech mechanism via the var-ious nerves which arise from either the base of the brain (cranial nerves) or spinal cord (spinal nerves). Likewise, language is also dependent on processes which occur in the brain, particularly in the cerebral cortex.

Gross anatomy of the nervous system

For the purposes of description, the nervous system can be arbitrarily divided into two large divisions: the central nervous system and the peripheral nervous system. The central nervous system comprises the brain and spinal cord, while the peripheral nervous system consists of the end organs, nerves and ganglia, which connect the central nervous system to other parts of the body. The major components of the peripheral nervous system are the nerves which arise from the base of the brain and spinal cord. These include 12 pairs of cranial nerves and 31 pairs of spinal nerves respectively. The peripheral nervous system is often further subdivided into the somatic and autonomic nervous systems, the somatic nervous system including those nerves involved in the control of skeletal muscles (e.g. the muscles of the speech mechanism) and the autonomic nervous system including those nerves involved in the regulation of involuntary structures such as the heart, the smooth muscles of the gastrointestinal tract and

exocrine glands (e.g. sweat glands). Although the autonomic nervous system is described as part of the peripheral nervous system, it is really part of both the central and peripheral nervous systems. It must be remembered, however, that these divisions are arbitrary and artificial and that the nervous system functions as an entity, not in parts. The basic organization of the nervous system is summarized in Figure 1.1.

Histology of the nervous system

Cell types

The nervous system comprises many millions of nerve cells, or neurones, which are held together and supported by specialized non-conducting cells known as neuroglia. The major types of neuroglia include astrocytes, oligodendrocytes and microglia. It is the neurones that are responsible for conduction of nerve impulses from one part of the body to another, such as from the central nervous system to the muscles of the speech mechanism to produce the movement of the lips, tongue and so on for speech production. Although there are a number of different types of neurones, most consist of three basic parts: a cell body (also known as a soma or perikaryon) which houses the

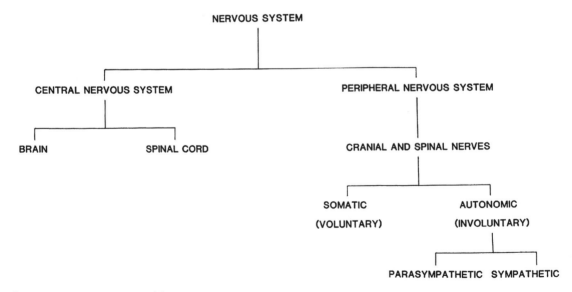

Figure 1.1 Basic organization of the nervous system.

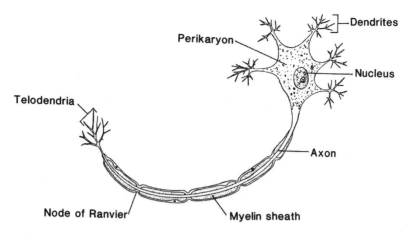

Figure 1.2 Structure of a typical motor neurone.

nucleus of the cell; a variable number of short processes (generally no more than a few millimetres in length) called dendrites (meaning 'tree-like') which receive stimuli and conduct nerve impulses; and a single, usually elongated, process called an axon, which in the majority of neurones is surrounded by a segmented fatty insulating sheath called the myelin sheath. A schematic representation of a neurone is shown in Figure 1.2.

The cytoplasm of a neurone contains the usual cell organelles (e.g. mitochondria) with the exception of the centrosome. Mature neurones cannot divide or replace themselves because of the lack of a centrosome. In addition to the usual organelles, however, the cytoplasm of nerve cells also contains two organelles unique to neurones: Nissl substance (chromidial substance) and neurofibrils. Seen with the light microscope Nissl substance (bodies) appears as rather large granules widely scattered throughout the cytoplasm of the nerve cell body. Nissl bodies specialize in protein synthesis, thereby providing the protein needs for maintaining and regenerating neurone processes and for renewing chemicals involved in the transmission of nerve impulses from one neurone to another. Seen with the light microscope neurofibrils are tiny tubular structures running through the cell body, axon and dendrites. Although the function of the neurofibrils is uncertain, it has been suggested that they may facilitate the transport of intracellular materials within the neurone.

In Alzheimer's disease, the neurofibrils become abnormally twisted, a feature used in the diagnosis of this condition (see Chapter 6).

In contrast to neurones, neuroglial cells (also often simply referred to as glial cells) contribute to brain function mainly by supporting neuronal functions. Although based on current evidence their role appears to be subordinate to that of the neurones, without glial cells the brain could not function properly. Astrocytes are the most numerous of the glial cells and are widely distributed in the central nervous system. These cells fill spaces between neurones and lie in close proximity to both neurones and capillaries. Evidence suggests that an essential role for astrocytes is the regulation of the chemical content of the extracellular space (e.g. astrocytes envelop synaptic junctions in the brain and thereby restrict the spread of neurotransmitter molecules released by neurones). Further, special proteins found within the membranes of astrocytes may be involved in the removal of many neurotransmitters from the synaptic cleft. In addition to regulating neurotransmitters, astrocytes also regulate the concentration of substances present within the extracellular space that have the potential to interfere with normal functioning of the neurones (e.g. astrocytes regulate the concentration of potassium ions in the extracellular fluid in the brain).

Oligodendrocytes and Schwann cells are two types of glial cells that form the insulation or myelin sheath that surrounds axons in the central and peripheral nervous systems respectively. Oligodendrocytes are only found in the central nervous system (i.e. brain and spinal cord), where they may wrap layers of membrane to form a myelin sheath around several axons. Schwann cells in contrast are located only in the peripheral nervous system, where they myelinate only a single axon. Periodical gaps in the myelin sheath are known as nodes of Ranvier. Nerve impulses travelling down myelinated axons jump from node to node, thereby increasing the speed of transmission, a process known as saltatory conduction.

Other neuroglial cells include ependymal cells and microglia. Ependymal cells provide the lining of fluid-filled cavities within the brain called the ventricles and thereby form a barrier between ventricular fluid and the neuronal substance of the brain. They also form the choroid plexuses, which produce cerebrospinal fluid. Microglia are few in number and small in size and function as phagocytes to remove debris left by dead or degenerating neurones and glial cells.

Synapses and neuroeffector junctions

The axon conducts nerve impulses away from the cell body to the next neurone or to a muscle or gland. The area where two neurones communicate with one another is called a synapse. It represents a region of functional but not anatomical continuity between the axon terminal of one neurone (the pre-synaptic neurone) and the dendrites, cell body or axon of another neurone (the post-synaptic neurone). The synapse is an area where a great degree of control can be exerted over nerve impulses. At the synapse, nerve impulses can be either blocked (inhibited) or facilitated. Axons branch repeatedly, forming anywhere from 1000 to 10 000 synapses. Consequently, there may be thousands of synapses on the surface of a single neurone. When one considers that there are billions of neurones, the complexity of the circuitry of the nervous system is staggering. It has been estimated that the number of synapses in the brain is possibly in the order of 100 trillion. Whether a specific neurone fires is dependent on the summation of the messages it receives from multiple sources.

Structurally, each synapse is made up as follows. As the terminal part of an axon approaches another neurone, it decreases in diameter, loses its myelin (if a myelinated fibre) and divides repeatedly forming small branches, termed telodendria. At the end of each telodendron is a small swelling called a bouton terminal or synaptic knob. The structure of the bouton terminal has been elucidated by electron microscopy. It contains a number of structures, in particular mitochondria and synaptic vesicles. The synaptic vesicles contain a neurotransmitter substance which is released when a nerve impulse arrives at the bouton. There are many kinds of neurotransmitter substance, some of which facilitate (excitatory transmitters) nerve impulse conduction in the post-synaptic neurone while others inhibit (inhibitory transmitters) nerve impulse conduction in the post-synaptic neurone. Some of the more common neurotransmitter substances include acetylcholine, norepinephrine, serotonin, dopamine and gamma aminobutyric acid (GABA).

When released from the synaptic knob the chemical transmitter diffuses across a gap called the synaptic cleft between the bouton and the membrane of the post-synaptic neurone to either excite or inhibit the post-synaptic neurone. As neurotransmitter substance is only located on the pre-synaptic side, a synapse can transmit in only one direction. In addition to the chemical synapses just described, in certain parts of the nervous system electrical synapses or gap junctions are present. In this type of synapse the membranes of the pre- and post-synaptic neurones lie in close proximity to one another and comprise a pathway of low resistance which allows current flow from the pre-synaptic neurone to act upon the post-synaptic neurone.

Neuroeffector junctions are functional contacts between axon terminals and effector cells. Structurally, neuroeffector junctions are similar to synapses with the exception that the post-synaptic structure is not a nerve cell but rather a muscle or gland. We will not concern ourselves greatly with junctions with smooth or cardiac muscles or glands, but will rather concentrate on junctions with skeletal muscles, as this is the type of muscle tissue that comprises the muscles of the speech mechanism.

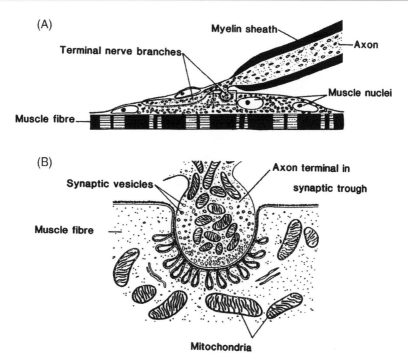

Figure 1.3 (A) Motor end plate. (B) Close-up of a motor end plate showing the relationship between structures in nerve cell and muscle.

In the case of skeletal muscles, the neuroeffector junction is termed a motor end plate. The structure of a typical motor end plate is shown in Figure 1.3.

Each motor nerve fibre branches at its end to form a complex of branching nerve terminals, each terminal innervating a separate skeletal muscle fibre. A single axon of a motor neurone, therefore, innervates more than one skeletal muscle fibre; the motor neurone plus the muscle fibres it innervates constitute a motor unit. The bouton of each terminal contains synaptic vesicles that contain neurotransmitter substance. The motor neurones running to skeletal muscles use acetylcholine as their transmitter substance. The arrival of a nerve impulse at the bouton causes release of acetylcholine from the vesicles in a similar manner to that for transmission at the synapse, only in this case the transmitter diffuses across the neuromuscular junction to cause contraction of the muscle fibre. In the condition called 'myasthenia gravis' there is a failure, possibly as a consequence of antibodies that interfere with the transmission of the acetylcholine. The result is that the mus-

cles of the body, including the muscles of the speech mechanism, fatigue very easily when active. Where the muscles of the speech mechanism are involved, this leads to a characteristic speech disorder which is described in Chapter 9.

Tissue types

Both parts of the central nervous system are composed of two types of tissue: grey matter and white matter. The grey matter is made up mainly of neurone cell bodies and their closely related processes, the dendrites. White matter comprises primarily bundles of long processes of neurones (mainly axons), the whitish appearance resulting from the lipid insulating material (myelin). Cell bodies are lacking in the white matter. Both the grey and white matter, however, contain large numbers of neuroglial cells and a network of blood capillaries. Within the white matter of the central nervous system, nerve fibres serving similar or comparable functions are often collected into bundles called tracts or pathways. Tracts are usually named according to their origin and destination (e.g. corticospinal tracts). By contrast, the nerve cell processes that leave the central nervous system are collected into bundles that form the various nerves. In fact, the term 'nerve' is reserved for groups of fibres that travel together in the peripheral nervous system. Any one nerve may contain thousands of nerve fibres of various sizes.

In the brain, most of the grey matter forms an outer layer surrounding the cerebral hemispheres. This layer, which varies from around 1.5 to 4 mm thick is referred to as the cerebral cortex ('cortex' meaning 'rind' or 'bark'). Within the spinal cord the distribution of grey and white matter is largely the reverse to that seen in the brain, the grey matter forming the central core of the spinal cord which is surrounded by white matter. In some parts of the central nervous system, notably the brainstem (see below), there are regions that contain both nerve cell bodies and numerous myelinated fibres. These regions therefore comprise diffuse mixtures of grey and white matter.

The central nervous system

The brain

The brain is that part of the central nervous system contained within the skull. It is the largest and most complex mass of nerve tissue in the body and in the average human weighs approximately 1400 g. The brain is surrounded by three fibrous membranes collectively called the meninges and is suspended in fluid called cerebrospinal fluid. Within the brain are a series of fluid-filled cavities called the ventricles. (The meninges and ventricles are described in detail later in this chapter.)

The nervous system begins development in the embryo as the neural tube. At the rostral end of the neural tube develop three swellings called the primary brain vesicles. These vesicles are the prosencephalon, mesencephalon and rhombencephalon which eventually become the fore-brain, midbrain and hind-brain respectively. Shortly after the appearance of the three primary brain vesicles, the prosencephalon divides into the telencephalon (which becomes the cerebral hemispheres) and the diencephalon (which gives rise to the thalamus and hypothalamus). In addition, the rhombencephalon is divided by a fold into a rostral part called the metencephalon (which becomes the pons and cerebellum) and the myelencephalon (which forms the medulla oblongata). The mesencephalon remains undivided and becomes the midbrain of the adult brain. The adult brain, or encephalon, can be divided into three major parts: the cerebrum, the brainstem and the cerebellum (Figure 1.4).

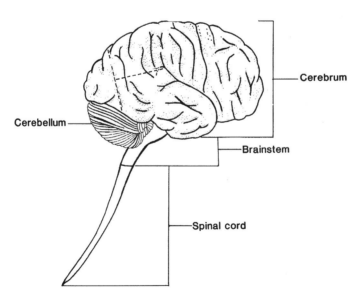

Figure 1.4 Major parts of the brain.

The cerebrum. The cerebrum is the largest portion of the brain, representing approximately seven-eighths of its total weight. Centres which govern all sensory and motor activities (including speech production) are located in the cerebrum. In addition, areas which determine reason, memory and intelligence as well as the primary language centres are also located in this region of the brain.

The surface of the cerebrum is highly folded or convoluted. The convolutions are called gyri (sing. gyrus) while the shallow depressions or intervals between the gyri are referred to as sulci (sing. sulcus). If the depressions between the gyri are deep, they are then called fissures. A very prominent fissure, called the longitudinal fissure, is located in the mid-sagittal plane and almost completely divides the cerebrum into two separate halves or hemispheres, called the right and left cerebral hemispheres. The longitudinal fissure can be viewed from a superior view of the brain, as shown in Figure 1.5.

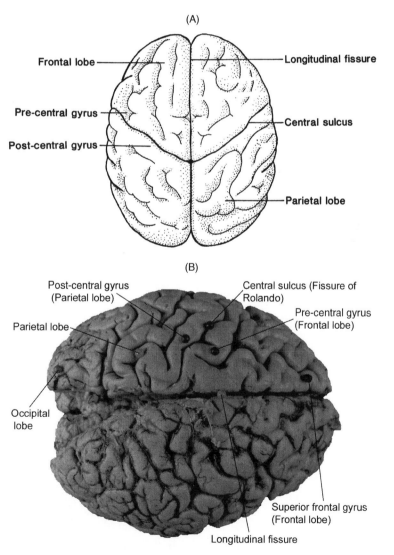

Figure 1.5 (A) Diagrammatic representation of a superior view of the brain (longitudinal fissure located vertically). (B) Superior view of the brain (longitudinal fissure located horizontally).

The cerebral cortex is the convoluted layer of grey matter covering the cerebral hemispheres. The cerebral cortex comprises about 40% of the brain by weight and it has been estimated that it contains in the region of 15 billion neurones. The cellular structure of the cerebral cortex itself is not uniform over the entire cerebrum and many researchers in the past have suggested that areas of the cortex with different cell structures also serve different functional roles. Inference concerning structure and function has been largely drawn from observations on animals, especially monkeys and chimpanzees, as well as from studies of humans undergoing brain surgery. Such studies have shown that some specific functions are localized to certain general areas of the cerebral cortex. These functional areas of the cortex have been mapped out as a result of direct electrical stimulation of the cortex or from neurological examination after portions of the cortex have been removed (ablated). Although several systems for mapping the various areas of the cerebral cortex have been developed, the number system developed by Brodmann in the early 1900s has been the most widely used. The Brodmann number system is shown in Figure 1.6.

In compiling this system, Brodmann attempted to correlate the structure and function of the cerebral cortex and arrived at a numerical designation of regions showing differential morphology. As a result, the cerebral cortex can be divided into motor, sensory and association areas (Figure 1.6). The motor areas control voluntary muscular activities while the sensory areas are involved with the perception of sensory impulses (e.g. vision and audition). Three primary sensory areas have been identified in each hemisphere, one for vision, one for hearing and one for general senses (e.g. touch). The association cortex (also called the uncommitted cortex because it is not obviously devoted to some primary sensory function such as vision, hearing, touch, smell, etc. or motor function) occupies approximately 75% of the cerebral cortex. It used to be believed that the association areas received information from the primary sensory areas to be integrated and analysed in the association cortex and then fed to the motor areas. It has been established, however, that they receive multiple inputs and outputs, many of them independent of the primary sensory and motor areas. Three main association areas are recognized: pre-frontal, anterior temporal and parietal temporal occipital area. Overall, they are involved in a variety of intellectual and cognitive functions.

Beneath the cerebral cortex, each cerebral hemisphere consists of white matter within which there is located a number of isolated patches of grey matter. These isolated patches of grey matter are referred to as the basal nuclei (a nucleus is a mass of grey matter in the central nervous system) or often as the basal ganglia (strictly speaking, however, a ganglion is a group of nerve cells located outside the central nervous system). The basal nuclei, or ganglia, serve important motor functions and when damaged are associated with a range of neurological disorders including Parkinson's disease, chorea, athetosis and dyskinesia (see Chapter 10), all of which may have associated motor speech deficits. The anatomy of the basal ganglia is described and their possible role in language discussed in Chapter 3.

The white matter underlying the cerebral cortex consists of myelinated nerve fibres arranged in three principal directions. First, there are association fibres. These transmit nerve impulses from one part of the cerebral cortex to another part in the same cerebral hemisphere.

One bundle of association fibres that is important for language function is the arcuate fasciculus (a fasciculus is a bundle of nerve fibres in the central nervous system). The arcuate fasciculus

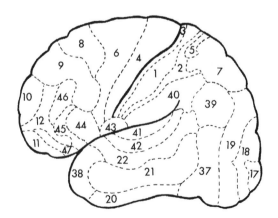

Figure 1.6 Brodmann number system.

connects a language area in the temporal lobe with a language region in the frontal lobe and when damaged is thought to cause a language disorder called 'conduction aphasia' (see Chapter 2). The second fibre group are known as commissural fibres. These transmit nerve impulses from one cerebral hemisphere to the other. The third group of fibres which make up the subcortical white matter are projection fibres. These form the ascending and descending pathways that connect the cerebral cortex to the lower central nervous system structures such as the brainstem and spinal cord.

In overall appearance each cerebral hemisphere is a 'mirror-twin' of the other and each contains a full set of centres for governing the sensory and motor activities of the body. Each hemisphere is also largely associated with activities occurring on the opposite (contralateral) side of the body. For instance, the left cerebral hemisphere is largely concerned with motor and sensory activities occurring in the right side of the body. Although each hemisphere has a complete set of structures for governing the motor and sensory activities of the body, each hemisphere tends to specialize in different functions. For example, speech and language in most people is largely controlled by the left cerebral hemisphere. The left hemisphere also specializes in hand control and analytical processes. The right hemisphere specializes in such functions as stereognosis (the sense by which the form of objects is perceived, e.g. if a familiar object such as a coin or key is placed in the hand it can be recognized without looking at it) and the perception of space. The cerebral hemisphere which controls speech and language is referred to as the dominant hemisphere. The concept of cerebral dominance is discussed further in Chapter 5.

Although almost completely separated by the longitudinal fissure, the two cerebral hemispheres are connected internally by a number of commissures. By far the largest commissure is the corpus callosum, a mass of white matter which serves as the major pathway for the transfer of information from one hemisphere to the other. The anterior portion of the corpus callosum is called the genu, while the posterior part is referred to as the splenium. Between the genu and the sple-

nium is located the body of the corpus callosum. In addition to the corpus callosum, three lesser commissures also connect the two hemispheres. These include the fornix, the anterior commissure and the posterior commissure. The location of these various commissures can be seen from a mid-sagittal section of the brain as shown in Figure 1.7.

Each cerebral hemisphere can be divided into six lobes. These include the frontal, parietal, occipital, temporal, central (also called the insula, or Island of Reil) and limbic lobes. The six lobes are delineated from each other by several major sulci and fissures, including the lateral fissure (Fissure of Sylvius), central sulcus (Fissure of Rolando), cingulate sulcus and the parieto-occipital sulcus. A superior view of the brain reveals two lobes, the frontal and parietal, separated by the central sulcus (Figure 1.5).

Four lobes, namely the frontal, parietal, temporal and occipital lobes, can be seen from a lateral view of the cerebrum (Figure 1.8). The boundaries of the lobes on the lateral cerebral surface are as follows: the frontal lobe is located anterior to the central sulcus and above the lateral fissure; the parietal lobe is located posterior to the central sulcus, anterior to an imaginary parieto-occipital line (this runs parallel to the parieto-occipital fissure which is found on the medial surface of the hemisphere in the longitudinal fissure – Figure 1.9) and above the lateral fissure and its imaginary posterior continuation towards the occipital pole; the temporal lobe is located below the lateral fissure and anterior to the imaginary parieto-occipital line.

The central lobe, or insula, is not visible from an external view of the brain. It is hidden deep within the lateral fissure. To view the central lobe the lateral fissure must be held apart or the operculae removed (Figure 1.10). Those parts of the frontal, parietal and temporal lobes which cover the external surface of the insula are called the frontal operculum, parietal operculum and temporal operculum respectively.

The limbic lobe is a ring of gyri located on the medial aspect of each cerebral hemisphere. The largest components of this limbic lobe include the hippocampus, the parahippocampal gyrus and the cingulated gyrus, some of which can be

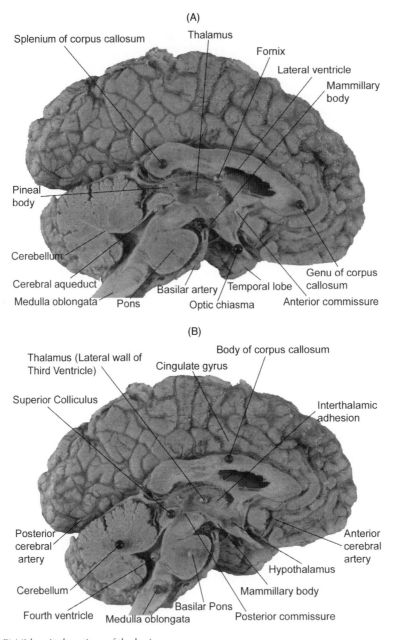

Figure 1.7 (A and B) Mid-sagittal sections of the brain.

examined from a mid-sagittal view of the brain (Figures 1.7 and 1.9).

The boundaries of the lobes on the medial cerebral surface are as follows: the frontal lobe is located anterior to the central sulcus and above the line formed by the cingulate sulcus; the parietal lobe is bounded by the central sulcus, cin-gulate sulcus and parieto-occipital sulcus; the temporal lobe is located lateral to the parahip-pocampal gyrus; the occipital lobe lies posterior to the parieto-occipital sulcus; the limbic lobe comprises the gyri bordered by the curved line formed by the cingulate sulcus and the collateral sulcus.

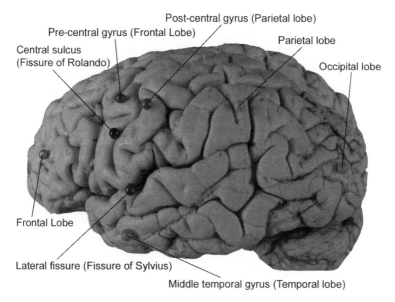

Figure 1.8 Lateral view of the left cerebral hemisphere.

Although there is considerable overlap in the functions of adjacent cerebral lobes, each lobe does appear to have its own speciality. For instance, located in the frontal lobes are the centres for the control of voluntary movement, the so-called motor areas of the cerebrum.

Immediately anterior to the central sulcus is a long gyrus called the pre-central gyrus (Figure 1.8). This gyrus (Brodmann area 4), also known as the primary motor area or motor strip, represents the point of origin for those nerve fibres which carry voluntary nerve impulses from the cerebral cortex to the brainstem and spinal cord. In other words, the nerve cells in this area are responsible for the voluntary control of skeletal muscles on the opposite side of the body. Electrical stimulation of the primary motor area causes the contraction of muscles primarily on the

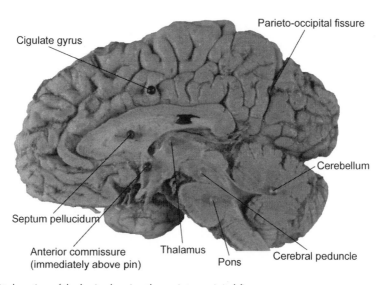

Figure 1.9 Mid-sagittal section of the brain showing the parieto-occipital fissure.

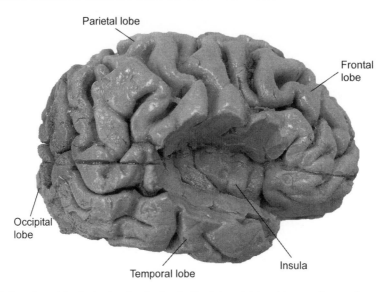

Parietal lobe

Frontal lobe

Occipital lobe

Temporal lobe

Insula

Figure 1.10 Lateral dissection of the brain showing the insula (frontal, parietal and temporal operculae removed).

opposite or contralateral side of the body. The nerve fibres which leave the primary motor area and pass to either the brainstem or spinal cord form what are known as the direct activation, or pyramidal, pathways. (These pathways are discussed in more detail in Chapter 9.)

All parts of the body responsive to voluntary muscular control are represented along the pre-central gyrus in something of a sequential array. A map showing the points in the primary motor cortex that cause muscle contractions in different parts of the body when electrically stimulated is shown in Figure 1.11. These points have been determined by electrical stimulation of the human brain in patients having brain operations under local anaesthesia.

The map as shown is referred to as the motor homunculus. It will be noted that the areas of the body are represented in an almost inverted fashion, the motor impulses to the head region originating from that part of the pre-central gyrus closest to the lateral sulcus, while impulses passing to the feet are initiated from an area located within the longitudinal fissure. The size of the area of pre-central gyrus devoted to a particular part of the body is not strongly related to the size of that body part. Rather, larger areas of the motor strip are devoted to those parts of the body which have a capacity for finer and more highly

controlled movement. Consequently, the area devoted to the hand is larger than that given to the leg and foot. Likewise, because the muscles of the larynx are capable of very discrete and precise movements, the area of pre-central gyrus devoted to their control is as large or larger than the area given to some of the big leg muscles, which are capable of only more gross movements.

In addition to the primary motor area, several other motor areas have been located in the frontal

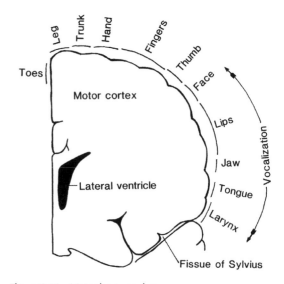

Figure 1.11 Motor homunculus.

lobes by stimulation studies. These latter areas include the pre-motor area (Brodmann area 6), the supplementary motor area, the secondary motor area and the frontal eye field (Brodmann area 8). The pre-motor area lies immediately anterior to the pre-central sulcus. Not only does it contribute fibres to the descending motor pathways, including the pyramidal pathways, it also influences the activity of the primary motor area. Electrical stimulation of the pre-motor area elicits complex contractions of groups of muscles. Occasionally, vocalization occurs, or rhythmic movements such as alternate thrusting of a leg forwards or backwards, turning of the head, chewing, swallowing or contortion of parts of the body into different postural positions. It is believed that the pre-motor area programmes skilled motor activity and thereby directs the primary motor area in its execution of voluntary muscular activity. Therefore, whereas the primary motor area controls the contraction of individual muscles and acts as the primary output source from the cerebral cortex for voluntary motor activities, the pre-motor area functions in the control of coordinated, skilled movements involving the contraction of many muscles simultaneously.

The secondary motor area is located in the dorsal wall of the lateral fissure immediately below the pre-central gyrus. Its functional significance is unknown. The supplementary motor area is an extension of Brodmann area 6 and is located within the longitudinal fissure on the medial aspect of the hemisphere immediately anterior to the leg portion of the primary motor area. Some researchers consider it a second speech area. The frontal eye field (Brodmann area 8) lies anterior to the pre-motor cortex (Brodmann area 6) (Figure 1.6). It controls volitional eye movements. Stimulation of the frontal eye field results in conjugate (joined) movements of the eyes to the opposite sides.

Another important area of the frontal lobe is Broca's area (Brodmann areas 44 and 45) (Figure 1.6). Also known as the motor speech area, Broca's area is one of two major cortical areas that have been identified as having specialized language functions. Broca's area is located in the inferior (third) frontal gyrus of the frontal lobe and appears to be necessary for the production of fluent, well-articulated speech. The importance of Broca's area to language production is outlined in more detail later in this chapter and the relationship between lesions of this region and the occurrence of specific speech-language disturbances is discussed in Chapter 2.

The parietal lobe is involved in a wide variety of general sensory functions. The sensations of heat, cold, pain, touch, pressure and position of the body in space and possibly some taste sensation all reach the level of consciousness here. The primary sensory area for general senses (also called the somesthetic area or sensory strip) occupies the post-central gyrus (areas 3, 1 and 2 of the Brodmann cytoarchitectural map) (Figure 1.6). Each sensory strip receives sensory signals almost exclusively from the opposite side of the body (a small amount of sensory (touch) information comes from the same, or ipsilateral, side of the face). As in the case of the motor strip, the various parts of the body can be mapped along the post-central gyrus to indicate the area devoted to their sensory control. This map is referred to as the sensory homunculus and is shown in Figure 1.12.

It can be seen that some areas of the body are represented by large areas in the post-central gyrus. The size of the area devoted to a particular part of the body is directly proportional to

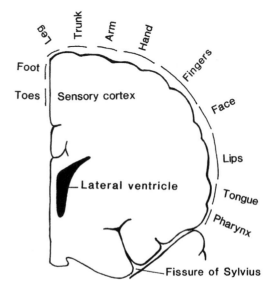

Figure 1.12 Sensory homunculus.

the number of specialized sensory receptors contained in that part of the body. In other words, the proportion of the sensory strip allocated to a particular body part is determined by the sensitivity of that part. Consequently, a large area of the post-central gyrus is assigned to highly sensitive areas such as the lips and hand (particularly the thumb and index finger) and a smaller area assigned to less sensitive areas such as the trunk and legs.

In addition to the post-central gyrus, two other gyri in the parietal lobe are also of importance to speech-language pathologists. These are the supramarginal gyrus and the angular gyrus (Figure 1.13). The supramarginal gyrus wraps around the posterior end of the lateral fissure while the angular gyrus lies immediately posterior to the supramarginal gyrus and curves around the end of the superior temporal gyrus. In the dominant hemisphere (usually the left), these two gyri form part of the posterior language centre, an area involved in the perception and interpretation of spoken and written language. The relationship between damage to these two gyri and the occurrence of specific language deficits is discussed in Chapters 2 and 8.

The temporal lobe is concerned with the special sense of hearing (audition), and at least some of the neurones concerned with speech and language are located here. The primary auditory area is not visible from a lateral view of the brain because it is concealed within the lateral fissure. The floor of the lateral fissure is formed by the upper surface of the superior temporal gyrus. This surface is marked by transverse temporal gyri. The two most anterior of these gyri, called the anterior temporal gyri or Heschl's convolutions, represent the primary auditory area (Brodmann areas 41 and 42). The posterior part of the superior temporal gyrus (Brodmann area 22) which is evident on the lateral surface of the temporal lobe together with that part of the floor of the lateral fissure that lies immediately behind the primary auditory area (an area called the planum temporal) constitute the auditory association area. In the dominant hemisphere the auditory association area is also known as Wernicke's area, another important component of the posterior language centre. The pathological effects on language lesions in Wernicke's area are discussed in Chapter 2.

The occipital lobe is primarily concerned with vision. The primary visual area (Brodmann area 17) surrounds the calcarine sulcus, which is located in the longitudinal fissure on the medial surface of the occipital lobe.

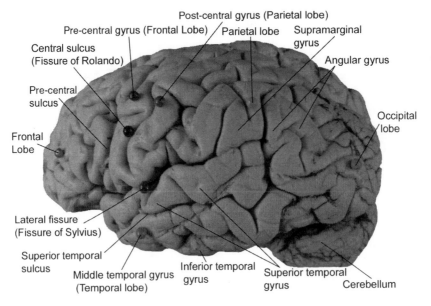

Figure 1.13   Lateral view of the left cerebral hemisphere.

The limbic lobe, also known as the rhinencephalon (smell brain), is associated with olfaction, autonomic functions and certain aspects of emotion, behaviour and memory. Although the functions of the central lobe are uncertain, it is believed that it also operates in association with autonomic functions.

The brainstem. If both the cerebral hemispheres and the cerebellum are removed from the brain, a stalk-like mass of central nervous system tissue remains: the brainstem. The brainstem comprises four major parts. From rostral (head) to caudal (tail), these include the diencephalon, midbrain (mesencephalon), pons (metencephalon) and medulla oblongata (myelencephalon). The relationship of these components to one another can be seen in Figure 1.14. (Note: in some classification systems the diencephalon is included as part of the cerebrum.)

The diencephalon. The diencephalon (or tweenbrain) lies between the cerebral hemispheres and the midbrain. It consists of two major components: the thalamus and hypothalamus. The thalamus is a large rounded mass of grey matter measuring about 3 cm antero-posteriorly and 1.5 cm in the two other directions. Located above the midbrain, it is not visible in surface views of the brain. It can be seen, however, from a mid-sagittal section of the brain (Figure 1.7). The thalamus is almost completely divided into right and left thalami by the third ventricle. In most people, however, the two large ovoid (egg-shaped) thalami of both sides are connected to one another by a band of grey matter called the interthalamic adhesion (intermediate mass) (Figure 1.7b). Each thalamic mass contains over 30 nuclei which enable it to perform important sensory and motor functions. In particular, the thalamus is one of the major sensory integrating centres of the brain and is sometimes referred to as the gateway to the cerebral cortex. All of the major sensory pathways with the exception of the olfactory pathways pass through the thalamus on their way to the cerebral cortex. The thalamus, therefore, receives sensory information via the sensory pathways, integrates that information and then sends it on to the cerebral cortex for further analysis and interpretation.

In addition to its sensory activities, the thalamus is functionally interrelated with the major motor centres of the cerebral cortex and can facilitate or inhibit motor impulses originating from the cerebral cortex. In recent years, a number of researchers have also documented the occurrence of language disorders following thalamic lesions, thereby suggesting that the thalamus may play a role in language function. A more complete

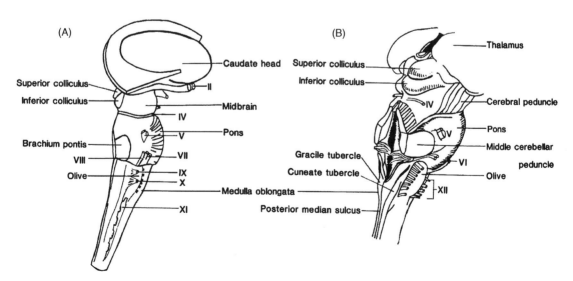

Figure 1.14   (A) Lateral view of the brainstem. (B) Dorsolateral view of the brainstem.

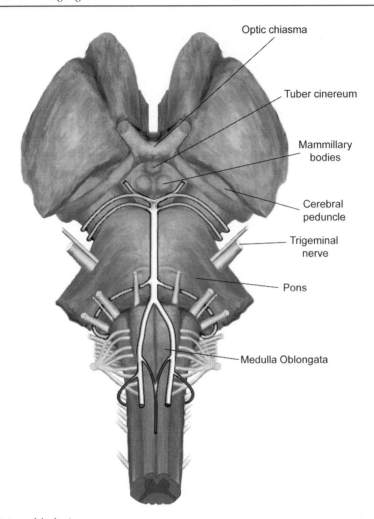

Figure 1.15 Ventral view of the brainstem.

description of the neuroanatomy of the thalamus together with a discussion of thalamic aphasia is presented in Chapter 3.

The hypothalamus lies below the thalamus (see Figure 1.7b) and forms the floor and the inferior part of the lateral walls of the third ventricle. When examined from an inferior view of the brain (Figure 1.15) the hypothalamus can be seen to be made up of the tuber cinereum, the optic chiasma, the two mammillary bodies and the infundibulum. The tuber cinereum is the name given to the region bounded by the mammillary bodies, optic chiasma and beginning of the optic tracts. The infundibulum, to which is attached the posterior lobe of the pituitary gland, is a stalk-like structure which arises from a raised portion of the tuber cinereum called the median eminence. The median eminence, the infundibulum and the posterior lobe of the pituitary gland together form the neurohypophysis (posterior pituitary gland). The mammillary bodies are two small hemispherical projections placed side by side immediately posterior to the tuber cinereum. They contain nuclei important for hypothalamic function. The optic chiasma is a cross-like structure formed by the partial crossing over of the nerve fibres of the optic nerves. Within the optic chiasma the nerve fibres originating from the nasal half of each retina cross the midline to enter the optic tract on the opposite side.

Although the hypothalamus is only a small part of the brain, it controls a large number of important body functions. The hypothalamus controls and integrates the autonomic nervous system, which stimulates smooth muscle, regulates the rate of contraction of cardiac muscle and controls the secretions of many of the body's glands. Through the autonomic nervous system, the hypothalamus is the chief regulator of visceral activities (e.g. it controls the heart rate, the movement of food through the digestive system and contraction of the urinary bladder). The hypothalamus is also an important link between the nervous and endocrine systems and regulates the secretion of hormones from the anterior pituitary gland and actually produces the hormones released from the posterior pituitary.

The hypothalamus is the centre for 'mind over body' phenomena. When the cerebral cortex interprets strong emotions, it often sends impulses over tracts that connect the cortex with the hypothalamus. The hypothalamus responds either by sending impulses to the autonomic nervous system or by releasing chemicals that stimulate the anterior pituitary gland. The result can be a wide range in changes of body activity. The hypothalamus controls other aspects of emotional behaviour such as rage and aggression. It also controls body temperature and regulates water and food intake and is one of the centres that maintains the waking state. The hypothalamus also has a role in the control of sexual behaviour.

The midbrain. The midbrain is the smallest portion of the brainstem and lies between the pons and diencephalon. The midbrain is traversed internally by a narrow canal called the cerebral aqueduct (Aqueduct of Sylvius), which connects the third and fourth ventricles and divides the midbrain into a dorsal and ventral portion. A prominent elevation lies on either side of the ventral surface of the midbrain (Figure 1.15). These two elevations are known as the cerebral peduncles (basis pedunculi) and consist of large bundles of descending nerve fibres.

The region between the two cerebral peduncles is the interpeduncular fossa. Cranial nerve III (the oculomotor nerve) arises from the side of this fossa. The floor of the fossa is known as

the posterior perforated substance owing to the many perforations produced by blood vessels that penetrate the midbrain.

The dorsal portion of the midbrain contains four rounded eminences, the paired superior and inferior colliculi (collectively known as the corpora quadrigemina) (Figures 1.14 and 1.16). The four colliculi comprise the roof, or tectum, of the midbrain. The superior colliculi are larger than the inferior colliculi, and are associated with the optic system. In particular, they are involved with the voluntary control of ocular movements and optic reflexes such as controlling movement of the eyes in response to changes in the position of the head in response to visual and other stimuli. The major role of the inferior colliculi, on the other hand, is as relay nuclei on the auditory pathways to the thalamus. Cranial nerve IV (the trochlear nerve) emerges from the brainstem immediately caudal to the inferior colliculus and then bends around the lateral surface of the brainstem on its way to the orbit (Figures 1.14 and 1.16).

The internal structure of the midbrain as seen in a transverse section at the level of the superior and inferior colliculus is shown in Figures 1.17 and 1.18 respectively.

Each cerebral peduncle is divided internally into an anterior part, the crus cerebri and a posterior part, the tegmentum, by a pigmented band of grey matter called the substantia nigra. The crus cerebri consists of fibres of the pyramidal motor system (see Chapter 9) (including corticospinal, corticobulbar and cortico-mesencephalic fibres) as well as fibres which connect the cerebral cortex to the pons (corticopontine fibres). The substantia nigra is the largest single nucleus in the midbrain. It is a motor nucleus concerned with muscle tone and has connections to the cerebral cortex, hypothalamus, spinal cord and basal ganglia. Another important motor nucleus found in the tegmentum of the midbrain is the red nucleus (Figure 1.17), so called because of its pinkish colour in fresh specimens. The red nucleus is located between the cerebral aqueduct and the substantia nigra. Large bundles of sensory fibres such as the medial lemniscus also pass through the tegmentum of the cerebral peduncles on their way to the thalamus from the spinal cord. In

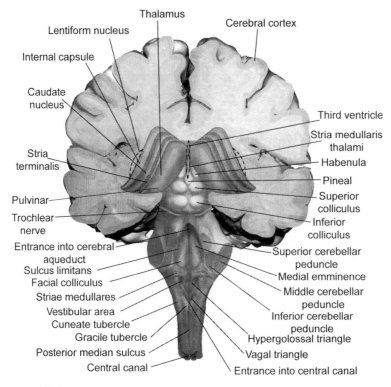

Figure 1.16 Dorsal view of the brainstem.

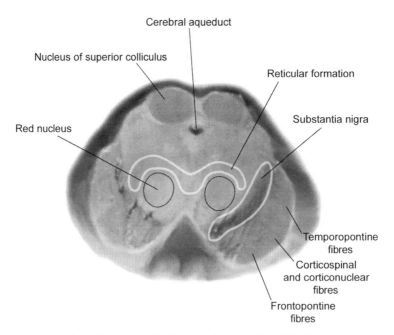

Figure 1.17 Transverse section of the midbrain through the level of the superior colliculi.

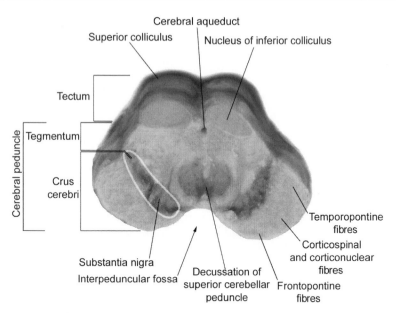

Figure 1.18   Transverse section of the midbrain at the level of the inferior colliculi, showing division of the midbrain into the tectum and the cerebral peduncles.

addition, the nuclei of cranial nerves III and IV are also located in the tegmentum of the midbrain.

The pons. The pons lies between the midbrain and medulla oblongata and anterior to the cerebellum, being separated from the latter by the fourth ventricle. The term 'pons' means 'bridge'; the pons takes its name from the appearance of its ventral surface, which is essentially that of a bridge connecting the two cerebellar hemispheres.

As in the case of the midbrain, the pons may also be divided into a dorsal and ventral portion. The dorsal portion is continuous with the tegmentum of the midbrain and is also called the tegmentum. The ventral portion of the pons is the basilar pons. The basilar pons is a distinctive brainstem structure, presenting as a rounded bulbous structure (Figures 1.14 and 1.15). It contains mainly thick, heavily myelinated fibres running in a transverse plane. These fibres connect the two halves of the cerebellum and run into the cerebellum as the brachium pontis or middle cerebellar peduncle. Cranial nerve V (the trigeminal nerve) emerges from the lateral aspect of the pons. Each trigeminal nerve consists of a smaller motor root and a larger sensory root. In the groove

between the pons and medulla oblongata (the ponto-medullary sulcus) there emerge from medial to lateral, cranial nerves VI (the abducens nerve), VII (the facial nerve) and VIII (the vestibulocochlear or auditory nerve). As in the case of the trigeminal nerve, the facial nerve emerges from the brainstem in the form of two distinct bundles of fibres of unequal size. The larger motor root is the motor facial nerve proper. The smaller bundle contains autonomic fibres and is known as the nervus intermedius.

The internal structure of the pons as seen in a transverse section at the level of the trigeminal nuclei and the level of the facial colliculus is shown in Figures 1.19 and 1.20 respectively.

The dorsal and ventral portions of the pons are separated by the trapezoid body which comprises transverse auditory fibres. Although the pons consists mainly of white matter, it does contain a number of nuclei. Nuclei located in the tegmentum include the motor and sensory nuclei of the trigeminal nerve, the facial nucleus and the abducens nucleus. A nucleus involved in the control of respiration, the pneumotaxic centre, is also located in the pons. Major sensory fibres also ascend through the tegmentum of the pons via the medial and lateral lemniscus. The basilar

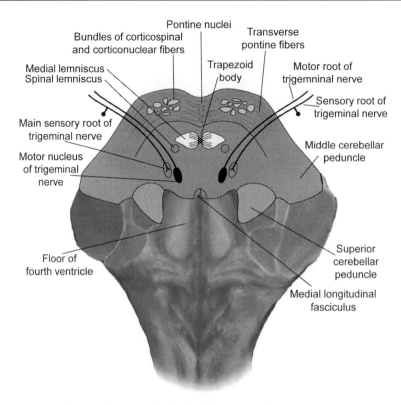

Figure 1.19   Transverse section through the pons at the level of the trigeminal nuclei.

pons near the midline contains small masses of nerve cells called the pontine nuclei. The cortico-pontine fibres of the crus cerebri of the midbrain terminate in the pontine nuclei. The axons of the nerve cells in the pontine nuclei in turn give origin to the transverse fibres of the pons, which cross the midline and intersect the corticospinal and corticobulbar tracts (both components of the pyramidal motor system – see Chapter 9), breaking them up into smaller bundles. Overall, the basal portion of the pons acts as a synaptic or relay station for motor fibres conveying impulses from the motor areas of the cerebral cortex to the cerebellum. These pathways are described more fully in Chapter 11.

The medulla oblongata. The medulla oblongata is continuous with the upper portion of the spinal cord and forms the most caudal portion of the brainstem. It lies above the level of the foramen magnum and extends upwards to the lower portion of the pons. The medulla is composed mainly of white fibre tracts. Among these tracts are scattered nuclei that either serve as controlling centres for various activities or contain the cell bodies of some cranial nerve fibres.

On the ventral surface of the medulla in the midline is the anterior median fissure. This fissure is bordered by two ridges, the pyramids (Figure 1.21). The pyramids are composed of the largest motor tracts that run from the cerebral cortex to the spinal cord, the so-called corticospinal tract (pyramidal tracts proper). Near the junction of the medulla with the spinal cord, most of the fibres of the left pyramid cross to the right side and most of the fibres in the right pyramid cross to the left side. The crossing is referred to as the decussation of the pyramids and largely accounts for the left cerebral hemisphere controlling the voluntary motor activities of the right side of the body and the right cerebral hemisphere the voluntary motor activities of the left side of the body.

Dorsally, the posterior median sulcus and two dorsolateral sulci can be identified on the medulla

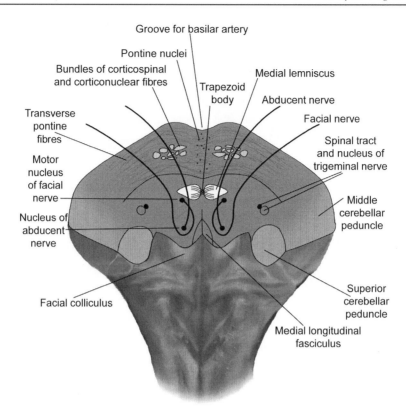

Figure 1.20 Transverse section through the caudal part of the pons at the level of the facial colliculus.

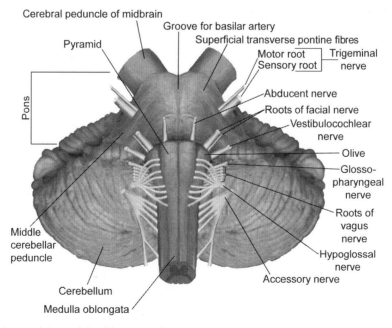

Figure 1.21 Ventral view of the medulla oblongata and pons.

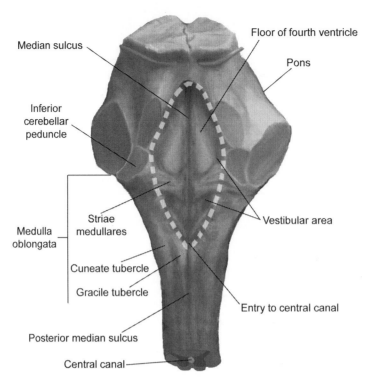

Figure 1.22   Dorsal view of the medulla oblongata.

(Figures 1.14, 1.16 and 1.22). On either side of the posterior median sulcus is a swelling, the gracile tubercle, and just lateral to this is a second swelling, the cuneate tubercle (see Figure 1.22). Both of these swellings contain important sensory nuclei, the gracile nucleus and cuneate nucleus respectively. These nuclei mark the point of termination of major sensory pathways called the fasciculus gracilis and fasciculus cuneatus, which ascend in the dorsal region of the spinal cord.

The ventrolateral sulcus can be identified on the lateral aspect of the medulla. Between this sulcus and the dorsolateral sulcus at the rostral end of the medulla is an oval-swelling called the olive (see Figure 1.14 and 1.21) which contains the inferior olivary nucleus. Posterior to the olives are the inferior cerebellar peduncles which connect the medulla to the cerebellum. In the groove between the olive and the inferior cerebellar peduncle emerge the roots of the IXth (glossopharyngeal nerve) and Xth (vagus) nerves and the cranial roots of the XIth (accessory) nerve. The XIIth (hy-poglossal) nerve arises as a series of roots in the groove between the pyramid and olive.

The internal structure of the medulla oblongata as seen from transverse sections at the level of the middle olivary nuclei and at the level of the decussation of the medial lemnisci are shown in Figures 1.23 and 1.24 respectively.

The medulla contains a number of important cranial nerve nuclei including the nucleus ambiguus (which gives rise to the motor fibres which are distributed to voluntary skeletal muscles via the IXth, Xth and cranial portion of the XIth nerves) and hypoglossal nucleus (which gives rise to the motor fibres which pass via the XIIth nerve to the muscles of the tongue). As well as containing the nuclei for various cranial nerves, the medulla also contains a number of nuclei that initiate and regulate a number of vital activities such as breathing, swallowing, regulation of heart rate and the calibre of smaller blood vessels.

Located in the central region, or core, of the brainstem, stretching through the medulla, pons

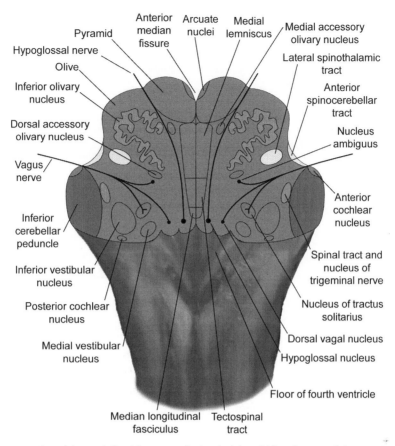

Figure 1.23 Transverse section of the medulla oblongata at the level of the middle olivary nuclei.

and midbrain to the lower border of the thalamus is a diverse collection of neurones collectively known as the reticular formation. The reticular formation receives fibres from the motor regions of the brain and most of the sensory systems of the body. Its outgoing fibres pass primarily to the thalamus and from there to the cerebral cortex. Some outgoing fibres pass to the spinal cord. Stimulation of most parts of the reticular formation results in an immediate and marked activation of the cerebral cortex leading to a state of alertness and attention. If the individual is sleeping, stimulation of the reticular formation causes immediate waking. The upper portion of the reticular formation plus its pathways to the thalamus and cerebral cortex have been designated the reticular activating system because of its importance in maintaining the waking state. Damage to the brainstem reticular activating system, as might

occur as a result of head injury, leads to coma, a state of unconsciousness from which even the strongest stimuli cannot arouse the subject.

The cerebellum. The cerebellum (small brain) lies behind the pons and medulla and below the occipital lobes of the cerebrum (Figure 1.7). Grossly, it may be seen to be composed of two hemispheres, the cerebellar hemispheres, which are connected by a median portion called the vermis. The cerebellum is attached to the brainstem on each side by three bundles of nerve fibres called the cerebellar peduncles.

In general terms, the cerebellum refines or makes muscle movements smoother and more coordinated. Although it does not in itself initiate any muscle movements, the cerebellum continually monitors and adjusts motor activities which originate from the motor area of the brain or peripheral receptors. It is particularly important for

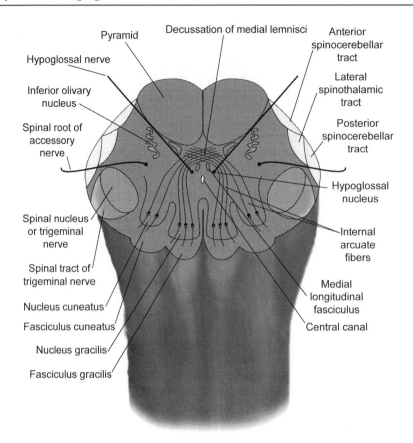

Pyramid
Hypoglossal nerve
Inferior olivary nucleus
Spinal root of accessory nerve
Spinal nucleus or trigeminal nerve
Spinal tract of trigeminal nerve
Nucleus cuneatus
Fasciculus cuneatus
Nucleus gracilis
Fasciculus gracilis

Decussation of medial lemnisci

Anterior spinocerebellar tract
Lateral spinothalamic tract
Posterior spinocerebellar tract
Hypoglossal nucleus
Internal arcuate fibers
Medial longitudinal fasciculus
Central canal

Figure 1.24 Transverse section of the medulla oblongata at the level of the decussation of the medial lemnisci.

coordinating rapid and precise movements such as those required for the production of speech.

The anatomy of the cerebellum together with the effects of cerebellar lesions on speech production are described and discussed in more detail in Chapter 11.

The spinal cord

The spinal cord is that part of the central nervous system that lies below the level of the foramen magnum. Protected by the vertebral column, the spinal cord lies in the spinal or vertebral canal and, like the brain, is surrounded by three fibrous membranes, the meninges. It is cushioned by cerebrospinal fluid and held in place by the denticulate ligaments. It comprises well-demarcated columns of motor and sensory cells (the grey matter) surrounded by the ascending and descending tracts which connect the spinal cord with the

brain (the white matter). A transverse section of the spinal cord shows that the grey matter is arranged in the shape of the letter 'H', with anterior and posterior horns and a connecting bar of grey matter (Figure 1.25). A lateral horn of grey matter is also present in the thoracic part of the cord. A narrow cavity called the central canal is located in the connecting bar of grey matter.

The spinal cord is divided into five regions, each of which takes its name from the corresponding segment of the vertebral column. These regions include (from top to bottom) the cervical, thoracic, lumbar, sacral and coccygeal regions. There are 31 pairs of spinal nerves arise from the spinal cord: eight of these nerves arise from the cervical region, 12 from the thoracic, five each from the lumbar and sacral regions and one from the coccygeal region. Each spinal nerve is formed by the union of a series of dorsal and ventral roots, the dorsal roots carrying only sensory fibres

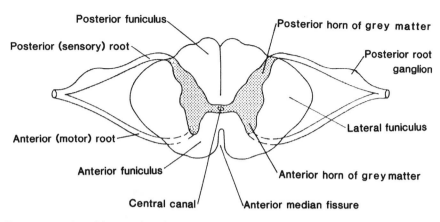

Figure 1.25 Transverse section of the spinal cord.

which convey information from peripheral receptors into the spinal cord, and the ventral roots containing only motor fibres which act as a final pathway for all motor impulses leaving the spinal cord.

The segments of the spinal cord in the adult are shorter than the corresponding vertebrae. Consequently, the spinal cord in the adult does not extend down the full length of the vertebral canal. Rather, the spinal cord extends only from the foramen magnum to the level of the first or second lumbar vertebra. The lower-most segments of the cord are compressed into the last 2–3 cm of the cord, a region known as the conus medullaris. Owing to the relative shortness of the spinal cord compared with the vertebral column, the nerve roots arising from the lower segments of the cord have a marked downward direction in the lower part of the vertebral canal forming a leash of nerves known as the cauda equina (horse's tail).

The white matter of the spinal cord is arranged into funiculi ('funiculus' meaning 'cord-like') (Figure 1.25). A posterior median septum divides the white matter into two (right and left) posterior funiculi in the dorsal portion of the spinal cord. The white matter between the dorsal and ventral nerve roots on each side is called the lateral funiculus. The ventral portion of the spinal cord is divided by the anterior median fissure into two anterior funiculi. Each funiculus contains tracts of ascending and descending fibres. The approximate positions of the various tracts are shown in Figure 1.26.

The peripheral nervous system

Nerve impulses are conveyed to and from the central nervous system by the various parts of the peripheral nervous system. Afferent or sensory nerve fibres carry nerve impulses arising from the stimulation of sensory receptors (e.g. touch receptors) towards the central nervous system. Those nerve fibres that carry impulses from the central nervous system to the effector organs (e.g. muscles and glands) are called efferent or motor fibres. The terms 'afferent' and 'efferent' are also used to describe fibres in the central nervous system as well as in the peripheral nervous system. When applied to central nervous system fibres, however, the term 'afferent' describes fibres taking nerve impulses to a particular structure (e.g. afferent supply of cerebellum), while the term 'efferent' refers to fibres taking impulses away from a particular structure (e.g. efferent supply of cerebellum).

Some nerve fibres are associated with the structures of the body wall or extremities, such as skeletal muscles, skin, bones and joints. These fibres are called somatic fibres and may of course be either sensory or motor. Other nerve fibres, which may be either sensory or motor, are more closely associated with the internal organs such as the smooth muscles found in the gastrointestinal tract and blood vessels and so on. These fibres are referred to as visceral fibres.

The nerves of the peripheral nervous system are made up of bundles of individual nerve fibres. In

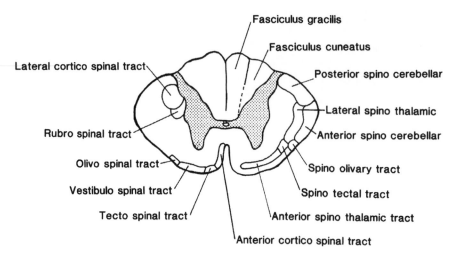

Figure 1.26 Transverse section of the spinal cord showing the general arrangement of the major ascending and descending tracts.

most cases these nerves contain all of the types of nerve fibres described above (i.e. somatic afferent and somatic efferent, visceral afferent and visceral efferent). Consequently, although it may be correct to speak of sensory or motor nerve fibres, it is rarely correct to speak of sensory or motor nerves. Only in the case of some cranial nerves is it possible to speak of sensory or motor nerves per se. For example, cranial nerve II (the optic nerve) is entirely a sensory nerve. On the other hand, cranial nerve XII (the hypoglossal nerve) is often regarded as a motor nerve.

The three principle components of the peripheral nervous system are the cranial nerves, the spinal nerves and the peripheral portions of the autonomic nervous system. These three morphologic subdivisions are not independent functionally, but combine and communicate with each other to supply both the somatic and visceral parts of the body with both afferent and efferent fibres.

The cranial nerves

Twelve pairs of cranial nerves arise from the base of the brain. With only one exception, the olfactory nerves, which terminate within the olfactory bulbs, all cranial nerves either originate from or terminate within the brainstem (Figure 1.21). The cranial nerves are numbered by Roman numerals according to their position on the brain

from anterior to posterior. The names given to the cranial nerves indicate either their function or destination. Some cranial nerves are both sensory and motor. Others, however, are either sensory or motor only. Table 1.1 summarizes the principal features of the 12 cranial nerves including their names and peripheral connections.

Cranial nerves are important to the speech-language pathologist in that they are responsible for the control of the majority of muscles comprising the speech mechanism. In particular, cranial nerves V, VII, IX, X, XI and XII are vital for normal speech production, and for this reason the anatomy of these nerves is described in more detail in Chapter 9.

The spinal nerves

As mentioned previously, each of the 31 pairs of spinal nerves is formed by the union of the dorsal and ventral nerve roots which emerge from each segment of the spinal cord. Once formed in this manner, each spinal nerve leaves the vertebral canal through its intervertebral foramen (opening) and ends soon after by dividing into a dorsal ramus (branch) and ventral ramus. The dorsal rami of the spinal nerves segmentally supply the deep back muscles and the skin of the posterior aspect of the head, neck and trunk. The ventral rami are larger than the dorsal rami and behave quite differently. Whereas the dorsal rami show

Table 1.1 Summary of the cranial nerves.

Nerve		Function
I	Olfactory	Smell
II	Optic	Vision
III	Oculomotor	Four extrinsic eye muscles (medial, inferior and superior recti, inferior oblique) and levator palpebrae. Parasympathetic to iris diaphragm of eye (constriction) and ciliary muscles of eye (lens accommodation)
IV	Trochlear	One extrinsic eye muscle (superior oblique)
V	Trigeminal	
	Motor root	Muscles of mastication and tensor typani
	Sensory root	Cranial facial sensation
VI	Abducens	One extrinsic eye muscle (lateral rectus)
VII	Facial	
	Motor root	Muscles of facial expression and stapedius
	Intermediate root	Parasympathetic innervetion of submandibular and sublingual salivary glands
VIII	Vestibulocochlear nerve	
	Vestibular nerves	Balance
	Cochlear nerve	Hearing
IX	Glossopharyngeal	Stylopharyngeus muscle. Parasympathetic innervation to parotid salivary gland. Sensation from pharynx and taste from posterior one-third of tongue
X	Vagus	Pharyngeal and laryngeal muscles and levator veli palatini. Parasympathetic innervation of thoracic and upper abdominal viscera
XI	Accessory	
	Cranial portion	Joins the vagus to supply the muscles of the larynx and pharynx
	Spinal portion	Sternocleidomastoid and trapezius muscles
XII	Hypoglossal	All intrinsic and most extrinsic tongue muscles

a segmental arrangement, the ventral rami in the cervical, lumbar and sacral regions form four extensive, intermingled networks of nerves called plexuses. Consequently, most nerves arising from these plexuses carry nerve fibres of neurones from more than one segment of the spinal cord. The ventral rami in the thoracic region course in the intercostal spaces to supply primarily the intercostal muscles and the skin overlying them. The four plexuses together with the major nerves arising from each are listed in Table 1.2.

The autonomic nervous system

The autonomic nervous system regulates the activity of cardiac muscle, smooth muscle and the glands of the body (particularly the exocrine glands). In this way the autonomic nervous system controls the activity of the visceral organs and, among other things, helps to regulate arte-

rial pressure, gastrointestinal motility and secretion, urinary output, sweating, body temperature and various other functions. Normally, the autonomic nervous system is an involuntary system that functions below the conscious level.

Although the visceral organs are supplied with both afferent and efferent nerve fibres, most authors when describing the components of the autonomic nervous system only include the efferent (motor) fibres that connect the central nervous system to effector organs such as smooth muscles, glands and so on in their description. One reason for this is that the sensory fibres coming from the visceral organs are similar to those of the somatic nervous system (i.e. similar to those that come from the skin and voluntary muscles). In both, the sensory fibres run all the way from the receptor to the central nervous system without synapsing. On the other hand, the efferent pathways that supply smooth muscles are arranged

Table 1.2   Spinal plexuses.

Plexus	Origin	Peripheral nerves arising from plexus
Cervical	Ventral rami of first and fourth cervical nerves and part of the fifth cervical nerve	Phrenic nerve[a]
Brachial	Ventral rami of fifth and eighth cervical nerves and first thoracic nerve	Axillary, median, radial and ulnar nerves
Lumbar	Ventral rami of first, second, third and greater part of fourth lumbar nerves	Femoral nerve
Sacral	Ventral rami of fourth and fifth lumbar nerves and first four sacral nerves	Sciatic nerve

[a] This nerve is important for speech production in that it supplies the respiratory diaphragm.

very differently from those that supply the skeletal muscles. Anatomically, the efferent pathways of the autonomic nervous system are unique in the following ways: whereas a skeletal muscle fibre is innervated by a neurone with its cell body in the central nervous system and its axon extending without interruption to the muscles, smooth muscle, cardiac muscle and glands are innervated by a two-neurone chain comprised of a pre-ganglionic neurone and a post-ganglionic neurone which synapse in a ganglion outside the central nervous system.

Anatomically and functionally, the autonomic nervous system can be divided into two major divisions: the sympathetic nervous system and the parasympathetic nervous system. Most visceral organs are innervated by both divisions, each of which has an opposite effect on the organ involved. The sympathetic or thoracolumbar division of the autonomic nervous system arises from all of the thoracic spinal nerves and the first two or three lumbar spinal nerves. The parasympathetic or craniosacral division of the autonomic nervous system is located within cranial nerves III, VII, IX and X and sacral spinal nerves 2, 3 and 4. All of these nerves also carry somatic motor fibres.

The parasympathetic fibres in the oculomotor nerve (III) supply the ciliary muscles of the lens of the eye and the sphincter of the pupil. Parasympathetic fibres distributed via the facial nerve (VII) regulate the secretion of saliva from the submandibular and sublingual glands, while secretion from the parotid salivary gland is controlled by the parasympathetic fibres of the glossopharyngeal nerve (IX). The vagus nerve provides parasympathetic innervation for most visceral organs contained in the thorax and abdomen and is the single most important nerve of the parasympathetic division. Vagal activity maintains the normal heart rate and a reduction in vagal tone causes the heart to beat more rapidly. The vagal fibres cause constriction of the bronchi and air passages of the lungs and supply the digestive tract as far as the transverse colon. The sacral parasympathetic outflow supplies the lower part of the digestive tract not supplied by the vagus as well as the bladder musculature and the erectile tissue of the external genitalia.

Under normal conditions, both divisions of the autonomic nervous system work together to maintain homeostasis. In times of stress, however, the sympathetic nervous system accelerates various body activities and prepares the body for 'flight or fight'. Some of the body changes that occur as a result of the actions of the sympathetic nervous system are shown in Box 1.1.

Following a period of stress, the parasympathetic nervous system tends to slow down body activities and bring the body back to its normal state. Parasympathetic action stimulates those functions of the body that are most appropriate

Box 1.1   Actions of the Sympathetic Nervous System

1. Dilates the pupils of the eyes to allow more light to enter.
2. Increases the heart rate and the force of contraction of the heart muscle.
3. Increases the respiratory rate.
4. Dilates the airways into the lungs.
5. Elevates the blood pressure through increased vasoconstriction and an increase in heart rate.
6. Inhibits digestion – the motility of the gastrointestinal system is decreased and blood is diverted from the gut to the skeletal muscles.
7. Stimulates the sweat glands to produce more sweat.

to times of relaxation (e.g. digestion, bladder and bowel emptying and sexual function).

The autonomic nervous system is closely integrated with the body's metabolism and with the endocrine system. Although it is influenced by the individual's emotional state, it operates without voluntary control. Many parts of the autonomic nervous system are able to function on a spinal basis. However, the activity of the autonomic nervous system is normally under the control of centres located in the medulla oblongata and hypothalamus.

The ventricular system

The ventricular system is a series of cavities within the brain which contain a fluid known as cerebrospinal fluid. These cavities develop from the canal within the cranial portion of the neural tube as the latter structure develops into the brain. The system includes two lateral ventricles, the third ventricle, the cerebral aqueduct (Aqueduct of Sylvius) and the fourth ventricle. The shapes and locations of the various brain ventricles are shown in Figure 1.27.

One lateral ventricle extends into each of the cerebral hemispheres. They lie below the corpus callosum, each extending in a large 'C' shape from the frontal lobe to the temporal lobe, though with a small spur (posterior horn) extending into the occipital lobe. The lateral ventricles communicate with one another and with the third ventricle through a pair of foramina known as the Foramina of Munro (interventricular foramina). The lateral ventricles are separated medially by a membranous partition known as the septum pellucidum.

The third ventricle is a small slit-like cavity in the centre of the diencephalon. The lateral walls of this cavity are formed mainly by the thalamus and to a lesser extent by the hypothalamus. It is connected posteriorly to the fourth ventricle by the cerebral aqueduct. The cerebral aqueduct is a narrow channel running within the midbrain between the corpora quadrigemina and the cerebral peduncles. The fourth ventricle is a cavity which lies between the pons and medulla on one side and the cerebellum on the other. It continues below into a narrow channel, the central canal, which is present in the lower medulla oblongata and throughout the length of the spinal cord. Cerebrospinal fluid escapes from the ventricular system through three foramina that are present in the roof and walls of the fourth ventricle. There are two lateral openings known as the Foramina of Luschka and a medial opening called the Foramen of Magendie. The location of the various components of the ventricular system as seen in a mid-sagittal section of the brain are indicated in Figure 1.7.

The ventricles and the central canal are lined by ependymal cells. In each of the four ventricles there are complex tufts of small blood vessels and modified ependymal cells which form what are known as choroid plexuses. These plexuses are concerned with the formation of cerebrospinal fluid.

The meninges

Three membranes, collectively known as the meninges, surround and protect the brain and spinal cord. From the outside these are the dura mater, arachnoid and pia mater. All three envelop the brain and spinal cord.

The dura mater is a tough, inelastic outer membrane, made of strong white fibrous connective tissue. In the head it is composed of two layers.

(A)   (B)

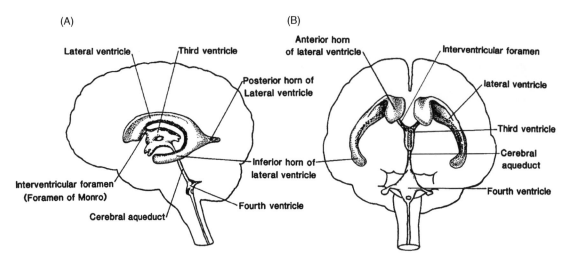

Figure 1.27   (A) Lateral view of the ventricles. (B) Frontal view of the ventricles.

The outer layer lines and adheres to the skull and is actually the periosteum of the cranial bones. The inner layer of the dura mater covers the brain and in certain locations extends down into the major fissures of the brain, where, in doing so, it forms three major folds which divide the skull cavity into adjoining compartments. First, it extends down into the longitudinal fissure and then is reflected back on itself, forming a membranous septum between the two cerebral hemispheres known as the falx cerebri. This septum is actually a double thickness or fold of the inner layer of the dura. A similar, but smaller, fold of the inner dura, called the tentorium cerebelli, extends between the occipital lobes of the cerebral hemispheres and the cerebellum in such a way as to form a roof or tent over the cerebellum. The tentorium cerebelli separates the posterior cranial fossa from the anterior and middle cranial fossae. Those parts of the brain that lie above the tentorium cerebelli, which include the paired frontal, parietal, temporal and occipital lobes of the cerebral hemispheres, the basal ganglia, thalamus, hypothalamus and cranial nerves I (olfactory) and II (optic), are referred to as supratentorial structures. Brain structures located below the tentorium cerebelli are located in the posterior crania fossa and include components of the brainstem (the midbrain, pons and medulla oblongata, and the origins of cranial nerves III through XII).

The brainstem passes through a hole in the tentorium cerebelli called the tentorial hiatus. Conditions leading to increased intracranial pressure in the supratentorial region (e.g. extradural haemorrhage resulting from traumatic head injury) may cause portions of the temporal lobes to be herniated through the tentorial hiatus leading to compression of the brainstem. Tentorial herniation, and its life-threatening consequences, is discussed more fully in Chapter 4. Finally, another fold of the inner dura extends between and separates the two cerebellar hemispheres. This latter fold is known as the falx cerebelli.

In certain areas within the skull, the two layers of the dura mater are separated from one another, forming spaces called cranial venous sinuses. These sinuses are filled with blood that flows from the brain to the heart. As we will see later, these sinuses are important in the absorption of cerebrospinal fluid into the blood stream.

In the vertebral canal, the dura mater is separated from bone (i.e. the vertebrae) by an interval, the epidural space, which contains fat and many small veins. It should be noted that the vertebrae have their own periosteal lining and thus the dura mater in the spinal canal is only a single layer. A comparable space to the epidural space is not found in the cranial cavity, except when artificially produced (e.g. by bleeding between the skull and dura mater following head trauma –

extradural haemorrhage). The main blood supply to the dura mater is the middle meningeal artery, which is a branch of the external carotid artery. Extradural haemorrhage classically follows traumatic rupture of middle meningeal artery.

Immediately deep to the dura mater is the second or middle meninge called the arachnoid. The arachnoid is a thin, avascular, delicate, transparent, cobwebby layer. It does not follow each indentation of the brain but rather skips from gyrus to gyrus. The small space between the arachnoid and the dura mater is known as the subdural space. This space is ordinarily filled with small amounts of lymph-like material. The arachnoid is loosely attached to the inner meninge (the pia mater) by a fine network of connective-tissue fibres (trabeculae), so that a space is created between the arachnoid and the pia mater. This space is called the subarachnoid space. Cerebrospinal fluid circulates through the subarachnoid space. Several large spaces called cisterns represent enlargements in the subarachnoid space. The cisterna magna (cerebral medullaris) is located dorsal to the medulla and inferior to the cerebellum. The pontine and interpeduncular cisterns are located to the anterior brainstem, and the superior cistern is located posterior to the midbrain.

The fourth ventricle of the brain communicates with the subarachnoid space via the Foramina of Luschka and Foramen of Magendie mentioned above. Cerebrospinal fluid circulates through the ventricles, enters the subarachnoid space via these foramina and is eventually absorbed into the venous system. We will look more at this circulation shortly. The arachnoid sends tuft-like extensions up through the inner layer of the dura mater into the venous sinuses. These extensions are called arachnoid villi, and they aid in the return of cerebrospinal fluid to the blood.

The pia mater is the innermost meninge and is intimately attached to the brain and spinal cord. It is composed of delicate connective tissue and contains the blood vessels that nourish the neural tissue of the brain and spinal cord. The cerebral blood vessels are adherent to the external surface of the pia mater. Unlike the other two membranes, it dips down into the invaginations of all the sulci of the brain and closely follows the convolutions of the gyri. The pia mater

together with the arachnoid are known as the leptomeninges. Inflammation of the meninges is called 'meningitis', which most often involves the leptomeninges.

In head injuries (see Chapter 4) bleeding may occur into the subarachnoid space (subarachnoid haemorrhage), into the subdural space (subdural haemorrhage) and between the outer dura mater and the skull (extradural haemorrhage). An extradural haemorrhage may result from bleeding meningeal vessels after a fracture of the skull, caused by a blow to the head. A subdural haemorrhage can be caused by the tearing of veins crossing the subdural space, which may follow after the sudden movement of the cerebral hemispheres relative to the dura and skull (e.g. as caused by head striking an immovable object such as a wall). A subarachnoid haemorrhage may result from the rupture of an aneurysm in a branch of the internal carotid or vertebral arteries. The presence of blood-stained cerebrospinal fluid obtained from a lumbar puncture is confirmatory of subarachnoid haemorrhage.

The cerebrospinal fluid

Cerebrospinal fluid is a clear, colourless fluid, which is found in the ventricular system and the subarachnoid space. The brain and spinal cord actually float in the medium. Most of the cerebrospinal fluid is produced by the choroid plexuses of the ventricles of the brain. The volume of cerebrospinal fluid in the ventricles and subarachnoid space is about 120–140 ml, with approximately 23 ml in the ventricular system and 117 ml in the subarachnoid space. It has been estimated that cerebrospinal fluid is replaced about once every six hours. To maintain a constant volume, therefore, cerebrospinal fluid has to constantly move into the venous sinuses, and hence into the blood stream, via the arachnoid villi.

Cerebrospinal fluid produced in each of the lateral ventricles flows through the interventricular foramen (Foramen of Munro) into the third ventricle. More fluid is produced in the third ventricle and all of it flows through the cerebral aqueduct (Aqueduct of Sylvius) to the fourth ventricle, where more fluid is added. From the fourth ventricle, the fluid escapes into the subarachnoid space through one of the three foramina mentioned above. It then circulates around the brain and spinal cord and eventually reaches the arachnoid villi, where, by a process of osmosis, it is emptied into the great venous dural sinuses, particularly the superior sagittal sinus.

An obstruction to the passage of cerebrospinal fluid results in a back-up of cerebrospinal fluid and an increase in intracranial pressure. This condition, in which there is an accumulation of cerebrospinal fluid in either the ventricular system or subarachnoid space, is called 'hydrocephalus' (water on the brain). If the obstruction to the flow is within the ventricular system itself (e.g. midbrain tumours often cause constriction of the cerebral aqueduct leading to accumulation of cerebrospinal fluid in the lateral and third ventricles), the condition is called 'obstructive, or non-communicating, hydrocephalus'. If the cerebrospinal fluid can get out of the ventricular system, but owing to a blockage in the subarachnoid space cannot then circulate properly to reach the arachnoid villi, the condition is called 'communicating hydrocephalus'. This latter form of hydrocephalus can occur if there are adhesions in the subarachnoid space owing to past inflammation (e.g. meningitis) or may be due to haemorrhage into the subarachnoid space.

Hydrocephalus can occur in either adults or children but is most commonly associated with infants who have a congenital abnormality that blocks the flow of cerebrospinal fluid. The cerebral aqueduct and foramina of the fourth ventricle are common sites of obstruction. The flexibility of the infant skull causes the head to enlarge in response to the increased intracranial pressure. Initially, therefore in infant cases the compression of neural tissue is moderate. Surgical intervention is usually required whereby a tube (shunt) is placed in a ventricle above the blockage and the excess fluid shunted into one of several areas distal to the block including the cisterna magna, jugular vein or atrium of the heart. Hydrocephalus can also occur in adults as a result of tumours, meningitis and traumatic haemorrhage. As the skull is inflexible in adults, brain tissue can be rapidly compressed and immediate

surgical procedures may be necessary to save the patient's life.

The normal functions of the cerebrospinal fluid are still uncertain. The fluid undoubtedly cushions the brain and spinal cord and minimizes damage that might otherwise result from sudden movements or from blows to the head and spine. The fluid plays a role in the diffusion of materials into and away from the brain, and it might well transport specific substances such as neurohormones from one part of the central nervous system to another.

Cerebrospinal fluid can be sampled by a procedure known as lumbar puncture and a variety of tests carried out to aid the medical diagnosis of a number of neurological disorders. The same procedure can be used to inject drugs to combat infections.

The blood supply to the brain

Disruption to the blood supply to the brain is a major cause of acquired neurological speech-language disorders with the features of the associated communicative disorder being largely determined by the specific cerebral blood vessel(s) involved. Consequently, an understanding of the blood supply to the brain is of fundamental importance to understanding the origins of many of the clinically recognized forms of motor speech-language disorders associated with cerebrovascular pathologies.

Arterial blood supply

The arterial blood supply of the contents of the cranial cavity is derived from the aortic arch in the thorax and then passes to the brain via the paired internal carotid and vertebral arteries. The internal carotid arteries supply blood to the greater part of the cerebral hemispheres. However, the occipital lobes get their chief supply via the vertebral arteries, which also feed the brainstem and cerebellum. The internal carotid artery gives rise to the ophthalmic, anterior cerebral, anterior choroidal, middle cerebral and posterior communicating arteries. The vertebral artery gives rise to the posterior inferior cerebellar artery, the

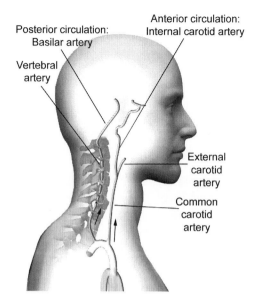

Posterior circulation:
Basilar artery

Anterior circulation:
Internal carotid artery

Vertebral
artery

External
carotid
artery

Common
carotid
artery

Figure 1.28 Extracranial and cranial courses of the vertebral, basilar and carotid arteries.

anterior and posterior spinal arteries and the basilar artery. The basilar artery in turn gives rise to the anterior inferior cerebellar artery, the superior cerebellar artery and the posterior cerebral arteries.

The common carotid arteries ascend in the neck (Figure 1.28). At the level of the thyroid cartilage each divides into an external and an internal carotid artery. Each internal carotid artery enters the cranial cavity through a canal (the carotid canal) in the base of the skull, emerges alongside the optic chiasma and divides into an anterior and middle cerebral artery. The two anterior cerebral arteries are united by a small communicating branch called the anterior communicating artery. Prior to dividing into the anterior and middle cerebral arteries, the internal carotid gives rise to the ophthalmic, posterior communicating and anterior choroidal arteries. The ophthalmic artery is the first branch of the internal carotid. It enters the orbit to supply the optic nerve and eye. The posterior communicating artery connects the internal carotid with the posterior cerebral artery and has branches which help supply parts of the hypothalamus, subthalamus, thalamus, internal capsule and midbrain. The anterior choroidal artery usually arises from the internal carotid distal to the posterior communicating artery. It helps supply the choroid plexuses of the lateral ventricles, optic tract, midbrain, globus pallidus, posterior limb of the internal capsule and thalamus (for details see Chapter 3).

The vertebral arteries ascend in foramina (openings) in the transverse processes of the cervical vertebrae (Figure 1.28) and enter the cranial cavity through the foramen magnum. On the ventral surface of the brainstem they join to form a single arterial stem, the basilar artery. This artery ascends in front of the brainstem and ends by dividing into two posterior cerebral arteries. Each of these is joined to the corresponding internal carotid artery by a communicating branch (posterior communicating arteries). This forms what is known as the Circle of Willis, that is a circle of arteries consisting of the two posterior cerebral arteries, the two anterior cerebral, the two internal carotid arteries and the posterior and anterior communicating arteries (Figure 1.29). Although the Circle of Willis provides a link between the major arteries that supply the brain, under normal conditions there is little exchange of blood between the main arteries through the slender anterior and posterior communicating arteries, since the arterial pressure in the internal carotid arteries is similar to that in the basilar artery. The Circle of Willis, however, provides alternative routes for blood when one of the major arteries leading into it is occluded. For example, if one of the posterior cerebral arteries is occluded where it branches from the basilar artery, the pressure distal to the occlusion will drop allowing blood from the internal carotid on the same side to flow into the posterior cerebral via the posterior communicating artery. These anastomoses (an anastomosis is a connection between two tubular organs), however, are frequently inadequate, especially in older people where the communicating arteries may be narrowed by vascular disease (atherosclerosis). Unfortunately, the Circle of Willis and its immediate branches are also common sites for aneurysms (sacs in blood vessel walls).

The regions of the cerebral hemisphere supplied by the various cerebral arteries are shown in Figure 1.30.

The middle cerebral artery, the largest branch of the internal carotid, travels laterally in the

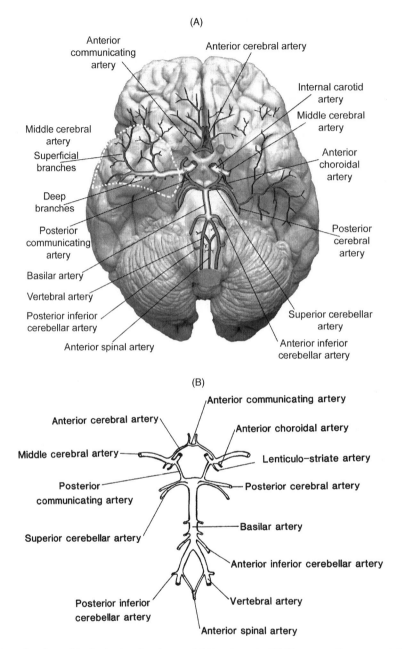

Figure 1.29 (A) Ventral surface of the brain showing the arterial blood supply. (B) Diagrammatic representation of the Circle of Willis.

lateral fissure. Eventually, it emerges from the lateral fissure onto the lateral surface of the cerebral hemisphere, as can be seen from Figure 1.30. Branches of the middle cerebral artery supply almost the entire lateral surface of the hemisphere, including the motor and sensory areas for the face, hand, arm, shoulder, trunk and pelvis. In the dominant hemisphere the region supplied by the middle cerebral artery also includes the major speech-language centres, making it the most important artery involved in pathologies associated with the occurrence of aphasia. While in the

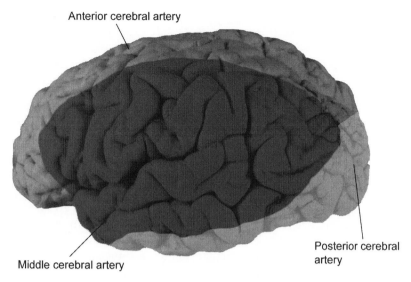

Anterior cerebral artery

Middle cerebral artery

Posterior cerebral artery

Figure 1.30 Lateral view of the left cerebral hemisphere showing the distribution of the major cerebral arteries.

lateral fissure, the middle cerebral artery gives off several branches which supply structures such as the cortex of the insula and various subcortical structures. One branch, the lateral striate artery, supplies components of the basal ganglia such as parts of the caudate and lenticular nuclei and the internal capsule. (The blood supply to subcortical structures is described in further detail in Chapter 3.)

The anterior cerebral artery branches off the internal carotid artery near the olfactory tract. It travels along the corpus callosum in the longitudinal fissure and supplies all the medial surface of the cerebral cortex as far back as the parieto-occipital sulcus including the foot and leg areas of the motor strip. A branch of the anterior cerebral artery called the medial striate artery supplies part of the caudate nucleus, lenticular nucleus and internal capsule. The anterior cerebral artery also supplies the undersurface of the frontal lobe.

The posterior cerebral artery branches off the basilar artery at its terminal bifurcation and curves laterally around the midbrain and then dorsally to the temporal and occipital lobes. It supplies the medial and inferior surface of the temporal lobe and the medial surface and pole of the occipital lobe. Branches of the posterior cerebral artery, which include the posterior choroidal arteries, the thalamoperforating branches and the

thalamogeniculate branches, also supply parts of the midbrain, the majority of the thalamus and part of the internal capsule.

Whereas the cerebrum is supplied primarily by branches of the internal carotid artery, the brainstem and cerebellum receive their arterial supply via branches of the basilar and vertebral arteries. The posterior spinal artery arises from the vertebral artery at the mid-medullary level and descends along the dorsal surface of the lower medulla and spinal cord. It helps supply the dorsal region of the medulla, including the nuclei cuneatus and gracilis and the dorsal portion of the spinal cord.

Two anterior spinal arteries arise from the vertebral arteries at the level of the olive. They unite almost immediately to form a single anterior spinal artery which descends in the anterior median fissure of the medulla and spinal cord (Figure 1.29). It supplies a medial wedge of the medulla including the hypoglossal nucleus, and the anterior portion of the spinal cord.

The posterior inferior cerebellar artery branches off the cerebral artery at the level of the mid-medulla and courses dorsally along the medulla and then curves upwards along the inferior surface of the cerebellum. It supplies the dorsolateral part of the medulla which contains the spinothalamic and rubrospinal tracts, the nucleus ambiguus, the dorsal motor nucleus of the vagus and the inferior cerebellar peduncle. It also supplies parts of the inferior vermis as well as the inferior surface of the cerebellar hemisphere and the deep nuclei of the cerebellum. Branches of this artery also supply portions of the choroid plexus of the fourth ventricle.

The anterior inferior cerebellar artery branches off the basilar artery at the level of the caudal pons and passes caudally and laterally to reach the inferior surface of the cerebellum. It helps to supply the tegmentum of the caudal pons, parts of the inferior vermis and the inferior surface of the cerebellar hemisphere and deep nuclei of the cerebellum.

Numerous small branches of the basilar artery form the major supply to the pons. These branches include paramedian branches that supply the medial portion of the pons, excluding the tegmentum and circumferential arteries that curve backward to supply the lateral and dorsal portions of the pons.

The superior cerebellar artery branches off the basilar artery at the level of the midbrain just below the point where it bifurcates into the two posterior cerebral arteries. It then passes back to the superior surface of the cerebellum. It contributes branches to the circumferential arteries that supply central and lateral parts of the crus cerebri and substantia nigra and lateral parts of the midbrain tegmentum. It also supplies the superior vermis, superior surface of the cerebellar hemisphere and the deep nuclei of the cerebellum.

Venous blood supply

The brain is drained by two sets of veins, both of which empty into the dural venous sinuses, which, in turn, empty into the internal jugular veins. These two sets of veins are known as the deep or great cerebral veins and the superficial cerebral veins. Before dealing with each of these, however, it is necessary to have an understanding of the dural venous sinuses.

The major dural venous sinuses include the superior sagittal sinus, which runs along the superior portion of the longitudinal fissure at the junction of the falx cerebri and the cranial dura and the inferior sagittal sinus, which runs deep within the longitudinal fissure along the deep margin of the falx cerebri. These two sinuses are joined together by the straight sinus, which runs along the midline crest of the tentorium cerebelli at its junction with the falx cerebri. The straight sinus empties into the transverse sinus. The two transverse sinuses pass laterally from the junction of the straight sinus and superior sagittal sinus and course downwards to leave the cranium through the jugular foramina and become the internal jugular veins. Another important venous sinus, the cavernous sinus, is a large, rather diffuse, sinus located around the sella turcica. It drains eventually into the transverse sinuses and jugular veins via the superior and inferior petrosal sinuses. A sinus known as the occipital sinus runs in the falx cerebri. It opens into the confluence of sinuses where the straight, transverse and superior sagittal sinuses meet.

The cerebral veins themselves have very thin walls, no muscular layer and no valves. As suggested above, they are found on the surface of the brain or in the substance of the central nervous system. The superficial cerebral veins lie in the sulci and are more external than the arteries. Those draining the cerebral hemispheres can be divided into superior, middle and inferior cerebral veins. A variable number of superior cerebral veins drain the superior surface of the cerebral cortex and empty into the superior sagittal sinus. The middle cerebral veins drain most of the lateral and inferior surface of the cerebral hemispheres. These vessels are found in the lateral fissure and empty into the cavernous sinus. The inferior cerebral veins drain the lateral occipital gyrus and part of the temporal lobe. These vessels drain into the transverse sinuses. All dural sinuses receive blood from their immediate vicinity.

The deep cerebral veins conduct blood from the centre of the cerebrum and converge upon a single large vein called the great cerebral vein or vein of Galen. The vein of Galen empties into the straight sinus. The veins that drain the brain stem and cerebellum also drain into the dural sinuses, some via the great cerebral vein.

Although most of the venous blood coming from the brain eventually leaves the cranial cavity via the internal jugular veins, other exits from the cranial cavity also exist. Some dural sinuses connect with the veins superficial to the skull by emissary veins. For example, the cavernous sinus is connected with emissary veins, including the ophthalmic vein, which extends through the orbit. A number of such communications via emissary veins exist between the dural sinuses and extracranial veins.

The blood–brain barrier

There is a free and rapid passage of substances between the brain tissue and the cerebrospinal fluid, but there is a barrier between the blood and brain tissue, the blood–brain barrier. This maintains a constant milieu for brain metabolism and is a protection against noxious substances present in the circulation (e.g. urea). The barrier is equally effective against antibiotics except when inflammation changes its characteristics.

The capillary network of the central nervous system is extensive, especially in the grey matter. The capillaries in the central nervous system have permeability characteristics that are fundamentally different, however, from those of capillaries elsewhere in the body. The endothelial cells in brain capillaries form a continuous rather than a fenestrated layer. The capillaries form the blood–brain barrier, which is a major obstacle

to the free movement of substances from the blood to the brain. In fact, the diffusion of most substances is definitely limited, except for lipid-soluble compounds and water. The importance of the barrier is that it may prevent potentially therapeutic drugs from reaching the brain. In such cases, these drugs may be administered directly into the cerebrospinal fluid via lumbar puncture.

Speech-language centres of the brain

Within the dominant hemisphere, two major cortical areas have been identified as having specialized language functions. These two areas are located in the perisylvian region (region surrounding the Fissure of Sylvius) and include the anterior or motor speech-language area (usually referred to as Broca's area) and the posterior or sensory speech-language area (usually called Wernicke's area) (Figure 1.31).

The two major speech-language areas have been largely identified by the study of patients in whom these areas were damaged by either occlusion of blood vessels or by war injuries. Until relatively recently, the most reliable information concerning the areas of the brain important for language has come from the results of long-term

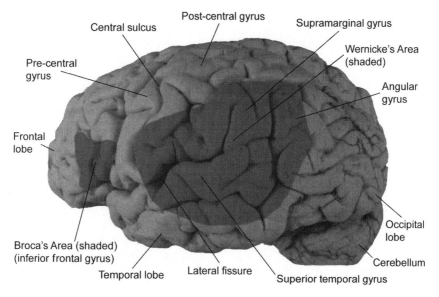

Figure 1.31 Lateral view of the left cerebral hemisphere showing the major speech-language areas.

studies of language-disordered patients whose lesions were identified at post-mortem examination. Since the mid-1970s, computer tomography has been extensively used to localize lesions associated with various types of language disorders. Using this technique, investigators were able to study for the first time the relationship between regions of brain damage and disturbances in language function in the living subject, particularly in those cases where the lesions involved deep cerebral structures below the level of the cortex. More recently introduced neuroimaging techniques such as positron emission tomography (PET) scanning and magnetic resonance imaging (MRI) scanning have further expanded the ability of researchers to localize lesions associated with specific language disorders in living subjects.

The anterior speech-language area was first identified by Paul Broca in the mid-nineteenth century and is, therefore, commonly referred to as Broca's area. Broca's area occupies the pars opercularis and pars triangularis of the inferior frontal gyrus (also called the third frontal convolution), which represents Brodmann areas 44 and 45 and lies immediately in front of that part of the cortical motor strip devoted to the peripheral organs of speech.

The posterior speech-language area lies posterior to the Fissure of Rolando. The existence of this area was first indicated by Carl Wernicke in the 1870s. Reports in the literature on the location and extent of the posterior speech-language area vary widely. Wernicke originally indicated that the auditory association cortex (Brodmann area 22) of the dominant hemisphere (Wernicke's area) acts as a language centre. Subsequent authors have modified and extended this area to include a greater part of the temporal lobe and parts of the parietal lobe. Currently, most descriptions of the posterior speech-language area include within its boundaries the lower half of the post-central gyrus, the supramarginal and angular gyri, the inferior parietal gyrus and the upper part of the temporal lobe, including parts of the superior and second temporal gyri and Wernicke's area.

In the majority of people (approximately 96%) the language areas are located in the left cerebral hemisphere. The anterior and posterior speech-language areas communicate with one another via the arcuate fasciculus, a bundle of association fibres that travel as part of a long association tract called the superior longitudinal fasciculus. The arcuate fasciculus sweeps around the insular region, and its fan-shaped ends connect parts of the temporal and frontal lobes.

It appears from observations of the speech-language deficits of patients with known lesion sites that the posterior language area is devoted to those tasks having to do mainly with the recognition, comprehension and formulation of language. As this region of the cerebral hemisphere also deals with the reception of sensory stimuli through the auditory, visual and somatosensory (body sensations) systems, it is believed that language data, which are transmitted through these same modalities, are processed in this area of the hemisphere. In contrast to the posterior area, the anterior language area is involved with the programming and execution of overt acts, such as those that result in speaking, writing or gesturing.

Obviously, the anterior and posterior language areas do not function separately. Rather, for normal language function to occur, the anterior and posterior areas must be in communication. As described above, the two areas are connected primarily by the arcuate fasciculus, although other connections through subcortical structures such as the thalamus also exist. It is believed, therefore, that information concerning the spoken or written word is decoded and translated in the posterior language area and, as a consequence of this, damage to the posterior area results in impairment of the ability to comprehend the written or spoken word.

Comprehension of speech takes place when auditory impulses are transmitted to the auditory cortex of both hemispheres and subsequently relayed to the posterior language area in the dominant hemisphere for translation. Comprehension of written words, on the other hand, takes place when visual impulses are transmitted to the visual cortex in the occipital lobes of each hemisphere and are subsequently relayed to the posterior language area. Following translation in the posterior area, information is then passed to the anterior area via the arcuate fasciculus for the complex programming of the speech organs in order to make a verbal response. Damage to the anterior language area, therefore, results in language production problems involving planning and execution. The anterior area feeds information to the primary motor cortex of each hemisphere and from there instructions are sent via the motor pathways to the muscles of the speech mechanism to produce a verbal response.

In addition to the above two areas, a third cortical area has been identified which may be involved in speech-language functions. This third area is small and lies mainly in the medial surface of the frontal lobe (i.e. within the longitudinal fissure) immediately anterior to the foot region of the primary motor strip. It is known as the secondary speech area or the supplementary motor area. Lesions in this area often lead to temporary aphasias and difficulty in producing rapidly alternating movements such as those required in the oral region during speech. The entire secondary speech area can be excised, however, without causing a permanent language disorder.

Although the centres described above, including the anterior and posterior language areas and the secondary speech area, comprise the primary speech-language centres of the brain, it is evident that other brain structures also play a role in language function. In particular, these other areas include the parietal, temporal and occipital association areas and various subcortical structures such as the basal ganglia. (For further discussion of the role of subcortical structures in language see Chapter 3.)

Neurologically based communication disorders – definitions

Speech sounds are produced by regulating the exhaled airstream as it passes from the lungs to the atmosphere. This regulation is brought about by movements of the jaw, lips, tongue, soft palate, pharynx and vocal cords, which vibrate the air column and alter the shape of the vocal tract. The movements are brought about by the contraction of skeletal muscles, which in turn are regulated by nerve impulses. The entire process of speech production is, of course, controlled by the central nervous system.

Box 1.2 Basic Processes Involved in Speech Production

1. A concept of the speech output has to be formed and symbolically formulated for expression as speech – disruption at this level is associated with APHASIA.
2. The symbolically formulated concept of speech output has to be externalized as speech through the concurrent motor functions of respiration, phonation, resonance, articulation and prosody – disruption at this level is associated with DYSARTHRIA.
3. Prior to externalization as speech, a programme has to be developed which determines the sequence of muscle contractions required to produce individual sounds and words that comprise the intended speech output – disruption at this level leads to APRAXIA OF SPEECH.

The efficient execution of speech production requires the smooth sequencing and coordination of three basic neurological processes (Box 1.2).

Impairment of each of these three processes results in a distinctive communication disorder. Impairment in the first process involving the organization of concepts and their symbolic formulation and expression is caused by pathological processes that damage the cerebral hemisphere that contains the speech-language centres, thereby leading to aphasia. Aphasia has been defined as the loss or impairment of language function caused by brain damage. Aphasia is due to brain injury and is an impairment of the capacity to interpret and formulate language symbols. Aphasia is a multimodality disorder (i.e. it manifests in difficulties in speaking, reading and writing) and involves a reduction in the capacity to decode (interpret) and encode (formulate) meaningful linguistic elements (i.e. words, or 'morphemes', and larger syntactical units such as sentences). The aphasic patient is impaired in the comprehension, formulation and expression of language although the relative amount of loss in each of these areas varies between one type of aphasia and another (see Chapter 2). All aphasic patients do, however, show some loss in all three of these areas.

Impairment in the second process involving the motor production of speech is associated with dysarthria, a group of speech disorders resulting from interference with any of the basic motor processes involved in speech production (a more complete definition of 'dysarthria' is given in Chapters 9). Damage located at a number of different sites in the nervous system including the cerebrum, brainstem or cerebellum can be associated with dysarthria, in each case a different type of dysarthria results (see Chapters 9, 10 and 11).

Impairment of the third process involving the programming of motor actions involved in speech production is caused by damage to those circuits located in the cerebrum devoted to the selection and sequencing of sensorimotor programmes that determine the sequence of muscle contractions required to produce speech. Such impairment leads to a communication disorder called 'apraxia of speech' (or verbal apraxia). Apraxia of speech is, therefore, a 'phonetic-motoric disorder of speech production caused by inefficiencies in the translation of well-formed and filled phonological frames into previously learned kinematic information used for carrying out intended movements' (McNeil, Robin and Schmidt, 2008, p. 264). The condition manifests, primarily, as errors in the articulation of speech and, secondarily, by what are thought by many researchers to be compensatory alterations of prosody (e.g. pauses, slow rate, equalization of stress). It is a disorder in which, although the muscles of the speech mechanism are neither paralysed nor weak, the individual has difficulty speaking because of a cerebral lesion that prevents executing voluntarily and on command the complex sequence of muscle contractions involved in speaking. The clinical features and neurological basis of apraxia of speech are described and discussed in detail in Chapter 8.

Whereas aphasia is considered a language disorder, dysarthria and apraxia of speech are motor speech disorders involving disruption of the motor control of speech. Although each of these three disorders is distinctive, it should be remembered that they can occur in combination and consequently a neurologically disordered patient may exhibit the characteristics of more than one of these disorders. Many aphasic patients, for instance, may exhibit some apraxic elements and some type of dysarthria.

Neuropathological substrate of neurogenic speech-language disorders

Any type of neuropathology capable of producing structural alterations in an appropriate portion of the brain, whether that be the cerebral cortex, subcortical structures, brainstem or cerebellum, is capable of producing a communication deficit in the form of either a speech or language disorder, or both. Widely diverse disease processes affecting particular brain structures may produce similar abnormalities in brain function. Consequently, it is the neuroanatomic location of the brain damage rather than the causative agent that largely determines the nature of the communicative deficit. The specific causative disease, however, can usually be identified by certain characteristics of the patient's history, the specific pattern of neurological dysfunction and by appropriate laboratory and/or clinical examinations.

The major diseases of the nervous system that produce speech-language disorders are cerebrovascular disease, neoplastic disorders, head trauma, degenerative disease, toxic conditions, demyelinating disorders and infectious diseases.

Cerebrovascular disorders

Disorders in which one or more of the blood vessels of the brain are primarily involved in the pathological process are the most common form of neurogenic disease. Consequently, in peacetime cerebrovascular disorders are the most common cause of brain damage relating to the occurrence of neurogenic speech-language disorders.

When the blood supply to the brain is seriously disturbed spontaneously (i.e. not owing to trauma or surgical ligation of cerebral vessels), the condition is referred to as a 'cerebrovascular accident' or 'stroke'. By definition, a cerebrovascular accident or stroke represents a syndrome characterized by the acute onset of a neurological deficit that persists for at least 24 hours, reflects focal involvement of the central nervous system and is the result of a disturbance of the cerebral circulation. The three major characteristics of cerebrovascular accidents include: (1) an abrupt onset of focal brain dysfunction; (2) the disability produced (including any speech or language deficit) is worst at onset or within a short period of onset; (3) if the patient survives, the disability tends to improve, in some cases partially, in others almost totally. Approximately 750 000 new cerebrovascular accidents occur in the United States each year with the incidence increasing with age. About two-thirds of all strokes occur in persons over 65 years of age, with the incidence being slightly higher in men than in women. However, even young children on occasions suffer from cerebrovascular accidents. Risk factors for cerebrovascular accidents include systolic or diastolic hypertension, hypercholesterolaemia, cigarette smoking, heavy alcohol consumption and oral contraceptive use. Genetic factors may also be important in some cases, but the cause of cerebrovascular accidents in most cases is likely to be multifactorial, involving both polygenic and environmental influences.

Cerebrovascular accidents can be divided into two major types: ischaemic strokes and haemorrhagic strokes. Ischaemic strokes occur when the supply of blood to part of the brain suddenly becomes inadequate for the brain cells to function. Haemorrhagic strokes occur when a blood vessel ruptures and blood either rushes through the brain tissue destroying it (intracerebral haemorrhage) or collects outside the brain in one of the spaces between the meninges causing compression of the brain within the skull.

Ischaemic stroke. Ischaemic strokes can arise in two ways: first, through occlusion of the vessel by thrombus formation (cerebral thrombosis) and, second, through occlusion of the vessel by an embolus (cerebral embolism). Approximately two-thirds of ischaemic strokes are caused by thrombosis, while one-third are attributed to embolism. Thrombosis is most commonly associated with atherosclerotic changes in the blood vessel wall. However, it can also be associated with inflammatory disorders which affect the blood vessels such as giant cell arteritis, syphilitic endarteritis and systemic lupus erythematosus among others. Atherosclerosis of the large extracranial arteries in the neck and at the base of the brain is the underlying cause of focal cerebral ischaemia in the great majority of cases of cerebrovascular accident. Although the pathogenesis of atherosclerosis is incompletely understood, the condition involves the formation of fibrous plaques in the walls of the blood vessels which may occlude the lumen of the affected vessel or give rise to atheromatous or platelet emboli. Within the cerebral circulation, the sites of predilection for the formation of atherosclerotic plaques are the origin of the common carotid artery, the internal carotid artery just above the common carotid bifurcation and within the cavernous sinus, the origin of the middle cerebral artery, the vertebral artery at its origin and just above where it enters the skull, and the basilar artery. Giant cell arteritis (also called temporal arteritis) produces inflammatory changes that affect branches of the external carotid, cervical internal carotid, posterior ciliary, extracranial vertebral and intracranial arteries. These inflammatory changes in the arterial wall may stimulate platelet adhesion and aggregation on damaged surfaces within the blood vessel leading to thrombosis or distal embolism. Syphilitic arteritis occurs within five years after a primary syphilitic infection and primarily affects medium-sized penetrating blood vessels leading to punctuate areas of infarction in the deep white matter of the cerebral hemispheres. In contrast, systemic lupus erythematosus is associated with a vasculopathy that involves small cerebral blood vessels and leads to multiple microinfarctions.

Thrombotic stroke usually develops abruptly, often during sleep or shortly after rising. In some cases, however, it may be preceded by transient warning signs, in which case it has a step-wise onset over several hours or days. Thrombotic strokes are the most common type of cerebrovascular accident.

Embolic strokes are almost always abrupt in onset and the patient is only rarely forewarned by transitory symptoms. Embolism is now well recognized as a frequent and important source of stroke. The potential sources of emboli are remarkably widespread. For a long time it was believed that almost all emboli came from the heart, as a result of small pieces of mural thrombosis (from the walls of the heart) becoming dislodged from the cardiac wall by atrial fibrillation or other cardiac arrhythmia. Angiography has demonstrated that calcified plaques associated with atherosclerosis, particularly in the carotid vessels, are also frequent sources of cerebral emboli. Cardiac surgery and bacterial endocarditis are less common but also real sources of emboli. Consequently, disorders such as rheumatic heart disease with atrial fibrillation, atrial fibrillation with coronary heart disease, recent myocardial infarction with mural thrombus formation or bacterial endocarditis all predispose to brain damage embolism. Occasionally, emboli emanate from the lungs or even the great veins and on rare occasions emboli of tumour cells may become lodged in the vessels of the brain.

Of central importance in both types of ischaemic stroke is the fact that they deprive brain tissue of needed oxygen. Both thrombosis and embolism cause acute ischaemia in the tissues receiving their vascular supply from the occluded vessel which, in turn, produces an area of cell death (infarct). Embolic infarctions develop much more rapidly than thrombotic infarcts. Both neurones and the myelinated pathways are affected but the white matter is considerably less sensitive to ischaemia than grey matter (i.e. the cortex). The centre of an infarct will be totally destroyed, but towards the periphery there may be preservation of white matter pathways and there is often a surrounding zone of lesser ischaemia in which cells cease to function on a temporary basis, but cell death does not occur. In time, some of these injured neurones recuperate sufficiently to resume function and many white matter pathways survive to carry impulses again. This delayed return of function to certain areas within an infarct provides one explanation (but not the only one, e.g. reduction in degree of associated oedema is another) of the spontaneous recovery so often seen in many types of aphasias. The outcome of an infarct is a cyst-like area from which both neurones and white matter have disappeared, surrounded by a scarred, sclerotic zone of glia.

Ischaemic attacks vary in their severity. At one extreme, a major vessel may be almost totally occluded by thrombosis or by a major embolism. At the other extreme, the ischaemic attack may be only transient and therefore may not deprive the brain tissue of oxygen for long enough to cause permanent brain damage. Transient ischaemic attacks tend to involve repetitive stereotyped attacks of focal neurological function followed by complete recovery (usually within 30 minutes). Formerly considered to be caused by episodic narrowing, or 'spasming', of blood vessels, it is now thought that transient ischaemic attacks are produced by repeated embolization of small particles from proximally located atherosclerotic plaques in the large vessels of the neck (e.g. the internal carotid arteries). Although transient ischaemic attacks do not themselves produce lasting neurological dysfunction, they are clinically important in that about one-third of patients who suffer these attacks go on to have a cerebrovascular accident within five years, a risk that my be reduced with appropriate treatment.

Haemorrhagic stroke. Haemorrhagic stroke may have a sudden onset with evolution to maximum deficit occurring in a smooth fashion over several hours. Cerebral haemorrhage, when the result of vascular disease (as opposed to trauma), is most often associated with hypertension but it may occur with a variety of pathologies affecting the cerebral vessels such as aneurysm, angioma, arteriovenous malformation, blood dyscrasia or arteritis. Anticoagulant therapy (e.g. warfarin therapy) is acknowledged as a frequent cause of cerebral haemorrhage which can lead to the production of speech-language disorders.

Most haemorrhages occur during activity and without warning. Onset therefore is abrupt and is associated with severe headache, vomiting and often loss of consciousness. The most common site for intracerebral haemorrhages is the region of the internal capsule, in which case the patient suddenly complains of something wrong in the head, followed by headache, dysarthria and/or aphasia, paralysis down the opposite side of the body and variable alterations in consciousness. With brainstem haemorrhage there is usually rapid loss of consciousness and often death in a short time. Cerebellar haemorrhages are associated with vertigo, nausea and ataxia followed by coma and often death. Overall, the prognosis for recovery for haemorrhagic strokes is poorer than it is for ischaemic strokes.

Intracerebral haemorrhages usually involve deeper structures of the brain than the cerebral cortex and produce brain damage both by local destruction and by compression of surrounding brain tissue. The force of blood coming from a ruptured blood vessel directly damages the brain tissue. This extravasated blood forms a clot, called a 'haematoma', which increases in size and displaces surrounding brain tissue. As the skull is a fixed box, the intracranial pressure increases as the clot develops causing compression of the brain tissue. Secondary rupture into the ventricular system or subarachnoid space may also occur. Emergency evacuation of the intracerebral clot is of value in aiding the relief of symptoms in some cases.

In addition to hypertension, rupture of an intracranial aneurysm is another major cause of haemorrhagic strokes. An aneurysm is a thin-walled enlargement of a blood vessel usually found in the Circle of Willis or its major branches. Aneurysms tend to occur at junctions, or bifurcations, and are believed to represent congenital deficiencies in the development of the vessel wall. They tend to increase in size and may produce cranial nerve palsies or focal seizures by compression of adjacent structures prior to rupture. Rupture usually occurs during activity and produces severe headache, collapse and unconsciousness. Generally, bleeding occurs into the subarachnoid space but may also occur into the brain tissue forming an intracerebral haemorrhage. In the latter case, prolonged unconsciousness and focal signs such as hemiplegia, hemianaesthesia and aphasia may also occur.

Neoplasms

Intracranial tumours (neoplasms) are the third-most-common disorder of the nervous system after cerebrovascular diseases and infections. Although they are, in general, a less frequent cause of speech-language disorders than cerebrovascular accidents, intracranial tumours are nonetheless not uncommon as aphasia-producing lesions. Such tumours may be either benign or malignant. Tumours affecting the central nervous system are said to be primary tumours if they grow from cells within the cranial cavity itself, or secondary (metastases) if they travel to the brain from a pri-

mary tumour elsewhere in the body (e.g. breasts, lungs, etc.).

Brain tumours produce symptoms in three ways. First, because tumours are space-occupying lesions, as they develop they cause the intracranial pressure to rise, leading to compression and distortion of surrounding brain structures. Second, as tumours grow they may disrupt the blood supply to specific regions of the brain or may interrupt the circulation of cerebrospinal fluid, such as by compressing the ventricles or occluding the cerebral aqueduct, thereby leading to increased intracranial pressure. Third, the tumour may directly damage the brain tissue in a localized area. The direct effect produces symptoms and signs (e.g. paralysis down one side of the body, epileptic fits, etc.) which become gradually worse and more extensive as the tumour grows, in complete contrast to the sudden onset of a cerebrovascular accident. Tumours growing in the dominant hemisphere may cause progressively increasing aphasia.

Intracranial tumours can be divided into two major types, namely intracerebral tumours and extracerebral tumours. Intracerebral tumours are those that directly involve the cerebral tissues, while extracerebral tumours arise from tissues outside the brain itself (e.g. the meninges and skull bones). By far the majority of intracerebral neoplasms are gliomas, which develop from the supporting tissue of the brain (i.e. the neuroglial cells), tumours of nerve cells being rare. The various types of glioma take their names from the particular neuroglial cells involved and include astrocytomas, oligodendrocytomas and microgliomas. Some intracerebral tumours called 'ependymomas' develop from the cells lining the ventricles (ependymal cells), while others called 'medulloblastomas' develop from primitive cells in the roof of the fourth ventricle. Any variety of intracerebral tumour is capable of producing a speech and/or language disturbance dependent upon its location in the brain. On the other hand, language disorders are rarely caused by extracranial tumours which include among others those growing from the meninges (meningiomas), sheaths of peripheral nerves (neurofibromas, e.g. acoustic neuromas), the skull bones (osteomas) and the pituitary gland (e.g. various adenomas).

These tumours are mostly benign and do not directly cause destruction of cerebral tissues as in the case of intracerebral tumours but instead may produce abnormal neurological signs as a result of distortion or displacement of cerebral tissue.

Although intracerebral tumours cause language disorders more often than extracerebral tumours, in neither variety does aphasia usually become a major complaint until late in the course of the disease. The reason why aphasic symptoms usually only appear late in the disorder is that intracerebral neoplasms infiltrate the cerebral tissues widely before producing focal destruction. Further, extracerebral tumours tend to develop slowly, allowing considerable accommodation by the cerebral tissues with only minimal disruption of functions until late in the course of the disorder. If aphasic symptoms do appear early in the development of a tumour, it is usually because the tumour has either disrupted the cerebral blood supply or interfered with the circulation of cerebrospinal fluid. Although the particular neurological signs, including any speech or language disorder, associated with the presence of a tumour may give some indication as to the location of that tumour in the brain, owing to the local effects of the tumour, it must be remembered that distortion and/or compression of cerebral tissue may actually occur at a distance from where the tumour is located. Consequently, the particular speech-language deficit exhibited may have no direct relationship with the location of the tumour itself.

Some intracranial tumours occur more frequently in persons belonging to a particular age group. Others produce characteristic syndromes because of their predilection for certain sites. In particular, tumours located in the posterior cranial fossa (i.e. infratentorial tumours involving the cerebellum, fourth ventricle and/or brainstem) occur more commonly in childhood than supratentorial neoplasms, accounting for up to 70% of all paediatric intracranial neoplasms. However, it has been reported that supratentorial tumours have a higher incidence in children less than three years of age. The most common posterior fossa tumours are astrocytomas, medulloblastomas and ependymomas. (For a more complete discussion of paediatric brain tumours, see Chapter 12.) Meningiomas, neurofibromas of cranial nerves, gliomas of the cerebral hemispheres and pituitary tumours are more common in the middle decades. Metastatic tumours are most common in the later decades of life.

Surgical removal of tumours may also be the cause of speech and/or language deficits. Often, such surgery requires destruction of both the grey and white matter that has been infiltrated by the tumour. In addition, there is evidence to suggest that radiotherapy and chemotherapy often given as part of the treatment of intracranial tumours may cause damage to the nervous tissue, which may manifest several years later as impaired language and cognitive abilities.

Head trauma

Traumatic head injury is a common cause of speech and/or language disorders, particularly in young adult males. Although head injury can result from a variety of different incidents, in peacetime the majority of head injuries are caused by motor vehicle accidents. Over the years, traumatic head injury cases, particularly subjects with brain injury resulting for war wounds, have provided an important source of language-disordered patients for academic study. The nature of the speech-language deficits seen in association with traumatic head injury are discussed in detail in Chapter 4.

Degenerative disorders

Degenerative diseases of the nervous system include a broad range of disorders all of which are characterized clinically by progressive deterioration of neurological function and pathologically by cellular depletion with atrophy of nervous tissue. Those affecting the cerebrum and particularly the cerebral cortex are characterized by progressive dementia in the middle or later decades of life and include disorders such as Alzheimer's disease and Pick's disease. Both of these conditions are associated with an initial dulling of intellectual abilities with impairment of memory and confusion. Language impairment has also been reported to be a common occurrence in these disorders. Progressive deterioration occurs in months or years, leading to profound dementia, immobility and death from secondary infections. Focal signs such as hemiparesis, hemianaesthesia, cranial nerve palsies and increased intracranial pressure do not occur. The language disorders associated with the major clinically encountered forms of dementia are discussed in Chapter 6.

In addition to those disorders characterized by atrophy of the cerebral cortex, some degenerative disorders are associated with degeneration primarily of the region of the basal ganglia. Examples of the latter conditions include Huntington's disease and Parkinson's disease. Huntington's disease is a dominantly inherited disorder characterized by mental deterioration and choreiform movements, which may involve the muscles of the speech mechanism causing a speech disturbance called 'hyperkinetic dysarthria'. The characteristics of hyperkinetic dysarthria are described in Chapter 10. Parkinson's disease is considered a degenerative disease with prominent motor system involvement and minimal organic mental symptoms. Tremor, muscular rigidity, bradykinesia (slowness and lack of movement), a mask-like face, stooped-flexed posture, a shuffling gait and hypokinetic dysarthria are characteristic features of the disorder (see Chapter 10).

Toxic disorders

Toxins are poisons which may be either produced within the body (e.g. when the kidneys fail) or may be introduced from outside. A wide range of different substances may interfere with the normal functioning of the nervous system including a large number of drugs (e.g. barbiturates, tranquilizers, some antibiotics, some antidepressants, etc.), heavy metals (e.g. lead, mercury, arsenic, etc.), organic phosphates (widely used in insecticides) and alcohol. Some toxic disorders of the nervous system are capable of producing a speech or language deficit as part of their overall neurological impairment. For example, tardive dyskinesia (see Chapter 10), a toxic disorder resulting from long-term treatment with antipsychotic drugs, has as one of its symptoms a hyperkinetic dysarthria.

Probably the best-known toxic disorder of the nervous system is Wernicke–Korsakoff syndrome (Chapter 6). This is a well-known complication of chronic alcoholism characterized by paralysis of eye movements, ataxia, variable alterations of consciousness, confusion, disorientation and memory loss. These patients also have a tendency to confabulate, often in an elaborate and colourful manner. Most of these patients have a polyneuritis (inflammation of many nerves).

Demyelinating disorders

Demyelinating diseases comprise a group of chronic disorders in which spontaneous degeneration of the myelin sheaths of nerve fibres in the central nervous system is the primary pathological alteration. Multiple (disseminated) sclerosis (see Chapter 7) is the most important disorder in this category of disease. In a typical case of multiple sclerosis, various symptoms of focal damage to the central nervous system appear and disappear over a prolonged period owing to numerous scattered areas of demyelination in almost any area of the central nervous system, including the cerebrum, brainstem and cerebellum.

Multiple sclerosis has been reported to be associated with language disorders that primarily involve high-level language abilities. More specifically, individuals with multiple sclerosis may present with impaired naming, word fluency, repetition, sentence construction and comprehension abilities. Significant problems completing verbal reasoning tasks such as defining words, making inferences and explaining absurdities, ambiguities and metaphors have also been identified. Patients with multiple sclerosis also often exhibit a speech deficit in the form of a mixed dysarthria (see Chapter 11).

Infectious disorders

The nervous system and its coverings can be infected by the same microorganisms that affect other organs of the body. Infections of the nervous system are classified according to the major site of involvement and type of infecting organism. Infection of the meninges (usually the leptomeninges) is called 'meningitis' while inflammation of the brain is referred to as 'encephalitis'. In some cases both the meninges and brain may be infected, a condition called 'meningo-encephalitis'. Inflammation of the spinal cord is known as 'myelitis'.

There are three major types of meningitis. These include: pyogenic meningitis, caused by a pus-forming bacteria (e.g. meningococci, pneumococci and the influenza bacillus); tuberculous meningitis, caused by the tubercle bacillus; and viral meningitis, caused by a variety of different viruses (e.g. polio, mumps, etc.). Meningeal infections by common bacteria produce obvious systemic and neurologic symptoms which include pyrexia (fever), headache, nausea, vomiting, photophobia (avoidance of bright light), neck stiffness or rigidity, a positive Kernig's sign and alterations in the level of consciousness. Signs of focal damage to the nervous system are rare. Viral meningitis produces a similar but less severe clinical picture.

As in the case of meningitis, encephalitis may be caused by either pyogenic bacteria or viruses. In addition, in some regions of the world encephalitis may also be due to various forms of parasite acquired from animals (e.g. hydatid disease). The general features of encephalitis include moderate headache, vomiting, confusion, delirium and increasing drowsiness eventually leading to coma. Kernig's sign is negative and, unless the meninges are also involved, there is little neck stiffness.

Most varieties of intracranial infection produce rather widespread neurological symptomatology and any associated language disorder is, therefore, liable to be lost amongst other neurobehavioural and cognitive dysfunctions. Occasionally, however, a significant aphasia can be traced to a central nervous system infection. Currently, the most common infection reported to give rise to aphasia syndromes is herpes simplex encephalitis.

Aphasia can also result from the formation of intracerebral abscesses. A cerebral abscess is a pus-filled cavity in the brain which develops around a localized bacterial infection. Abscesses most commonly develop in the frontal and temporal lobes. Prior to antibiotic drugs, temporal lobe abscesses were a frequent source of aphasia secondary to chronic ear infections. In a manner similar to other types of space-occupying lesions such as intracerebral tumours, as it grows an abscess can produce symptoms by compressing and distorting surrounding brain structures and by interrupting the vascular supply or the flow of cerebrospinal fluid.

Summary

Speech-language function is dependent on processes that take place in the human nervous system. Consequently, damage to the nervous system, as might occur subsequent to cerebrovascular accidents, traumatic brain injury, brain tumours, infections and toxic conditions, among others, often results in impairments in speech-language abilities. These acquired communicative impairments include various forms of aphasia, dysarthria and apraxia. In order to understand the signs, symptoms and neurological mechanisms that underlie the various acquired speech-language disorders associated with lesions in the nervous system discussed in later chapters, the reader must first have a sound knowledge of the anatomy of the nervous system. The contents of the present chapter provide that knowledge. In those instances where damage to specific components of the nervous system is associated with the occurrence of particular acquired speech and/or language disorders, details of the neuroanatomy of those components are provided in the relevant chapter.

Reference

McNeil, M.R., Robin, D.A. and Schmidt, R.A. (2008) Apraxia of speech: definition and differential diagnosis, in *Clinical Management of Sensorimotor Speech Disorders* (ed. M.R. McNeil), Thieme, New York, pp. 249–264.

Aphasia syndromes 2

Introduction

Aphasia has been defined as the loss or impairment of language caused by brain damage (see Chapter 1). In by far the majority of cases seen in peacetime, aphasia is caused by ischaemic cerebrovascular accidents (see Chapter 1). Although aphasic disability is complex, many aphasic patients are clinically similar and fall into recurring identifiable groups. Over the years, a bewildering amount of nomenclature has been used to describe and classify the various aphasia syndromes. This vast amount of terminology serves to confuse the student of aphasiology in that, dependent upon their own individual concept and model of language, different authors have often used different terms to describe the same aphasic disturbance. For instance, at various times the aphasic disturbance associated with damage to the anterior language centre has been referred to as 'Broca's aphasia', 'motor aphasia', 'efferent motor aphasia' and 'verbal aphasia'.

In an attempt to unravel at least some of the terminological tangles associated with aphasia, prior to looking at the major contemporary aphasia classifications systems, it is useful to briefly review the history of aphasia in terms of the models of language that have been proposed by various authors. A brief look at the history of aphasia also allows a better appreciation of some of the controversy that still surrounds many aspects of aphasia, including arguments regarding the role of various speech-language areas and other brain structures in language.

Models of language – a brief history

Early history of aphasiology – Egyptian surgeons to Paul Broca (1861)

Although the earliest-known reference to aphasic phenomena comes from the so-called surgical papyrus of Edwin Smith (Prins and Bastiaanse, 2006) and many forms and symptoms of aphasia were described in the writing of the early Greeks and Romans, much of what is currently known about aphasia has come from the large amount of research into this area that has taken place since the middle of the nineteenth century, when Broca (1861) and Wernicke (1874) described the two classical forms of aphasia that bear their names. By the early nineteenth century, two clearly separate schools of thought regarding the brain's function in language had developed. One school comprised those investigators who believed that specific (mental) functions were subserved by specific areas of the brain. Investigators supporting this viewpoint became known as 'localizationists'. By correlating specific language disorders exhibited by individuals during life with lesions of specific brain structures determined at postmortem, the localizationists designated certain regions of the brain as centres responsible for specific language functions. Some localizationists even went as far as to denote specific areas of the brain as centres for mental functions such as love, pride and greed as well as speech. Opponents to the localizationist viewpoint, known as 'holists', believed that mental function was the product of the entire brain working as a unit and that mental ability was a reflection of total brain volume. This latter viewpoint became known as the 'holistic viewpoint'. Aphasia researchers over the past century or so can generally be divided into one or other of the above two schools. Many of the problems associated with the study of aphasia, such as the diverse terminology, have resulted from the controversy generated between the localizationists and the holists.

Franz-Joseph Gall and phrenological theory

The beginning of the nineteenth century saw a radical change in the ideas concerning the neuroanatomical basis of aphasic disorders. The commencement of this development was the phrenological theory proposed by a young Austrian neuroanatomist called Franz-Joseph Gall (1758–1828). Gall (1809), through his introduction of the concept of 'phrenology', was the first person to propose a systematic relationship between specific psychological components of human behaviour and specific cerebral regions. According to phrenological theory, complex behaviours such as language, mathematical ability, musical ability and various aspects of human character (e.g. ambition, charity, etc.) were regulated in specific locations in the cerebral cortex. These specific cortical locations were thought to correspond to surface regions of the skull and accordingly the exterior of the skull was partitioned

into regions that were believed to be the 'seat' of a 'faculty', with the size of these seats and the areas of the protuberances and lumps of the skull being innately determined in a given individual (Figure 2.1). Further, the area of each region was considered a measure of the complex behaviour or particular aspect of character regulated by that region. Although phrenology fell into disfavour, the underlying premise of phrenological theory – that all aspects of a complex behaviour (e.g. language) are regulated in an anatomically discrete, separable, area of the cerebral cortex – remained as an important component of influential models and theories of speech-language function (e.g. Wernicke–Lichtheim model) that dominated this field throughout the majority of the twentieth century.

Importantly, Gall was the first to relate speech to a particular area of the brain. In a description of what he called 'two speech-disordered patients', Gall postulated the existence of an organ for words and language in the anterior portions of the brain (i.e. the frontal lobes). One of the most prominent supporters of Gall's theory that the seat of language is situated in the frontal lobes was Jean-Baptiste Bouillaud (1796–1881). Bouillaud (1825) collected clinical as well as pathological evidence to support Gall's hypothesis. In a study of 850 cases, he found lesions in the frontal lobes of 116 patients who were speech-defective. He insisted that it was necessary to distinguish two different phenomena in the act of speech. First, the power of creating words (internal speech) as a sign of our ideas; and, second, the power of articulating these same words (external speech). On this basis, Bouillaud suggested that there are two causes which can lead to loss of speech, each in its own way, one by destroying the organ of memory of words, the other an impairment in the nervous principle which directs the movements of speech. The validity of Bouillaud's division of aphasic disorders into an articulatory and an amnesic category is still generally accepted under the rubric of non-fluent and fluent types of aphasia.

Opposed to this early localization point of view was Pierre Flourens (1794–1867) who stated that all parts of the brain were equipotential and that specific areas for specific purposes did not exist.

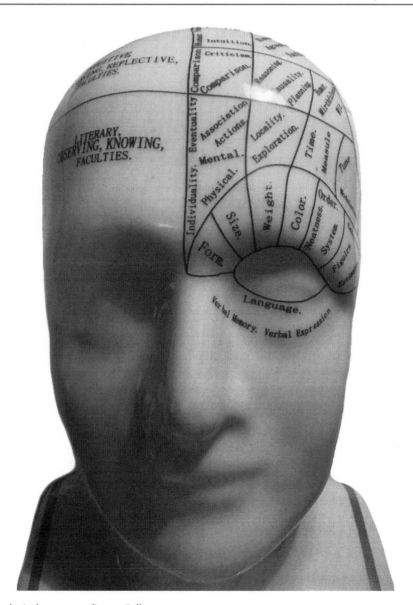

Figure 2.1 Phrenological map according to Gall.

He suggested that the effect of a brain lesion solely depended on its size and not on its location (Flourens, 1842). According to Flourens (1824), if an area of the brain was damaged due to disease or injury, any other area of the brain could take over that function. Although we now know that this may happen to some degree, it clearly does not occur, especially in adult patients, to the extent predicted by Flourens. For instance, most global aphasics remain severely language-impaired and do not exhibit the degree of recovery that could be expected if Flourens' hypothesis was correct.

Another opponent of Gall and Bouillaud was Andral (1797–1876). In a study of 37 patients with lesions in the frontal lobes (found at autopsy), Andral (1840) reported only 21 having speech disorders. In addition, he also reported having seen 14 cases of aphasia with lesions not involving the frontal lobes, but rather confined to post-rolandic areas. He concluded that loss of speech is not a necessary result of lesions in the anterior lobes and that speech disorders can also result from lesions not involving the frontal lobes.

Discovery of the 'speech centre' – Paul Broca (1861) and Carl Wernicke (1874)

The theory proposed by Gall and Bouillaud that different brain regions had different functions and that 'articulated speech' could be localized in the frontal lobes led to considerable debate in subsequent decades and ultimately laid the foundation for the discovery in 1861 of the so-called speech centre by a French neurologist named Paul Broca (1824–1880) (Figure 2.2). The paper published by Broca (1861) is widely regarded as having provided the major stimulus for the revolution in aphasia research that continued throughout the twentieth century to the present day. On the basis of the autopsy findings of two aphasic patients that Broca had cared for in the last months of their lives, Broca reported that the 'motor speech area' was located in the posterior part (pars triangularis) of the third frontal convolution even though the lesion not only included the third frontal gyrus but also extended to include the frontal, central and parietal opercula regions (Figure 2.3).

The two patients observed by Broca (Leborgne and Lelong) were able to understand language but were unable to produce any spontaneous speech, other than the perseverative utterance 'tan' in the former and a small set of monosyllables in the latter, in the absence of muscular paralysis, poor comprehension and reduced intelligence. Broca interpreted his findings as supporting the Gall–Bouillaud thesis that the seat of language was in the frontal lobes. He emphasized, however, that he did not mean to imply that all forms of aphasia were related to frontal lobe disease, only the motoric type, which he called 'aphemia' (or loss of speech) (the term 'aphasia' was coined by Trousseau in 1864 and was adopted in place of 'aphemia') and which was essentially the same as the articulatory aphasia proposed by Bouillaud. After further study in 1865, Broca made another important contribution to the study of language

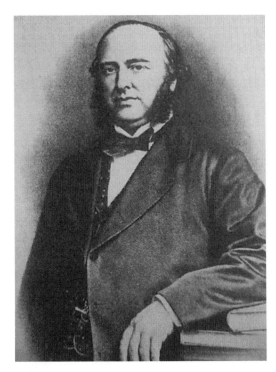

Figure 2.2 Paul Broca, French Neurologist (1824–1880).

and the brain when he was the first to draw attention to the fact that language is a function of the left cerebral hemisphere, having noted that in all of his right-handed aphasic patients the lesion was located in the left hemisphere. This discovery led to a major revolution in medical and physiological thinking. From a medical standpoint, aphasia was transformed from a minor curiosity to an important symptom of focal brain disease. (It is now generally accepted that the link between the left hemisphere and language was first reported by Dax (1836) in a presentation to a congress in Montpellier; however, Dax's findings were not published until three decades later by his physician son Gustav Dax in April (1865), six weeks prior to Broca's (1865) publication.)

The next major advance in aphasiology came from a German neuropsychiatrist, Carl Wernicke, who demonstrated that the occurrence of the other major type of aphasic disorder (i.e. the amnesic type) postulated by Bouillaud was related to disease of the left temporal lobe. In a publication in 1874, Wernicke described the

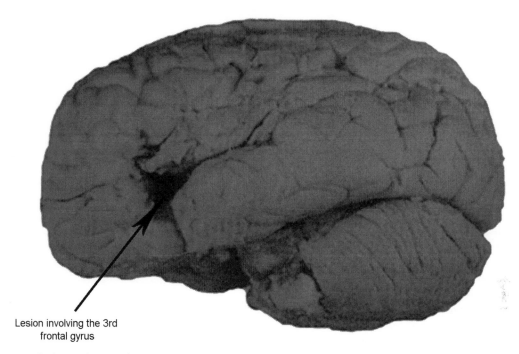

Lesion involving the 3rd
frontal gyrus

Figure 2.3 The brain of Broca's first patient showing a lesion in the third frontal gyrus of the left hemisphere and extending to include the frontal, central and parietal opercula.

major features of what he called 'sensory aphasia'. These features were fluent but disordered speech, with analogous disturbances in writing and reading (both oral and silent) and impaired understanding of oral speech. Wernicke determined that the lesion most commonly associated with this disorder was situated in the posterior part of the superior temporal gyrus (first temporal gyrus) of the left hemisphere (i.e. the auditory association cortex of the dominant hemisphere).

Wernicke further stated that the anterior portions of the brain were devoted to motor functions and the posterior areas to sensory functions. He accepted the existence of Broca's area and, on this basis, proposed the existence of two distinct types of aphasia: 'motor aphasia' and 'sensory aphasia'. Not only did Wernicke emphasize the importance of cortical centres in language performance, he also stressed the role played by the association fibre tracts which connect the cortical language centres. He postulated the existence of a bundle of fibres (now known to be the arcuate fasciculus) connecting Broca's area to the first temporal gyrus and suggested that lesions

here would produce 'conduction aphasia' (an entity now well recognized). In this way Wernicke was the first to propose that aphasia could be caused by cortical–cortical disconnections. From his simple neural model, Wernicke therefore not only accounted for aphasic syndromes known at this time but also correctly predicted the existence of syndromes that had not been described at the time.

The Wernicke–Lichtheim model

Following the publication of Wernicke's work, a large number of schemes and aphasia classification systems, based mainly on localizationist theories, were proposed by various authors. Among the most notable of these contributions were the works of Bastian (1898), Charcot (1877), Lichtheim (1885) and Nielson (1936). As an example of these works, Lichtheim (1885) elaborated Wernicke's model and postulated the existence of five interconnected cortical centres (Figure 2.4): a centre for the memory images of

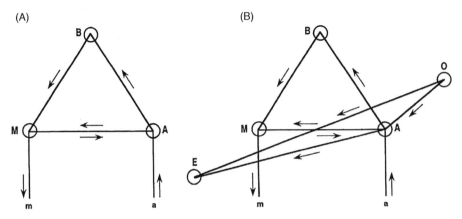

Figure 2.4 The Wernicke–Lichtheim model and the related disorders for spoken (A) and written (B) language. Centres: A = Audioverbal Centre (centre for auditory word representations), M = Expressive Speech Centre (centre for motor word representations), B = Concept Centre (centre for object concepts), a = auditory speech input, m = motor speech output, O = Visuoverbal Centre (centre for reading words), E = Writing Centre (centre for writing words). Disorders of spoken language by lesion in: M = cortical motor aphasia, A = cortical sensory aphasia, AM = conduction aphasia, BM = transcortical motor aphasia, AB = transcortical sensory aphasia, O = cortical alexia, E = cortical agraphia.

the movement patterns of oral speech (expressive speech centre) located in Broca's area in the frontal lobe, a centre for the memory images of word sounds (audioverbal centre) located in Wernicke's area in the temporal lobe, a centre for the memory images of the movement patterns of writing (writing centre), a centre for the memory images of written words (visuoverbal centre) and a centre in which concepts or ideas to be expressed are formulated (concept centre) located in the inferior part of the parietal lobe. According to Lichtheim's proposal, these centres were linked, not only with each other but also with other cortical and subcortical structures. For example, Lichtheim proposed that the audioverbal and visuoverbal centres were intimately associated with the primary cortical receptive areas for hearing and vision.

The model of the cortical speech centres developed by Lichtheim on the basis of Wernicke's proposals has become known as the Wernicke–Lichtheim model (or schema). Lichtheim agreed with Wernicke that a disruption of the connection between the audioverbal centre and the expressive speech centre would lead to a 'conduction aphasia'. Further, Lichtheim postulated that a break in the connection between the concept centre and the expressive speech centre would lead to a language disorder characterized

by impoverished spontaneous speech, since formulated ideas would not be able to be expressed verbally. At the same time, however, since the basic mechanisms of speech would remain intact in such a case, strictly linguistic performance such as repetitive speech and reading aloud would be preserved. The understanding of speech would be spared, since both the audioverbal centre and its connection with the expressive speech centre remain intact. The real existence of this syndrome, designated 'transcortical motor aphasia', together with conduction aphasia, has since been confirmed by more recent workers.

The Wernicke–Geschwind model

The original model of language processing proposed by Wernicke and Lichtheim has more recently been modified by Geschwind (1965a, b) to form a new model known as the Wernicke–Geschwind model. According to this latter model, language comprehension occurs when either spoken or written language is transferred from the primary auditory and visual cortices to Wernicke's area. Briefly, spoken language is passed from the medial geniculate body through the internal capsule to the primary auditory cortex (areas 41 and 42) and then via short association fibres to Wernicke's area. Written language passes from the primary visual cortex in the occipital lobe to the supramarginal and angular gyri which form part of Wernicke's area. Following comprehension in Wernicke's area, language information is passed to the pre-frontal cortex and Broca's area in the frontal lobes via the arcuate fasciculus. Coding for expressive speech occurs in Broca's area. Although the model is supported to some extent by functional neuroimaging studies, it has a number of limitations, including: the model does not account for the occurrence of language disturbances associated with subcortical lesions with the exception of those that involve the arcuate fasciculus leading to conduction aphasia; the model does not account for the often significant recovery of language function after stroke (e.g. compensation from other cortical regions); most aphasias often involve both comprehension as well as expressive components, suggesting that the sharp functional distinctions between cortical regions implied by the model may not exist.

Using the Wernicke–Geschwind model as an example, it is evident that the models of language proposed by the early localizationists were successful, at least in part, in predicting the existence of a number of now clinically recognized aphasia syndromes. Aphasia, however, is a complex disorder and, as will become evident later, the localizationist models of language have been only partly successful in explaining some of the curious combinations of symptoms often encountered in aphasic patients.

The non-localizationist 'holistic' view of language

Strongly opposed to the localizationist theories of the latter part of the nineteenth century was the English neurologist John Hughlings Jackson (1835–1911). Jackson considered aphasia from a dynamic, psychological viewpoint rather than as a static, neuroanatomical correlation. He was the founder of what is often called the 'cognitive school' in the field of aphasia and distinguished between two levels of speech: emotional (or automatic) and intellectual. He believed it was the intellectual level of utterance, involving the statement of what he termed 'propositions' that was impaired in the aphasic patients, considering that aphasics may show considerable preservation of automatic language in the form of interjections, oaths, clichés and recurring utterances. Jackson did not deny that Broca's area was frequently damaged in patients who suffered from aphasic disturbances, especially when motor speech involvements were manifest. He refused, however, to localize language function in Broca's area alone, and stressed the notion that language was a psychological rather than a physiological function. Jackson emphasized that for language, as well as for other intellectual functions, the brain operates as a functional unit.

The non-localizationist viewpoint was supported by the work of Pierre Marie (1853–1940). Marie (1906) presented a paper entitled 'The third frontal convolution plays no special role in the function of language', in which he rejected the notion of two distinct language centres as claimed by Wernicke, suggesting that the superior temporal gyrus was the only true language centre. Marie suggested that the language disorder known as Broca's (motor) aphasia was actually a Wernicke's (sensory) aphasia combined with 'anarthria'. Further, he proposed that there was only one true form of aphasia: Wernicke's (sensory) aphasia, which is characterized by poor comprehension, paraphasia, jargon and reading and writing difficulties. For a lesion in Broca's area to cause aphasia, Marie suggested it would be necessary for the lesion to extend posteriorly to involve Wernicke's area or its connections to the thalamus. Marie agreed with Jackson that, while localized lesions could not be held responsible for language and speech disturbances, lesions in certain cortical areas could more readily disturb speech than could lesions in other areas. Both he and Jackson emphasized the point that knowledge of pathological conditions which disturb and impair language function does not provide information per se as to how the function is normally controlled in the healthy individual. Jackson, in particular, emphasized the importance of observing the live patient rather than studying autopsy findings. Following the publication of Marie's work, the influence of the holistic approach on aphasia increased over the early part of the twentieth century, causing Wernicke's disconnectionist model of language to fall into some degree of disrepute. Major advocates of the holistic approach included Critchley (1970), Head (1926), Luria (1970), Pick (1931), Schuell, Jenkins and Jiminez-Pabon (1964) and Wepman (1951).

Although, as discussed above, it is generally possible to divide models of language proposed over the past century into those belonging to the anatomically based localizationist school and those belonging to the psychologically based holistic school, most clinicians at some time have observed language behaviours supportive of each of these two viewpoints. In addition, most contemporary aphasia researchers make use of both approaches in explaining and classifying the aphasia exhibited by their subjects. For example, the Soviet psychologists headed by Luria tend to lie between the strict localizationists and the holists promoting equipotentiality for all areas of the brain. Luria, sometimes described as a dynamic localizationist, considered that the material basis of the higher nervous processes (including language) is the brain as a whole. Further, however, Luria stated that he believed the brain to be a highly differentiated system whose parts are responsible for the different aspects of the unified whole. The work of Luria and his associates, based on a moderate localization position, features careful descriptions of aphasia syndromes often correlated with an anatomical localization of pathology. (Luria's aphasia classification system is discussed later in this chapter.) In this way, a better integration of the anatomical and psychological approaches to aphasia has resulted.

In 1965 Norman Geschwind reintroduced the disconnectionist approach to the study of language and aphasia first proposed by Wernicke. The publication of Geschwind's works subsequently provided a new impetus to the anatomical study of aphasia syndromes and has led to the revival of the Wernicke–Lichtheim model of language. Added to this, the introduction of new neuroimaging techniques since the mid-1970s, including computerized tomographic (CT) scanning, positron emission tomography (PET) scanning and magnetic resonance imaging (MRI) and regional cerebral blood flow studies, which allow the localization of aphasia producing lesions in the living subject, have better enabled clinicopathological studies of aphasia to be carried out. The results of studies that have utilized these techniques have, in general, tended to vindicate the Wernicke–Lichtheim model of language. The new neuroimaging techniques have, however, also verified the need expressed by many researchers over the years to expand the classical concept of the 'speech-language area' of the dominant hemisphere to include subcortical structures such as the components of the striato-capsular region and the thalamus. Consequently, in addition to the specific cortical centres and cortical–cortical connections (e.g. the arcuate fasciculus) specified in older language models, recently proposed models have been extended to acknowledge the importance of subcortical structures as centres relevant for language processes (Crosson, 1985). (The role of subcortical structures in language is discussed in Chapter 3.)

It should be stressed that the intent of the above brief history of aphasia was to provide some insight into the major approaches to aphasia over the past century or so and the controversies surrounding them. Consequently, only a very small proportion of the contributors to aphasiology have been mentioned. The works of many of the more recent researchers in aphasiology are referred to either later in this chapter or in subsequent chapters of this text.

Classification of aphasia

As a consequence of the complexity and variability of aphasia, over the years an extraordinarily large number of systems have been developed to classify the various aphasia syndromes. In general, each aphasia researcher has tended to develop their own terminology to differentiate the various types of aphasia based on their own idea of the nature of aphasia. Although the various authors have tended to agree to a greater extent than may be readily apparent on the major criteria that distinguish one aphasia type from another, they have used a diverse array of terminology to define the aphasia syndromes that they recognized. Consequently, it is difficult for the student of aphasiology to determine how the various aphasia syndromes as defined in the different classification systems are related. Further, because of the variability of the language disturbance seen from one aphasic patient to the next, clinicians often have difficulty when making a diagnosis as to where the boundaries between one aphasia type and another exist.

Simple dichotomies in aphasia classification

To avoid the confusion associated with a broad classification system, many authors make use of simple dichotomies to classify aphasia. The two most widely used dichotomies are the expressive/receptive division proposed by Weisenberg and McBride (1935) and the motor/sensory division originally introduced by Wernicke (1874). Two additional dichotomies also frequently used in the literature include the fluent/non-fluent (Benson, 1967) and anterior/posterior (Goodglass and Kaplan, 1972) dichotomies.

Expressive, or motor, aphasia is presumably associated with lesions involving the anterior language centre of the dominant hemisphere (i.e. Broca's area) and is therefore primarily related to an inability to translate speech concepts into meaningful sounds. In other words, the primary disturbance here is an inability to execute speech production. As a result, speech is non-fluent with pauses between words or phrases. Receptive, or sensory, aphasia is presumably associated with lesions in the posterior language area of the dominant hemisphere. It, therefore, is related to problems in the comprehension, formulation and so on of speech. The primary disturbance in the receptive aphasic patient is lack of comprehension of language. In that the expressive aspects of speech are dependent upon normal functioning of the receptive speech processes, however, the expression of language may also be disturbed in persons with sensory aphasia, with the production of jargon, substitution of words (parapha-

sia) and other expressive disturbances being evident in their spoken output. Speech, however, is generally fluent, although full of mistakes. Thus, the major differences between motor and sensory aphasia are: comprehension of language is only mildly affected in motor but severely affected in sensory aphasia, and that speech is usually non-fluent in motor aphasia but fluent in sensory aphasia.

As a modification of the expressive/receptive dichotomy, some authors, including Wernicke (1874) and Geschwind (1969, 1971), have divided aphasics into those with fluent speech (fluent aphasia) (able to effortlessly produce well-articulated, long phrases with a normal grammar, melody and rhythm) and those with non-fluent speech output (non-fluent aphasia) (able to produce only sparse speech that is uttered slowly with great effort and poor articulation). Wernicke (1874) suggested an anatomical correlation for the two different aphasic outputs. The significance of the dichotomy in aphasic verbal output has been re-emphasized by a number of recent studies which confirmed Wernicke's observations and showed that non-fluent aphasic patients have lesions involving structures anterior to the Fissure of Rolando, while fluent aphasic patients on the other hand have lesions posterior to the Fissure of Rolando (Benson, 1967; Poeck, Kerchensteiner and Hartje, 1972; Wagenaar, Snow and Prins, 1975).

Although each of the dichotomies has validity and a usefulness, none adequately characterizes the distinguishing features of most varieties of aphasia. For instance, pure forms of aphasia (i.e. pure motor or pure sensory) are not commonly encountered. This is especially the case with sensory aphasia, which is accompanied by some loss of motor speech. Thus, most aphasic patients will have some symptoms of both these types. Further, posterior lesions can produce disorders of expression, and anterior lesions can produce disorders of comprehension. In addition, aphasic disturbances can be caused by brain lesions which do not directly involve the cortical language centres of the dominant hemisphere. Studies in recent years, for instance, have shown that subcortical and even right-hemisphere structures contribute to language function.

Although the fluent/non-fluent dichotomy does offer significant anatomical localizing information, it should be pointed out that exceptions to the anterior/posterior correlation do exist. First, not all aphasics can be classified as fluent or non-fluent (Benson, 1967; Karis and Horenstein, 1976). Second, almost all children who become acutely aphasic are non-fluent (often they are mute) (see Chapter 12) and even with recovery almost never does a child develop a fully fluent, paraphasic, jargon type of output. Thus, the acquired aphasia of childhood does not fit into the fluent/non-fluent division. Finally, evaluation of fluency in the early stages of aphasia may be misleading. Many patients with freshly acquired aphasia show non-fluent characteristics at the onset. While some aphasics with lesions posterior to the Fissure of Rolando rapidly become fluent, others may be non-fluent for weeks before altering to a fluent output (Benson, 1979).

It is evident, therefore, that aphasic disturbances need to be divided into a greater number of types rather than simply being divided into one of the categories specified by the above dichotomies. Two major classification systems above all others have gained some degree of clinical acceptance in recent years. These include the Boston Aphasia Classification System (developed by the Speech Pathology Section, Aphasia Research Unit, Veterans Administration Hospital, Boston) and the Lurian Aphasia Classification System proposed by Luria (1970).

The Boston Classification System

According to a modified version of the Boston classification system (Benson, 1979), there are eight clinically recognizable aphasia syndromes. These include: (1) Broca's aphasia, (2) Wernicke's aphasia, (3) conduction aphasia, (4) global aphasia, (5) transcortical motor aphasia, (6) transcortical sensory aphasia, (7) isolation (mixed transcortical) aphasia and (8) anomic aphasia.

The suggested lesion sites, according to the Wernicke–Lichtheim model (Figure 2.4) for each of these aphasia types are as follows:

1   Broca's aphasia is associated with a lesion involving the expressive speech centre.

2   Wernicke's aphasia is caused by a lesion of the audioverbal centre.

3   Conduction aphasia results from a lesion involving the pathways connecting the audioverbal and expressive speech centres.

4   Global aphasia is produced by an extensive lesion involving both the audioverbal centre and the expressive speech centre.

5   Transcortical motor aphasia is associated with disruption of the pathways connecting the concept centre to the audioverbal centre.

6   Transcortical sensory aphasia results from lesions of the pathways connecting the audioverbal centre to the concept centre.

7   Isolation aphasia is caused by lesions which disconnect the concept centre from both the audioverbal centre and the expressive speech centre.

8   Anomic aphasia is produced by a lesion involving the pathways which connect the concept centre to the expressive speech centre or, in those cases where comprehension is also disturbed, by a lesion of the concept centre.

Each of the Bostonian aphasia syndromes is characterized by a particular group or cluster of language signs and symptoms. Consequently, allocation of language-disordered patients to each of these symptoms is carried out on the basis of the particular cluster of language symptoms exhibited by the patient. It is important to realize, however, that even though each syndrome has its own set of language characteristics, the particular set of language signs and symptoms associated with each syndrome is not fixed. Certainly, not every member of the set needs to be present in the patient before a diagnosis of that syndrome can be made. Likewise, occasionally, language findings not normally characteristic of a particular aphasia syndrome may be present among a group of signs and symptoms more typical of that aphasia syndrome. Consequently, clinicians need to allow some degree of flexibility in the membership of the language signs and symptoms they take to be indicative of specific aphasia syndromes.

Central and pericentral aphasias

The various Bostonian aphasias can be grouped a number of ways in order to assist localization.

Lesions in the central speech areas that bank the Fissure of Sylvius give rise to the central aphasias, which have in common loss of repetition. Central aphasias include Broca's aphasia, Wernicke's aphasia, and conduction and global aphasia. The pericentral aphasias – which include transcortical motor, transcortical sensory, anomic and isolation aphasias – are caused by lesions surrounding the central speech areas and have in common good repetition. Thus, a central aphasia can be distinguished from a pericentral aphasia by testing the repetition abilities of the patient. In fact, if repetition is not tested, the examiner will have difficulty in distinguishing between the following central and pericentral syndromes: Broca's from transcortical motor; Wernicke's from transcortical sensory; anomic from conduction; and global from isolation.

Differentiation between the perisylvian and the borderzone (pericentral) types of aphasia as determined by the ability to repeat is not only a valid localizing feature but also offers a clue as to the nature of the underlying pathology. When vascular disease is the aetiology, most aphasias with normal repetition are based on occlusive disease of the left internal carotid artery. Following acute occlusion of the carotid vessel, the limited arterial circulation available through the Circle of Willis, may be sufficient to perfuse only the immediate perisylvian cortex, allowing this area to remain viable but not providing enough oxygenated blood to maintain borderzone tissues. In contrast, a cerebrovascular accident producing an aphasia with repetition disturbance is most likely based on thrombotic or embolic vascular problems with involvement of one or more of the branches of the middle cerebral artery (Romanul and Abramowitz, 1961). (The various Bostonian aphasia syndromes are discussed in terms of their symptoms and lesion sites later in this chapter.)

The Lurian Classification System

Based on his studies of soldiers who had suffered head wounds in war, Luria distinguished seven main types of aphasia: sensory (acoustic) aphasia, acoustico-mnestic aphasia, semantic aphasia, efferent (kinetic) motor aphasia, pre-motor apha-

sia, afferent (apraxic) motor aphasia and frontal dynamic aphasia. (The symptoms and lesion sites of each of the Lurian aphasia syndromes are described later in this chapter.)

Bostonian Aphasia Syndromes

Broca's aphasia

Broca's aphasia is characterized by non-fluent speech output and poor repetition abilities. Auditory comprehension, however, is relatively spared. Speech output is slow, effortful, agrammatic and often telegrammatic (i.e. containing a predominance of content words such as nouns and action verbs and a paucity of adjectives, adverbs and prepositions giving the patient's speech a telegraphic style). The vocabulary of patients with Broca's aphasia is generally restricted in range. These patients may use words repetitively (perseveration) and long pauses may occur between words or phrases. A motor speech disorder in the form of an apraxia of speech (see Chapter 8) and/or dysarthria often accompanies Broca's aphasia.

As the more lateral portions of the primary motor strip are usually damaged by the causative lesion, Broca's aphasia is most often associated with either a right hemiplegia (paralysis down one side of the body) or right hemiparesis (muscle weakness down one side of the body) affecting the lower half of the face and the right arm more severely than the right leg. Hyperactive reflexes and pathological reflexes (e.g. a positive Babinski sign) are frequently present on the right-hand side. Ideomotor dyspraxia (see Chapter 8), an inability to carry out on command a task that can be performed spontaneously, frequently involves the 'non-pathological' left hand of Broca's aphasics. Although sensory deficits such as loss of pain and temperature sense are occasionally present, they are inconsistent findings in Broca's aphasia. Likewise, persistent visual-field deficits occur less frequently in association with Broca's aphasia than most other aphasia syndromes.

Writing in Broca's aphasia is usually similarly impaired to speech. Typically, the written material contains multiple misspellings and the omission of letters. Individual letters tend to be oversized and poorly formed, a situation made worse by the fact that because most Broca's aphasics have a concomitant hemiplegia, they are required to use their left hand for writing. Typically, these patients are better able to copy written material than they can write either to command or to dictation. Most Broca's aphasics read aloud poorly, while reading comprehension is usually similar to auditory comprehension.

The localization of lesions associated with Broca's aphasia has been an area of controversy since Broca's first description of the area to bear his name in 1861. For a long time, we were taught to associate the occurrence of Broca's aphasia to damage in Broca's area. Clinicopathological studies, using computerized tomography, however, have shown us that the localization of Broca's aphasia is less clearly defined, Broca's area being damaged in some cases but unharmed in others.

Mohr *et al.* (1978) carried out an extensive study of Broca's aphasia in which the lesions in 20 cases were documented by autopsy, computerized tomographic scan or arteriogram. They found that a lesion confined to Broca's area produced not aphasia but 'transient speech apraxia'. Their findings suggest that infarction affecting Broca's area and its immediate environs, even deep into the brain, causes a mutism that is replaced by a rapidly improving dyspraxic and effortful articulation, but that no significant disturbance in language function persists (Broca's area infarction syndrome). Rather than being confined to Broca's area, it would appear that Broca's aphasia required a large lesion to the sylvian region, encompassing much of the opercula, insula and subjacent white matter in the territory of the upper division of the middle cerebral artery, including Broca's area. As emphasized by Marie (1906) and Mohr (1976), the extensive lesion in Paul Broca's original case included much more than the posterior portion of the left frontal gyrus (Broca's area). Indeed, clinicopathological studies have shown that Broca's aphasia usually follows extensive cortical-subcortical damage of the left frontal parietal operculum (including both the inferior frontal gyrus and pre-central gyrus) with the lesion, in some cases, also involving the ante-

rior parts of the parietal and, sometimes, the temporal lobe (Naeser and Hayward, 1978; Mazzocchi and Vignolo, 1979; Murdoch *et al.*, 1986a). Mazzocchi and Vignolo (1979) also noted that all of their Broca's aphasics had lesions involving the lenticular nucleus and insula.

The involvement of Broca's area in Broca's aphasia remains somewhat controversial. Certainly from Mohr's work, lesions restricted to Broca's area itself do not appear to produce Broca's aphasia but rather Broca's area infarction syndrome (centred on apraxia of speech). (The relationship between apraxia of speech and Broca's aphasia is discussed further in Chapter 8.) Whether a lesion needs to involve Broca's area to produce a Broca's aphasia, however, is less clear. Functional neuroimaging techniques such as PET have provided considerable evidence that changes in the brain's metabolic activity outside of Broca's area contribute to the pattern of language impairment associated with Broca's aphasia (Metter *et al.*, 1989, 1992). For example, Metter *et al.* (1989) examined 11 patients with Broca's aphasia and compared their CT and PET findings. Although lesions demonstrated by CT showed consistent damage to the anterior internal capsule and lenticular nuclei with variable cortical changes, brain activity as estimated by glucose metabolism was found to be decreased throughout the cerebral hemisphere. Damasio (1998) summarizes the pathophysiology of Broca's aphasia: 'In general, it is fair to say that the lesions in Broca's area not only encompass the frontal operculum (Brodmann's area 44 and 45), but also pre-motor and motor regions immediately behind and above, in addition to extending to underlying white matter and basal ganglia as well as the insula. As might be expected, the extension of damage into these different regions correlate(s) with diverse accompanying deficits and with the extent of recovery' (p. 54).

Wernicke's aphasia

The major feature of the language disorder exhibited by patients with Wernicke's aphasia is an impairment in language comprehension. Consequently, these patients have a problem in understanding what is said to them and what they read. Some researchers have reported a bipolar tendency in the comprehension deficit of Wernicke's aphasia. Some Wernicke's aphasics have their greatest problem in understanding spoken words (word deafness) while others have more difficulty comprehending written words (word blindness). Elements of deficit in both areas are always present to some degree, however, in Wernicke's aphasics.

In addition to impaired comprehension abilities, Wernicke's aphasics also exhibit poor naming and poor repetition abilities. Unlike Broca's aphasics, however, the speech output of Wernicke's aphasics is fluent, the speech being well articulated with phrases of normal length and melody. Despite being fluent, however, the content of the spoken language is abnormal and is contaminated by the substitution of words (verbal paraphasia) or parts of words (literal paraphasia). As these patients are not capable of monitoring their own verbal expression owing to their comprehension difficulty, they often unknowingly invent new words (neologisms) as they speak and, although they speak in full sentences, the sentences mean nothing to others. Therefore, despite their fluent speech, Wernicke's aphasics fail to communicate their ideas to others and are commonly frustrated by their inability to make themselves understood. In severe cases, verbal confusion and the presence of paraphasic errors may result in a very disjointed language disorder in which the patient produces meaningless jargon.

Unlike patients with Broca's aphasia, those with Wernicke's aphasia rarely have a concomitant hemiplegia. Consequently, the handwriting of Wernicke's aphasics is usually satisfactory in terms of motor ability, the written output consisting of well-formed legible letters. As in the case of their spoken language, however, the content of the written language of Wernicke's aphasia is also abnormal. Although in their writing the individual letters are often arranged in the appearance of words, the letters are often combined in a meaningless manner. In some instances, the written output resembles the paraphasic spoken output.

Reading aloud and reading comprehension are both disturbed in Wernicke's aphasics, although,

as indicated above, reading comprehension may be better than auditory comprehension. Likewise, the naming abilities of these patients are also impaired, Wernicke's aphasics often failing totally or producing grossly paraphasic responses when asked to name objects, body parts and so on.

The results of a neurological examination are typically negative in the majority of Wernicke's aphasics, there being no indication of the presence of any associated neurological deficit. As indicated above, there is usually no concomitant hemiplegia or hemiparesis, and disturbances in general sensation are only rarely present. A visual-field deficit in the form of a quadrantanopsia (blindness in one fourth of the visual field) is present in some Wernicke's aphasics.

Classically, Wernicke's aphasia is believed to result from a temporal parietal lesion which invariably involves Wernicke's area itself. A number of studies based on neuroradiological findings have provided evidence to support this suggestion. For example, using CT scanning, Naeser and Hayward (1978) found the lesions associated with four cases of Wernicke's aphasia to primarily involve the post-rolandic and temporal parietal areas and included Wernicke's area in all cases. There was no pre-rolandic overlap or extension into Broca's area in any of their cases. Kertesz, Harlock and Coates (1979) also reported the case of a chronic Wernicke's aphasic (post-12 months) who had a post-rolandic lesion without extension into the frontal operculum. The findings of Chapman *et al.* (1989) pointed to damage in the dominant superior temporal gyrus as a common factor among patients deemed most seriously impaired by Wernicke's aphasia. However, in another study based on CT scans, Kertesz, Lau and Polk (1993) determined that persisting Wernicke's aphasia usually involves the supramarginal and angular gyri in addition to the superior temporal area.

Some authors, however, have reported that Wernicke's aphasia can be associated with lesions involving both pre- and post-rolandic structures (Kertesz, Harlock and Coates, 1979; Mazzocchi and Vignolo, 1979). Lesions restricted to areas anterior to the Fissure of Rolando fissure, however, do not appear from most reports to be capable of supporting a Wernicke's aphasia.

Basso *et al.* (1985) reported eight cases of Wernicke's aphasia (characterized by both comprehension and repetition disorders coexisting with fluent jargon) associated with extensive perisylvian lesions which might have been expected to produce global aphasia. These authors did not, however, document the involvement of subcortical structures in these lesions and the extent of subcortical damage is therefore unknown. The documentation of subcortical involvement in these cases would appear to be important in the light of the findings of Naeser *et al.* (1982) that Wernicke's aphasia can result from capsular/putaminal lesions with posterior white matter lesion extension across the auditory radiations in the temporal isthmus. In stark contrast to classical expectations, Basso *et al.* (1985) also reported four cases of Wernicke's aphasia associated with anterior only lesions. Such cases, however, seem to be rare exceptions and, although not commented on by Basso *et al.* (1985), their respective CT scans showed involvement of the subcortical structures deep to Broca's area in the lesion in all these cases. Mohr *et al.* (1978) also reported that one of their patients (case 3) with a lesion in the left inferior frontal region had Wernicke's aphasia characterized by a comprehension disorder, impaired repetition and fluent jargon. As in the four cases reported by Basso *et al.* (1985), however, the lesion also involved the subcortical structures deep to Broca's area and the depth of the subcortical white matter lesion may, therefore, be more critical to the occurrence of the language impairments observed in these cases than the cortical damage in Broca's area.

Post-rolandic lesions are recognized as being associated with fluent aphasias. Although fluent aphasias are associated with comprehension deficits (hence the terms 'receptive' and 'sensory' aphasias), the different subtypes of fluent aphasias are defined largely by the relative occurrence of two major errors in speech production: lexical semantic and phonological (phonemic) errors. There is some evidence that lexical errors occur primarily with lesions of the inferolateral temporal (middle and inferior temporal gyri) and parietal 'integration' cortices, and that lexical processing is more bilaterally organized (Cappa, Cavallotti and Vignolo, 1981). Phono-logical errors, on the other hand, occur with lesions of the left Wernicke area proper (posterior part of the superior temporal gyrus and supramarginal gyrus) (Cappa, Cavallotti and Vignolo, 1981). These findings raise the possibility of there being several different forms of Wernicke's aphasia.

Pure or subcortical word deafness (auditory aphasia) is a very rare and fractional language disorder closely related to Wernicke's aphasia. Although these patients distinguish words from other sounds, they cannot understand them. Consequently, their own speech sounds like a foreign language. Patients with this disorder cannot repeat words or write to dictation although spontaneous speech, writing and reading are unimpaired. The condition is thought to be caused by a lesion of the white matter deep to the posterior part of the left (dominant) superior temporal gyrus.

Conduction aphasia

Conduction aphasia is characterized by a disproportionate impairment in repetition relative to spontaneous speech and oral and written comprehension. Although the spontaneous speech output of conduction aphasics is relatively fluent, these patients have a problem in choosing and sequencing their phonemes so that their speech is contaminated by numerous paraphasic errors, typically of the literal type (i.e. involving use of incorrect phonemes within words). In addition, there may be a slight impairment of articulation and frequent pauses and hesitations associated with word-finding difficulties are usually present causing the speech output to be dysprodic.

The impairment in repetition is the most outstanding feature of this disorder and is most marked for multisyllabic words and sentences. It is during performance of repetition tasks that the literal paraphasic errors are most prominent in conduction aphasics. Most of these patients also demonstrate difficulty in confrontation naming. Auditory comprehension abilities are good.

Written spontaneous language is impaired similarly to spoken spontaneous language, although the motor aspects of handwriting are usually normal. Conduction aphasics are usually able to produce well-formed letters, but spelling is poor with omission, reversal and substitution of letters being present in their written output. Also, words in a sentence are frequently interchanged, misplaced or omitted. The ability to read aloud is also impaired, oral reading being paraphasic. These patients, however, often retain relatively good reading comprehension abilities.

The neurological examination of conduction aphasics shows considerable variation from case to case. Often, no associated neurological abnormality can be demonstrated. Significant hemiparesis is rare. When present, however, muscle weakness almost always involves the arm to a greater extent than the leg. Sensory findings are also variable, sensory abnormalities being totally absent in some patients and present in the form of a limited right-sided hemianaesthesia (loss of sensation down one side of the body) in others. Visual field defects involving either a hemianopia (loss of one half of the visual field) or quadrantanopsia are present in some conduction aphasics. Ideomotor dyspraxia is frequently, but not constantly, present. When asked to perform buccofacial or limb movements on command, the conduction aphasic may fail, even while protesting that they know what they want to do. Often, such commands result in an improper movement which nevertheless demonstrates that the patient has comprehended the command (e.g. waving the hand near the face when asked to salute). (Ideomotor dyspraxia is discussed more fully in Chapter 8.) The variation in neurological findings in conduction aphasia probably reflects involvement of different sites neighbouring the locus of pathology underlying this condition.

Wernicke (1874) proposed that conduction aphasia results from separation of the posterior language comprehension area and the anterior motor speech area of the left hemisphere. This proposal has since been supported by Geschwind (1965a, b) and the arcuate fasciculus has been the most frequently suggested site of such a disconnection.

Neuroradiological studies of patients with conduction aphasia have most frequently identified lesions involving the post-rolandic areas of the left cerebral hemispheres (Palumbo, Alexander and Naeser, 1992; Axer *et al.*, 2001). Lesions involving deep structures have also been reported (Palumbo, Alexander and Naeser, 1992). The two lesion sites most often associated with conduction aphasia are: (1) the supramarginal gyrus and the arcuate fasciculus of the left hemisphere and (2) the insula contiguous auditory cortex and underlying white matter of the left cerebral hemisphere.

In general, the findings of clinicopathological studies that have identified the location of the aphasia-producing lesion by CT scanning have tended to support the disconnection theory (Naeser and Hayward, 1978; Damasio and Damasio, 1980). For example, in the cases of conduction aphasia reported by Naeser and Hayward (1978), the lesions were either subcortical with lesions deep to, but not including, Wernicke's area or cortical with lesions extending from the surface of the supramarginal gyrus area to the body of the left lateral ventricle. In addition, the lesions were primarily post-rolandic but did not involve either Broca's or Wernicke's areas and were consistent with involvement of the posterior portions of the arcuate fasciculus.

Although involvement of the arcuate fasciculus has been proved in a number of cases of conduction aphasia, some authorities insist that involvement of the supramarginal cortex, not the underlying white matter, is the essential finding (Levine and Calvanio, 1982). Wernicke's and Geschwind's interpretation of the disturbance as a disconnection syndrome, therefore, has not been universally accepted. The arcuate fasciculus theory has been further challenged by reports of conduction aphasia occurring subsequent to lesions in the dominant Wernicke's area, suggesting that a cortical lesion, not a disconnection, is the crucial factor (Kleist, 1962; Mendez and Benson, 1985; Anderson *et al.*, 1999).

Mendez and Benson (1985) reported three atypical cases of conduction aphasia in which the lesions did not lie in the arcuate fasciculus. Two of their patients had left temporal parietal lesions, the other was a right-handed case with a right temporal parietal lesion (i.e. a crossed aphasic). They concluded, however, that even these atypical conduction aphasias are best explained by the disconnection concept, which they agreed remains the most tenable model for this language disturbance. Others discount the disconnection model based on metabolic studies of brain function (Metter *et al.*, 1989).

Kertesz (1979) proposed that there are actually two types of conduction aphasia, one he called 'efferent conduction aphasia' and the other 'afferent conduction aphasia'. Kertesz based this proposal on radioisotope localization studies (Kertesz, Lesk and McCabe, 1977). In the efferent type of conduction aphasia, the patients are less fluent and have more anterior lesions while, in the afferent type, the subjects are more fluent with more posterior lesions.

Global aphasia

In global or total aphasia, all major language functions are seriously impaired, including both the expressive and receptive components of language. In its most severe form, the patient does not communicate and verbal output is limited to expletives or a stereotypic repetitive utterance. Occasionally, however, these utterances are said quite fluently, with inflection and associated emotional expression conveying some meaning. Comprehension abilities are severely impaired, although they are frequently reported to be better than verbal output, possibly because global aphasics become skilled at interpreting non-verbal communication through gesture, facial expressions and so on. It is possible that this non-verbal comprehension will be mistaken by clinicians for comprehension of the spoken word. Repetition, naming, reading and writing are all severely, usually totally, disturbed.

In the majority of cases, global aphasics exhibit a range of concomitant neurological signs indicative of severe brain damage. These neurological signs may include hemiplegia, sensory loss, visual field defects and often an attention disturbance.

Most studies reported in the literature indicate that global aphasia results from an extensive left-hemisphere lesion involving both Broca's and Wernicke's areas (Hayward, Naeser and Zatz, 1977; Naeser and Hayward, 1978; Kertesz, Harlock and Coates, 1979; Murdoch *et al.*,

1986a). Although most studies have found the lesions associated with global aphasia to be large, involving the entire perisylvian region and subcortical structures in the frontal, parietal and temporal lobes, some authors have found that exceptions do exist (Mazzocchi and Vignolo, 1979; Naeser *et al.*, 1982; Basso *et al.*, 1985; Vignolo, Boccardi and Caverni, 1986). These last authors suggest that global aphasia does not necessarily result from large lesions involving both Broca's and Wernicke's areas. In particular, Wernicke's area may be spared even in chronic global aphasia with persisting comprehension deficit.

Global aphasia occurring without lesions of Wernicke's area was first described by Mazzocchi and Vignolo (1979). They suggested that the critical anatomical difference between global and Broca's aphasia might be related to the greater size of the lesion rather than to actual damage to Wernicke's area. However, this does not seem to be invariably true, since the lesions found in global aphasics are not always larger than those found in Broca's aphasics. An example of this can be found in the work of Basso *et al.* (1985), who reported 10 cases of global aphasia with spared Wernicke's area. Vignolo, Boccardi and Caverni (1986) reported a further eight cases of global aphasia with anterior lesions sparing Wernicke's area and three cases with posterior lesions sparing Broca's area. Further, Vignolo, Boccardi and Caverni (1986) described four cases of global aphasia with deep lesions centred on the insula and lenticular nucleus. It is apparent, therefore, that there is more than one type of lesion underlying global aphasia.

Naeser *et al.* (1982) reported the occurrence of global aphasia in association with small subcortical lesions. They described three cases of lasting global aphasia subsequent to capsular/putaminal lesions with both anterior/superior and posterior lesion extension and suggested that the severely limited speech output observed in these patients was probably the result of isolation of Broca's area due to disruption of the afferent and efferent pathways. A global aphasia was also described in four cases with striatocapsular lesions involving both the anterior and posterior limbs of the internal capsule by Murdoch *et al.* (1986b). It is evident therefore that, in addition to the large combined cortical and subcortical lesions reported in most studies, damage to subcortical structures such as the white matter pathways (including the internal capsule, extreme capsule, genu of the corpus callosum and temporal isthmus) can also be the cause of a global aphasia. Consequently, damage to both cortical and subcortical structures should be documented in any descriptions of lesions associated with global aphasia. Unfortunately, a number of authors, such as Basso *et al.* (1985), have concentrated their lesion descriptions primarily on involvement of the cerebral cortex and have largely ignored damage to subcortical structures.

Transcortical motor aphasia

The term 'transcortical aphasia' was coined by Wernicke (1908) to describe a group of aphasic syndromes characterized by retention of repetition out of all proportion compared to other language functions. Three types of transcortical aphasia are recognized: transcortical motor aphasia, transcortical sensory aphasia and mixed transcortical aphasia.

Transcortical motor aphasia is characterized by a marked reduction in the quantity and complexity of spontaneous speech in the presence of a retained ability to repeat. Preserved repetition is the most striking feature of this condition. The repetitions of transcortical motor aphasics, however, are not mandatory and therefore these patients cannot be regarded as echolalic (echolalia is the automatic repetition by a patient of what is said to them). Although transcortical motor aphasics may echo a word or phrase, they will correct grammatically incorrect statements they are asked to repeat and at the same time will reject nonsense syllables.

The limited spontaneous speech output of transcortical motor aphasics is non-fluent, the speech often being described as 'stumbling', 'repetitive' and 'stuttering-like'. Conversational verbalization is produced only with considerable effort and is in most cases agrammatic and highly simplified. Series speech is usually performed well once the patient is started.

Often these patients may require prompting for the first few numbers in a series but can then continue unhindered.

Comprehension of spoken and written language is relatively preserved. Reading aloud is almost invariably defective, a poorly articulated output being produced. The ability to write is affected in the majority of transcortical motor aphasics, the written language output featuring large, clumsily produced letters, poor spelling and agrammatic output. Transcortical motor aphasics usually perform poorly in confrontation naming tasks.

In general, the associated neurological signs exhibited by transcortical motor aphasics are similar to those found in Broca's aphasics. The majority of these patients have a right hemiplegia. Similarly, ideomotor dyspraxia is a common finding in the non-paralysed left hand of these patients. Neither sensory loss nor visual field defects, however, are characteristic of transcortical motor aphasia.

Most textbooks tell us that transcortical aphasias are associated with lesions in the arterial borderzone of the left hemisphere. Lesions in the anterior parts of the borderzone are usually said to be associated with transcortical motor aphasia, while those in the posterior parts are said to produce transcortical sensory aphasias (Benson, 1979). Isolation syndrome (mixed transcortical aphasia) results from lesions involving both the anterior and posterior parts of the borderzone (Benson, 1979).

Few studies have investigated lesions associated with transcortical motor aphasia (Naeser and Hayward, 1978; Mazzocchi and Vignolo, 1979; Ross, 1980). Naeser and Hayward (1978) reported the lesions associated with four cases of transcortical motor aphasia. In general, the lesions tended to be small and agree with the borderzone theory and reports based on radionuclide scans (Rubens, 1976) in that they were scattered primarily anteriorly and superiorly to Broca's area in the frontal lobe. Two patients, however, had lesions that included the superior portion of Broca's area. None of the four patients had lesions directly involving Wernicke's area. A single case of transcortical motor aphasia was also reported by Mazzocchi and Vignolo (1979). This case had a typical clinical picture with a CT scan showing a lesion in the frontal lobe ante-rior and superior to Broca's area. Two further cases of transcortical motor aphasia associated with infarction of the anterior cerebral artery were reported by Ross (1980). In both cases, the lesions were confined to the medial aspects of the left frontal lobe. In summary, when lesions are produced by vascular pathology, individuals with transcortical motor aphasia most typically have lesions representing the watershed region between the middle cerebral and anterior cere-bral arteries of the dominant hemisphere. How-ever, transcortical motor aphasia has also been reported to be caused by frontal pathology as-sociated with non-vascular pathologies such as trauma (Liu, Moore and Goldman, 1991), tu-mour, herpes simplex encephalitis (Brazzelli *et al.*, 1994) and progressive diseases (Kartsounis *et al.*, 1991).

Overall, it would appear that in transcorti-cal motor aphasia Broca's area may remain in-tact or be only slightly damaged. Transcortical motor aphasia has also been reported to follow unilateral subcortical damage, such as a lesion near the anterior horn of the left lateral ventricle (Damasio, 1981) or in the anterior capsu-loputaminal region, interrupting the thalamic–frontal connections (Sterzi and Vallar, 1978). (Aphasias associated with subcortical lesion sites are discussed more fully in Chapter 3.)

Transcortical sensory aphasia

Transcortical sensory aphasia is characterized by impaired comprehension abilities occurring in conjunction with preserved repetition and a fluent speech output. Comprehension of spoken language is severely disturbed in transcortical sensory aphasia, often to the point of total non-comprehension. This group of patients often in-corporate words and phrases uttered by the clini-cian into their ongoing speech output while at the same time failing to comprehend the meaning of these words and phrases. In fact, the most out-standing feature of transcortical sensory aphasia is the presence of echolalia. Unlike the situation in transcortical motor aphasia, the repetition of statements by transcortical sensory aphasics of-ten appears to be mandatory, the patient appar-ently being unable to omit from their utterances the statements made by the examining clinician. In contrast to patients with transcortical motor aphasia, those with transcortical sensory apha-sia repeat syntactically incorrect statements, non-sense words and even foreign phrases without apparent awareness of what is said and without appropriate correction.

Spontaneous speech, although fluent, is of-ten contaminated by paraphasic errors, including both neologistic and semantic (verbal) substitu-tions and by pauses associated with word-finding difficulties. Series speech, if initiated by the exam-iner, is good. Confrontation naming is seriously defective.

The ability to read aloud is better preserved in transcortical sensory aphasics than reading for comprehension. The latter is almost invariably defective in a similar way to that seen in Wer-nicke's aphasia.

The concomitant neurological problems evi-denced at neurological examination of transcor-tical sensory aphasics vary from case to case. The majority of patients with this condition show no elementary neurological deficit. Others, however, show a mild and usually transient hemiparesis. Sensory deficits, although not common, are found in some transcortical sensory aphasics.

Transcortical sensory aphasia is a syndrome characterized by poor comprehension but ex-cellent repetition. The most extensive localiza-tion study of transcortical sensory aphasia, to date, is that carried out by Kertesz, Sheppard and Mackenzie (1982). Their findings were in agreement with the borderzone theory, the le-sions being primarily located in the inferior parietal–temporal–occipital area.

Kertesz, Sheppard and Mackenzie (1982) found that the lesions separated into two groups, one group being located in a more medial, in-ferior and posterior position in the territory of the posterior cerebral artery. In the other group, the lesion was located in a relatively more lat-eral, superior and anterior position in the wa-tershed (borderzone) area between the distribu-tions of the middle and posterior cerebral arteries. It appears, therefore, that transcortical sensory aphasia is most often seen in association with infarction in the territory of posterior cerebral artery or subsequent to watershed area lesions that involve the territory between the posterior cerebral and middle cerebral arteries, in the posterior temporal parietal region.

Isolation aphasia (mixed transcortical aphasia)

Isolation aphasia is a rare aphasia syndrome characterized by preserved repetitional abilities occurring in association with a marked reduction in spontaneous speech and impaired comprehension of language. The most outstanding feature of this disorder is the loss of the voluntary aspects of language, including spontaneous speech and the ability to initiate and actively participate in conversation. The verbal output of patients with isolation aphasia is almost entirely limited to what has been said to them. Consequently, these patients tend to speak only when spoken to. Isolation aphasics, however, usually exhibit the completion phenomenon (i.e. if told the beginning of a common phrase, the patient may not only repeat what has been said but also continue the phrase to completion). Although the ability of isolation aphasics to repeat is dramatically preserved compared to other language functions, it is limited compared to the repetition abilities of normal individuals. For instance, the number of words in a phrase that can be repeated may be limited to three or four only.

The articulation of phonemes during repetition is good and isolation aphasics demonstrate preserved series speech (e.g. counting) abilities once they are started. Reading aloud as well as reading comprehension and writing are all severely disturbed in this disorder. Isolation aphasics also have severe difficulties in naming, often producing no response at all but occasionally producing neologisms or semantic paraphasias in naming tasks. In many ways, therefore, isolation aphasics resemble global aphasics, with the major exception that the former group are able to repeat what has been said.

The results of neurological examination of these patients are variable. Some exhibit bilateral upper motor neurone paralysis producing

a severe quadriplegia or quadriparesis. Others exhibit unilateral motor disturbances such as right hemiplegia. A significant sensory loss is also frequently present. A visual-field deficit in the form of a hemianopia has been reported in some cases.

Only a limited number of studies have documented the results of a comprehensive clinicopathological analysis of this condition (Geschwind, Quadfasel and Segarra, 1968; Whitaker, 1976; Chenery and Murdoch, 1986). Only two studies using CT localization have been reported (Ross, 1980; Chenery and Murdoch, 1986). The studies by Geschwind, Quadfasel and Segarra (1968) and Whitaker (1976) relied on autopsy evidence which suggested involvement of both the anterior and posterior aspects of the vascular borderzone between the distributions of the major cerebral arteries. However, in the case reported by Chenery and Murdoch (1986), CT scans revealed no focal lesions to be present, only mild cerebral atrophy indicated by prominent cortical sulci and dilated ventricles. Ross (1980) documented a case of mixed transcortical aphasia with infarction involving the left anterior cerebral artery. In the case in question, the lesion extended beyond the left motor and sensory cortices to involve the anterior precuneus lobule of the left parietal lobe. This finding led Ross to suggest that the 'supplementary' sensory area of the left medial parietal lobe participates in receptive language functions.

The full spectrum of the anatomical basis of isolation syndrome remains unknown. It has been argued that comprehension and spontaneous speech are lost in this syndrome because the central speech area no longer has access to other cortical areas necessary for these functions, whereas those functions that can be carried out by the central speech area such as repetition and completion of well-learnt phrases are preserved. Maeshima *et al.* (1996) reported a case of mixed transcortical aphasia associated with a left-hemisphere lesion. A single-photon emission computed tomography (SPECT) scan revealed an area of low perfusion involving the entire left hemisphere except for the perisylvian speech areas. These latter findings support the notion of 'functional isolation' of the left posterior perisylvian language-processing regions in mixed transcortical aphasia.

Anomic aphasia

Anomia, the name given to a word-finding difficulty in confrontational naming tasks and in spontaneous speech, is a symptom common to all types of aphasia. When, however, anomia is the most prominent feature of an aphasic disorder, the condition is referred to as an 'anomic aphasia'.

Anomic aphasia is a commonly encountered form of aphasia in which the patient has little expressive or receptive difficulty. Spontaneous speech is produced easily and fluently, although at times there is an emptiness resulting from a lack of substantive words. In addition, the speech output at times is very circumlocutory (circuitous) as a result of replacement of specific words (names) by generalizations (e.g. 'thing', 'it', 'them', etc.) which often fail to communicate the message satisfactorily. As a result, the speech of anomic aphasics is often described as being vague. The degree of word-finding difficulty varies widely from case to case, some patients showing only a mild naming disturbance on confrontation naming tasks while in others confrontation naming is severely disturbed.

Anomic aphasics have good repetitional abilities and near normal auditory and written comprehension. Their ability to read aloud is also relatively good in most cases. Writing is near normal in some cases and impaired in others. Anomic aphasia is often the result of recovery from other aphasic syndromes such as Wernicke's or conduction aphasia. Anomia remains the complaint of many well-recovered aphasics.

The associated neurological findings vary widely in anomic aphasia. Many cases of this disorder exhibit no associated neurological signs at all. On the other hand, hemiparesis, hemiplegia, hemisensory loss and visual field defects may occur in some of these patients.

Anomic aphasia is regarded as a non-localizing aphasia syndrome. In general, the lesion site cannot be readily localized to a particular cortical area. Gloning, Gloning and Hoff (1963), in a study of the location of pathology in patients with various aphasia syndromes, found that 60% of their patients with anomic aphasia had a dominant hemisphere parietal–temporal junction lesion. The other 40% of their anomic patients, however, had lesions scattered over a wide area. CT studies have come up with similar findings. For example, Hayward, Naeser and Zatz (1977) reported that, although there was some concentration of lesions in the region of the angular gyrus, in general the lesions in anomic aphasia were scattered about the left hemisphere with a lack of specific location involvement.

Subcortical aphasia syndromes

Since the introduction of CT scanning in the 1970s, with its ability to demonstrate deep-structured brain pathology in the living subject, it has become increasingly recognized that aphasia syndromes can be caused by damage to subcortical structures as well as cortical lesions. In particular, it has been suggested that aphasia can be produced by lesions involving the region of the basal ganglia or thalamus. For this reason, in recent years an increasing number of researchers have advocated the addition of subcortical aphasia syndromes to the list of clinically recognized aphasic disturbances. The various subcortical aphasias are discussed in Chapter 3.

Lurian aphasia syndromes

Based on an extensive study of patients who exhibited speech-language disorders subsequent to traumatic brain injuries, Luria (1970) described seven major types of aphasia including: (1) efferent (kinetic) motor aphasia, (2) frontal dynamic aphasia, (3) pre-motor aphasia, (4) afferent (apraxia) aphasia, (5) sensory (acoustic) aphasia, (6) acoustico-mnestic aphasia and (7) semantic aphasia. By careful mapping of the sites of injury in wounded soldiers and examining their associated speech-language disorder, Luria was able to establish with some confidence the correlation between the above aphasia syndromes and the territory in which the brain was damaged. Unfortunately, few studies using modern localization methods such as CT scanning have been carried out in order to either confirm or refute Luria's proposals. Remembering that Luria formed his classification on shrapnel wounds, such studies are needed to confirm the relevance of his classification system to cerebrovascular accident cases.

Luria proposed that there are three principal functional units of the brain whose participation is necessary for any type of mental activity (including speech-language function). These three units include: a unit for regulating tone and waking and mental states; a unit for receiving, analysing and storing information; and a unit for programming, regulation and verification of activity. Luria suggested that damage to either of the last two units listed above could cause aphasia. Damage to the second functional unit, which comprises the primary receptive areas for vision, hearing and general senses and the association areas of the parietal, temporal and occipital lobes, may lead to the various receptive aphasias including sensory (acoustic) aphasia, acoustico-mnestic aphasia, afferent (apraxic) motor aphasia and semantic aphasia. On the other hand, lesions of the third functional unit, located in the cerebral hemispheres anterior to the pre-central sulcus, cause the various expressive aphasias including pre-motor, efferent (kinetic) motor aphasia and frontal dynamic aphasia.

Efferent (kinetic) motor aphasia

Patients with efferent motor aphasia have difficulty in formulating their thoughts in language. Although these patients are able to pronounce individual sounds easily, they fail when required to produce those same sounds as part of a whole word. In particular, efferent motor aphasics have difficulty in shifting from one articulatory position to another and therefore their speech disorder becomes most apparent when pronouncing multisyllabic words or combinations of words.

According to Luria, there are two essential components to efferent motor aphasia, the first involving the loss of serial organization of speech and the second a disturbance in inner speech. Inner speech mediates the transition of thought to external speech. As part of the formulation of inner speech, the predicative structure or dynamic schema of the speech output to follow is determined. Disruption of inner speech in these patients, therefore, makes the formulation of sentences impossible. Sentences, therefore, are absent in the everyday speech of efferent motor aphasics. Likewise, the loss of inner speech causes disruption of the dynamic schema of words leading to a loss of the predicative significance of words and causing the articulation of words to also become impossible.

Efferent motor aphasics exhibit a writing disturbance similar to the disturbance in speech. In addition, most of these patients have a concomitant right hemiparesis. The lesion associated with this disorder involves the inferior pre-motor region of the left hemisphere.

Frontal (dynamic) aphasia

Although patients with frontal (dynamic) aphasia are able to utter words (e.g. repetition tasks) and distinguish speech sounds, they are deprived of spontaneous speech and seldom use it for purposes of communication. It is thought that these patients have lost the ability to formulate thoughts into sentences (propositionizing) and consequently show no spontaneity of speech and are unable to use speech for generalizing or expressing thoughts or desires.

Writing is disturbed in a similar manner to speech. Although these patients are able to follow simple instructions, comprehension is also disturbed. Reading aloud is disturbed. A right hemiplegia or hemiparesis is a common finding in this type of aphasia. According to Luria, the lesion is usually located in the inferior part of the left frontal lobe just anterior to Broca's area.

Pre-motor aphasia

Pre-motor aphasia is caused by lesions in the upper and middle portions of the pre-motor area. It is characterized by a loss of smoothness of speech, agrammatism, disturbed comprehension and intonation and perseveration.

Patients with pre-motor aphasia pronounce individual sounds and words haltingly. Long pauses occur in the transition from one word to another and each word is produced with considerable effort. Pre-motor aphasia, however, does not simply represent a motor speech disorder. Rather a disturbance of inner speech is present. In particular, the patient appears unable to store the schemata of inner speech which in turn leads to the halting speech and a reduction in the grammatical complexity of sentences produced. The vocal and written speech of these patients is characterized by short sentence fragments. Pre-motor aphasics speak in monotone and are unable to suppress articulatory patterns once created, leading to perseveration. Comprehension is also disturbed and statements may need to be presented several times to these patients before they are understood. Even then, complex statements may only be understood in part.

Luria (1970) suggested that the basic disorder in patients with pre-motor aphasia is not an impairment in their ability to create new speech articulations but rather a disturbance in the automaticity of continuous speech as a result of a disturbance in the schema of speech. A right hemiparesis is a concomitant finding in the majority of these cases.

Afferent (apraxic) motor aphasia

The most outstanding feature of afferent (apraxic) motor aphasia is the patient's inability to determine immediately the positions of the components of the speech mechanism (e.g. lips and tongue) necessary to articulate the required sounds of speech. Consequently, a given individual sound may be articulated differently depending upon the syllables in which it occurs. This difficulty is present in both spontaneous speech and repetitive speech.

According to Luria (1970), the disturbance in expressive speech involves difficulty finding the articulatory movements necessary for the pronunciation of individual sounds and sound sequences which go to make up words and phrases.

In other words, the disorder involves an apraxic disturbance of the speech organs. Unlike the three Lurian syndromes associated with pre-motor lesions described above, the dynamic aspects of speech are not disturbed in afferent motor aphasia. Although in severe cases the patient may not know where to put the tongue, lips and so on to produce necessary sounds, in more mild cases the patient may only confuse the positions for similar articulemes leading to substitution of phonemes within words (i.e. literal paraphasias).

Deficits in writing and reading are also present in this disorder. An ideomotor dyspraxia of the oral, lingual and pharyngeal musculature is a common finding. A right hemiparesis affecting the arm more than the leg is present in some cases. According to Luria, the lesion associated with afferent motor apraxia is located in the lower parts of the post-central area of the left hemisphere (i.e. the left inferior parietal region).

Sensory (acoustic) aphasia

Sensory (acoustic) aphasia is associated with lesions of the superior parts of the temporal lobe. The major symptoms include a disturbance of phonemic hearing, loss of meaning of words, difficulty naming objects, the presence of literal and verbal paraphasias and a writing disturbance.

The major factor underlying this condition is a disturbance in phonemic hearing, which in turn leads to a breakdown in those linguistic tasks requiring sound discrimination. These tasks include the understanding of speech, the naming of objects and the recalling of words. Difficulty in understanding spoken speech (i.e. the loss of the meaning of words) arises from the loss of the ability to discriminate between closely sounding phonemes. Likewise, because they no longer have a differentiated phonemic system of language, the sensory aphasic finds it difficult to name objects and to recall necessary words, thereby leading to the substitution of incorrect words or phonemes (i.e. paraphasia errors). As a result of a deficient phonemic system of language, these patients are unable to monitor their own speech and are therefore unaware of the defects in their speech. Consequently, they are unable to correct for these deficits so that their speech becomes converted into empty jargon in which the nominative components (the substantives) are lacking and their output is reduced to consisting of interjections or habitual expressions. The melodic and intonational aspects of their speech, however, remain intact.

In addition to the loss of phonemic hearing, the semantic aspect of language is also profoundly disturbed in these patients.

Acoustico-mnestic aphasia

Lesions in the posterior inferior part of the temporal lobe cause a disturbance in audioverbal memory, which in turn gives rise to a condition called 'acoustico-mnestic aphasia'. Patients with acoustico-mnestic aphasia have difficulty in retaining word series. Although typically these patients can retain single words and repeat them after several minutes, they cannot retain a short series of words presented aloud, being able to repeat only the first or last word in most cases.

Although in the acute stage post-onset, these patients may have difficulty understanding the speech of others, this symptom usually clears rapidly. Unlike patients with sensory (acoustic) aphasia, phonemic hearing is preserved in acoustico-mnestic aphasia and literal paraphasias are absent. Writing is also usually intact.

Semantic aphasia

Semantic aphasia is caused by lesions of the temporal parietal occipital region of the left hemisphere. The language disorder seen in this condition is based on neither a hearing nor a memory deficit. Rather, it represents a disturbance in the understanding of logico-grammatical relationships. Semantic aphasia is characterized by an inability to synthesize isolated simultaneous events into a meaningful unity.

Patients with semantic aphasia experience an inner loss of the semantic structure of words. They have no difficulty in hearing or understanding individual words and speak fluently. Their phonemic hearing is intact and they show no signs of having forgotten the primary meaning of words. Often, the only language disturbance noted by an outside observer is an impairment in naming objects. Careful testing, however, reveals that even though patients with semantic aphasia appear to understand the general meaning of speech, they are unable to see the grammatical relationship between words because they can no longer see the entire complex of associations of words. Consequently, these patients are unable to process or decode information according to the logico-grammatical rules of language. Therefore, although there is a preserved ability to understand isolated words, semantic aphasics are unable to grasp the meaning of an entire sentence.

Semantic aphasics often exhibit a concomitant disturbance in spatial orientation. Difficulties with computation (acalculia) are also a frequent finding. Writing is disturbed in a similar manner to speech.

Hier *et al.* (1980) documented the lesions associated with three cases of semantic aphasia using CT scanning. In all cases, the lesions involved the left temporal–parietal–occipital junction in agreement with Luria's suggestion (one case actually had bilateral damage involving both the left and right temporal–parietal–occipital junction).

Methods of lesion localization in aphasia

Since the middle of the last century, many investigators have attempted to prove or disprove the theory that the various aphasia syndromes and lesions of specific anatomic sites of the brain are correlated. The general methods used to investigate this theory have been to: obtain indices of the site and size of brain lesions, measure the features and characteristics of the aphasic patient's clinical presentation and attempt correlation of the above two parameters.

While these basic procedures have been followed, many of the studies have used different kinds of specific instrumentation to measure both the pathological and the clinical parameters of the various aphasia syndromes. Prior to the 1970s, the most commonly used methods of ascertaining lesion localization have been post-mortem examination, post-traumatic skull defects, cerebral angiography, cortical stimulation, electroencephalography, regional cerebral blood flow and radioisotope brain scans.

Unfortunately, all of these localization techniques have important limiting factors which restrict their validity for making correlations between site of pathology and aphasia type. Post-mortem examination, although an accurate localizing technique, by its very nature, prevents direct correlation of clinical findings with the location of pathology in the living subject. Post-traumatic skull defects do not necessarily reflect specific site or extent of brain lesion and, indeed, may be quite misleading, owing to 'contre-coup' effect. Similarly, cerebral angiography indicates only the vessel occluded, not the specific part of the brain infarcted. Electroencephalograms also lack localizing precision. Cortical stimulation has provided important information about the localization of some language functions, for example naming, repetition, reading and writing (Ojemann and Whitaker, 1978). It does not, however, give information about the coordination and integration of these functions. Regional cerebral blood flow provides accurate two-dimensional information, but gives no indication of depth of lesion, nor, as in the case of angiography, is it conducted without some risk to the patient. A number of studies have, however, correlated language and other cognitive behaviours with regional cerebral blood flow. The findings of these studies suggest that, in addition to the classic language areas, many other parts of the brain are also activated during speech production and comprehension.

Radioisotope brain scanning is safe and relatively effective, and is probably the best method of localization of those mentioned above. However, it also has some technical limitations. An accurate three-dimensional picture (i.e. information about depth of lesion) cannot be obtained, because the area of isotope uptake may not necessarily conform to the boundaries of the lesion and all areas of damaged brain tissue are not necessarily shown. Radioisotope scans lack clear definition and do not differentiate between ischaemic and haemorrhagic lesions. In addition, positive readings for identifying brain lesions are only evident in radioisotope scans taken within a limited time post-onset.

The most commonly used method for localizing aphasia-producing lesions has been CT scanning.

Structural neuroimaging techniques

Computerized tomography

Since the mid-1970s, a number of new neuroimaging techniques have been introduced that have greatly increased the accuracy of lesion localization, thereby enabling a greater understanding of the neuropathophysiological basis of various aphasia syndromes. These techniques include computerized tomographic (CT) scanning, magnetic resonance imaging (MRI), positron emission tomography (PET), single-photon emission computed tomography (SPECT) and functional magnetic resonance imaging (fMRI). CT scanning and MRI represent techniques for detecting structural changes in the living brain, while PET, SPECT and fMRI represent functional neuroimaging techniques.

CT scanning has a number of advantages compared to the previously used methods of lesion localization. Most importantly, it was the first technique to allow visualization of deep-structured pathology (i.e. subcortical lesions) in the living subject. Further, CT scanning is useful for viewing a wide variety of different brain pathologies, including tumours, haematomas, infarcts and the effects of trauma.

Briefly, CT scanning is the product of applying computer technology and techniques of image reconstruction to modern radiological equipment. An X-ray source produces a narrow beam which transverses the head of the patient. This source is coupled to a radiation detector system, both of which move across the head in a linear fashion. Each point in the brain is investigated from 180 angles. That is to say, the X-ray beam has to complete a semicircle so that the object is transversed 180 times. The computer then analyses the information obtained and generates an image on the cathode ray tube. The brightness of the image is proportional to the density of the brain tissue at that point.

The examination starts at the base of the skull (the plane may be horizontal (axial) or angled, often parallel to the orbitomeatal line) and extends up the cranium in a series of about 10 slices. Scan slices are usually 8–10 mm thick. Within the brain, CT scans can define structures such as the ventricles, the sulci, the cisterns, the putamen and thalamus, the choroid plexus, the eye, optic nerve, eye muscles, pineal gland, pituitary fossa, nasopharynx, cranial bone structures, venous structures, foramen magnum and so on.

CT scanning permits the detection of structural intracranial abnormalities with precision and speed and can be used in the evaluation of patients with focal neurological deficits (e.g. strokes) as well as those with progressive neurological disorders (e.g. dementia). It is particularly useful in the evaluation of strokes in that it can distinguish infarction from intracranial haemorrhage. The procedure is important in the evaluation of patients following traumatic head injury where it can detect traumatic subarachnoid, extradural and intracerebral haemorrhage and bony injuries. It also provides a more precise delineation of associated skull fractures than do plain X-rays. CT scans are also able to demonstrate the site of a brain tumour, whether the tumour is cystic or solid and whether it has displaced midline or other normal anatomic structures. Intravenous administration of an iodinated contrast agent improves the ability of CT scanning to detect and define lesions such as tumours and abscesses associated with a disturbance of the blood–brain barrier.

As an aphasia localization technique, CT scanning has been used in research investigating clinicopathological correlations of aphasia for approximately the past three decades. Although this technique has provided considerable evidence to support an anatomically based model and classification of aphasia, it is evident that we cannot assume that the area of brain damage identified on CT scans is solely responsible for concomitant disturbances in language function. There are many cases of aphasia reported in the literature with unexpected computerized tomographic le-

sions, which point to limitations of anatomical analysis to fully explain the neuropathology of language. In addition, the reported findings of studies based on more recently introduced brain-scanning methods have indicated that structural brain damage, as indicated by CT scanning, is associated with modifications to brain metabolism in areas distant to the lesion. It is possible that these distant effects will also influence language behaviour.

The findings of studies based on CT scanning have forced a revision of the classical concept of language function. Although in previous years it was thought that the occurrence of aphasia was associated with damage to the speech-language area (including Broca's and Wernicke's area) of the dominant hemisphere, CT scanning has demonstrated the need to extend that area to include subcortical as well as cortical structures.

Magnetic resonance imaging

Magnetic resonance imaging (MRI) used to be called 'nuclear magnetic resonance imaging'. Overall, the magnetic resonance scanner bears a similar resemblance to the CT scanner.

Unlike CT scanning, MRI does not involve the use of ionizing radiation. Rather, in this technique, the objects of study are the nuclei of atoms that have an odd number of protons (e.g. hydrogen-1, phosphorus-31, carbon-13, sodium-23). The nucleus that yields the strongest magnetic resonance signal is hydrogen. It is also the most abundant atom in biological tissue and has consequently received the greatest attention in magnetic resonance techniques. These atomic nuclei are of interest because they have a property called 'spin' (or magnetic moment) that makes them behave like small bar magnets spinning around their axes. Normally, these nuclei assume a random alignment. When we place the head in the strong magnetic field of the magnetic resonance unit, the spinning protons become aligned with the magnetic field (i.e. reach a state of equilibrium). A short burst of radio waves at specific frequencies is then introduced which causes the aligned protons to be 'tipped' in a controlled way. After the burst of radio waves, the protons return to their equilibrium point but, as they do, emit electromagnetic signals whose frequency and duration can be measured by a receiver and, subsequently, used to generate spatial coordinates and a visual image using computerized methods similar to those employed for CT scanning. The signal intensity depends upon the concentration of mobile hydrogen nuclei (or nuclear-spin density) of the tissues. Spin-lattice (T1) and spin-spin (T2) relaxation times are mainly responsible for the relative differences in signal intensity of the various soft tissues. The images produced largely represent the distribution of hydrogen (or other proton, e.g. sodium) through the brain or other body region being examined. Different tissues have characteristic differences in hydrogen atom (water) concentrations. Abnormalities can be detected by observing differences between the concentrations of hydrogen atoms (water) found and those expected. Pulse sequences with varying dependence on T1 and T2 selectively alter the contrast between the soft tissues. Intravenous injection of gadopentetate dimeglumine (gadolinium) is an effective enhancing agent for MRI that can be used for the detection of some structural abnormalities such as small tumours that may otherwise be missed by unenhanced scans.

MRI provides an image which correlates with anatomy and can distinguish grey from white matter to a greater extent than can CT scanning. MRI can also detect the presence of tumour, oedema, atrophy, arteriovenous malformation, haematoma and infarcts, and can identify the effects of demyelinating disease. Because MRI is free of bony artefacts, the procedure is superior to CT scanning for visualizing abnormalities (e.g. tumours) in the posterior cranial fossa and spinal cord. The procedure is also superior for the early detection of ischaemic brain infarcts following stroke. Such infarcts may fail to be detected by CT scans in the first 48 hours post-stroke. In contrast, intracranial haemorrhage is not easily detected by MRI within the first 36 hours and CT scanning is more reliable for this purpose. Consequently, CT scanning without contrast is usually preferred for the initial examination of patients with acute stroke, in order to determine whether haemorrhage has occurred. Haematomas of more than 2–3 days' duration, however, are better visualized by MRI.

Factors that preclude the use of MRI include the presence of ferromagnetic surgical clips (e.g. aneurysm clips), metallic foreign bodies in the eye or elsewhere, pacemakers, cochlear implants and conditions requiring close monitoring of the patient. Patients with claustrophobia, gross obesity, uncontrolled movement disorders or respiratory disorders that require assisted ventilation or carry any risk of apnea may also be difficult to image. The recent development of MRI compatible monitoring equipment, ventilators and so on, however, has made the procedure available to a larger range of patients.

The relative advantages and disadvantages of MRI compared to CT scanning are summarized in Table 2.1.

Functional neuroimaging techniques

While the technical details of the three major forms of functional neuroimaging differ, these procedures detect changes in regional blood flow and by inference measure the varying levels of metabolic activity in different areas of the brain during different types of mental activity. More simply, these techniques indirectly measure neuronal activity by measuring increases in blood flow to active areas of the brain. The basic principle is simple. Neurones that are active demand more oxygen and glucose. The brain vasculature responds to neural activity by directing more blood to the active areas. Thus, by detecting changes in blood flow, functional neuroimaging techniques reveal the regions of the brain that are most active under differing circumstances. In recent years, numerous studies have utilized functional neuroimaging techniques to examine aspects of language processing in both normal and aphasic individuals and to determine possible brain mechanisms involved in language recovery subsequent to acquired brain damage (e.g. stroke). (For recent reviews see Cao *et al.*, 1998; Pizzamiglio, Galati and Committeri, 2001; Kuest and Karbe, 2002; Wise, 2003; Demonet, Thierry and Cardebat, 2005; Price and Crinion, 2005; Zahn, Schwarz and Huber, 2006; Van Lancker Sidtis, 2007).

Table 2.1 Summary of the relative advantages and disadvantages of magnetic resonance imaging.

Advantages	Disadvantages
■ MRI is non-invasive ■ Does not require use of ionizing radiation ■ Has very good resolution in transverse, coronal and sagittal planes ■ Unlike computerized tomography, bone does not induce artefacts in the image. The posterior cranial fossa can therefore be viewed in detail ■ Distinguishes grey and white matter better than CT scans ■ Sensitive to early changes associated with stroke ■ Sensitive to changes associated with demyelinating disease ■ Because there are no known hazardous effects, can be repeated in a serial manner if necessary	■ High capital outlay and running costs ■ Narrow gantry causes claustrophobia in some patients. Patient may require sedation ■ Potential hazards related to ferromagnetic surgical clips or prostheses and effects on patients with cardiac pacemakers ■ Because of the high magnetic field, ferrous instruments etc. in proximity to the MRI unit may become airborne missiles

Positron emission tomography (PET)

This is a non-invasive functional neuroimaging technique which utilizes positron-emitting radionuclides to measure brain metabolism. It is a technique which estimates functional damage rather than structural damage as in CT scanning. PET involves computerized techniques the same as CT scanning to generate visual images, and uses the same brain slices. The method involves measurement of the metabolism of radioactively labelled molecules (positron emitters) such as ^{18}FDG (fluorodeoxyglucose), $^{15}O_2$ and so on. In most reported studies so far, ^{18}FDG has been the most commonly utilized molecule.

The radioactive material (e.g. ^{18}FDG) is injected intravenously into the patient and accumulates in the brain over a 45-minute period. Accumulation of ^{18}FDG is proportional to the rate of glucose metabolism. As the isotope decays, positrons are emitted. The emitted positrons quickly combine with nearby electrons and the two particles annihilate each other, producing gamma rays. By surrounding the patient's head with a ring of gamma ray detectors, it is possible to localize the positron-emitting isotope within the brain. In addition to ^{18}FDG, a range of different compounds can be labelled with positron-emitting isotopes, making it possible to map out not only glucose metabolism but also oxygen con-sumption, blood flow and the location of receptors for neurotransmitters and hormones. It is also possible to combine PET and MRI scans to map functional changes in blood flow onto high-quality structural images of the brain.

PET has become an important tool with which to investigate the functional involvement of different cerebral areas in behavioural and cognitive tasks, including language processing. A number of studies have been reported which have utilized PET scans to localize lesions associated with aphasia. Most of these have been conducted by Metter and his co-workers in California. In general, their data suggest that reliance on CT scanning in delineating the extent of brain lesions in aphasia or other neuropsychological defects can be misleading. The reason for this is that PET scans usually reveal that cerebral metabolic activity is diminished in an area larger than the area of the infarction demonstrated by CT scanning. This suggests that function (metabolism) in non-structurally damaged tissue is not normal and that consequently the observed language impairment may not be solely attributable to the structural brain damage evident in the CT scan.

In addition, it has been found that in some cases PET scans reveal metabolic lesions to be present that might account for aphasia in patients where CT scans revealed no structural deficit to be present.

Although PET has proven to be a useful technique, it has several limitations. The spatial resolution is only 5–10 mm^3 and consequently the images show the activity of many thousands of neurones. Further, a single PET scan may take many minutes. This, combined with concerns regarding radiation exposure, limits the number of scans that can be obtained from one person in a reasonable period.

Functional magnetic resonance imaging (fMRI)

The fMRI method takes advantage of the fact that oxyhaemoglobin (the oxygenated form of haemoglobin in the blood) has a different magnetic resonance than deoxyhaemoglobin (haemoglobin that has donated its oxygen). The fMRI technique detects the locations of increased neural activity in relation to the performance of specific mental tasks (e.g. language tasks) by measuring the ratio of oxyhaemoglobin to deoxyhaemoglobin. Basically, active areas of the brain receive an even greater increase in blood flow than they need, so blood leaving active areas actually has a higher concentration of oxygen than blood leaving inactive areas. Hence, MRI scans that reflect oxyhaemoglobin/deoxyhaemoglobin ratios can provide a measure of regional changes in blood flow.

Although fMRI is the newest of the functional neuroimaging techniques, it has rapidly emerged as the method of choice for functional neuroimaging because the scans can be made relatively quickly, they have better spatial resolution (3 mm^3) and are described as being non-invasive.

Single-photon emission computed tomography (SPECT)

SPECT involves the intravenous administration of gamma-emitting isotopes that emit single gamma ray photons in order to image the brain. A scan utilizing a ring of gamma-ray detectors and tomographic calculations similar to those used in CT scanning to determine the radiopharmaceutical uptake is performed several hours later. The isotope is taken up by areas of increased blood flow, theoretically associated with the activity being investigated. SPECT has been used, in partic-

ular, for perfusion studies, the investigation of receptor distribution and the detection of areas of increased brain metabolism such as might occur with seizures or the performance of various cognitive tasks. The major limitation of SPECT is that the technique has low spatial resolution (approximately 10 mm^3). Additionally, certain logistic issues occur, including the need for personnel to prepare the radioisotope and administer it with appropriate timing.

Summary

The term 'aphasia' is used to describe those language impairments caused by brain damage. Over the years, several opposing views as to the neurological basis of aphasia have been proposed with researchers in this field, in general, being labelled as either 'localizationists' or 'holists'. The controversy over the neurological basis of aphasia has led to the application of a large array of nomenclature and terminology to describe aphasic disorders. Although a number of different models of language function have been proposed, the most influential model over the past century has been the Wernicke–Lichtheim model.

Owing to the complexity and variability of aphasia syndromes, a large number of systems have been devised to classify the various forms of aphasia. The classification system used in most contemporary clinical settings is that devised by the Speech Pathology Section, Aphasia Research Unit at the Veterans Administration Hospital in Boston, more commonly known as the Bostonian Classification System. This system recognizes eight clinically recognisable aphasia syndromes, namely: Broca's aphasia, Wernicke's aphasia, conduction aphasia, global aphasia, transcortical motor aphasia, transcortical sensory aphasia, mixed transcortical (isolation) aphasia and anomic aphasia. An alternative aphasia classification used by some clinicians and researchers is that devised by the Russian neurologist Luria, on the basis of his examination of the language abilities of soldiers with war injuries to the head. The Lurian classification system recognizes seven major types of aphasia, including: efferent (kinematic) motor aphasia, frontal dynamic aphasia, pre-motor aphasia, afferent (apraxic) aphasia, sensory (acoustic) aphasia, acoustico-mnestic aphasia and semantic aphasia.

Although prior to the 1970s lesion localization was limited to imprecise techniques such as radioisotope scanning and basic X-ray techniques, since that time the introduction of accurate structural imaging techniques such as CT scanning and MRI have greatly enhanced our ability to examine the relationship between specific aphasia syndromes and the localization of associated brain lesions *in vivo*. More recently, the application of functional neuroimaging techniques such as PET, fMRI and SPECT have enabled the examination of changes in regional cerebral blood flow and by inference changes in brain activity in both normal and aphasic individuals while performing various language tasks. In this way functional neuroimaging techniques have provided important information on possible brain mechanisms involved in recovery from aphasia.

References

Anderson, J., Gilmore, R., Roper, S. *et al.* (1999) Conduction aphasia and the arcuate fasciculus: a re-examination of the Wernicke–Geschwind model. *Brain and Language*, **70**, 1–12.

Andral, G. (1840) *Clinique Médicale*, Fortin Masson et Cie, Paris.

Axer, H., von Keyserlingk, A., Berks, G. and von Keyseringk, D. (2001) Supra- and infrasylvian conduction aphasia. *Brain and Language*, **76**, 317–331.

Basso, A., Lecours, A.R., Morashini, S. and Vanier, M. (1985) Anatomo-clinical correlations of the aphasias as defined through computed tomography: exceptions. *Brain and Language*, **26**, 201–229.

Bastian, H.C. (1898) *Aphasia and Other Defects*, H. K. Lewis, London.

Benson, D.F. (1967) Fluency in aphasia: correlation with radioactive scan localization. *Cortex*, **3**, 373–394.

Benson, D.F. (1979) *Aphasia, Alexia and Agraphia*, Churchill Livingstone, New York.

Bouillaud, M.J. (1825) Recherches cliniques propres à démontrer que la perte de la parole correspond à la lésion des lobules antérieurs du cerveau, et à con-firmer l'opinion de M. Gall, sur le siège de l'organe du langage articulé. *Archives Générals de Médecine*, **3**, 22–45.

Brazzelli, M., Colombo, N., Della Sala, S. and Spinnler, H. (1994) Spared and impaired cognitive abilities after bilateral frontal damage. *Cortex*, **30**, 27–51.

Broca, P. (1861) Portée de la parole: Ramollissement chronique et destruction partielle du lobe antérieur gauche du cerveau. *Bulletins de la Société d'anthropologie de Paris*, **2**, 219.

Broca, P. (1865) Sur le siège de la faculté du langage articulé. *Bulletins de la Société d'anthropologie de Paris*, **36**, 337–393.

Cao, Y., George, P., Ewing, J.R. *et al.* (1998) Neuroimaging of language and aphasia after stroke. *Journal of Stroke and Cerebrovascular Diseases*, **7**, 230–233.

Cappa, S.F., Cavallotti, G. and Vignolo, L. (1981) Phonemic and lexical errors in fluent aphasia: correlation with lesion site. *Neuropsychologia*, **19**, 171–177.

Chapman, S.B., Pool, K.D., Finitzo, T. and Hong, C.T. (1989) Comparison of language profiles and electrocortical dysfunction in aphasia, in *Clinical Aphasiology*, vol. **18** (ed. T.E. Prescott), College Hill Press, Boston, pp. 41–59.

Charcot, J.M. (1877) *Lectures on the Diseases of the Nervous System*, New Sydenham Society, London.

Chenery, H.J. and Murdoch, B.E. (1986) A case of mixed transcortical aphasia following drug overdose. *British Journal of Disorders of Communication*, **21**, 381–392.

Critchley, M. (1970) *Aphasiology*, Edward Arnold, London.

Crosson, B. (1985) Subcortical functions in language: a working model. *Brain and Language*, **25**, 257–292.

Damasio, H. (1981) Cerebral localization of the aphasias, in *Acquired Aphasia* (ed. M.T. Sarno), Academic Press, New York, pp. 25–40.

Damasio, H. (1998) Neuroanatomic correlates of the aphasias, in *Acquired Aphasia* (ed. M.T. Sarno), Academic Press, New York, pp. 43–68.

Damasio, H. and Damasio, A.R. (1980) The anatomical basis of conduction aphasia. *Brain*, **103**, 337–350.

Dax, M. (1836) Lésions de la moitié gauche de l'encéphale coïncidant avec l'oubli des signes de la pensée. Paper presented at the Congrés Méridional, Montpellier, 1836.

Dax, M. (1865) Lésions de la moitié gauche de l'encéphale coïncidant avec l'oubli des signes de la pensée. Lu au Congrés Méridional tenu à Montpellier en 1836, par la docteur Marc Dax. *Gazette hebdomadaire de médecine et de chirurgie*, **227** (4), April 28, 259–262.

Demonet, J.F., Thierry, G. and Cardebat, D. (2005) Renewal of the neurophysiology of language: functional neuroimaging. *Physiological Reviews*, **85**, 49–95.

Flourens, P. (1824) *Recherches Expérimentales sur les Propriétés et les Fonctions du Système Nerveux*, Bailliére, Paris.

Flourens, P. (1842) *Examen de la Phrénologie*, Hachette, Paris.

Gall, F.J. (1809) *Recherches sur le Système Nerveux*, Bailliére, Paris.

Geschwind, N. (1965a) Disconnection syndromes in animals and man. Part 1. *Brain*, **88**, 237–294.

Geschwind, N. (1965b) Disconnection syndromes in animals and man. Part 2. *Brain*, **88**, 585–644.

Geschwind, N. (1969) Anatomical understanding of the aphasias, in *Contribution to Clinical Neuropsychology* (ed. A.L. Benton), Aldine Publishing, Chicago, pp. 24–36.

Geschwind, N. (1971) *Aphasia. New England Journal of Medicine*, **284**, 654–656.

Geschwind, N., Quadfasel, F.A. and Segarra, J.M. (1968) Isolation of the speech area. *Neuropsychologia*, **6**, 327–340.

Gloning, I., Gloning, K. and Hoff, H. (1963) Aphasia: a clinical syndrome, in *Problems of Dynamic Neurology* (ed. L. Halpern), Hebrew University, Jerusalem, pp. 63–70.

Goodglass, H. and Kaplan, E. (1972) *The Assessment of Aphasia and Related Disorders*, Lea and Febiger, Philadelphia.

Hayward, R.W., Naeser, M.A. and Zatz, L.M. (1977) Cranial computed tomography in aphasia. *Radiology*, **123**, 653–660.

Head, H. (1926) *Aphasia and Kindred Disorders*, Cambridge University Press, London.

Hier, D.B., Mogil, S.I., Rubin, N.P. and Komros, G.R. (1980) Semantic aphasia: a neglected entity. *Brain and Language*, **10**, 120–131.

Karis, R. and Horenstein, S. (1976) Localization of speech parameters by brain scan. *Neurology*, **26**, 226–231.

Kartsounis, L.D., Crellin, R.F., Crewes, H. and Toone, B.K. (1991) Primary progressive non-fluent aphasia: a case study. *Cortex*, **27**, 121–129.

Kertesz, A. (1979) *Aphasia and Associated Disorders: Taxonomy, Localization and Recovery*, Grune & Stratton, New York.

Kertesz, A., Harlock, W. and Coates, R. (1979) Computer tomographic localization of lesion size and prognosis in aphasia and nonverbal impairment. *Brain and Language*, **8**, 34–50.

Kertesz, A., Lau, W.K. and Polk, M. (1993) The structural determinants of recovery in Wernicke's aphasia. *Brain and Language*, **44**, 153–164.

Kertesz, A., Lesk, D. and McCabe, P. (1977) Isotope localization of infarcts in aphasia. *Archives of Neurology*, **34**, 590–601.

Kertesz, A., Sheppard, A. and Mackenzie, R. (1982) Localization in transcortical sensory aphasia. *Archives of Neurology*, **39**, 475–478.

Kleist, K. (1962) *Sensory Aphasia and Amusia*, Pergamon Press, London.

Kuest, J. and Karbe, H. (2002) Cortical activation studies in aphasia. *Current Neurology and Neuroscience Reviews*, **2**, 511–515.

Levine, D.N. and Calvanio, R. (1982) Conduction aphasia, in *Neurolinguistics: the Neurology of Aphasia*, vol. **12** (eds H.S. Kirshner and F.R. Freeman), Swets and Zeitlinger, Amsterdam, pp. 79–111.

Lichtheim, L. (1885) On aphasia. *Brain*, **7**, 433–484.

Liu, G.T., Moore, M.R. and Goldman, H. (1991) Transcortical motor aphasia due to a subdural hematoma. *American Journal of Emergency Medicine*, **9**, 620–622.

Luria, A.R. (1970) *Traumatic Aphasia*, Mouton, The Hague.

Maeshima, S., Uematsu, Y., Terada, T. *et al.* (1996) Transcortical mixed aphasia with left frontoparietal lesions. *Neuroradiology*, **38**, S78–S79.

Marie, P. (1906) The third frontal convolution plays no special role in the function of language. *Semaine Médicale*, **26**, 241–247.

Mazzocchi, F. and Vignolo, L.A. (1979) Localization of lesions in aphasia: clinical-CT scan correlations in stroke patients. *Cortex*, **15**, 627–654.

Mendez, M.F. and Benson, D.F. (1985) Atypical conduction aphasia: a disconnection syndrome. *Archives of Neurology*, **42**, 886–891.

Metter, E.J., Jackson, C.A., Kempler, D. and Hanson, W.R. (1992) Temporo-parietal cortex and recovery of language comprehension in aphasia. *Aphasiology*, **6**, 349–358.

Metter, E.J., Kempler, D., Jackson, C. *et al.* (1989) Cerebral glucose metabolism in Wernicke's, Broca's and conduction aphasia. *Archives of Neurology*, **46**, 27–34.

Mohr, J.P. (1976) Broca's area and Broca's aphasia, in *Studies in Neurolinguistics*, vol. **1** (eds H. Whitaker and H.A. Whitaker), Academic Press, New York, pp. 29–38.

Mohr, J.P., Pessin, M., Finkelstein, S. *et al.* (1978) Broca aphasia: pathologic and clinical. *Neurology*, **28**, 311–324.

Murdoch, B.E., Afford, R.J., Ling, A.R. and Ganguley, B. (1986a) Acute computerized tomographic scans: their value in the localization of lesions and as prognostic indicators in aphasia. *Journal of Communication Disorders*, **19**, 311–345.

Murdoch, B.E., Thompson, D., Fraser, S. and Harrison, L. (1986b) Aphasia following non-haemorrhagic lesions in the left striato-capsular region. *Australian Journal of Human Communication Disorders*, **14**, 5–21.

Naeser, M.A., Alexander, M.P., Helm-Estabrooks, M. *et al.* (1982) Aphasia with predominantly subcortical lesion sites. *Archives of Neurology*, **39**, 2–12.

Naeser, M.A. and Hayward, R.W. (1978) Lesion localization in aphasia with cranial computed tomography and the BDAE. *Neurology*, **28**, 545–551.

Nielson, J.M. (1936) *Agnosia, Apraxia and Aphasia: Their Value in Cerebral Localization*, Hafner, New York.

Ojemann, G.A. and Whitaker, H.A. (1978) Language localization and variability. *Brain and Language*, **6**, 239–260.

Palumbo, C., Alexander, M. and Naeser, M. (1992) CT scan lesion sites associated with conduction aphasia, in *Conduction Aphasia* (ed. S. Kohn), Lawrence Erlbaum, Hillsdale, NJ, pp. 51–75.

Pick, A. (1931) *Aphasia*, Charles C. Thomas, Springfield, IL.

Pizzamiglio, L., Galati, G. and Committeri, G. (2001) The contribution of functional neuroimaging to recovery after brain damage: a review. *Cortex*, **37**, 11–31.

Poeck, K., Kerchensteiner, M. and Hartje, W. (1972) A qualitative study on language understanding in fluent and nonfluent aphasia. *Cortex*, **8**, 299–304.

Price, C.J. and Crinion, J. (2005) The latest on functional imaging studies of aphasic stroke. *Current Opinions in Neurology*, **18**, 429–434.

Prins, R. and Bastiaanse, R. (2006) The early history of aphasiology: from the Egyptian surgeons (*c*.1700BC) to Broca (1861). *Aphasiology*, **20**, 762–791.

Romanul, F.C.A. and Abramowitz, A. (1961) Changes in brain and pial vessels in arterial borderzones. *Archives of Neurology*, **11**, 40–49.

Ross, E.D. (1980) Left medial parietal lobe and receptive language functions: mixed transcortical aphasia and left anterior cerebral artery infarction. *Neurology*, **30**, 144–151.

Rubens, A.B. (1976) Transcortical motor aphasia, in *Studies in Neurolinguistics*, vol. **1** (eds H. Whitaker and H.A. Whitaker), Academic Press, New York, pp. 293–304.

Schuell, H., Jenkins, J. and Jiminez-Pabon, E. (1964) *Aphasia in Adults*, Harper and Row, New York.

Sterzi, R. and Vallar, G. (1978). Frontal lobe syndrome as a disconnection syndrome: report of a case. *Acta Neurologica*, **33**, 419–425.

Van Lancker Sidtis, D. (2007). Does functional neuroimaging solve the questions of neurolinguists? *Brain and Language*, **102**, 200–214.

Vignolo, L.A., Boccardi, E. and Caverni, L. (1986). Unexpected CT scan findings in global aphasia. *Cortex*, **22**, 55–69.

Wagenaar, W., Snow, C. and Prins, R. (1975). Spontaneous speed of aphasic patients: a psycholinguistic analysis. *Brain and Language*, **2**, 281–303.

Weisenberg, T.S. and McBride, K.L. (1935) *Aphasia*, Hafner, New York.

Wepman, J.M. (1951) *Recovery from Aphasia*, Ronald, New York.

Wernicke, C. (1874) *Der Aphasische Symptomencomplex*, Cohn and Weigert, Breslau.

Wernicke, C. (1908) The symptom-complex of aphasia, in *Modern Clinical Medical Diseases of the Nervous System* (ed. A. Church), Appleton-Century-Crofts, New York, pp. 265–324.

Whitaker, H. (1976) A case of isolation of the language function, in *Studies in Neurolinguistics*, vol. **2** (eds H. Whitaker and H.A. Whitaker), Academic Press, New York, pp. 1–58.

Wise, R.J. (2003) Language systems in normal and aphasic human subjects: functional imaging studies and inferences from animal studies. *British Medical Bulletin*, **65**, 95–119.

Zahn, R., Schwarz, M. and Huber, W. (2006) Functional activation studies of word processing in the recovery from aphasia. *Journal of Physiology – Paris*, **99**, 370–385.

Subcortical aphasia syndromes 3

Introduction

Aphasia has traditionally been described as a language disorder resulting from damage to the cerebral cortex. Recent advances in our understanding of the connectivity of subcortical structures such as the basal ganglia and cerebellum with the cerebral cortex, combined with the development and introduction of advanced neuroimaging techniques, have, since the 1990s, forced a rethink of our concepts of the contribution of subcortical structures to speech-language function. In particular, there has been a growing realization that subcortical structures such as the thalamus, caudate nucleus, globus pallidus, subthalamic nucleus, substantia nigra and cerebellum among others, not only contribute to the regulation and coordination of the motor aspects of speech production but also are important components of the neural circuits that regulate cognitive and linguistic function. Consequently, there is now much greater acceptance that subcortical structures participate in the regulation of language to a greater extent than proposed by various localizationist models of language function (e.g. Wernicke–Lichtheim model) that had their origins in phrenological theory in the early 1800s

and the post-mortem studies of Broca (1861), Wernicke (1874) and Lichtheim (1885), each of which dominated our thinking in relation to language function throughout the twentieth century.

The first person to propose a systematic relationship between specific psychological components of human behaviour and specific cerebral regions was Gall (1809) through his introduction of the concept of phrenology. Although phrenology fell into disfavour, the underlying premise of phrenological theory that all aspects of a complex behaviour (e.g. language) are regulated in an anatomically discrete, separable, area of the cerebral cortex remained as an important component of influential models and theories of speech-language function (e.g. Wernicke–Lichtheim model). For example, Broca (1861) adhered to phrenological theory when he concluded that speech production was regulated in the anterior cortical region of the left cerebral hemisphere on the basis of his observation of a patient with a lesion in this region who was unable to speak except for the production of a single monosyllable.

Unfortunately, Broca overlooked the fact that his patient also had extensive subcortical damage and extensive non-linguistic motor impairment. Likewise, on the basis of his observation that patients who had suffered lesions in the second temporal gyrus of the cortex in the posterior left hemisphere had difficulty comprehending speech, Wernicke (1874) concluded that receptive linguistic ability was located in the posterior region of the left temporal gyrus. Lichtheim (1885) proposed a hypothetical pathway connecting Broca's and Wernicke's areas of the cerebral cortex, his revision of the Broca–Wernicke model, later recognized as the Wernicke–Lichtheim model persisting in textbooks and research literature to the present day. Importantly, the Wernicke–Lichtheim model down-plays the importance of subcortical structures in language function, and implies that subcortical lesions only disrupt language if they cause disconnection between the major language centres of the cerebral cortex, as occurs for instance with disruption of the arcuate fasciculus in conduction aphasia.

More recently, localizationist models such as the Wernicke–Lichtheim model that neglect the contribution of subcortical structures to speech and language have been challenged, primarily because of their failure to account for emerging knowledge of the computational architecture of the human brain. Clinical evidence is now available to show that permanent loss of language does not occur without subcortical damage, even when Broca's and Wernicke's areas have been destroyed by lesions. For example, patients with extensive damage to Broca's area generally recover linguistic ability, unless subcortical damage also occurs (Stuss and Benson, 1986; Dronkers *et al.*, 1992; D'Esposito and Alexander, 1995). Also, patients suffering from brain damage that involves subcortical structures but that leaves Broca's area alone can also manifest the signs and symptoms of Broca's aphasia (Alexander, Naeser and Palumbo, 1987; Mega and Alexander, 1994). The case for Wernicke's aphasia appears to be similar, with reports of pre-morbid linguistic skills being recovered after complete destruction of Wernicke's area (Lieberman, 2000). Also, although the locus for brain damage associated with Wernicke's aphasia includes the posterior region of the left temporal gyrus (Wernicke's area), it often extends to the supramarginal and angular gyrus

including involvement of the white matter below. As stated by D'Esposito and Alexander (1995), a purely cortical lesion that can produce Broca's or Wernicke's aphasia has never been documented. In contrast, numerous clinico-neuroradiological correlation studies reported in recent years have documented the occurrence of aphasic syndromes in association with subcortical lesions that apparently spare the cerebral cortex. Further details of the latter studies are outlined below.

Rather than being regulated by specific cortical sites, it is now recognized that complex behaviours such as talking, walking and so on are mediated by neural circuits that link anatomically segregated populations of neurones in both subcortical and cortical regions of the human brain. In other words, complex behaviours such as talking, walking and so on are regulated by neural circuits that constitute networks linking activity in many parts of the brain at both the cortical and subcortical levels; these networks therefore constitute the neural basis of complex behaviours. As Mesulam (1990) states, 'complex behaviour is mapped at the level of multifocal neural systems rather than specific anatomical sites, giving rise to brain–behaviour relationships that are both localized and distributed' (p. 588). Although 'local operations' occur in particular areas of the brain (e.g. specific areas of the cerebral cortex or specific components of the basal ganglia system), these areas in themselves do not constitute an observable behaviour such as talking, walking and so on. Rather, these local processes form part of the neural 'computations' that when linked together in complex neural circuits (e.g. cortico-striato-thalamo-cortical loops; cerebrocortico-ponto-cerebellocortico-dentato-thalamo-cerebrocortical loops) manifest in behaviours such as talking, auditory comprehension, walking and so on. For example, the corpus striatum (caudate nucleus plus the lenticular nucleus), although best recognized for its role in the regulation of motor activities, is known to receive input from most areas of the cerebral cortex. In turn, output from the striatum is targeted not only at the primary motor cortex but also at specific areas of the pre-motor and pre-frontal cortex, suggesting that the corpus striatum has the ability to influence not only motor control but also several types of cognitive, language and limbic functions. Similarly, it has been hypothesized that output from the lateral deep cerebellar nucleus (the dentate) influences not only motor areas of the cerebral cortex but also areas of the pre-frontal cortex involved in language and cognition (Fabbro, 2000; Marien *et al.*, 2001).

Evidence to support this functional diversity of the basal ganglia and cerebellum comes from several sources, including: neuroanatomical studies documenting the presence of extensive connections between the basal ganglia and cerebral cortex; animal studies reporting a range of behavioural correlates documented by single-cell recordings from basal ganglia neurones; observations of the behavioural effects of disease-induced lesions in the basal ganglia; clinico-neuroradiological studies documenting the presence of speech disorders and other behavioural deficits in association with subcortical lesions; the findings of studies based on functional neuroimaging, including positron emission tomography (PET) and functional magnetic resonance imaging (fMRI), and, more recently, observations of the behavioural effects of deep brain stimulation and surgically induced lesions in the globus pallidus (pallidotomy), thalamus (thalamotomy) and subthalamic nucleus, carried out as part of the treatment for Parkinson's disease and other basal ganglia syndromes.

Role of subcortical structures in language: historical perspective

As outlined above, ever since the era of 'phrenological science' the cerebral cortex has been considered the neural substrate of higher psychological function, including language. In keeping with this view, the standard 'associationist' anatomo-functional model of language organization was deeply rooted in cortical areas and their fibre connections (Lichtheim, 1885; Wernicke, 1874). According to this still influential model, linguistic representations are stored in discrete cortical areas and consequently subcortical brain lesions were thought to only produce language deficits if they disrupted the white matter fibres that connect the various cortical language centres.

Despite the emphasis on the cerebral cortex, speculation has existed since the end of the nineteenth century that subcortical brain structures have a role in language processing. More than a century ago, Broadbent (1872) proposed that words were 'generated' as motor acts in the basal ganglia. Marie (1906) challenged the traditional view of aphasia and described a clinical syndrome that he called 'anartria' secondary to dysfunction of a specific subcortical region involving the caudate nucleus, putamen, internal capsule and thalamus (Marie's quadrilateral space). Monakow (1914) also championed the participation of the lentiform nucleus in the pathogenesis of aphasia. Perusal of the monumental anatomo-clinical summaries published in the early twentieth century, such as those by Moutier (1908), Henschen (1922) and Nielsen (1946), also reveals a number of cases of language disturbance associated with lesions apparently limited to subcortical structures. Unfortunately, these empirical data were subjected to radically different interpretations by the various authors. Moutier supported the 'quadrilatère' proposed by his teacher Pierre Marie. In contrast, Nielsen explicitly denied any role of subcortical structures in mental activities, interpreting his observations in strict adherence to the traditional Wernicke–Lichtheim model. Later, Fisher (1959) described aphasia as a clinical feature in a patient with left thalamic haemorrhage. Penfield and Roberts (1959) suggested that the thalamus had an integrative function in language processing.

Since the late 1970s, the traditional view of language processing in the brain has been challenged by the findings of an increasing number of clinico-neuroradiological correlation studies that have documented the occurrence of adult language disorders in association with apparently subcortical vascular lesions. The introduction in recent decades of new neuroradiological methods for lesion localization *in vivo*, including computerized tomography (CT) scanning in the 1970s and more recently magnetic resonance imaging (MRI), has led to an increasing number of reports in the literature of aphasia following subcortical lesions (for reviews of *in vivo* correlation studies see Alexander, 1989; Cappa and Vallar, 1992; Murdoch, 1996). In particular, these new neuroimaging techniques have allowed more precise identification and localization of subcortical lesion parameters (Alexander, Naeser and Palumbo, 1987; Cappa and Wallesch, 1994) and hence the ability to evaluate the influence of specific lesions in producing motor and cognitive anomalies. Therefore, although the concept of subcortical aphasia remains somewhat controversial, recent years have seen a growing acceptance of a role for subcortical structures in language and the development of a range of models that attempt to explain the nature of that role. Prior to discussing models of subcortical participation in language, however, it is necessary to first review the relevant subcortical neuroanatomy and the reported clinical features of subcortical aphasia syndromes.

Neuroanatomy of the subcortical region

The basal ganglia, thalamus, subcortical white matter pathways and cerebellum represent the subcortical structures which have been afforded the most consideration within contemporary models of subcortical participation in language. More recently, studies based on deep brain stimulation have also suggested a possible role for the subthalamic nucleus in language processes (Whelan, Murdoch and Theodoros, 2003; Whelan *et al.*, 2004a). Further, a role for the cerebellum in language has also been suggested (Leiner, Leiner and Dow, 1993; Docking, Murdoch and Ward, 2003).

Neuroanatomy of the striatocapsular region

The striatocapsular region occupies the deep, central portion of each cerebral hemisphere and comprises the basal ganglia and internal capsule. The basal ganglia are a collection of subcortical nuclei which process motor information in parallel with the cerebellum.

Anatomically, the basal ganglia consist of the caudate nucleus, the putamen, the globus pallidus and the amygdaloid nucleus. Collectively, the globus pallidus and the putamen are referred to as the lenticular nucleus (lentiform nucleus). Some neurologists also include another nucleus, the claustrum, as part of the basal ganglia. Clinically, the basal ganglia represent a functional system of interconnected components which typically include the caudate nucleus, putamen and internal (GPi) and external (GPe) segments of the globus pallidus, the subthalamic nucleus and substantia nigra (pars compacta (SNPC) and pars reticulata (SNPR)).

The relative positions of the basal ganglia to other structures within the cerebral hemispheres are shown in Figures 3.1 and 3.2.

The caudate nucleus is the most medial part of the basal ganglia. It is an elongated mass of grey matter, which is bent over on itself and throughout its length follows the lateral ventricle. The nucleus is divided into a head, body and tail. The head of the caudate nucleus bulges into the anterior horn of the lateral ventricle and lies rostral to the thalamus. The body extends along the dorsolateral surface of the thalamus. The remainder of the caudate nucleus is drawn out into a highly arched tail that, conforming to the shape of the lateral ventricle, turns into the temporal lobe and terminates in relation to the amygdaloid nucleus (Figure 3.3). Throughout much of its extent, the caudate nucleus is separated from the lenticular nucleus by the internal capsule.

The lenticular nucleus is located in the midst of the cerebral white matter. Its shape is somewhat similar to that of a biconvex lens, hence the name lenticular or lentiform (Figure 3.3). The largest portion of the lenticular nucleus is the putamen, which is a rather thick, convex mass, located just lateral to the globus pallidus and internal capsule. Its lateral surface is separated from the cortex by the claustrum, the external capsule and the extreme capsule (Figures 3.1 and 3.2). The globus pallidus is the smaller and most medial part of the lenticular nucleus. It is traversed by numerous bundles of white fibres, which make it appear lighter in colour than the putamen. The globus pallidus is subdivided into medial and lateral parts by a small band of white fibres called

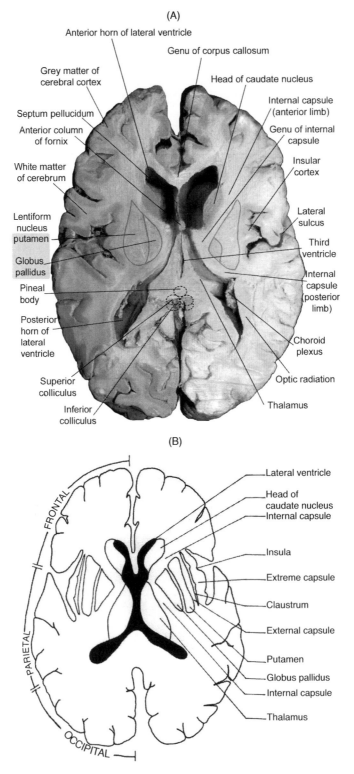

Figure 3.1   (A) Horizontal section of the cerebral hemispheres showing the anatomy of the striatocapsular region. (B) Diagrammatic representation of a horizontal section of the cerebral hemispheres showing the anatomy of the striatocapsular region.

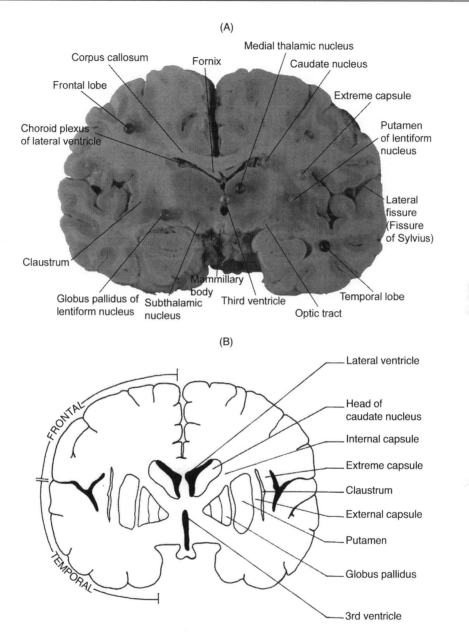

Figure 3.2 (A) Coronal section of the cerebral hemispheres at the level of the mammillary bodies showing the anatomy of the striatocapsular region. (B) Diagrammatic representation of a coronal section of the cerebral hemispheres at the level of the optic chiasma showing the anatomy of the striatocapsular region.

the medial medullary lamina. The medial palli-dal segment in turn is divided by the accessory medullary lamina into outer and inner portions. The lenticular nucleus combined with the cau-date nucleus make up what is known as the corpus striatum, so named because of the stri-

ated (striped) nature of this region. The func-tion of the corpus striatum is concerned with so-matic motor functions. The term extrapyramidal motor system is used by neurologists to group together the corpus striatum and certain brain-stem nuclei considered to subserve these somatic

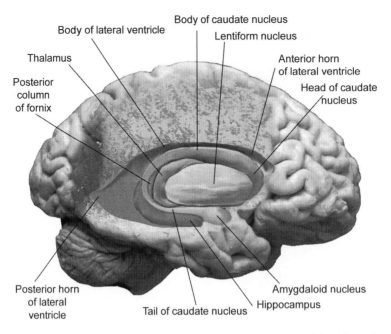

Figure 3.3   Lateral view of the right cerebral hemisphere dissected to show the position of the different basal ganglia.

motor functions. The extrapyramidal system is discussed more fully in Chapter 10.

The claustrum is a thin layer of grey matter which lies between the insular cortex and the lenticular nucleus (Figures 3.1 and 3.2). It is separated from the more medial putamen by the external capsule and from the insular cortex by the extreme capsule. Both the external and extreme capsules carry association fibres. The amygdaloid nucleus (body) is a small, spherical grey mass located in the temporal lobe in the roof of the inferior horn of the lateral ventricle.

Connections exist between the various individual nuclei of the basal ganglia and between the nuclei and other brain structures, which include the cerebral cortex, thalamus, red nucleus and reticular formation. These connections are extremely complex and, as yet, have not been fully determined in humans. Briefly, the afferent inflow to the corpus striatum is mainly from the massive corticostriatal pathways which project fibres to the caudate nucleus and putamen from nearly all parts of the cerebral cortex, but especially from the motor areas. From the caudate nucleus and putamen, the input is relayed to the globus pallidus. Other less significant inputs come from

the thalamus via the thalamostriatal pathways and brainstem nuclei including the substantia nigra (nigrostriatal tracts). Output from the basal ganglia occurs primarily through the globus pallidus. It sends massive bundles of inhibitory fibres mainly to the thalamus (pallidothalamic tracts), particularly to the ventral anterior nucleus of the thalamus, but also to the brainstem. Since the ventral anterior nucleus of the thalamus projects its output to the motor and pre-motor cortex, an important circuit is established between the motor cortex, basal ganglia, thalamus and motor cortex again. In general, therefore, the basal ganglia can be considered to comprise a group of 'input structures' (the caudate nucleus, putamen and ventral striatum) that receive direct input essentially from all areas of the cerebral cortex and 'output structures' (the internal segment of the globus pallidus, the substantia nigra pars reticulata and the ventral pallidum) that project back to the cerebral cortex via the thalamus. Contemporary thinking is that the striatum acts as a 'multilaned' throughway which forms part of a series of multisegmented circuits connecting the cerebral cortex, basal ganglia and thalamus (Alexander, De Long and Strick, 1986; Graybiel and Kimura,

1995; Middleton and Strick, 2000). Thus, basal ganglia anatomy is characterized by their participation in multiple 'loops', with the cerebral cortex each of which follows the basic route of:

$$cortex \rightarrow striatum \rightarrow globus\ pallidus/$$
$$substantia\ nigra \rightarrow thalamus \rightarrow cortex$$

in a unidirectional fashion. As explained further below, within contemporary theories of subcortical participation in language, it has been suggested that the basal ganglia mediate linguistic processes by way of these cortico-striato-pallido-thalamo-cortical pathways (Crosson, 1985; Wallesch and Papagno, 1988). Consequently, these loops constitute the neuroanatomical basis of subcortical participation in language.

Lesions of the basal ganglia are associated with several extrapyramidal syndromes including Parkinson's disease, chorea, athetosis, dystonia and hemiballismus. These syndromes are discussed in Chapter 10 in relation to hypo- and hyperkinetic dysarthria.

The internal capsule is composed of afferent fibres to and efferent fibres from the cerebral cortex, diverging from and converging towards the brainstem. In horizontal section (Figure 3.1), the internal capsule in each hemisphere is 'V'-shaped with the apex pointing medially. Two distinct parts of the internal capsule are evident in horizontal sections: an anterior limb and a posterior limb which meet at the genu (the apex of the 'V'). The larger limb, the posterior limb, is bordered medially by the diencephalon and laterally by the lenticular nucleus. The anterior limb lies between the caudate nucleus and the putamen.

Efferent fibres in the internal capsule arise from cells in various regions of the cerebral cortex and project to specific nuclei in the brainstem and spinal cord. In so doing they form a number of tracts which include the corticothalamic, corticorubral, corticopontine, corticoreticular, corticobulbar and corticospinal tracts. On the other hand, the afferent fibres in the internal capsule arise mainly from the thalamus and project to almost all regions of the cerebral cortex. These afferent fibres are referred to as the thalamocortical radiations and together with the corticothalamic fibres form the thalamic radiations. The location

of the various efferent and afferent tracts in the internal capsule is shown in Figure 3.4.

The anterior thalamic radiation (or peduncle) and the frontal pontine tract are located in the anterior limb. The genu contains corticobulbar and corticoreticular fibres. Within the posterior limb are found the corticospinal fibres, the superior and posterior thalamic radiations and relatively smaller numbers of corticotectal, corticorubral and corticoreticular fibres.

Because of the high concentration of nerve fibres, more widespread disability is produced by lesions in the internal capsule than in any other region of the nervous system. Most injuries to the internal capsule are of vascular origin arising, in most cases, from either thrombosis or haemorrhage of branches of the middle cerebral artery. Unilateral lesions of the posterior limb may result in contralateral hemianaesthesia of the head, trunk and limbs owing to injury of the thalamocortical fibres en route to the sensory cortex. A contralateral hemiplegia is also present owing to the involvement of the corticospinal tracts.

Neuroanatomy of the thalamus

The thalamus is a large mass of grey matter located above the midbrain. It forms part of the diencephalon. Although almost completely separated by the third ventricle into right and left thalami, the thalamic mass in each hemisphere is connected in most cases to that in the opposite hemisphere by a band of grey matter called the intermediate mass or interthalamic adhesion. In horizontal section (Figure 3.1), the thalamus can be seen to lie medial to the posterior limb of the internal capsule.

The thalamus has multiple connections with both higher and lower structures in the nervous system, such as the cerebral cortex and spinal cord, and acts as an important relaying and integrating centre for both sensory and motor impulses. The majority of sensory impulses arriving at the cerebral cortex (with the exception of olfactory impulses) have travelled through one or more nuclei in the thalamus. The thalamus receives sensory stimuli from the peripheral receptors via the sensory pathways, integrates and organizes this

Anterior limb
[1] Anterior thalamic peduncle
[2] Frontopontine tract

Genu

Posterior limb
Lenticulothalamic part
[3] Superior thalamic peduncle
[4] Pyramidal tract

Sublenticular part
[5] Ansa peduncularis
[6] Thalamotemporal radiations
[7] Auditory radiations
[8] Optic radiations

Retrolenticular part
[9] Posterior thalamic peduncle
[10] Temporoparietopontine tract
[11] Corticotectotegmental tract

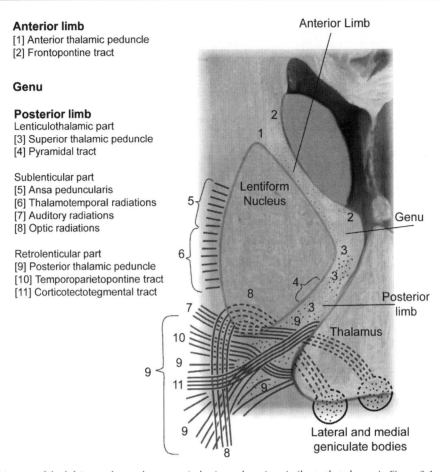

Figure 3.4 Diagram of the left internal capsule as seen in horizontal section similar to that shown in Figure 3.1.

information and then relays the stimulus to the appropriate sensory area of the cerebral cortex. Visual stimuli, for instance, are relayed by the thalamus to the cortex of the occipital lobe for interpretation.

The thalamus also contributes to emotional responses to sensory experience. The posterior end of the thalamus is an expanded prominence called the pulvinar, which overhangs the superior colliculus of the midbrain. It is the largest nucleus in the thalamus. Attached to the pulvinar are two smaller prominences: the lateral geniculate body, which receives the optic tract and projects to the visual cortex, and the medial geniculate body, which receives the ascending auditory fibres and projects to the auditory cortex of the temporal lobe. Internally, the grey matter of the thalamus is divided by a 'Y'-shaped vertical sheet of white

matter, the internal medullary lamina, into three parts. The anterior part of the thalamus lies between the two limbs of the Y and the medial and lateral parts lie on the sides of the stem of the Y. The internal medullary lamina consists of nerve fibres which connect the various parts of the thalamus.

The thalamus contains more than 30 nuclei some of which have been indicated as important in language. The locations of some of the major thalamic nuclei mentioned in the speech-language literature together with their cortical projections are shown in Figure 3.5.

The pulvinar interconnects with many other thalamic nuclei and is connected reciprocally with the supramarginal gyri, the angular gyri, the superior parietal lobule and the occipital and posterior temporal regions. The ventral lateral

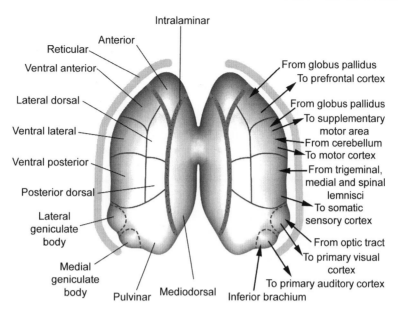

Figure 3.5   Thalamic nuclei viewed from above.

nucleus and the ventral anterior nucleus are specific motor nuclei in the sense that they receive information from the cerebellum, corpus striatum and substantia nigra and project to motor areas in the frontal lobe via the anterior limb of the internal capsule. The ventral posterior nucleus is a specific sensory nucleus and functions as a thalamic relay for general sensations. It receives input from ascending sensory systems and projects fibres to the primary somesthetic cortex located on the post-central gyrus via the posterior limb of the internal capsule. Where appropriate, the thalamic nuclei are discussed below in relation to models proposed that have attempted to explain the role of subcortical structures in language.

Lesions in the thalamus are, in most cases, the result of thrombosis or haemorrhage of one of the branches of the posterior cerebral artery. Neurological signs of damage to the thalamus include contralateral hemianaesthesia (especially if the ventral posterior nucleus is damaged), contralateral hemiplegia and emotional disturbances. Some or all of these concomitant neurological signs may be evident in patients with thalamic aphasia. Although impairment of all forms of sensation may occur, some pain and temperature sensation from the contralateral side may

be retained. Some patients may experience thalamic syndrome, a condition in which there is an overreaction to sensation such that mild sensory stimuli (e.g. light touch) may trigger exaggerated sensory responses which may lead to intractable pain.

A contralateral upper motor neurone paralysis (spastic paralysis) usually accompanies thalamic lesions owing to involvement of the adjacent internal capsule. Emotional instability may also occur with spontaneous laughing and crying being evident in some patients. Neurosurgical destruction of the ventral anterior thalamic nuclei interrupt connections between the basal ganglia and motor areas of the cerebral cortex and serve to decrease rigidity and tremor in patients with Parkinson's disease.

Blood supply to the striatocapsular region and thalamus

In most reported cases of subcortical aphasia, the language disturbance has occurred secondary to a cerebrovascular accident, usually a haemorrhage. As the particular vessel involvement determines which of the subcortical structures will be

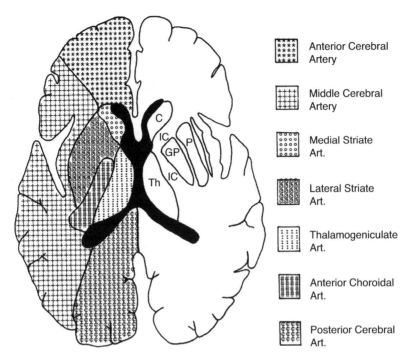

Figure 3.6 Horizontal section of the cerebral hemispheres showing the subcortical distribution of the anterior, middle and posterior cerebral arteries and branches. Th = thalamus; P = putamen; IC = internal capsule; GP = globus pallidus; C = caudate nucleus.

involved in the area of lesion and consequently influences the expected language disturbance, it is important that the reader has some knowledge of the vascular supply to the striatocapsular region and thalamus prior to looking in detail at the variety of language disorders reported to occur in association with lesions in these two areas.

The distribution of the anterior, middle and posterior cerebral arteries and their deep branches to the subcortical region is shown in Figure 3.6.

The medial and lateral striate (also called lenticulostriate) and the anterior choroidal arteries provide the blood supply to the internal capsule. The anterior limb is supplied primarily by the lateral striate branches of the middle cerebral artery, the medial striate (also called the recurrent artery of Heubner) from the anterior cerebral supplying the rostral medial tip. Blood supply to the genu comes via some direct branches from the internal carotid or from the lateral striate arteries. The posterior limb of the internal capsule is supplied partly by the anterior choroidal artery

(internal carotid) and partly by the lateral striate arteries.

Arterial supply to the corpus striatum is mainly provided by the lateral striate arteries. Part of the head of the caudate nucleus, however, is provided with nourishment by the medial striate artery. Most of the putamen and body of the caudate is supplied by the lateral striate arteries, while the tail of the caudate and posterior portion of the putamen receive blood from the anterior choroidal artery. The majority of the globus pallidus is also supplied by this latter artery.

Whereas the striatocapsular region is supplied by branches of the middle and anterior cerebral arteries, branches of the posterior cerebral artery provide the major blood supply to the thalamus. The medial and anterior regions of the thalamus are supplied by the thalamoperforating branches while the pulvinar (posterior portion of the thalamus) and lateral aspects of the thalamus are nourished by the thalamogeniculate branches. The dorsal part of the thalamus is supplied by the posterior choroidal branches of the posterior cerebral artery. Some branches of the anterior choroidal artery are thought to pass to the lateral geniculate body.

Neuroanatomy of the cerebellum

The cerebellum is located in a dorsal position to the pons and medulla oblongata and occupies the majority of the posterior cranial fossa. It is kept separate from the cerebral cortex by a fold in the dura mater called the tentorium cerebelli (cerebellar tentorium). Similar to the cerebrum, it consists of two highly convoluted hemispheres connected at the midline by the vermis. The cerebellar hemispheres are divided into three lobes: anterior, posterior and flocculonodular. The external surface of the cerebellum comprises grey matter and the internal structure consists primarily of white matter. Within this internal white matter are embedded four bilaterally paired masses of grey matter known as the intracerebellar (or deep) nuclei, namely the dentate, emboliform, globose and fastigial nuclei. Axonal inputs and outputs enter and exit the cerebellum via three fibre bundles or peduncles, namely the superior, middle and inferior peduncles. A detailed description of the neuroanatomy of the cerebellum and its connections is presented in Chapter 11.

Aphasia syndromes associated with striatocapsular and thalamic lesions

The primary avenue for investigating the role of subcortical brain structures in language has involved observation of 'experiments in nature', namely the clinico-neuroanatomical study of language function in individuals with vascular lesions involving the subcortical regions of the dominant hemisphere. Cerebrovascular accidents involving the subcortical region may be centred on either the striatocapsular region (head of the caudate nucleus, putamen, anterior limb of the internal capsule) or thalamus, as these two areas have differing blood supplies (see below). Consequently, the majority of studies which have attempted to explore the notion of subcortical

participation in language have investigated the impact of vascular thalamic and striatocapsular lesions on linguistic abilities (Murdoch, 1990), giving rise to syndromes of thalamic and striatocapsular aphasia. Despite the fact that the aphasic symptom complex associated with thalamic lesions appears to approximate a more uniform syndrome than its striatocapsular counterpart, heterogeneity within each aphasic category has been documented with respect to language profiles and recovery rates (Murdoch, 1996). This inconsistency has been partly attributed to methodological limitations, including the wide-ranging scope of language assessments utilized and experimental designs employed.

Kennedy and Murdoch (1990) emphasized that general measures of language function typically utilized in the assessment of subcortical aphasia may have lacked the requisite sensitivity to detect more subtle, high-level linguistic deficits within this population. Furthermore, it has been suggested that the complexity of circulatory dynamics and the protean nature of spontaneous vascular lesions may also have contributed to the inherent variability of symptoms observed (Graff-Radford *et al.*, 1984).

Thalamic aphasia

The first clinicopathological study of thalamic stroke was published by Dejerine and Roussy (1906), who emphasized sensorimotor disturbances. Twenty years later, cognitive deficits after isolated thalamic lesions were described by Hillemand (1925) and subsequently by Lhermitte (1936) with 'atypical' aphasia reported in patients with left thalamic lesions. Since that time, evidence to support a role for the thalamus in language function has come from studies of language changes owing to surgical destruction and stimulation of thalamic targets as well as from observations of language disturbances following spontaneous thalamic lesions, including neoplastic, infectious and vascular lesions. In most reported cases of thalamic aphasia, the language disorder has been associated with thalamic haemorrhage (Fisher, 1959; Ciemens, 1970; Mohr, Watters and Duncan, 1975; Kirshner and

Kistler, 1982; Murdoch, 1987). A smaller number of cases have also been reported in association with thalamic tumours (Smyth and Stern, 1938; Cheek and Taveras, 1966), thalamic abscesses (Panchal, Parikh and Karapurkar, 1974) and, more recently, induced thalamic lesions (thalamotomy) for the treatment of Parkinson's disease (Whelan *et al.*, 2002). Because most of these disorders (i.e. thalamic haemorrhage, tumour and abscess) are associated with a considerable mass effect, a number of authors have suggested that the accompanying language deficit may not be directly attributable to the localized damage to the thalamus per se (Mohr, Watters and Duncan, 1975). Rather, the observed language abnormalities may be the products of the effects of pressure and oedema on the other areas of the brain, particularly the left cerebral hemisphere where the known speech-language centres are located. In other words, the aphasia associated with localized thalamic lesions reported in many studies may not be the direct product of thalamic destruction but rather the secondary product of pressure effects on other parts of the brain.

To some extent, the influence of extraneous factors such as pressure effects can be reduced by studying patients with ischaemic infarcts in the thalamus as these are associated with much smaller mass effects. Although rare, several authors have documented such cases of ischaemic infarcts of the thalamus (Gorelick *et al.*, 1984; Graff-Radford *et al.*, 1984) in association with language disorders. These findings lend support to the suggestion that aphasia subsequent to thalamic lesions is the direct result of thalamic damage rather than the product of associated pressure effects. Added to this, left thalamotomy has been reported to impact negatively on high-level linguistic abilities and possibly semantic processing skills (Whelan *et al.*, 2002). Further, thalamic aphasia is more frequently found in lesions of the dominant tuberothalamic (polar) and interpeduncular profunda (paramedian thalamic) arteries, and as they are small vessels, there is a low probability that some associated cortical dysfunction may exist (Crosson and Nadeau, 1998).

Language impairment associated with thalamic lesions appears to be much more homogeneous than the language profile associated with stria-

tocapsular lesions. Although some variability in the language profile does exist, a number of authors believe that thalamic aphasia has enough defining characteristics to warrant its identification as a 'new' aphasia syndrome. Despite this, thalamic aphasia does not fit neatly into any of the currently accepted cortical aphasias.

Clinical characteristics of thalamic aphasia

Overall, the language disturbance resulting from lesions of the thalamus resembles a transcortical aphasia (Crosson, 1992; Murdoch, 1996), and is characterized by word-finding difficulties, paraphasia (predominantly semantic), neologisms, perseveration, circumlocution, impaired writing abilities and reduced spontaneous speech output in the presence of relatively preserved repetition and variable, but often good, auditory comprehension abilities (Crosson, 1985; Murdoch, 1987). This profile, however, has been reported to vary, including reports of normal language abilities in individuals following thalamic haemorrhage (Cappa *et al.*, 1986).

In particular, it is the relative preservation of repetition that indicates similarities between thalamic and transcortical aphasia. The relatively intact repetition abilities of thalamic aphasics in the presence of semantic impairment (semantic paraphasias) suggests that the system for semantic monitoring involves the thalamus, while that involved in the transmission of phonological linguistic information for repetition is separate and does not involve thalamic structures. Crosson (1985) suggested that the arcuate fasciculus is involved in phonological processing. Preservation of repetition further suggests that the aphasia associated with thalamic lesions is not due to compression of adjacent or surrounding brain structures such as the temporal isthmus, as damage to these structures is known to cause aphasia syndromes in which repetition abilities are not preserved (e.g. Wernicke's and conduction aphasia).

Because of the similarities to transcortical aphasia (particularly transcortical sensory aphasia), it has been suggested that the language deficits observed in cases of thalamic aphasia may possibly be due to compression of the internal carotid artery intracranially, or its middle and anterior cerebral branches, or both. Such restriction of the internal carotid is known to produce diffuse ischaemic damage in the arterial borderzone of the left hemisphere, a condition known to be associated with transcortical aphasias. This theory, however, does not explain why auditory comprehension abilities of thalamic aphasics are often reported to be relatively good whereas in transcortical sensory aphasia, comprehension of spoken language is severely defective. Further, as indicated previously, thalamic infarcts are generally caused by occlusion of the posterior cerebral arteries (or their branches) which represent branches of the basilar artery and therefore supplied by the vertebral artery system rather than the internal carotid system. Although similar therefore to transcortical aphasia, thalamic aphasia does show some differences especially in comprehension abilities. Thalamic aphasics exhibit greater retention of the phonemic level of verbal behaviour than the semantic level, as evidenced by the high number of semantic paraphasic errors present in their speech. The preserved repetition abilities of thalamic aphasics suggest that integrity of the thalamus is not crucial for intentional speech and the phonemic level of verbal behaviour.

Lateralization and thalamic aphasia

The results of studies of patients following surgical intervention in the thalamus are also suggestive of a role for the thalamus in language. These include studies of the effects of surgical ablation of the thalamus (thalamotomy) (Whelan *et al.*, 2002) and thalamic stimulation (Ojemann, 1977; Cappa and Vignolo, 1979). Based on conclusions drawn from these studies, several authors have suggested that thalamic involvement with language is entirely a left thalamic function. For example, the single left thalamotomy case studied by Whelan *et al.* (2002) was reported to exhibit significant post-operative declines in performance on tasks of verbal memory, construction of syntax with contextually constrained boundaries, comprehension of written logical semantic relationships, category-specific generative naming (with an advantage for inanimate concepts) and the temporal processing of words coded for

number of meanings and meaning relatedness. In contrast, the right thalamotomy case examined by Whelan *et al.* (2002) demonstrated no significant post-operative changes in language abilities. According to Lhermitte (1984), neither ablation nor stimulation of the right thalamus has been reported to produce effects on language. The lesion has primarily involved the left thalamus rather than the right in most reported cases of acquired thalamic aphasia (Cappa and Vignolo, 1979). Karussis, Leker and Abramsky (2000) reported that the incidence of aphasia subsequent to left thalamic stroke was 87.5%. Other more traditional researchers advocate a dominant hemisphere thalamic function. Language disorders have been reported after right thalamic haemorrhage in right-handed (Murdoch, 1987) and left-handed (Kirshner and Kistler, 1982; Chesson, 1983) patients, thereby lending support to the suggestion that thalamic involvement in language is a dominant hemisphere function.

Role of the thalamus in language

The function of the thalamus in language has been described in terms of an integrative role (Penfield and Roberts, 1959; Schuell, Jenkins and Jimenez-Pabon, 1965), arousal mechanism (Riklan and Cooper, 1975; Luria, 1977; McFarling, Rothi and Heilman, 1982), modulation and integration of cortical areas to permit language processing (Ojemann, 1983), semantic verification of formulated cortical language segments in verbal production (Cappa and Vignolo, 1979; Wallesch and Papagno, 1988) and managing of verbal memory (Reynolds *et al.*, 1979). More recently, studies have put forward the hypothesis of a thalamic involvement in a mechanism of selective engagement of cortical areas required to perform verbal tasks (Nadeau and Crosson, 1997a,b). This latter concept is close to that of an alerting system activating a mosaic of specific discrete cortical areas appropriate to a particular language-processing mechanism suggested by Ojemann (1983) on the basis of the findings of electrical stimulation studies of the thalamus. According to this view, the thalamus would intervene not only in activating the cortical area required for a given language task but also in maintaining other cortical areas in a state of relative disengagement.

Mechanisms of thalamic aphasia

Despite the above theories, the precise mechanism of thalamic aphasia remains controversial, with several explanations for language impairment occurring subsequent to thalamic lesions having been proposed. As indicated earlier, thalamic lesions may induce cortical dysfunction by mass effect leading to direct compression of the cortex or via a compromise of the vascular supply to the cortex. Although this explanation may apply in cases of thalamic haemorrhage or tumours, it is unlikely that well-demarcated ischaemic infarcts reported in some cases of thalamic aphasia (e.g. Karussis, Leker and Abramsky, 2000) could compromise functioning of the cortical language centres by this mechanism. Alternatively, thalamic lesions may lead to metabolic depression of the cerebral cortex by way of diaschisis. This entails a transient functional depression of activity occurring at a distance from a focal lesion. Studies based on techniques such as positron emission tomography (PET) have demonstrated hypoperfusion subsequent to thalamic infarction in the cerebral cortex and subcortical grey matter in addition to the infarcted area of the thalamus (Baron *et al.*, 1986; De Reuck *et al.*, 1995). The severity of aphasia has also been reported to correlate with the severity of cortical hypoperfusion documented by PET scans following left thalamotomy, suggesting that the cortical hypoperfusion is not the outcome of cerebral artery stenosis (Baron *et al.*, 1986, 1992). Rather, it is likely due to diaschisis, particularly since the hypoperfusion is observed in the thalamocortical projections from the intralaminar, anterior, medial and lateral nuclei of the thalamus. Recovery of both aphasia and cortical perfusion likely reflects re-establishment of input to cortical areas owing to synaptic reorganization (Baron *et al.*, 1986, 1992).

Currently, thalamic aphasia is primarily considered to represent a disconnection syndrome between the cortical language areas and the thalamus. Several authors have emphasized the possibility of frontal lobe dysfunction as a prominent disturbance in thalamic stroke (Sandson *et al.*, 1991; Bogousslavsky, 1994). Nagaratnam, McNeil and Gilhotra (1999) also proposed that the akinetic mutism and mixed transcortical aphasia observed in their case with left thalamo-mesencephalic infarction was the result of an interruption to frontal subcortical circuitry.

Prognosis for language disorders associated with thalamic lesions

The reported prognosis for thalamic aphasia varies, some authors reporting a good prognosis for some of their patients and a poor prognosis for others. Riklan and Levita (1970) found that speech disorders associated with left unilateral thalamotomy for Parkinson's disease tended to recover well. Benson (1979) suggested that the language findings following thalamic haemorrhage are transient, 'recovery often beginning within days or weeks and except in cases complicated by widespread damage, the course is usually one of consistent improvement over a few weeks or months' (p. 96). Although several cases of aphasia following left thalamic haemorrhage have been reported to recover completely, or have been left with only mild deficits, some reports suggest that persistent language deficits, particularly naming problems, may occur (Chesson, 1983; Murdoch, 1987).

Striatocapsular aphasia

As directed previously, the striatocapsular region occupies the deep, central portion of each cerebral hemisphere and comprises the basal ganglia (the caudate nucleus, putamen, globus pallidus) and the anterior limb of the internal capsule. With regard to the current state of understanding of the relationship between structures of the striatocapsular region and language function, Kinnier Wilson's (1925) original characterization of the basal ganglia as the dark basements of the brain still rings true today. Various possible functional attributes of these structures have been illuminated through studies of individuals with subcortical vascular lesions, surgical lesions and electrical stimulation during neurosurgical procedures and more recently through functional neuroimaging studies. Despite these findings, the question of whether the structures comprising the striatocapsular region play any role in language functions remains a point of controversy.

The occurrence of language disturbances subsequent to lesions in the striatocapsular region is well documented (Alexander and Lo Verme, 1980; Crosson, 1985; Murdoch *et al.*, 1986; Kennedy and Murdoch, 1993; Nadeau and Crosson, 1997a). Although these *in vivo* correlation studies have documented beyond reasonable doubt that language impairments may occur in association with lesions confined to the striatocapsular region of the dominant hemisphere, manifestations of language pathology subsequent to lesions of the basal ganglia and internal capsule have failed to establish a homogeneous symptom complex with no unitary striatocapsular aphasia identified (Crosson, 1985; Kennedy and Murdoch, 1993; Nadeau and Crosson, 1997a). Furthermore, the effects of striatocapsular lesions on language abilities appear, in general, to be more enduring than the impact associated with thalamic lesions (Wallesch *et al.*, 1983). Indeed, reported language profiles extend from normal to severe impairments on the parameters of auditory and reading comprehension, spontaneous speech, repetition, naming and writing (Alexander and Lo Verme, 1980; Damasio *et al.*, 1982; Vallar, Papagno and Cappa, 1988).

Characteristics of striatocapsular aphasia

The classification of language deficits subsequent to striatocapsular lesions in terms of existing classical aphasia syndromes has been reported to be of limited value. For example, Weiller *et al.* (1993) reported that of 15 aphasic patients with striatocapsular infarcts, four had a Broca's-type aphasia, three exhibited a Wernicke's aphasia, four were anomic, two appeared global and two were unclassifiable. Basso, Della Sala and Farabola (1987) and Cappa *et al.* (1983) also reported cases with striatocapsular lesions fitting all of the classical aphasia syndromes. The considerable number of striatocapsular cases which have presented with an atypical constellation of language deficits (Alexander and Lo Verme,

1980; Damasio *et al.*, 1982; Cappa *et al.*, 1983; Wallesch, 1985) also suggests that an insistence on describing language deficits associated with striatocapsular lesions in terms of classical aphasia syndromes may be of limited benefit.

Despite the documented variability of language disturbances associated with striatocapsular aphasia, some researchers have identified a distinct pattern of impairment which conforms to the anterior-non-fluent/posterior-fluent cortical dichotomy (Cappa *et al.*, 1983). In one of the first systematic studies of this nature, Naeser *et al.* (1982) noted that patients with capsuloputaminal lesions extending into the anterior superior white matter typically had good comprehension and slow but grammatical speech. In contrast, those with capsuloputaminal lesions, including posterior white matter extension, showed poor comprehension and fluent Wernicke's-type speech, while those with both anterior superior and posterior white matter involvement were globally aphasic. Similarly, D'Esposito and Alexander (1995) found that patients with striatocapsular lesions extending anteriorly into the deep frontal white matter were non-fluent, while patients with lesions extending posteriorly into the temporal white matter showed comprehension deficits.

Cappa *et al.* (1983) provided further support for this anterior–posterior distinction by describing an atypical non-fluent aphasia associated with anterior capsuloputaminal lesions (putamen and anterior limb of the internal capsule) and a mild fluent aphasia sometimes associated with posterior striatocapsular involvement (putamen and posterior limb of the internal capsule). Similarly, Murdoch *et al.* (1986) found that patients with striatocapsular lesions involving the anterior limb of the internal capsule exhibited a non-fluent aphasia with semantic paraphasias, while lesions involving the posterior limb of the internal capsule and the posterior putamen resulted in a mild fluent Wernicke's-type aphasia. Damasio *et al.* (1982) also reported that patients with lesions involving the head of the caudate nucleus, the anterior limb of the internal capsule and putamen commonly exhibited semantic paraphasias, but noted that subjects were varied in terms of fluency, comprehension, repetition and the presence of phonemic paraphasias.

Despite this apparent consensus, several other studies have questioned the accuracy and utility of the anterior–posterior dichotomy by describing a number of cases in which the patterns of language impairment could not be accounted for in terms of this anatomical distinction (Wallesch, 1985; Kennedy and Murdoch, 1993). For example, Wallesch (1985, 1997) reported that patients with anterior striatocapsular lesions exhibited a Wernicke's-type aphasia with semantic and phonemic paraphasias and later suggested that anterior striatocapsular lesions may be associated with fluent or non-fluent paraphasic output, impaired comprehension and intact repetition. Puel *et al.* (1984) demonstrated the variability in this area by describing fluent aphasia with semantic paraphasia in patients with anterior putaminocapsular haemorrhage and a non-fluent aphasia with phonemic and semantic paraphasia subsequent to a haemorrhage involving the head of the caudate nucleus and anterior limb of the internal capsule.

Nadeau and Crosson (1997a) comprehensively reviewed findings of anterior striatocapsular infarction (involving the head of the caudate nucleus, the putamen and the anterior limb of the internal capsule) and revealed a diverse range and pattern of language deficits in subjects. Findings included fluent paraphasic patients with impaired comprehension, repetition and naming in a syndrome which is more typically associated with posterior cortical lesions, as well as non-fluent cases with or without comprehension deficits.

Accounts also exist of patients with posterior striatocapsular lesions whose language function differs from the symptoms previously noted following lesions of this area (Naeser *et al.*, 1982; Cappa *et al.*, 1983; Murdoch *et al.*, 1986). For example, Weiller *et al.* (1993) cited 12 cases with posterior striatocapsular lesions presenting with no aphasia. Further, Nadeau and Crosson (1997a) observed that infarcts of the head of the caudate nucleus, the putamen and the anterior limb of the internal capsule which extend posteriorly to involve the temporal stem result in more significant impairments in comprehension, repetition and naming than in patients without this extension.

Consequently, despite numerous attempts at delineating specific patterns of language impairment subsequent to circumscribed striatocapsular lesions, this area still defies any clear clinicoanatomical picture. As a case in point, Weiller *et al.* (1993) concluded that aphasic syndromes did not differ accordingly to the involvement of particular striatocapsular structures in a study of 57 cases, again bringing into question the validity of any anterior–posterior distinction.

Levels of language processing compromised in striatocapsular aphasia

The different levels of language processing compromised following striatocapsular lesions is somewhat difficult to interpret given that the majority of studies in this area have reported language function only in broad terms of fluency, comprehension, repetition, naming and the presence of paraphasias. Although, as indicated above, the performance of patients with striatocapsular lesions reportedly varies widely on these parameters, some trends are evident. Following striatocapsular lesions, the phonological system (as assessed minimally by repetition and the presence of phonemic paraphasias) may be impaired (Damasio *et al.*, 1982; Naeser *et al.*, 1982; Cappa *et al.*, 1983) but is often spared (Alexander and Lo Verme, 1980; Wallesch, 1985; Murdoch *et al.*, 1986). Repetition of phrases of increasing length and complexity may be compromised (Naeser *et al.*, 1982; Kennedy and Murdoch, 1989). In a more detailed test of phonological discrimination and phonologically based short-term storage, patients with lesions centred on the striatocapsular region performed within normal limits (Vallar, Papagno and Cappa, 1988). Minimal phonemic errors have also been reported in naming tasks (Vallar, Papagno and Cappa, 1988; Kennedy and Murdoch, 1990).

Auditory comprehension may be impaired to varying degrees (Damasio *et al.*, 1982; D'Esposito and Alexander, 1995) but also is reported to remain intact in other patients (Naeser *et al.*, 1982; Mega and Alexander, 1994). Alexander (1992) reported that subjects in the post-acute phase had no major problems with basic auditory comprehension tasks such as word discrimination, sentence-length requests or two element commands, whereas difficulties were revealed on more complex comprehension tasks. Vallar, Papagno and Cappa (1988) described mild impairment in sentence comprehension and concluded that this performance might relate to a syntactic or lexical semantic deficit. Other studies have reported deficits where subjects were required to follow complex sequential commands and comprehend complex instructions (Kennedy and Murdoch, 1993; Mega and Alexander, 1994).

Fluency varies greatly among patients with dominant striatocapsular lesions and Alexander (1992) makes an important distinction between non-fluent speech and non-fluent language production in this population. Non-fluent speech is characterized by impaired articulatory agility, disturbed melodic line and hypophonia, while non-fluent language is indicated by decreased phrase length and agrammatism. Applying these criteria to 13 subjects with non-thalamic subcortical lesions, Alexander (1992) found that 12 subjects exhibited fluent language using complex grammatical forms and a phrase length greater than seven words, although responses were frequently truncated. In contrast, these subjects exhibited characteristically non-fluent speech. This disassociation between intact language fluency and impaired speech fluency is supported by common findings of grammatical language following striatocapsular lesions (Naeser *et al.*, 1982; Kirk and Kertesz, 1994), although agrammatism has been reported in several instances (Kennedy and Murdoch, 1989; Fabbro, Clarici and Bava, 1996).

Evidence suggests that, while other aspects of language vary greatly among patients with striatocapsular lesions, lexical semantic processing is commonly affected (Vallar, Papagno and Cappa, 1988; Wallesch and Papagno, 1988). There have been numerous reports of confrontation naming deficits, semantic paraphasias and word-finding difficulties subsequent to striatocapsular lesions (Cappa *et al.*, 1983; Wallesch, 1985; Kennedy and Murdoch, 1990, 1993; Mega and Alexander, 1994). Impaired performance on word-fluency and picture description tasks (Vallar, Papagno and Cappa, 1988; Kennedy and Murdoch, 1989,

1990; Mega and Alexander, 1994) may also indicate a lexical semantic deficit, although extra linguistic factors may be involved in the case of word-list generation (Kennedy and Murdoch, 1989).

In summary, a large degree of variability still appears to exist in the reported language profiles of patients with striatocapsular lesions. However, some core features may be present with Mega and Alexander (1994) proposing the existence of a profile of striatocapsular aphasia comprising impaired generative language accompanied by a naming deficit of varying severity. It is possible that the severity of this profile may vary depending on the extent of damage caused by the lesion and the time post-onset of the lesion.

Cortical dysfunction as an explanation for striatocapsular aphasia

Although, as outlined above, language disorders are common subsequent to dominant hemisphere striatocapsular lesions, it has been suggested that the more overt language symptoms in such cases may be related to concomitant cortical dysfunction via various pathophysiological mechanisms (Nadeau and Crosson, 1997a,b). Nadeau and Crosson (1997a,b) described five potential mechanisms of aphasia associated with subcortical strokes. These included: (1) a direct effect of the subcortical lesions indicating that the basal ganglia and other subcortical structures are essential components of the brain networks involved in language function (Damasio *et al.*, 1982); (2) disconnection of cortical structures by white matter lesions that are essential for language (Alexander, Naeser and Palumbo, 1987); (3) impaired 'release' of language segments formulated in the cortex into output (Crosson, 1985, 1992); (4) diaschisis, in which the subcortical lesion 'cuts off' neural input to a remote area of the brain, causing dysfunction of the remote area, as first proposed by Von Monakow (1914) (Metter *et al.*, 1983; Perani *et al.*, 1987) and (5) stenosis or occlusion of the large cerebral vessels that independently cause the subcortical stroke and hypoperfusion of the cortex. Several studies utilizing techniques such as PET and single-photon emission computed tomography (SPECT) have demonstrated cortical hypoperfusion in patients with aphasia associated with striatocapsular lesions (Skyhoj-Olsen, Bruhn and Öberg, 1986; Vallar, Papagno and Cappa, 1988; Radanovic and Scaff, 2003). However, it is not clear in these cases if the cortical hypoperfusion is due to the subcortical infarct (through diaschisis, as proposed by Metter *et al.* (1983)) or an independent phenomenon caused by large vessel stenosis or occlusion.

Nadeau and Crosson (1997a) argued strongly that a direct or indirect effect of the striatocapsular lesion itself should result in a consistent aphasia syndrome. They therefore suggested that the variable aphasias reported in association with striatocapsular lesions (as outlined above) were most likely due to stenosis or occlusion of the large vessels supplying the language cortex, which causes hypoperfusion of a variety of cortical regions and also causes the striatocapsular infarct by occluding a lenticulostriate artery or the recurrent artery of Heubner. This suggestion is consistent with the wide range of cortical regions that have been shown to be hypoperfused on SPECT after subcortical stroke (Radanovic and Scaff, 2003). Further evidence to support the proposal of Nadeau and Crosson (1997a) comes from the findings of Hillis *et al.* (2002). Based on a study of a consecutive series of patients with acute strokes limited to subcortical tissue using magnetic resonance perfusion-weighted imaging as well as diffusion-weighted imaging, these latter authors reported cortical hypoperfusion in all 28 of their aphasic patients and none of their 12 non-aphasic patients. Further, they reported that, in those cases in which blood flow could be restored to the cortex within a few days from onset, reperfusion was associated with immediate resolution of aphasia. In a further study, Hillis *et al.* (2004) reported that in their patients with acute left caudate stroke, the variation of speech-language deficits observed could be accounted for by variation in the region of cortical hypoperfusion as demonstrated by magnetic resonance perfusion imaging conducted the same day as language testing. Further, not only did the presence and type of aphasia reflect the regions of hypometabolism, they generally followed predictions based on chronic lesion studies regarding

anatomical lesions associated with classic aphasia types.

Although the notion that overlying cortical dysfunction via hypoperfusion is the critical determinant of language impairments associated with striatocapsular lesions has been argued forcefully (Nadeau and Crosson, 1997a; Hillis *et al.*, 2004), there are other views counter to this position (Wallesch and Papagno, 1988; Mega and Alexander, 1994; D'Esposito and Alexander, 1995). Han *et al.* (2003) proposed that aphasia associated with subcortical stroke is due to small infarcts in the cerebral cortex that are not visible on computed tomographic or conventional magnetic resonance imaging (MRI) scans, but are seen on diffusion-weighted or delayed conventional MRI. While this explanation of aphasia would account for the variety of aphasia types observed in patients with so-called subcortical strokes, it does not account for patients with acute aphasia and no cortical infarct on diffusion-weighted imaging.

It remains that the relationship between the structured site and aetiology of the subcortical lesions, time post-onset, the extent of cortical hypometabolism and hypoperfusion, and associated language function, remains to be fully elucidated. Further, the question of whether language deficits associated with striatocapsular lesions are the sequelae of cortical or subcortical dysfunction should not be considered as necessarily mutually exclusive. Concomitant cortical dysfunction may result in overlying language deficits that mask more subtle changes in language function which relate directly to basal ganglia dysfunction. Indeed, Metter *et al.* (1983) provided evidence that striatocapsular structural damage may have direct and indirect (through hypometabolism) effects on certain aspects of language function.

Prognosis of striatocapsular aphasia

Reports in the literature vary as to the prognosis of aphasic disturbances resulting from striatocapsular lesions. Performance on standard aphasia batteries indicates that striatocapsular lesions may result in a transient aphasia or resolve to a mild aphasia (Basso, Della Sala and Farabola, 1987; Vallar, Papagno and Cappa, 1988; Mega and Alexander, 1994). Other studies have identified long-lasting deficits resulting from left striatocapsular lesions. These latter deficits include the presence of semantic paraphasias and word-finding difficulties in spontaneous speech (Damasio *et al.*, 1982; Murdoch *et al.*, 1986; Kennedy and Murdoch, 1989). Further, although basic auditory comprehension may be intact (Damasio *et al.*, 1982), more subtle long-term deficits have been documented in understanding constructions (Murdoch *et al.*, 1986; Vallar, Papagno and Cappa, 1988; Kennedy and Murdoch, 1993). Likewise, repetition may be either intact (Damasio *et al.*, 1982; Mega and Alexander, 1994) or impaired in the long-term only for low-probability items or sentences (Murdoch *et al.*, 1986; Kennedy and Murdoch, 1989). Confrontation naming may be either normal or chronically impaired (Damasio *et al.*, 1982; Kennedy and Murdoch, 1989; Mega and Alexander, 1994).

Language disorders associated with cerebellar lesions

Investigation of a possible role for the cerebellum in the mediation of cognitive processes, including language, has historically been overshadowed by research interest in cerebellar coordination of motor control. Over the past two decades, however, the question of a possible participation of the cerebellum in language processing itself has come to the forefront. In particular, recent advances in our understanding of the neuroanatomy of the cerebellum combined with evidence from functional neuroimaging, neurophysiological and neuropsychological research has, however, extended our view of the cerebellum from that of a simple coordinator of autonomic and somatic motor function. Rather, it is now more widely accepted that the cerebellum, and in particular the right cerebellar hemisphere, participates in modulation of cognitive functioning, especially to those parts of the brain to which it is reciprocally connected (Marien *et al.*, 2001). Indeed, the discovery of major reciprocal neural pathways between the cerebellum and the frontal areas of the language-dominant hemisphere, includ-

ing Broca's area and the supplementary motor area, was a major impetus in the development of the concept of cerebellar involvement in non-motor linguistic processes.

Much of the credit for this development goes to Leiner, Leiner and Dow, who wrote a series of articles reviewing the potential role of the cerebellum in cognition. In their first publication (Leiner, Leiner and Dow, 1986), they reviewed long-neglected evidence that portions of the lateral cerebellar hemispheres and dentate nuclei were greatly expanded in humans. They hypothesized that these cerebellar regions project to pre-frontal and other association cortices in humans and higher primates, forming corticocerebellar loops used for certain types of cognitive skills. The primary loops thought to be involved in the regulation of voluntary movements and cognitive/linguistic functions are the cerebrocortico-ponto-cerebellocortico-dentalo-thalamo-cerebrocortical loop (Bloedel and Bracha, 1997; Middleton and Strick, 1997) and the cerebrocortico-rubro-olivo-neodentato-cerebrocortical loop (Leiner, Leiner and Dow, 1991, 1993). Importantly, in both loops, each cerebellar hemisphere sends information to, and receives it from, primarily the contralateral cerebral hemisphere. Therefore, the right cerebellar hemisphere is connected to the left cerebral hemisphere and conversely.

In support of this hypothesis, non-motor behavioural deficits associated with cerebellar damage or abnormalities were reported by several investigators, and functional neuroanatomical studies using PET during the late 1980s demonstrated the selective activation of some cerebellar structures during language tasks (Petersen *et al.*, 1989). In the early 1990s, Fiez *et al.* (1992) described a patient with an extensive right cerebellar lesion who presented with language disturbances. Since that time numerous studies have identified the presence of disturbed language processing in association with primary lesions of various aetiologies involving both the right (Marien *et al.*, 2001) and left (Murdoch and Whelan, 2007) cerebellar hemispheres. In particular, clinical investigations of both adults and children with cerebellar pathology using sensitive linguistic tests capable of detecting subtle, high-level language impairments (Cook *et al.*, 2004; Docking, Murdoch and Suppiah, 2007; Murdoch and Whelan, 2007) have demonstrated the presence of a variety of linguistic impairments in association with cerebellar pathology, including problems in verbal fluency, word retrieval, syntax, reading, writing and metalinguistic abilities.

Several different theories have been proposed relating to possible neuropathological mechanisms involved in the occurrence of language disorders subsequent to cerebellar lesions. First, it has been suggested that crossed cerebello-cerebrocortical diaschisis reflecting a functional depression of supratentorial language areas owing to reduced input to the cerebral cortex via cerebello-cerebrocortical pathways may represent the neuropathological mechanism responsible for linguistic deficits associated with cerebellar pathology (Broich *et al.*, 1987; Marien *et al.*, 2001). In support of this suggestion, functional neuroimaging studies based on SPECT, PET or fMRI have consistently revealed regions of contralateral cortical hypoperfusion in relation to the orientation of the cerebellar lesion (e.g. Silveri, Leggio and Molinari, 1994; Beldarrain *et al.*, 1997). According to the cerebello-cerebrocortical diaschisis model, therefore, the cerebellum is not involved in the generation of language (which remains a supratentorial activity) but rather modulates language function via segregated, multicomponent neural circuits the major pathways of which include the cerebrocortico-ponto-cerebellocortico-dentato-thalamic-cerebrocortical loop and the cerebro-cortico-rubro-olivo-neodentato-cerebrocortical loop. In this way, the cerebellum acts as an important relay in the neural circuits responsible for language in much the same way as other subcortical structures such as the basal ganglia form important components of the segregated, multicomponent neural circuits that enable those structures to also influence frontal lobe activities.

A second theory proposed to explain cerebellar involvement in linguistic function is the timing hypothesis, which proposes that the cerebellum has no direct influence on linguistic processes but plays an important role in the timing of linguistic functions represented on a supratentorial

level (Keele and Ivry, 1991; Silveri, Leggio and Molinari, 1994). A third hypothesis relating to the role of the cerebellum in language proposes a direct cerebellar contribution via the topographically organized reciprocal connections with the cerebral cortex. According to this theory, the cerebellum does not act as a sole modulator of language but is actively involved in the organization, construction and execution of linguistic processes. As yet, however, the precise role of the cerebellum in language is not clear. Further studies that rely on a combination of neuroanatomical, neuroimaging and neurolinguistic investigations are needed to further elucidate the nature of the role of this complex and somewhat neglected and underestimated part of the brain in language function.

Models of subcortical participation in language

The possible existence of subcortical aphasia as a clinical entity has catalysed the development of contemporary language theories which suggest functional roles for subcortical nuclei, including the striatum, globus pallidus and thalamus. These theoretical constructs specifically promote a network model of language organization (Cappa and Vallar, 1992), whereby cortico-subcortical-cortical pathways represent the neural basis of linguistic processing, in preference to exclusive cortical–cortical connections.

The work of Alexander and colleagues (Alexander, De Long and Strick, 1986; Alexander, Crutcher and De Long, 1990) provides the basis for our understanding of the anatomical and functional organization of cortico-subcortical-cortical circuits. Seminal schemas proposed parallel yet functionally segregated basal ganglia–thalamocortical pathways to underlie skeletomotor, occulomotor, cognitive and limbic functions. To date, the skeletomotor circuit has proffered the greatest contribution to the conceptualization of basal ganglia–thalamocortical organizational substrates. As such, contemporary models of subcortical participation in language have largely evolved from theories of motor control, the foundations of which were established within studies of basal ganglia dysfunction in primates with experimentally induced 1-methyl-4-phyl-1,2,3,6-tetrahydropyridine (MPTP) toxicity (Starr, Vitek and Bakay, 1998).

Based on clinicoanatomical evidence thus far, three major basal ganglia–thalamocortical circuits have been speculated to participate in the mediation of linguistic processes (Cappa and Vallar, 1992): (1) the anterior 'complex' loop (i.e. dorsolateral pre-frontal and lateral orbitofrontal circuits (Alexander, De Long and Strick, 1986): frontal association cortex–caudate nucleus–globus pallidus–ventroanterior thalamus–frontal association cortex; (2) the anterior 'motor' loop (i.e. skeleton-motor circuit (Alexander, De Long and Strick, 1986): sensory motor cortex–putamen–globus pallidus–ventrolateral thalamus–sensory motor cortex and (3) the posterior loop (Van Buren and Borke, 1969): temporal parietal cortex–pulvinar–temporal parietal cortex. The anterior 'complex' and 'motor' pathways were hypothesized to mediate lexical semantic expression and articulation respectively and the posterior loop to facilitate auditory comprehension (Cappa and Vallar, 1992). Additional subcortical–cortical pathways have also been postulated to participate in the regulation of language (Cappa and Vallar, 1992), including: temporal auditory cortex–caudate nucleus pathway facilitating auditory comprehension (Damasio *et al.*, 1982; Van Hoesen, Yeterian and Lavizzo-Mourey, 1981); amygdala–temporal neocortex–dorsomedial thalamus (Cappa and Sterzi, 1990) and caudate nucleus–supplementary motor area–anterior (Naeser *et al.*, 1989) regulating speech production. The functional specificity of language-dedicated subcortical circuits to date has been largely restricted to the elementary linguistic faculties of auditory comprehension and verbal expression (Alexander, De Long and Strick, 1986). It is anticipated, however, that contemporary research may serve to expose functional subdivisions within non-motor basal ganglia–thalamocortical circuits, which reflect a similar level of organizational complexity to that of the somatotopic channels identified within subcortical motor circuitry

(Alexander, De Long and Strick, 1986). Indeed, this disclosure may potentially involve the elucidation of the neural substrates underpinning language at both single-word and sentential levels of processing.

Several theories have attempted to explicate the subcortical neural mechanisms underlying receptive and expressive linguistic abilities. These include: the Subcortical White Matter Pathways (Alexander, Naeser and Palumbo, 1987), Response–Release/Semantic Feedback (Crosson, 1985), Lexical Decision Making (Wallesch and Papagno, 1988) and Selective Engagement (Nadeau and Crosson, 1997a) models.

Subcortical white matter pathways model

The Subcortical White Matter Pathways model (Alexander, Naeser and Palumbo, 1987) dismisses a role for the subcortical nuclei in language and advocates corticocortical, corticostriatal, thalamocortical and corticobulbar white matter pathways as critical to the facilitation of auditory comprehension and verbal expression. The fulcrum of this theoretical schema developed from a series of robust clinico-neuroradiological studies which highlighted an array of receptive and expressive language deficits in individuals with large striatal lesions, extending into the surrounding white matter pathways (Alexander, Naeser and Palumbo, 1987). This profile was in stark contrast to that observed in patients with relatively circumscribed lesions of the putamen and caudate nucleus, which resulted in covert or nominal disturbances to language such as mild word-finding difficulties and hesitant verbal output. This finding consequently supported a minimal function hypothesis for basal ganglia participation in language and directed discussion towards the white matter pathways linking cortical-cortical and subcortical-cortical regions (Figure 3.7).

Vascular lesions of the striatum that extended beyond the lateral boundary of the anterior limb of the internal capsule, incorporating the anterior, extra anterior, anterior superior,

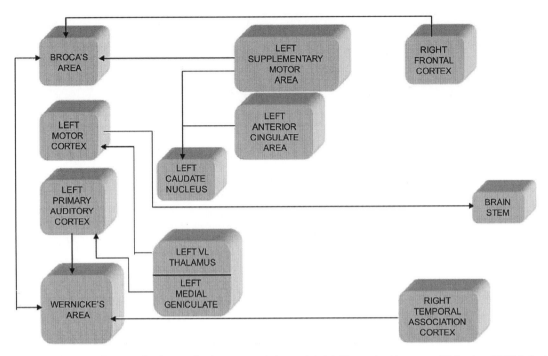

Figure 3.7 Schematic diagram of Subcortical White Matter Pathways Model (Alexander, Naeser and Palumbo, 1987) (adapted from Crosson (1992)). VL = ventral lateral nucleus.

superior or posterior periventricular white matter (PVWM), temporal isthmus, insular cortex and/or external capsule, were documented to produce a range of expressive and receptive language deficits (Alexander, Naeser and Palumbo, 1987). More specifically, non-thalamic lesions with extensions into the anterior superior PVWM were reported to result in transcortical motor aphasia, largely evidenced as sparse verbal output and difficulty initiating speech. This symptom complex was hypothesized to result from damage to the fibre pathways connecting the supplementary motor area and Broca's area (Figure 3.7). Anterior superior PVWM pathway disconnection was postulated to restrict limbic inputs to cortical language centres, resulting in reduced speech drive. Repetition deficits were reported to arise from lateral and/or superior lesion extensions relative to the putamen, which implicate the external and extreme capsules and, potentially, the arcuate fasciculus.

In relation to speech motor control, corticobulbar fibres within the superior PVWM and genu of the internal capsule, in addition to cortico-

cerebellar and thalamocortical fibres within the anterior portion of the superior PVWM and anterior limb of the internal capsule, were inculpated. The temporal isthmus, linking the medial geniculate nucleus of the thalamus to the primary auditory association cortex and the auditory association callosal pathway connecting Wernicke's area and the right temporal association cortex were identified as the subcortical white matter pathways integral to auditory comprehension. Posterior striatal lesion extension incorporating these structures typically resulted in comprehension deficits and neologistic output. Furthermore, wide-ranging lesion extension relative to the putamen, including the anterior limb of the internal capsule, extra anterior PVWM, anterior PVWM, anterior superior PVWM and temporal isthmus was reported to result in global language impairment. Alexander, Naeser and Palumbo (1987) avoided attributing a role in language functioning to the thalamus on the basis that language deficits resulting from thalamic and putaminal lesions are subserved by disparate pathophysiological mechanisms.

Given that white matter pathways provide the means by which components of the language system communicate with each other, the importance given to these pathways in the model proposed by Alexander, Naeser and Palumbo (1987) would, on the surface, appear reasonable. However, the findings of subsequent studies refute the notion that white matter pathway disconnection provides a valid datum for clinical manifestation of subcortical damage (Cappa and Vallar, 1992).

Response–release semantic feedback model

A postulated thalamocortical alerting system (Ojemann, 1976) represents the plinth of the Response–Release Semantic Feedback (RRSF) (Crosson, 1985) model (Figure 3.8). The model proposes a role for subcortical structures in regulating the release of pre-formulated language segments from the cerebral cortex. According to

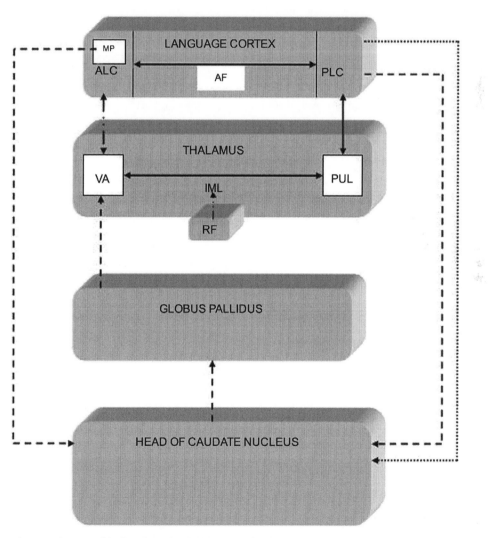

Figure 3.8 Schematic diagram of the basal ganglia–thalamocortical Response-Release Semantic Feedback Model (adapted from (Crosson, 1985, 1992)). ALC = anterior language centre; PLC = posterior language centre; MP = motor programming cortex; AF = arcuate fasciculus; RF = reticular formation; VA = ventral anterior thalamic nucleus; IML = internal medullary lamina; PUL = pulvinar; ──▶ = excitatory pathway; ----▶ = inhibitory pathway; ·······▶ = disinhibitory pathway.

this model, the conceptual, word-finding and syntactic processes that fall under the rubric of language formulation occur in the anterior cerebral cortex. The monitoring of anteriorly formulated language segments, as well as the semantic and phonological decoding of incoming language, occurs in the posterior temporal parietal cortex. Language segments are conveyed from the anterior language formulation centre to the posterior language centre via the thalamus prior to release for motor programming. This operation allows the posterior semantic decoding centres to monitor the language segment for semantic accuracy. If an inaccuracy is detected, then the information required for correction is conveyed via the thalamus back to the anterior cortex. If the language segment is found to be accurate during monitoring, then it is released from a buffer in the anterior cortex for subsequent motor programming. In addition to subcortical structures participating in the pre-verbal semantic monitoring process, the model also specifies that the striato-capsular structures are involved in the release of the formulated language segment for motor programming. Specifically, it is suggested that this release occurs through the cortico-striato-pallido-thalamo-cortical loop in the following way. Once the language segments have been verified for semantic accuracy, the temporal parietal cortex releases the caudate nucleus from inhibition. The caudate nucleus then serves to weaken inhibitory pallidal regulation of thalamic excitatory outputs in the anterior language centre, which in turn arouses the cortex to enable generation of the motor programmes for semantically verified language segments. According to this model, Crosson (1985) hypothesized that subcortical lesions within the cortico-striato-pallido-thalamo-cortical loop would produce language deficits confined to the lexical semantic level.

The original conception of the response–release mechanism in Crosson's (1985) model has since been revised and elaborated in terms of the neural substrates involved (Crosson, 1992). Although the actual response–release mechanism in the modified version resembles that in the original conception, the route for this release is altered (Figure 3.9). The formulation of a language segment causes frontal excitation of the caudate, which increases inhibition of specific fields within the globus pallidus. However, this level of inhibition alone is not sufficient to alter pallidal output to the thalamus. An increase in posterior language cortex excitation to the caudate, which occurs once a language segment has been semantically verified posteriorly, provides a boost to the inhibition of the pallidum. The pallidal summation of this anterior and posterior inhibitory input allows the release of the ventral anterior thalamus from inhibition by the globus pallidus, causing the thalamic excitation of the frontal language cortex required to trigger the release of the language segment for motor programming. Overall, the revised model provides an integrated account of how subcortical structures might influence language output through a neuroregulatory mechanism that is consistent with knowledge of cortical-subcortical neurotransmitter systems and structural features.

Lexical Decision Making Model

In line with the RRSF model, the Lexical Decision Making (LDM) model (Wallesch and Papagno, 1988) also proposes a cortico-striato-pallido-thalamo-cortical loop as the neural platform for linguistic operations, including a specific thalamocortical arousal mechanism, consistent with Ojemann's (1976) theorem. Despite evident parallels, however, distinct incongruities prevail between these theoretical constructs with respect to functional cortical organization viewpoints, and the nature of proposed subcortical mechanisms.

Wallesch and Papagno (1988) postulated that the subcortical components of the loop constitute a 'frontal lobe system' comprising parallel modules with integrative and decision-making capabilities rather than the simple neuroregulatory function proposed in Crosson's (1985) model (Figure 3.10). Specifically, the basal ganglia system and thalamus were hypothesized to process situational as well as goal-directed constraints and lexical information from the frontal cortex and posterior language area, and to subsequently participate in the process of determining the appropriate lexical item, from a range of cortically

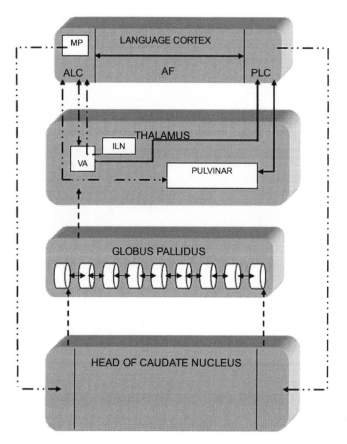

Figure 3.9 Schematic diagram of the revised basal ganglia–thalamocortical Response-Release Semantic Feedback Model (adapted from (Crosson, 1985, 1992)). ALC = anterior language centre; PLC = posterior language centre; MP = motor programming cortex; AF = arcuate fasciculus; VA = ventral anterior thalamic nucleus; PUL = pulvinar; ──▶ = excitatory pathway; ----▶ = inhibitory pathway; 〇 = disc-shaped dendritic fields; ↔ = spatial summation properties.

generated lexical alternatives, for verbal production. The most appropriate lexical alternative is then released by the thalamus for processing by the frontal cortex and programming for speech. Cortical processing of selected lexical alternatives is made possible by inhibitory influences of the globus pallidus on a thalamic gating mechanism. This most appropriate lexical alternative has an inhibitory effect on the thalamus, promoting closure of the thalamic gate, resulting in activation of the cerebral cortex and production of the desired response. Cortical processing of subordinate alternatives is suppressed as a consequence of pallidal disinhibition of the thalamus, and the inhibition of cortical activity.

Selective Engagement Model

Selective Engagement (SE) theory represents the most contemporary schema of subcortical participation in language and principally proposes a frontal inferior thalamic peduncle (ITP) nucleus reticularis (NR) centrum medianum (CM) system to subserve the 'engagement' of cortical components which mediate attentional and behavioural processes, including language (Nadeau and Crosson, 1997a) (Figure 3.11). This proposed linguistic frontal lobe system complied with the tenets of the LDM model, with the exception of two distinct anomalies. In particular, selective engagement theory disputes a role

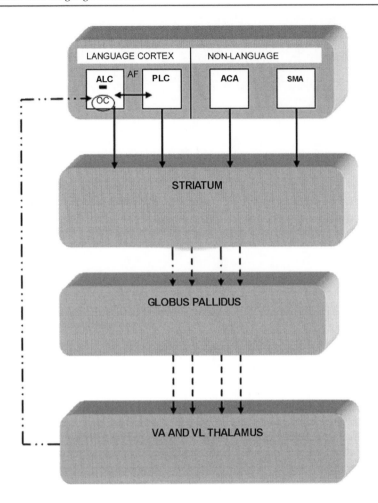

Figure 3.10 Schematic diagram of the basal ganglia-thalamo-cortical Lexical Decision Making Model (adapted from (Crosson, 1992)). ALC = anterior language centre; PLC = posterior language centre; ACA = anterior cingulate area; SMA = supplementary motor area; AF = arcuate fasciculus; VA = ventral anterior nucleus; VL = ventral lateral nucleus; OC = output channel; ▬ = inhibitory cortical interneurones; ----▶ = inhibitory pathway; ──▶ = excitatory pathway.

for the basal ganglia in language and redefines non-specific thalamic nuclei (i.e. NR, CM and parafascicular nucleus) as critical to the mediation of linguistic processes. Nadeau and Crosson (1997b) considered ventral anterior (VA) and ventral lateral (VL) thalamic participation in language an insolvent hypothesis. This postulate was largely fuelled by two lines of evidence: (1) an observed decline in the incidence of aphasia following surgically induced lesions of the VA and VL thalamus, concomitant with enhanced stereotactic technique accuracy (Fox, Ahlskog and Kelly, 1991) and (2) the fact that aphasia resulting

from tuberothalamic territory infarcts involving the VA nucleus typically resembles that following paramedian territory lesions, which spare the VA thalamus. Postulated thalamic engagement of the cortex, however, was in line with Ojemann's (1976) proposed ventral thalamic focal altering mechanism in addition to Crosson's (1985) VA response–release system, relative to the galvanization of verbal output channels. The expansion of these postulates to consider the activation of more extensive language-dedicated cortical mosaics (Ojemann, 1983), largely under NR control (Nadeau and Crosson, 1997a), accommodated

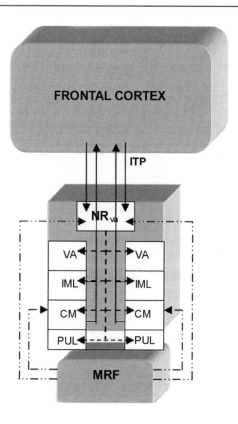

Figure 3.11 Schematic diagram of the frontal ITP–NR–CM system subserving the proposed engagement of cortical language mechanisms (adapted from Nadeau and Crosson, 1997a). ITP = inferior thalamic peduncle; NR_{va} = ventral anterior nucleus reticularis; VA = ventral anterior thalamus; IML = internal medullary lamina; CM = centre medianum, PUL = pulvinar; MRF = midbrain reticular formation; ----▶ = inhibitory pathway; ——▶ = excitatory pathway. Thalamocortical and corticothalamic pathways are largely unrepresented for the sake of clarity, with the exception of CM-frontal and frontal NR_{va} projections.

manifestations of receptive as well as expressive language deficits observed subsequent to lesions of the thalamus. The RRSF and LDM models previously discussed focused primarily on output versus input mechanisms, providing no discernible explanation for comprehension deficits. In contrast, the structural complexity of the neural system subserving SE mechanisms accommodates the spectrum of aphasic characteristics observed following lesions of the dominant thalamus (Nadeau and Crosson, 1997b), perhaps approximating a more cogent axiom of subcortical participation in language than its antecedents.

An important feature of the SE theory is that it discounts a role for the basal ganglia in language. A variable symptom complex with respect to observed manifestations of language pathology in the presence of classically defined striatocapsular lesions formed the basis of this postulate. In more detail, Nadeau and Crosson (1997a) analysed the linguistic profiles of 50 cases subsequent to relatively uniform striatocapsular infarctions, including the caudate head, putamen, anterior limb of the internal capsule and portions of the globus pallidus. Vast heterogeneity relative to the severity and incidence of language deficits including fluency, articulation, comprehension, repetition and naming was reported. Nadeau and Crosson (1997a) hypothesized that an integral role for the basal ganglia in language would be fortified by a coherent aphasic syndrome, in the event of uniform damage. Based on the above evidence, therefore, a minimal function hypothesis with respect to the contribution of the basal ganglia to language functions was promoted.

Nadeau and Crosson (1997a) largely attributed language disturbances subsequent to lesions of the basal ganglia to cortical hypoperfusion. Thrombotic or embolic occlusions primarily of the middle cerebral artery (MCA), or less commonly the internal carotid artery, were identified as precursors to striatocapsular infarction (Weiller *et al.*, 1990). More importantly, circulatory dynamics pertaining to the rate of arterial recanalization and the efficiency of anastomotic circulation following basal ganglia infarction were considered integral factors in determining the presence or absence of aphasia. Perisylvian cortex ischaemia by way of MCA occlusion-induced cystic infarction, neuronal drop out or generalized tissue dysfunction (Nadeau and Crosson, 1997a) provided a tenable explanation for the variable array of expressive and receptive language deficits associated with striatocapsular infarcts. Furthermore, haemorrhagic basal ganglia lesions were also postulated to disturb cortical circulatory dynamics relevant to language functions. Pressure effects inducing cortical ischaemia were held responsible for consequent manifestations of aphasia.

Evidence is available that disputes Nadeau and Crosson's (1997a) claim that lesions of the striatocapsular region fail to establish a homogeneous aphasic syndrome. A coherent aphasic syndrome relative to generative aspects of language, including verbal fluency, sentence generation and extended discourse has been reported (Mega and Alexander, 1994). This finding suggests a need to revisit the notion of basal ganglia aphasia, paying particular attention to the scope and sensitivity of linguistic assessments utilized in addition to circulatory dynamics (Crosson *et al.*, 1997). Indeed, this evidence supports a potential role for the basal ganglia in mediating linguistic processes. In all probability, this role may entail the regulation of thalamocortical engagement. One proposed mechanism involves the switching of engagement between neural nets (Malapani *et al.*, 1994).

Limitations of theoretical models of subcortical participation in language

Each of the models outlined above has a number of limitations and consequently no one model has achieved uniform acceptance. A major limitation of these models is that they fail to fully explain the considerable variability in clinical presentation of subcortical aphasia. According to Cappa (1997), a further problem is that the models suggest such extensive and widely distributed systems subserving lexical processing that specific predictions appear to be difficult to disprove on the basis of pathological evidence. In other words, these models do not lend themselves readily to empirical testing. Yet another limitation arises from the nature of the research on which these models are based. The available models of subcortical participation in language are largely based on the observation that certain contrasting deficits of language production arise in subjects with particular subcortical vascular lesions when tested on traditional tests of language function. These language measures were typically designed for taxonomic purposes regarding traditional cortical-based aphasia syndromes and may be inadequate for developing models of brain functioning. It has also been argued that language deficits associated with subcortical vascular lesions may actually be related to concomitant cortical dysfunction via

various pathophysiological mechanisms. For instance, owing to limitations inherent to currently available neuroimaging techniques, cortical infarction may not have been detected by neuroimaging. Consequently, inaccurate lesion parameters may have served to contaminate our conceptualization of subcortical aphasia thus far.

In addition to the recognized shortcomings of current neuroimaging techniques as outlined previously, a number of physiological mechanisms have also been proposed which potentially attribute manifestations of subcortical aphasia to cortical dysfunction. Subcortical lesions have been reported to exert distance effects upon the cerebral cortex, including cortical hypoperfusion and hypometabolism (Perani *et al.*, 1987). Reduced cerebral blood flow results in ischaemia-induced neuronal loss (Lassen *et al.*, 1983) and ischaemic penumbra (i.e. maintenance of tissue viability in the presence of neuronal dysfunction) both mechanisms having the potential to disable cortical activity. Also, subcortical lesions may result in diaschisis or the functional deactivation of distant, related cortical structures (Metter *et al.*, 1983). As yet, however, the relationship between the structural site and aetiology of subcortical lesions, the extent of diaschisis, cortical hypometabolism and hypoperfusion, and associated language function remains to be fully elucidated.

Overall, the validity of the aforementioned operative models of subcortical participation in language remains largely unattested owing primarily to a previous incapacity to strictly define the extent of vascular neuropathology. A further encumbrance to empirical ratification rests with the inadequacy of animal models in providing an appropriate linguistic platform for investigation (Crosson, 1992). The value of model-driven and theoretically founded studies of cognition cannot be overestimated in quests to extricate the subcortical-cortical mechanisms underpinning language (Cappa and Sterzi, 1990). The utilization of existing frameworks, however, in the context of advancing scientific techniques is considered critical to their ultimate interpretation. In line with this proposal, a recent resurgence in functional neurosurgery to treat the motor symptoms of Parkinson's disease, involving the generation of discrete surgically induced lesions of the subcortical nuclei, would appear to provide an unprecedented opportunity to empirically test contemporary theories of subcortical participation in language.

Role of subcortical structures in language: evidence from neurosurgical lesions

Over the course of the past decade or so, primate research has served to catalyse the development of a sound theoretical framework that has enhanced our understanding of the pathophysiology underlying movement disorders, such as those seen in Parkinson's disease. This, combined with advances in neuroimaging and neurosurgical techniques and a degree of disillusionment with drug treatments for movement disorders, has led to a revival of stereotactic neurosurgical procedures such as pallidotomy (involving lesioning of specific components of the globus pallidus) and thalamotomy (involving lesioning of specific nuclei in the thalamus) in the treatment of Parkinson's disease. In addition to their patent therapeutic value, the discrete circumscribed lesion sites provided by these procedures afford an unprecedented opportunity to empirically test contemporary subcortical language theories. More recently, as an alternative to ablative procedures such as pallidotomy and thalamotomy which overtly destroy neural tissue, deep brain stimulation (DBS) involving implantation of electrodes within a range of subcortical targets such as the subthalamic nucleus (STN) has gained increasing support as the preferred method of treatment for Parkinson's disease. In that DBS has been documented to simulate the effects of ablative lesions (i.e. block neuronal activity at the target site), this technique also provides an opportunity to test models that implicate structures such as the STN and thalamus in language.

The majority of studies reported to date pertaining to the impact of pallidotomy (Trepanier *et al.*, 1998; Lombardi *et al.*, 2000; Scott *et al.*, 2002), thalamotomy (Fukuda *et al.*, 2000)

on cognitive function have been largely neuropsychologically based. Assessment batteries have typically included measures of attention, memory, concentration, visuospatial abilities and executive functioning. In regard to language, the domains of confrontation naming, verbal learning, semantic and phonemic fluency have been afforded considerable scrutiny; however, in-depth linguistic analyses were not included. A series of studies by Whelan, Murdoch and colleagues have addressed this problem by utilising a battery of high-level language tests to examine the effects of pallidotomy (Whelan *et al.*, 2000, 2004b; Murdoch, Whelan and Theodoros, 2003), thalamotomy (Whelan *et al.*, 2002) and DBS of the STN (Whelan, Murdoch and Theodoros, 2003; Whelan *et al.*, 2004a) on linguistic function. Overall, these studies provided evidence to suggest that the concatenation of subcortical nuclei comprising basal ganglia–thalamocortical circuits play a fundamental role in high-level linguistic processes potentially underpinning the recruitment and directed interplay of frontal and temporal parietal cortical regions. With regard to the STN, the findings of Whelan *et al.* (Whelan, Murdoch and Theodoros, 2003; Whelan *et al.*, 2004a) highlighted the need to modify contemporary theories of subcortical participation in language to incorporate the STN. More specifically, the outcomes of their research challenged unilateral models of functional basal ganglia organization with the proposal of a potential interhemispheric regulatory function for the STN in the mediation of high-level linguistic processes. Indeed, the STN may contribute to the mediation of linguistic processes by indirectly regulating thalamocortical outputs within the cortical-subcortical-cortical language circuits.

Role of subcortical structures in language: evidence from functional neuroimaging

Further clarification of the role of subcortical structures in language is likely to come through the use of functional neuroimaging techniques and neurophysiological methods such as electrical and magnetic-evoked responses. Functional neuroimaging techniques such as functional magnetic resonance imaging (fMRI) and positron emission tomography (PET) enable brain images to be collected while the subject is performing various language production tasks (e.g. picture naming, generating nouns) or during language comprehension (e.g. listening to stories). These techniques therefore enable visualization of the brain regions involved in a language task, with a spatial resolution as low as a few millimetres. Although functional neuroimaging does therefore offer promise as a tool to unravel the role of subcortical structures in language, results from functional neuroimaging studies to date have proven less than definitive (Cabeza and Nyberg, 2000). These studies have, however, revealed a number of cortical and subcortical structures beyond the perisylvian cortex to be active during linguistic processing (Petersen *et al.*, 1989; Warburton *et al.*, 1996; Crosson *et al.*, 1999) providing support for a distributed network model of language organization (Mesulam, 2000). In particular, word-generation studies have shown consistent activation of the medial frontal cortex, usually near the boundary of pre-supplementary motor area (pre-SMA) and the rostral cingulated zone. Although the pre-SMA is known to have extensive subcortical connections, including projections to the striatal grey matter spanning the internal capsule and to the caudate nucleus and putamen as well as receiving connections from ventral anterior and dorsomedial thalamus in the majority of functional neuroimaging studies, these subcortical components have not shown consistent activity in functional neuroimaging studies of word generation. This reported inconsistency in activation of the basal ganglia and thalamus may be the product of limitations in numbers of subjects studied, number of trials during functional neuroimaging and experimental design. Crosson *et al.* (2003) using fMRI observed significant activity in the subcortical structures during word-generation tasks but not during nonsense syllable generation. They inferred the existence of a left pre-SMA–dorsocaudate–ventral anterior thalamic loop involved in lexical retrieval. Further, Crosson *et al.* (2003) hypothesized 'that

activity in this loop was related to maintaining a bias toward the retrieval of one lexical item versus competing alternatives for each response during word generation blocks' (p. 1075). Several PET studies have also demonstrated activation of the thalamus and basal ganglia during completion of language tasks such as picture naming (Price *et al.*, 1996a) and word repetition (Price *et al.*, 1996b).

In relation to the role of the cerebellum in language, functional neuroimaging studies have provided a possible explanation for the occurrence of language problems subsequent to cerebellar pathology. Specifically, studies based on functional neuroimaging techniques such as single-photon emission computed tomography (SPECT), PET and fMRI have consistently revealed regions of contralateral cortical hypoperfusion in relation to the orientation of the cerebellar lesion (Silveri, Leggio and Molinari, 1994; Beldarrain *et al.*, 1997), a phenomenon called 'crossed cerebello-cerebral diaschisis'. Several authors have proposed that this phenomenon, reflecting a functional depression of supratentorial language areas due to reduced input via cerebellocortical pathways, may represent the neuropathological mechanism responsible for language problems associated with cerebellar pathology (Broich *et al.*, 1987; Marien *et al.*, 2001).

Language disorders in degenerative subcortical syndromes

In past years, one argument often raised against a role for subcortical structures in language processing was an apparent lack of language impairment in individuals with degenerative subcortical syndromes such as Parkinson's disease and Huntington's disease. In recent years, however, studies that have utilized sufficiently sensitive tests have identified deficits in high-level language functions (i.e. those language functions more highly dependent on frontal lobe support) in persons with a range of degenerative subcortical conditions including Parkinson's disease and Huntington's disease.

Language disorders in Parkinson's disease

Parkinson's disease is a progressive, degenerative neurological condition resulting from nigrostriatal dopamine depletion and characterized primarily by motor symptoms such as tremor, bradykinesia, rigidity and postural instability. When James Parkinson first described Parkinsonism in 1817, he claimed that there were no mental manifestations of the disease. Today, however, it is widely acknowledged that even in the absence of global intellectual decline or dementia some individuals with Parkinson's disease will experience subtle deficits in a range of cognitive domains including memory, visuospatial abilities, executive planning, attention and language function (Cooper *et al.*, 1991; Dubois *et al.*, 1991; Levin and Katzen, 1995).

Support for the proposal that language may be compromised in Parkinson's disease comes from distributed processing models of neural function as well as proposals that implicate subcortical structures in both cognitive and linguistic functions (see models of subcortical participation in language above). While the potential role of dopamine as an important neuroregulator of cognitive functioning has been recognized (Nieoullon, 2002), disruption to the functioning of the striatum and the dopamine connections to the frontal lobes may also be expected to influence cognitive functioning. Consistent with this proposal, it has been suggested that cognitive deficits in Parkinson's disease may be consistent with a disturbance in frontal striatal function (Bondi *et al.*, 1993). Accordingly, given the role of dopamine and the striatum in cognitive function, it is highly likely that language function is also impaired in Parkinson's disease. Indeed, there have been some isolated reports of abnormal performance by persons with Parkinson's disease on language tasks such as naming, sentence repetition and auditory comprehension (Cummings *et al.*, 1988; Beatty and Monson, 1989; Blonder *et al.*, 1989; Lewis *et al.*, 1998).

Unfortunately, comprehensive investigations of language function in Parkinson's disease are limited. More common are studies that have focused on the impact of Parkinson's disease on specific aspects of language performance, such as sentence comprehension and verbal fluency. Early investigations of language functioning reported equivocal results of language assessment in Parkinson's disease. Studies of single word use and sentence processing based on traditional aphasiologic measures at times described mild deficits (Cummings *et al.*, 1988; Geyer and Grossman, 1994). Confrontation naming difficulties and compromised category naming fluency have been reported by some investigators (Matison *et al.*, 1982; Cooper *et al.*, 1991; Auriacombe *et al.*, 1993). Even in the absence of dementia, persons with Parkinson's disease exhibit subtle difficulties processing semantic language as evidenced by impaired performance on off-line tests of verbal fluency and naming (Beatty and Monson, 1989; Blonder *et al.*, 1989; Raskin, Sliwinski and Borod, 1992; Bayles *et al.*, 1993; Frank, McDade and Scott, 1996).

Lewis *et al.* (1998) identified subtle language impairments across a range of complex linguistic functions in a group of 20 subjects with idiopathic Parkinson's disease on a battery of measures selected to be sensitive to frontal lobe language function. More specifically, as a group the Parkinsonian group examined by Lewis *et al.* (1998) presented with impaired naming and definitional abilities and difficulties in interpreting ambiguity and figurative language. Further, Lewis *et al.* (1998) reported that, when the subjects with Parkinson's disease were divided into groups based on their score on a cognitive rating scale, those individuals with below normal cognitive status presented with a larger range of language impairments than those persons with normal cognitive status. The former group presented with deficits in naming, definition and multidefinition abilities, as well as problems in interpreting ambiguity and figurative language, sentence construction and semantic verbal fluency. In contrast, the subjects with Parkinson's disease and normal cognitive status presented with problems in providing definitions and in sentence construction alone. Based on their findings, Lewis *et al.* (1998) concluded that the difficulties inherent in idiopathic Parkinson's disease go well beyond the motoric sphere that affects ambulation and motor speech production.

Individuals with Parkinson's disease are, in general, able to perform basic receptive and expressive language functions such as the recognition and repetition of single words and simple sentences, and the naming of common objects, in a normal manner. However, language deficits are frequently observed on those tasks that place increasing demands on both the semantic and the syntactic subcomponents of the linguistic system. Indeed, researchers have demonstrated that the integrity of semantic processing may be compromised in Parkinson's disease (Bayles *et al.*, 1993; Randolph *et al.*, 1993). As previously mentioned, there is considerable evidence to suggest that verbal fluency and complex sentence comprehension are impaired in Parkinson's disease (Grossman, 1999; Gurd, Master and Oliveira, 2001). A number of researchers have reported reductions in the grammatical complexity and informative content of the sentences and discourse produced by non-demented persons with Parkinson's disease (Cummings *et al.*, 1988; Illes *et al.*, 1988; Murray, 1998). In addition, Parkinson's disease related performance decrements have been identified on tasks of verbal and semantic reasoning (Bayles, 1990; Cohen *et al.*, 1994; Lewis *et al.*, 1998; Portin *et al.*, 2000).

Although some language difficulty is evident, patients with Parkinson's disease do not exhibit a language disorder that resembles one of the classic aphasia syndromes seen after stroke. Since the turn of the century, a limited number of studies based on on-line semantic priming tasks have demonstrated the presence of impaired lexical semantic processing in individuals with Parkinson's disease possibly resulting from disruption to the neuromodulatory role of dopamine as an outcome of neural dopamine depletion (Arnott *et al.*, 2001; Angwin *et al.*, 2004). Collectively, these findings suggest that enlightened clinical management of individuals with Parkinson's disease should include an awareness, a sensitivity and perhaps an appropriate clinical intervention plan for the cognitive linguistic deficits that these individuals are likely to present.

Language disorders in Huntington's disease

Huntington's disease is an autosomal-dominant, neurodegenerative disorder associated with neuropathological changes that are most marked in the head of the caudate nucleus, and to a lesser extent the putamen and globus pallidus (Zakzanis, 1998), suggesting that at least part of any language impairments found in patients with this condition may result from non-thalamic subcortical pathology. The cause of the language impairment in Huntington's disease, however, has been a point of contention (Podoll *et al.*, 1988; Wallesch and Fehrenbach, 1988). Specifically, it has been suggested that language deficits in Huntington's disease are the result of the general cognitive impairment and/or dementia associated with the disease and it has been questioned whether the language disturbances in Huntington's disease are a consequence of damage to the subcortical structures.

Recent studies involving investigation of complex language tasks have demonstrated that the language profile in Huntington's disease is essentially the same as that observed in persons with striatocapsular lesions of vascular origin, suggesting that a signatory language impairment is associated with damage to the striatocapsular region of the brain irrespective of whether such damage results from acute focal lesions or degenerative conditions such as Huntington's disease. Chenery, Copland and Murdoch (2002) compared the language profiles of a group of patients with Huntington's disease with those of a group of persons with striatocapsular lesions due to cerebrovascular accidents. Both groups of subjects were administered a comprehensive battery of standardized language tests that assessed both primary and more complex language abilities. They reported that patients with Huntington's disease exhibited deficits on complex language tasks primarily involving lexical semantic operations, on both single-word and sentence-level generative tasks, and on tasks which required interpretation of ambiguous, figurative and inferential meaning. Further, Chenery, Copland and Murdoch (2002) reported that the difficulties that patients with Huntington's disease experienced with tasks assessing complex language abilities were strikingly similar, both qualitatively and quantitatively, to the language profile produced by subjects with striatocapsular vascular lesions. They concluded that their results provided evidence to suggest that a signature language profile is associated with damage to the striatocapsular region of the brain resulting from either focal neurological insult or a degenerative condition such as Huntington's disease. In a follow-up study designed to investigate the impact of subcortical disturbances on complex language formulation tasks, Jensen, Chenery and Copland (2006) also reported that the language profiles of patients with Huntington's disease and subjects with striatocapsular lesions of vascular origin were similar in nature and severity, with the only difference being the presence of a syntactic impairment in the group with Huntington's disease. These latter authors suggested that the syntactic deficit in the patients with Huntington's disease might have reflected a compensatory syntactic strategy related to the presence of dysarthria or generalized cognitive deficits associated with Huntington's disease rather than a primary language disturbance, but conceded that this explanation requires confirmation.

Summary

Although it has been recognized that lesions involving subcortical structures such as the basal ganglia and cerebellum are associated with motor impairments, including motor speech disorders, for more than a century, it is only relatively recently that attention has been directed at the potential role of these subcortical structures in language processing. Although controversy still exists as to whether the structures of the striatocapsular region and the cerebellum participate directly in language processing or play a role as supporting structures for language, contemporary theories suggest that, as in the case of motor functions, the role of subcortical structures in language is essentially neuroregulatory. Evidence based on neuroanatomical, clinical and functional neuroimaging studies indicates that speech-language functions are mediated by complex, segregated neural circuits that comprise networks linking activity in many parts of the brain, at both the cortical and subcortical level, with subcortical structures such as the basal ganglia and cerebellum representing important relays in these complex pathways.

In recent years, further evidence to support a role for subcortical structures in language function has come from studies of language function in patients with circumscribed surgical lesions in subcortical structures such as the globus pallidus and subthalamic nucleus. In addition, the recent identification of high-level language impairments in patients with degenerative subcortical conditions such as Parkinson's and Huntington's disease has added further to the body of evidence implicating subcortical structures in language processing.

References

Alexander, G.E., Crutcher, M.D. and De Long, M.R. (1990) Basal ganglia-thalamocortical circuits: parallel substrates of motor, oculomotor, prefrontal and limbic functions. *Progress in Brain Research*, **85**, 119–146.

Alexander, G.E., De Long, M.R. and Strick, P.L. (1986) Parallel organization of functionally segregated circuits linking basal ganglia and cortex. *Annual Review of Neuroscience*, **9**, 357–381.

Alexander, G.E., Naeser, M.A. and Palumbo, C.L. (1987) Correlations of subcortical CT lesion sites and aphasia profiles. *Brain*, **110**, 961–991.

Alexander, M.P. (1989) Clinico-anatomical correlations of aphasia following predominantly subcortical lesions, in *Handbook of Neuropsychology* (eds F. Boller and J. Grafman), Elsevier, Amsterdam, pp. 47–66.

Alexander, M.P. (1992) Speech and language deficits after subcortical lesions of the left hemisphere: a clinical CT and PET study, in *Neuropsychological Disorders Associated with Subcortical Lesions* (eds G. Vallar, S.F. Cappa and C.-W. Wallesch), Oxford University Press, Oxford, pp. 455–477.

Alexander, M.P. and Lo Verme, S.R. (1980) Aphasia after left hemisphere intra-cerebral hemorrhage. *Neurology*, **30**, 1193–1202.

Angwin, A.J., Chenery, H.J., Copland, D.A. *et al.* (2004) Dopamine and semantic activation: an investigation of masked direct and indirect priming. *Journal of the International Neuropsychological Society*, **10**, 15–25.

Arnott, W.L., Chenery, H.J., Murdoch, B.E. and Silburn, P.A. (2001) Semantic priming in Parkinson's disease: evidence for delayed spreading activation. *Journal of Clinical and Experimental Neuropsychology*, **23**, 502–519.

Auriacombe, S., Grossman, M., Carvell, S. *et al.* (1993) Verbal fluency deficits in Parkinson's disease. *Neuropsychology*, **7**, 182–192.

Baron, J.C., D'Antona, R., Pantano, P. *et al.* (1986) Effects of thalamic stroke on energy metabolism in the cerebral cortex. *Brain*, **109**, 1243–1259.

Baron, J.C., Levasseur, M., Mazoyer, B. *et al.* (1992) Thalamo-cortical diaschisis: PET study in humans. *Journal of Neurology, Neurosurgery and Psychiatry*, **55**, 935–942.

Basso, A., Della Sala, S. and Farabola, M. (1987) Aphasia arising from purely deep lesions. *Cortex*, **23**, 29–44.

Bayles, K.A. (1990) Language and Parkinson's disease. *Alzheimer's Disease and Associated Disorders*, **4**, 171–180.

Bayles, K.A., Trosset, M.W., Tomeoda, C.K. *et al.* (1993) Generative naming in Parkinson's disease. *Journal of Clinical and Experimental Neuropsychology*, **15**, 547–562.

Beatty, W.W. and Monson, N. (1989) Lexical processing in Parkinson's disease and multiple sclerosis. *Journal of Geriatric Psychiatry and Neurology*, **2**, 145–152.

Beldarrain, M.G., Garcia-Monco, J.C., Quintana, J.M. *et al.* (1997) Diaschisis and neuropsychological performance after cerebellar stroke. *European Neurology*, **37**, 82–89.

Benson, D.F. (1979) Neurologic correlates of anomia, in *Studies in Neurolinguistics* (eds H. Whitaker and H.A. Whitaker), Academic Press, New York, pp. 293–328.

Bloedel, J.R. and Bracha, V. (1997) Duality of cerebellar motor and cognitive functions, in *International Review of Neurobiology: the Cerebellum and Cognition*, vol. **41** (ed. J.D. Schmahmann), Academic Press, San Diego, pp. 613–634.

Blonder, L.X., Gur, R.E., Ruben, C.G. *et al.* (1989) Neuropsychological functioning in hemiparkinsonism. *Brain and Cognition*, **9**, 244–257.

Bogousslavsky, J. (1994) Frontal stroke syndromes. *European Neurology*, **34**, 306–315.

Bondi, M.W., Kaszniak, A.W., Bayles, K.A. and Vance, K.T. (1993) Contributions of frontal system dysfunction to memory and perceptual abilities in Parkinson's disease. *Neuropsychology*, **7**, 89–102.

Broadbent, G. (1872) *On the Cerebral Mechanism of Speech and Thought*, Longmans, London.

Broca, P. (1861) Remarques sur le siège de la faculté du langage articulé, suivies d'une observation d'aphémie (perte de la parole), *Bulletins de la Société d'anthropologie de Paris*, **2**, 235–238.

Broich, K., Hartmann, A., Biersack, H.J. and Horn, R. (1987) Crossed cerebro-cerebral diaschisis in a patient with cerebellar infarction. *Neuroscience Letters*, **83**, 7–12.

Cabeza, R. and Nyberg, L. (2000) Imaging cognition II: an empirical review of 275 PET and fMRI studies. *Journal of Cognitive Neuroscience*, **12**, 1–47.

Cappa, S.F. (1997) Subcortical aphasia: Still a useful concept? *Brain and Language*, **58**, 424–426.

Cappa, S.F., Cavallotti, G., Guidotti, M. *et al.* (1983) Subcortical aphasia: two clinical-CT scan correlation studies. *Cortex*, **19**, 227–241.

Cappa, S.F., Papagno, C., Vallar, G. and Vignolo, L.A. (1986) Aphasia does not always follow left thalamic hemorrhage: a study of five negative cases. *Cortex*, **22**, 639–647.

Cappa, S.F. and Sterzi, R. (1990) Infarction in the territory of the anterior choroidal artery: a cause of transcortical motor aphasia. *Aphasiology*, **4**, 213–217.

Cappa, S.F. and Vallar, G. (1992) Neuropsychological disorders after subcortical lesions: implications for neural models of language and spatial attention, in *Neuropsychological Disorders Associated with Subcortical Lesions* (eds G. Valler, S.F. Cappa and C-W. Wallesch), Oxford University Press, Oxford, pp. 7–41.

Cappa, S.F. and Vignolo, L.A. (1979) Transcortical features of aphasia following left thalamic haemorrhage. *Cortex*, **15**, 121–130.

Cappa, S.F. and Wallesch, C.-W. (1994) Subcortical lesions and cognitive deficits, in *Localisation and Neuroimaging in Neuropsychology* (ed. A. Kertesz), Academic Press, San Diego, pp. 545–566.

Cheek, W.R. and Taveras, J. (1966) Thalamic tumours. *Journal of Neurosurgery*, **24**, 505–513.

Chenery, H.J., Copland, D.A. and Murdoch, B.E. (2002) Complex language function and subcortical mechanisms: evidence from Huntington's disease and patients with non-thalamic subcortical lesions. *International Journal of Language and Communication Disorders*, **37**, 459–474.

Chesson, A.L. (1983) Aphasia following right thalamic hemorrhage. *Brain and Language*, **19**, 306–316.

Ciemens, V.A. (1970) Localized thalamic hemorrhage: a cause of aphasia. *Neurology*, **20**, 776–782.

Cohen, H., Baichard, S., Scherzer, P. and Whitaker, H. (1994) Language and verbal reasoning in Parkinson's disease. *Neuropsychiatry, Neuropsychology and Behavioral Neurology*, **7**, 166–175.

Cook, M., Murdoch, B.E., Cahill, L. and Whelan, B.-M. (2004) Higher-level language deficits resulting from left primary cerebellar lesions. *Aphasiology*, **18**, 771–784.

Cooper, J.A., Sagar, H.J., Jordan, N. *et al.* (1991) Cognitive impairment in early, untreated Parkinson's disease and its relationship to motor disability. *Brain*, **114**, 2095–2122.

Crosson, B. (1985) Subcortical function in language: a working model. *Brain and Language*, **25**, 257–292.

Crosson, B. (1992) *Subcortical Functions in Language and Memory*, The Guilford Press, New York.

Crosson, B., Benefield, H., Cato, M.A. *et al.* (2003) Left and right basal ganglia and frontal activity during language generation: contributions to lexical, semantic and phonological processes. *Journal of the International Neuropsychological Society*, **9**, 1061–1077.

Crosson, B. and Nadeau, S.E. (1998) The role of subcortical structures in linguistic processes: recent developments, in *Handbook of Neurolinguistics* (eds B. Stemmer and H.A. Whitaker), Academic Press, San Diego, pp. 431–445.

Crosson, B., Sadek, J.R., Bobholz, J.A. *et al.* (1999) Activity in the paracingulate and cingulate sulci during word generation: an fMRI study of functional anatomy. *Cerebral Cortex*, **9**, 307–316.

Crosson, B., Zawacki, T., Brinson, G. *et al.* (1997) Models of subcortical functions in language: current status. *Journal of Neurolinguistics*, **10**, 277–300.

Cummings, J.L., Darkins, A., Mendez, M. *et al.* (1988) Alzheimer's disease and Parkinson's disease: comparison of speech and language alternations. *Neurology*, **38**, 680–684.

Damasio, A.R., Damasio, H., Rizzo, M. *et al.* (1982) Aphasia with non-hemorrhagic lesions in the basal ganglia and internal capsule. *Archives of Neurology*, **29**, 15–20.

Dejerine, J. and Roussy, G. (1906) Le syndrome thalamique. *Revue Neurologique*, **14**, 521–532.

De Reuck, J., Decoo, D., Lemanhieu, U. *et al.* (1995) Ipsilateral thalamic diaschisis after middle cerebral artery infarction. *Journal of Neurological Science*, **134**, 130–135.

D'Esposito, M. and Alexander, M.P. (1995) Subcortical aphasia: distinct profiles following left putaminal hemorrhage. *Neurology*, **45**, 38–41.

Docking, K., Murdoch, B.E. and Suppiah, R. (2007) The impact of a cerebellar tumour on language function in childhood. *Folia Phoniatrica et Logopaedica*, **59**, 190–200.

Docking, K., Murdoch, B.E. and Ward, E.C. (2003) Cerebellar language and cognitive functions in childhood: a comparative review of the clinical research. *Aphasiology*, **17**, 1153–1161.

Dronkers, N.F., Shapiro, J.K., Redfern, B. and Knight, R.T. (1992) The role of Broca's area in Broca's aphasia. *Journal of Clinical and Experimental Neuropsychology*, **14**, 198.

Dubois, B., Boller, F., Pillon, B. and Agid, Y. (1991) Cognitive deficits in Parkinson's disease, in *Handbook of Neuropsychology*, vol. 5 (eds F. Boller and J. Grefman), Elsevier, New York, pp. 195–239.

Fabbro, F. (2000) Introduction to language and the cerebellum. *Journal of Neurolinguistics*, **13**, 83–94.

Fabbro, F., Clarici, A. and Bava, A. (1996) Effects of left basal ganglia lesions on language production. *Perceptual and Motor Skills*, **82**, 1291–1298.

Fiez, J.A., Petersen, S.E., Cheny, M.K. and Raichle, M.E. (1992) Impaired non-motor learning and error detection associated with cerebellar damage. *Brain*, **115**, 155–178.

Fisher, C.M. (1959) The pathologic and clinical aspects of thalamic hemorrhage. *Transections of the American Neurological Association*, **84**, 56–59.

Fox, M.W., Ahlskog, J.E. and Kelly, P.J. (1991) Stereotaxic ventrolateralis thalamotomy for medically refractory tremor in post-levodopa era Parkinson's disease patients. *Journal of Neurosurgery*, **75**, 723–730.

Frank, E.M., McDade, H.L. and Scott, W.K. (1996) Naming in dementia secondary to Parkinson's, Huntington's and Alzheimer's diseases. *Journal of Communication Disorders*, **29**, 183–197.

Fukuda, M., Kameyama, S., Yoshino, M. *et al.* (2000) Neuropsychological outcome following pallidotomy and thalamotomy for Parkinson's disease. *Stereotactic and Functional Neurosurgery*, **74**, 11–20.

Gall, F.J. (1809) *Recherches sur le Système Nerveux*, Baillière, Paris.

Geyer, H.L. and Grossman, M. (1994) Investigating the basis for the sentence comprehension deficit in Parkinson's disease. *Journal of Neurolinguistics*, **8**, 191–205.

Gorelick, P.B., Hier, D.B., Benevento, L. *et al.* (1984) Aphasia after left thalamic infarction. *Archives of Neurology*, **41**, 1296–1298.

Graff-Radford, N.R., Eslinger, P.J., Damasio, A.R. and Yamada, T. (1984) Non-haemorrhagic infarction of the thalamus: behaviour, anatomic and physiological correlates. *Neurology*, **34**, 14–23.

Graybiel, A.M. and Kimura, M. (1995) Adaptive neural networks in the basal ganglia, in *Models of Information Processing in the Basal Ganglia* (eds J.C. Houk, J.L. Davis and D.G. Beiser), MIT Press, Cambridge, pp. 103–116.

Grossman, M. (1999) Sentence processing in Parkinson's disease. *Brain and Cognition*, **40**, 387–413.

Gurd, J.M., Master, N. and Oliveira, R.M. (2001) A method for investigating the relationship between cognitive and motor functions in Parkinson's disease. *Journal of Neurolinguistics*, **14**, 45–57.

Han, M., Kang, D., Bae, H. *et al.* (2003) Aphasia in striatocapsular infarction may be explained by concomitant small cortical infarctions of cortical language zones. *Stroke*, **34**, 259.

Henschen, S.E. (1922) *Klinische und Anatomishe Beitrage zur Pathologic des Gehirns*, Almquisét and Wiksell, Stockholm.

Hillemand, P. (1925) *Contribution à l'étude des Syndromes Thalamiques*, Thèse, Paris.

Hillis, A.E., Barker, P.B., Wityk, R.J. *et al.* (2004) Variability in subcortical aphasia is due to variable sites of cortical hypoperfusion. *Brain and Language*, **89**, 524–530.

Hillis, A.E., Kane, A., Tuffiash, E. *et al.* (2002) Reperfusion of specific brain regions by raising blood pressure restores selective language function in subacute stroke. *Brain and Language*, **79**, 495–510.

Illes, J., Metter, E.J., Hanson, W.R. and Iritani, S. (1988) Language production in Parkinson's disease: acoustic and linguistic considerations. *Brain and Language*, **33**, 146–160.

Jensen, A.M., Chenery, H.J. and Copland, D.A. (2006) A comparison of picture description abilities in individuals with vascular subcortical lesions and Huntington's disease. *Journal of Communication Disorders*, **39**, 62–77.

Karussis, D., Leker, R.R. and Abramsky, O. (2000) Cognitive function following thalamic stroke: a study of 16 cases and review of the literature. *Journal of the Neurological Sciences*, **172**, 25–29.

Keele, S.W. and Ivry, R. (1991) Does the cerebellum provide a common computation for diverse tasks? A timing hypothesis, in *The Developmental and Neural Basis of Higher Cognitive Functions* (ed. A. Diamond), New York Academy of Sciences, New York, pp. 179–211.

Kennedy, M. and Murdoch, B.E. (1989) Speech and language disorders subsequent to subcortical vascular lesions. *Aphasiology*, **3**, 221–247.

Kennedy, M. and Murdoch, B.E. (1990) Cortical dysfunction subsequent to subcortical vascular lesions: An explanation for subcortical aphasia? *Journal of Neurolinguistics*, **5**, 31–54.

Kennedy, M. and Murdoch, B.E. (1993) Chronic aphasia subsequent to striato-capsular and thalamic lesions in the left hemisphere. *Brain and Language*, **44**, 284–295.

Kirk, A. and Kertesz, A. (1994) Cortical and subcortical aphasia compared. *Aphasiology*, **8**, 65–82.

Kirshner, H.S. and Kistler, K.H. (1982) Aphasia after right thalamic hemorrhage. *Archives of Neurology*, **39**, 667–669.

Lassen, N.A., Olsen, T., Hojgaard, K. and Skriver, E. (1983) Incomplete infarction: a CT negative irreversible ischaemic brain lesion. *Journal of Cerebral Blood Flow and Metabolism*, **3** (Suppl. 1), 602–603.

Leiner, H.C., Leiner, A.L. and Dow, R.S. (1986) Does the cerebellum contribute to mental skills? *Behavioural Neuroscience*, **100**, 443–454.

Leiner, H.C., Leiner, A.L. and Dow, R.S. (1991) The human cerebro-cerebellar system: its computing, cognitive and language skills. *Behavioral Brain Research*, **24**, 113–128.

Leiner, H.C., Leiner, A.L. and Dow, R.S. (1993) Cognitive language functions of the human cerebellum. *Trends in Neuroscience*, **16**, 444–447.

Levin, B.E. and Katzen, H.L. (1995) Early cognitive changes and nondementing behavioral abnormalities in Parkinson's disease. *Behavioral Neurology of Movement Disorders*, **65**, 85–95.

Lewis, F.M., La Pointe, L.L., Murdoch, B.E. and Chenery, H.J. (1998) Language impairment in Parkinson's disease. *Aphasiology*, **12**, 193–206.

Lhermitte, J. (1936) Symptomatologie de l'hémorragie du thalamus. *Revue Neurologique*, **65**, 89–93.

Lhermitte, J. (1984) Language disorders and their relationship to thalamic lesions. *Advances in Neurology*, **42**, 99–113.

Lichtheim, L. (1885) On aphasia. *Brain*, 7, 433–484.

Lieberman, P. (2000) *Human Language and our Reptilian Brain: the Subcortical Bases of Speech, Syntax and Thought*, Harvard University Press, Cambridge, MA.

Lombardi, W.J., Gross, R.E., Trepanier, L.L. *et al.* (2000) Relationship of lesion location to cognitive outcome following microelectrode-guided pallidotomy for Parkinson's disease: support for the existence of cognitive circuits in the human pallidum. *Brain*, 123, 746–758.

Luria, A.R. (1977) On quasi-aphasic speech disturbances in lesions of the deep structures of the brain. *Brain and Language*, 4, 432–459.

Malapani, C., Pillon, B., Dubois, B. and Agid, Y. (1994) Impaired simultaneous cognitive task performance in Parkinson's disease: a dopamine-related dysfunction. *Neurology*, 44, 319–326.

Marie, P. (1906) The third left frontal convolution plays no special role in the function of language, in *Pierre Marie's Papers on Speech Disorders* (eds M.F. Cole and M. Cole), Hafner, New York, 1971.

Marien, P., Engelborghs, S., Fabbro, F. and DeDeyn, P.P. (2001) The lateralized linguistic cerebellum: a review and a new hypothesis. *Brain and Language*, 79, 580–600.

Matison, R., Mayeux, R., Rosen, J. and Fahn, S. (1982) 'Tip of the tongue' phenomenon in Parkinson's disease. *Neurology*, 32, 567–570.

McFarling, D., Rothi, L.J. and Heilman, K.M. (1982) Transcortical aphasia from ischaemic infarcts of the thalamus: a report of two cases. *Journal of Neurology, Neurosurgery and Psychiatry*, 45, 107–112.

Mega, M.S. and Alexander, M.P. (1994) Subcortical aphasia: the core profile of capsulostriatal infarction. *Neurology*, 44, 1824–1829.

Mesulam, M.M. (1990) Large-scale neurocognitive networks and distributed processing for attention, language and memory. *Annals of Neurology*, 28, 597–613.

Mesulam, M.M. (2000) Behavioural neuroanatomy: large scale networks, association cortex, frontal syndromes, the limbic system, and hemispheric specialisations, in *Principles of Behavioural and Cognitive Neurology* (ed. M. Mesulam), Oxford University Press, Oxford, pp. 1–120.

Metter, E.J., Riege, W.H., Hanson, W.R. *et al.* (1983) Comparison of metabolic rates, language and memory in subcortical aphasias. *Brain and Language*, 19, 33–47.

Middleton, F.A. and Strick, P.L. (1997) Dentate output channels: motor and cognitive components. *Progress in Brain Research*, 114, 555–568.

Middleton, F.A. and Strick, P.L. (2000) Basal ganglia output and cognition: evidence from anatomical, behavioural and clinical studies. *Brain and Cognition*, 42, 183–200.

Mohr, J.P., Watters, W.C. and Duncan, G.W. (1975) Thalamic hemorrhage and aphasia. *Brain and Language*, 2, 3–17.

Monakow, C. (1914) *Die Lokalisation in Grosshirn*, Bergmann, Wiesbaden.

Moutier, F. (1908) *L'aphasie de Broca*. Doctoral dissertation, Paris.

Murdoch, B.E. (1987) Aphasia following right thalamic hemorrhage in a dextral. *Journal of Communication Disorders*, 20, 459–468.

Murdoch, B.E. (1990) *Acquired Speech and Language Disorders: a Neuroanatomical and Functional Neurological Approach*, Chapman & Hall, London.

Murdoch, B.E. (1996) The role of subcortical structures in language: clinico-neuroradiological studies of brain damaged subjects, in *Evaluating Theories of Language: Evidence from Disordered Communication* (eds B. Dodd, R. Campbell and L. Worrall), Whurr Publishers, London, pp. 137–160.

Murdoch, B.E., Theodoros, D., Fraser, W. and Harrision, L. (1986) Aphasia following non-haemorrhagic lesions in the left striato-capsular region. *Australian Journal of Human Communication Disorders*, 14, 5–21.

Murdoch, B.E. and Whelan, B-M. (2007) Language disorders subsequent to left cerebellar lesions: a case for bilateral cerebellar involvement in language? *Folia Phoniatrica et Logopaedica*, 59, 184–189.

Murdoch, B.E., Whelan, B.-M. and Theodoros, D.G. (2003) Subcortical aphasia: evidence from stereotactic surgical lesions, in *The Sciences of Aphasia: from Theory to Therapy* (eds I. Papathanasiou and R. De Bleser), Pergamon, Oxford, pp. 65–92.

Murray, L. (1998) Productive syntax in adults with Huntington's or Parkinson's disease: preliminary analyses. *Brain and Language*, 65, 36–39.

Nadeau, S.E. and Crosson, B. (1997a) Subcortical aphasia. *Brain and Language*, 58, 355–402.

Nadeau, S.E. and Crosson, B. (1997b) Subcortical aphasia: response to reviews. *Brain and Language*, 58, 436–458.

Naeser, M.A., Alexander, G.E., Helm-Estabrooks, N. *et al.* (1982) Aphasia with predominantly subcortical lesion sites: description of three capsular/putaminal aphasia syndromes. *Archives of Neurology*, **39**, 2–14.

Naeser, M.A., Palumbo, C.L., Helm-Estabrooks, N. *et al.* (1989) Severe non-fluency in aphasia: role of the medial subcallosal fasciculus and other white matter pathways in the recovery of spontaneous speech. *Brain*, **112**, 1–38.

Nagaratnam, N., McNeil, C. and Gilhotra, J.S. (1999) Akinetic mutism and mixed transcortical aphasia following left thalamo-mesencephalic infarction. *Journal of Neurological Sciences*, **163**, 70–73.

Nielsen, J.M. (1946) *Agnosia, Apraxia, Aphasia*, Hoeber, New York.

Nieoullon, A. (2002) Dopamine and the regulation of cognition and attention. *Progress in Neurobiology*, **67**, 53–83.

Ojemann, G. (1976) Subcortical language mechanisms, in *Studies in Neurolinguistics* (eds H.A. Whitaker and H. Whitaker), Academic Press, New York, pp. 103–138.

Ojemann, G. (1977) Asymmetric function of the thalamus in man. *Annals of the New York Academy of Science*, **299**, 380–396.

Ojemann, G. (1983) Brain organization for language from the perspective of electrical stimulation mapping. *Behavioural and Brain Sciences*, **2**, 189–230.

Panchal, V.G., Parikh, V.R. and Karapurkar, A.P. (1974) Thalamic abscesses. *Neurology (India)*, **22**, 106–110.

Penfield, W. and Roberts, L. (1959) *Speech and Brain Mechanisms*, Princeton University Press, Princeton.

Perani, D., Vallar, G., Cappa, S.F. *et al.* (1987) Aphasia and neglect after subcortical stroke: a clinical/cerebral perfusion correlation study. *Brain*, **110**, 1211–1229.

Petersen, P.M., Fox, P.T., Posner, M.I. *et al.* (1989) Positron emission tomographic studies of the processing of single words. *Journal of Cognitive Neuroscience*, **1**, 153–170.

Podoll, K., Caspary, P., Lange, H.W. and North, J. (1988) Language functions in Huntington's disease. *Brain*, **111**, 1475–1503.

Portin, R., Laatu, S., Revonsuo, A. and Rinne, U.K. (2000) Impairment of semantic knowledge in Parkinson's disease. *Archives of Neurology*, **57**, 1338–1343.

Price, C.J., Moore, C., Humphreys, G.W. *et al.* (1996a) The neural signs sustaining object recognition and naming. *Proceedings of the Royal Society of London, B*, **263**, 1501–1507.

Price, C.J., Wise, R.J., Warburton, E.A. *et al.* (1996b) Hearing and saying: the functional neuroanatomy of auditory word processing. *Brain*, **119**, 919–931.

Puel, M., Demonet, J.F., Cardebat, D. *et al.* (1984) Aphasies sous-corticales: etude neurolinguistique avec scanner X de 25 cas. *Revue Neurologique*, **140**, 695–710.

Radanovic, M. and Scaff, M. (2003) Speech and language disturbances due to subcortical lesions. *Brain and Language*, **84**, 337–352.

Randolph, C., Braun, A.R., Goldberg, T.E. and Chase, T.N. (1993) Semantic fluency in Alzheimer's, Parkinson's and Huntington's disease: dissociation of storage and retrieval failures. *Neuropsychology*, **7**, 83–88.

Raskin, S.A., Sliwinski, M. and Borod, J.C. (1992) Clustering strategies on tasks of verbal fluency in Parkinson's disease. *Neuropsychologia*, **30**, 95–99.

Reynolds, A.F., Turner, P.T., Harris, A.B. *et al.* (1979) Left thalamic hemorrhage with dysphasia: a report of five cases. *Brain and Language*, **7**, 62–73.

Riklan, M. and Cooper, I.S. (1975) Psychometric studies of verbal functions following thalamic lesions in humans. *Brain and Language*, **2**, 45–64.

Riklan, M. and Levita E. (1970) Psychological studies of thalamic lesions in humans. *Journal of Nervous and Mental Disorders*, **150**, 251–265.

Sandson, T.A., Daffner, K.R., Carvalho, P.A. and Mesulam, M.M. (1991) Frontal lobe dysfunction following infarction of the left-sided medial thalamus. *Archives of Neurology*, **48**, 1300–1303.

Schuell, H., Jenkins, J.J. and Jimenez-Pabon, E. (1965) *Aphasia in Adults*, Harper Row, New York.

Scott, R.B., Harrison, J., Boulton, C. *et al.* (2002) Global attentional-executive sequelae following surgical lesions to globus pallidus interna. *Brain*, **125**, 565–574.

Silveri, M.C., Leggio, M.G. and Molinari, M. (1994) The cerebellum contributes to linguistic production: a case of agrammatic speech following a right cerebellar lesion. *Neurology*, **44**, 2047–2050.

Skyhøj-Olsen, T., Bruhn, P. and Öberg, R.G. (1986) Cortical hypoperfusion as a possible cause of subcortical aphasia. *Brain*, **106**, 393–410.

Smyth, G.E. and Stern, K. (1938) Tumours of the thalamus: a clinicopathological study. *Brain*, **61**, 339–360.

Starr, P.A., Vitek, J.L. and Bakay, R.A.E. (1998) Ablative surgery and deep brain stimulation for Parkinson's disease. *Neurosurgery*, **43**, 989–1105.

Stuss, D.T. and Benson, D.F. (1986) *The Frontal Lobes*, Raven, New York.

Trepanier, L.L., Saint-Cyr, J.A., Lozano, A.M. and Lang, A.E. (1998) Neuropsychological consequences of posteroventral pallidotomy for the treatment of Parkinson's disease. *Neurology*, **51**, 207–215.

Vallar, G., Papagno, C. and Cappa, S.F. (1988) Latent dysphasia after left hemispheric lesions: a lexical-semantic and verbal memory deficit. *Aphasiology*, **2**, 463–478.

Van Buren, J.M. and Borke, R.C. (1969) Alterations in speech and the pulvinar: a serial section study of cerebrothalamic relationships in cases of acquired speech disorders. *Brain*, **92**, 255–284.

Van Hoesen, G.W., Yeterian, E.H. and Lavizzo-Mourey, R. (1981) Widespread cortico-striate projections from temporal cortex of the Rhesus monkey. *Journal of Comparative Neurology*, **199**, 205–219.

Von Monakow, C. (1914) *Die Lokalisation im Grosshirn und der Abbau der Funktionen Durch Corticale Herde*, Bergmann, Wiesbaden.

Wallesch, C.-W. (1985) Two syndromes of aphasia occurring within ischaemic lesions involving the left basal ganglia. *Brain and Language*, **25**, 357–361.

Wallesch, C.-W. (1997) Symptomatology of subcortical aphasia. *Journal of Neurolinguistics*, **10**, 267–275.

Wallesch, C.-W. and Fehrenbach, R.A. (1988) On the neurolinguistic nature of language abnormalities in Huntington's disease. *Journal of Neurology, Neurosurgery and Psychiatry*, **51**, 367–373.

Wallesch, C.-W., Kornhuber, H.H., Brunner, R.J. *et al.* (1983) Lesions of the basal ganglia, thalamus and deep white matter: differential effects on language function. *Brain and Language*, **20**, 286–304.

Wallesch, C.-W. and Papagno, C. (1988) Subcortical aphasia, in *Aphasia* (eds F.C. Rose, R. Whurr and M.A. Wyke), Whurr Publishers, London, pp. 256–287.

Warburton, E., Wise, R.J.S., Price, C.J. *et al.* (1996) Noun and verb retrieval by normal subjects: studies with PET. *Brain*, **119**, 159–179.

Weiller, C., Ringelstein, E.B., Reiche, W. *et al.* (1990) The large striatocapsular infarct: a clinical and pathological entity. *Archives of Neurology*, **47**, 1085–1091.

Weiller, C., Willmes, K., Reiche, W. *et al.* (1993) The case of aphasia or neglect after striatocapsular infarction. *Brain*, **116**, 1509–1525.

Wernicke, C. (1874) *De Aphasische Symtomencomplex*, Cohn & Weigert, Breslau.

Whelan, B.-M., Murdoch, B.E. and Theodoros, D.G. (2003) Defining a role for the subthalamic nucleus with operative theoretical models of subcortical participation in language. *Journal of Neurology, Neurosurgery and Psychiatry*, **74**, 1543–1550.

Whelan, B.-M., Murdoch, B.E., Theodoros, D.G. *et al.* (2002) Role for the thalamus in language? A linguistic comparison of 2 cases subsequent to unilateral thalamotomy procedures in the dominant and non-dominant hemispheres. *Aphasiology*, **16**, 1213–1226.

Whelan, B.-M., Murdoch, B.E., Theodoros, D.G. *et al.* (2004a). Re-appraising contemporary theories of subcortical participation in language: proposing an interhemispheric regulatory function for the subthalamic nucleus in the mediation of high level linguistic processing. *Neurocase*, **10**, 345–352.

Whelan, B.-M., Murdoch, B.E., Theodoros, D.G. *et al.* (2004b). Redefining functional models of basal ganglia organization: a role for the posteroventral pallidum in linguistic processing. *Movement Disorders*, **19**, 1267–1278.

Whelan, B.-M., Murdoch, B.E., Theodoros, D.G. *et al.* (2000) Towards a better understanding of the role of subcortical nuclei participation in language. The study of a case following bilateral pallidotomy. *Asia Pacific Journal of Speech, Language and Hearing*, **5**, 93–112.

Wilson, S.A.K. (1925) Disorders of motility and muscle tone with special reference to the striatum. *Lancet*, **2**, 1–10.

Zakzanis, K.K. (1998) The subcortical dementia of Huntington's disease. *Journal of Clinical and Experimental Neuropsychology*, **20**, 565–578.

Speech-language disorders associated with traumatic brain injury

4

Introduction

Traumatic brain injury (TBI) has been defined as 'an insult to the brain, not of the degenerative or congenital nature, but caused by an external force, that may produce a diminished or altered state of consciousness' (National Head Injury Foundation, 1985). According to this definition, TBI occurs only in those cases where the brain damage is caused by an external force and thereby excludes brain insult resulting from other neurological conditions such as cerebrovascular accidents, tumours, degenerative brain diseases (e.g. Parkinson's disease), demyelinating conditions (e.g. multiple sclerosis) and infectious disorders (e.g. encephalitis). TBI, therefore, is the consequence of a head injury in which the severity has been of sufficient magnitude to cause damage to the brain. Head injuries incurred in road traffic accidents, falls, sporting and industrial accidents or assaults are the most frequent causes of TBI in peacetime.

Communication impairments are commonly reported sequelae of TBI. Depending on the location of the damage in the nervous system, TBI may be associated with a variety of communication problems, including speech disorders, language disorders or both (Figure 4.1).

When present, communication impairments in the form of speech and/or language disorders have important negative implications for the long-term quality of life of survivors of TBI. Some authors have suggested that communication abilities may play the pivotal role in determining the quality of survival after head trauma (Najenson *et al.*, 1978). Certainly, the presence of a communication disorder reduces the individual's ability to function in situations that require normal receptive and expressive language abilities as well as understandable, efficient and natural-sounding speech (e.g. vocational positions that require independent interaction with the public). Put simply, the presence of a communication disorder in an adult following TBI may impede the successful return of the individual to study, work or general social activities, leading to academic failure, loss of vocational standing and social isolation. In the case of a child, following TBI, a communication disorder may affect the developmental process of the individual, leading to impairment of further acquisition of speech, language and social skills.

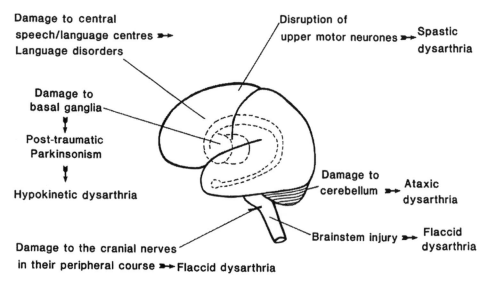

Figure 4.1 Speech and language disorders associated with traumatic brain injury.

Classification of traumatic brain injury

Brain injuries arising from head trauma are generally classified into two broad types: non-penetrating (closed) injuries and penetrating (open) brain injuries. In non-penetrating injuries, the membranes (meninges) covering the brain remain intact, even though the skull may be fractured. Penetrating, or open brain injuries, on the other hand, occur when the coverings of the brain are ruptured as a result of tearing of the dura mater by skull fragments, as may occur in depressed fractures of the skull or when the brain is penetrated by some missile such as a bullet or is lacerated by a depressed bone fragment(s). Non-penetrating brain injuries tend to be associated with diffuse brain pathology and represent by far the majority of traumatic head injuries incurred in civilian life. In contrast, penetrating head trauma tends to be associated with more focal brain pathology, although diffuse effects can also be observed, and is more common in wartime.

Historically, most of what we know about the effects of head injury on speech-language function has come from studies of patients who have sustained penetrating missile wounds in wartime (Russell and Espir, 1961; Luria, 1970). In most cases, these descriptions sought to connect a par-ticular speech or language disorder to a specific lesion site in the central nervous system. Reports in the literature have indicated that the prevalence of communication disorders in large groups of patients with open head trauma ranges from 14 to 23% (Hillbom, 1959; Teuber, 1975). In contrast to the open head wounds characteristic of war injuries, however, the majority of traumatic head injuries in civilian life are of the closed type, stemming mainly from motor vehicle accidents and affecting predominantly young adult males (Annegers *et al.*, 1980). Owing to the nature of the pathology, a number of authors have suggested that there may also be differences in the associated communication deficit between open versus closed head injuries (Hagen, Malkmus and Burditt, 1979). Luria (1970) reviewed 800 head injury cases and compared the speech-language deficits exhibited by closed head injury cases with those observed in patients with open head injuries. He concluded that there was no significant difference in the language abilities of each group immediately post-trauma. Groher (1983), however, conducted a closer analysis of Luria's results and found they indicated that open head injured patients exhibited language deficits for a longer period than did closed head injured patients. Further, the re-analysis showed that, in the initial period post-trauma, the patients with

Table 4.1   Glasgow Coma Scale (adapted from Teasdale and Jennett, 1974).

Eye Openings		Best Verbal Response		Best Motor Response	
4.	Spontaneous	5.	Orientated	6.	Responds to verbal commands
3.	Non-specific reaction to speech	4.	Confusion, disorientation	5.	Localized movement to terminate painful stimulus
2.	Response to painful stimulus	3.	No sustained or coherent conversation	4.	Withdrawal from painful stimulus
1.	No response	2.	No recognizable words	3.	Decorticate posture
		1.	No response	2.	Decerebrate posture
				1.	No response

closed head injury as a group suffered fewer communication deficits than patients with penetrating head wounds. From this re-analysis, it can be implied that closed head injured patients with communication deficits exhibit greater and faster improvement than those with open head injuries. Darley (1982) also reported a better prognosis for the language disorder following closed head injury than for the communication deficit associated with open head wounds.

TBI is also classified according to the level of severity, based on the level of altered consciousness experienced by the patient following the trauma. Altered-consciousness levels post trauma may vary from transient disorientation at one extreme to a deep coma at the other. A patient can be classified as having a mild, moderate or severe TBI, according to where their level of consciousness fits on this continuum. To date, however, medical professionals have not been able to agree on the measure of altered consciousness to be used in assigning severity levels to TBI. The most commonly used scale, the Glasgow Coma Scale (GCS), (Table 4.1) was developed by Teasdale and Jennett (1974, 1976) and involves estimation of the depth of coma as a measure of severity, within the first 24 hours of the trauma. The patient is assigned a score of between 3 and 15 on the GCS, with points being assigned in the categories of eye opening (ranging from four points for spontaneous eye opening to one point for no response), best motor response (from six points for obeying commands to one point for no response) and best verbal response (from five

points for oriented to one point for no response). The greater the score on the GCS, the more conscious the patient, with a total score of 13–15 representing a mild TBI, a score of 9–12 indicating a moderate TBI and a score of eight or less indicating a severe TBI.

As an alternative to the GCS, the severity of TBI is estimated by some medical personnel on the basis of the duration of post-traumatic amnesia (PTA) (Russell, 1932). PTA represents the period from the time the patient regains consciousness, but is still in a disoriented and confused state, until the time the patient's memory for ongoing events becomes reliable and accurate. According to the PTA classification system devised by Russell (1932), a mild TBI is one in which the period of coma plus subsequent PTA is less than one hour, a moderate TBI involves a period of coma and PTA of 1–24 hours' duration, a severe TBI involves a period of coma and PTA extending greater than seven days.

Epidemiology of traumatic brain injury

In a review of incidence studies carried out within the United States, Canada, Norway, Great Britain, China and Australia during the 1960s and 1980s, Naugle (1990) consistently found that an annual incidence rate of TBI of approximately 200 per 100 000 population was reported. Fortunately, it has been estimated that in the majority (82%) of head injury cases, the associated brain damage is either mild or non-existent (Kraus *et al.*, 1984), with the annual incidence of moderate or severe TBI being between 12–14/100 000 and 15–20/100 000 population respectively (Kraus *et al.*, 1984; Tate, McDonald and Lulham, 1998).

Research into the factors associated with the frequency with which TBI occurs, or the epidemiology of TBI, has identified a number of activities that are conducive to TBI (Naugle, 1990). Motor vehicle accidents appear to be the leading cause of TBI, followed by falls, assaults, sports and recreational activities (Naugle, 1990). For each of the causes, different age groups have been identified as being most susceptible. There appear to be three age groups associated with a peak in incidence of TBI (Beukelman and Yorkston, 1991; Finlayson and Garner, 1994). The first peak is early in life, below five years of age, with another peak in the elderly population, particularly in those over 75 years of age. Both peaks appear to be largely the result of falls (Naugle, 1990; Yorkston and Beukelman, 1991; McDonald, Togher and Code, 1999). The third, but most prominent peak in incidence has consistently been found to be in the age range of mid-adolescence to mid-twenties (Naugle, 1990; McDonald, Togher and Code, 1999), with the leading causes of TBI in this group being motor vehicle accidents and assaults (Naugle, 1990; McDonald, Togher and Code, 1999). Despite the fact that motor vehicle accidents may not be the most common cause of head injuries in children, reports are available to suggest that road traffic accidents may be the cause of most of the long-term morbidity and nearly all of the mortality in the paediatric population. In fact, it appears that in all age groups including both adults and children, the most common cause of head injury associated with acute neurological injury is a motor vehicle accident (Vernon-Levett, 1991). It is also noteworthy that the type of road traffic accidents experienced by children differ from those of adolescents and adults. Whereas this latter group are primarily involved in high-velocity motor vehicle accidents as drivers, children less than two years of age are almost exclusively injured as occupants of motor vehicles, while older children are primarily injured as pedestrians or cyclists.

Across all activities and across the entire age range, males appear to be at greater risk of TBI than females. The male to female ratio estimated in various studies has ranged from approximately 2 : 1 up to 4 : 1 as reviewed by Yorkston, Beukelman and Bell (1988), Naugle (1990) and McDonald, Togher and Code (1999). An especially high male/female ratio of 3–4 : 1 has been noted during mid-adolescence to early adulthood (Klauber *et al.*, 1981).

Biomechanics of head injury

Brain damage following traumatic head injury may be either focal, multifocal or diffuse in nature and may involve any part of the brain. Consequently, brain damage following head injury can be associated with a variety of communicative deficits depending primarily upon the location and extent of the lesion. In general, closed head injuries tend to produce more diffuse pathology, while open head injuries are usually associated with the more focal pathology.

The communication disorders, frequently associated with TBI are the result of complex biomechanical processes associated with a head injury. In order to understand the neuropathophysiological basis of these deficits, therefore, it is necessary to understand the basic mechanical forces involved in causing brain damage subsequent to closed head trauma. Briefly, the biomechanical forces involved in closed head injury include compression, acceleration/deceleration and rotational acceleration, which result in brain tissue being compressed, torn apart by the effects of tension and sheared by rotational forces (Murdoch, 1990).

According to Gennarelli (1993), the application of force to the head results in mechanical loading which sets off a cascade of physiological events. Mechanical loading can be initiated by either static or dynamic forces. Static loading results from slow or rapid forces applied to a stationary head so that it is crushed (e.g. compression of the head). The more common type of head injury, however, occurs following dynamic loading. This results from a very brief insult which has either been applied directly to the moveable head (impact) or by impacting elsewhere on the body causing a sudden movement of the head (impulsive) (e.g. whiplash injury sustained in rear-end motor vehicle collisions). Thus, a significant TBI can occur without the victim sustaining a direct blow to the head (Jennett, 1986).

Dynamic loading produces two main mechanical phenomena responsible for pathological changes in closed head injury: contact and inertial loading (acceleration) (Katz, 1992; Gennarelli, 1993). Contact loading is a direct result of an impact to the head and leads to local skull distortions or fractures, and contusions or laceration of the brain at the point of contact (i.e. coup contusions). The propagation of shock waves throughout the skull and brain can also occur and may result in small intracerebral haemorrhages in certain vulnerable areas.

Inertial loading (or acceleration), results from head motion generated by either impact or impulsive forces. This event results in translational or rotational acceleration (Pang, 1985; Gennarelli, 1993). Translational acceleration occurs when all parts of the body are similarly accelerated and there is no resultant relative movement taking place among the constituent parts of the brain (Pang, 1985). There is, however, differential movement between the brain and the skull during which the cortex may repeatedly impact against the sharp internal structures of the skull. The predominant injuries resulting from this mechanism are brain contusions which occur directly opposite the point of impact (i.e. contrecoup contusions).

Rotational acceleration occurs when the head receives a force which does not pass through its centre of gravity. This results in the head assuming an angular acceleration and rotating around its own centre of gravity. Such acceleration of the head results in a twisting motion between the brain and the skull and causes shear-strain or distortion of the brain tissue (Pang, 1985; Bigler, 1990). Such distortion of the brain tissue results in the permanent stretching or rupturing of neuronal fibres that interconnect different brain regions. The resultant damage is referred to as 'diffuse axonal injury' (DAI) and is widely distributed with most lesions occurring in deep white matter areas of the cerebral hemispheres and in the brainstem (Bigler, 1990).

The biomechanics of closed head injury are largely determined by the physical and structural properties of the skull and contents (Holbourn, 1943). The brain is a relatively mobile mass of material within a rigid container. Holbourn (1943) considered the most important physical properties of the brain to be its comparatively uniform density, its extreme incompressibility, its small resistance to change in shape and its high susceptibility to shear-strain damage. During rotational acceleration of the head, the brain does not compress but readily changes shape or distorts, in an attempt to follow the motion of the skull as it rotates about the brain resulting in shear-strain damage to the brain tissue. Holbourn (1943) described shear-strain distortion as the 'type of deformation which occurs in a pack of cards when it is deformed from a neat rectangular pile into an oblique-angled pile' (p. 438). He expounded the view that, following impacts that cause rotational acceleration of the head, shearing distortion takes place in all parts of the brain as it tries to follow the motion of the skull.

At the time of impact, as a result of external forces, the brain moves within the skull, making contact with its rigid walls, with the greatest degree of contact occurring between the soft frontal and temporal lobes and the bony prominences of the skull (e.g. sphenoidal ridge). Consequently, the skull–brain interface also has an important influence on the mechanics of head injury, particularly in relation to sites of lesion (Bigler, 1990). Anatomically, the skull is a spherical vault, with its anterior and middle cranial fossae having rough and irregular bases. The sharp, lesser wing of the sphenoid bone intervenes between these two fossae. The anterior ventral aspect of both frontal lobes of the brain is separated by a bony protuberance of the ethmoid bone called the crista galli. In adults, the surfaces of the skull in the regions of both the lesser wing of the sphenoid bone and the ethmoid bone are jagged and rough. Many authors view these structures as being directly responsible for 'bruising' of surrounding brain tissues following a closed head injury (Adams, 1975; Bigler, 1990). Holbourn (1943) suggested that the anatomical structures in these areas allow the skull to get a good 'grip' on the brain during rotational acceleration.

Differences in the physical and structural properties of children's heads and adult heads have been implicated as at least part of the explanation for the better prognosis for recovery from TBI reported to occur in children compared to adults (Levin, Ewing-Cobbs and Benton, 1983). These latter authors attributed the greater capacity of young children to survive severe closed head injury, as compared with adults, to anatomical and physical features of head injury that differ between the two populations. Jellinger (1983) also suggested that the morphology of cranial injuries and childhood is different from that in adults. As indicated earlier, according to Holbourn (1943), the type of brain damage that results from a severe head injury depends on the physical properties of the individual's brain and skull. These physical properties are known to differ in a number of ways between children and adults, thereby contributing to different patterns of brain injury following head trauma in each group (Lindenberg and Freytag, 1969). First, an infant's brain weight at birth is 15% of body weight, progressing through to only 3% of body weight in adults (Friede, 1973). By the end of the second year of life, brain weight is 75% of the adult brain weight and reaches 90% of adult brain weight by the end of the sixth year (Jellinger, 1983). Second, the existence of unfused sutures and open fontanelles makes the skull of an infant and young child more pliable. Some authors have suggested that, because of its elasticity and greater degree of deformation, the skull of an infant absorbs the energy of the physical impact and thereby protects the brain better than the skull of an adult (Menkes and Till, 1995). Other authors, however, believe the greater pliability of the heads of infants makes them more susceptible to external forces than older children and adults. According to Menkes and Till (1995), although deformation of the head absorbs much of the energy of the impact, thereby reducing the effects of acceleration/deceleration, it adds to the risk of tearing blood vessels. A third anatomical difference in the skulls of children versus adults that may aid a better prognosis in the former group is that, unlike adults, the floors of the middle cranial fossa and the orbital roofs in children are relatively smooth and offer little resistance to the shifting brain.

Alternatively, the differences reported in the prognosis for recovery following TBI between children and adults may also be related to the different nature of the impacts causing head injury in these two groups (Hendrick, Hardwood-Nash and Hudson, 1964). As described earlier in this chapter, most childhood accidents result from child abuse, falls or low speed (30–60 km/hr) pedestrian or bicycle accidents that involve a motor vehicle. Consequently, many paediatric head injuries are associated with a lesser degree of rotational acceleration and, therefore, presumably a lesser amount of brain damage (Levin, Benton and Grossman, 1982). Adults, on the other hand, as well as persons in their late teenage years, are more likely to sustain TBI as a result of high-speed motor vehicle accidents, which by their nature are likely to yield greater diffuse brain injury.

Neuropathophysiology of traumatic brain injury

A knowledge of the neuropathophysiology of closed head injury provides a framework for predicting and understanding the resultant clinical behaviours and contributes insight into brain–behaviour relationships. The principal pathologies associated with closed head injury have been categorized in various ways. Typically, the divisions involve differentiating focal or diffuse lesions, as well as those that are primary (immediate on impact) injuries and those that are secondary phenomena not attributable to the impact itself. There is evidence, however, that primary and secondary pathologies combine to form a marked heterogeneity of injury (Levin, Benton and Grossman, 1982; Pang, 1985). The frequent neuropathophysiological sequelae of closed head injury are summarized in Table 4.2 and discussed further below.

Primary neuropathophysiological effects of traumatic brain injury

Primary brain damage occurs at the moment of impact and is the result of the instantaneous

Table 4.2 Primary and secondary brain injury after closed head injury.

Lesion	Injury
Primary diffuse	Diffuse axonal injury
Primary focal	Contusions
	Laceration
	Basal ganglia haemorrhage
	Cranial nerve lesions
Secondary diffuse	Cerebral oedema
	Raised intracranial pressure
	Ischaemia
	Brain shift and herniation
	Cerebral atrophy and ventricular enlargement
Secondary focal	Haematoma:
	• extradural
	• subdural
	• intracranial

events caused by the blow. This damage frequently constitutes the limiting factor for ideal neurological recovery (Pang, 1985) and includes DAI, contusions, laceration, basal ganglia haemorrhage and cranial nerve lesions.

Primary diffuse lesions

Diffuse cerebral injury, in the form of widespread damage to the axons in the white matter of the brain, produced at the moment of impact is widely considered to be the primary mechanism of brain damage in individuals with closed head injury, and a more important factor in determining outcome than the presence of focal lesions (Strich, 1956, 1961, 1969; Adams *et al.*, 1977; Gennarelli *et al.*, 1982). This pathological state, also referred to as 'diffuse axonal injury' (DAI), was first described by Strich (1956), who determined the presence of diffuse degeneration of the cerebral white matter in the absence of focal pathology in the brains of four survivors of TBI who were quadriplegic and in a profoundly demented or vegetative state. Strich (1956, 1961) concluded that the severe neurological deficit manifest in these cases was the result of axonal damage produced by mechanical forces shearing the fibres at the moment of impact.

A number of different areas of the brain have been reported to be commonly affected by DAI subsequent to traumatic head injury, including the subcortical white matter of the cerebral hemispheres, the upper brainstem, the superior cerebellar peduncles and the basal ganglia (Strich, 1969; Adams *et al.*, 1982). The interface between the grey and white matter is also commonly involved because of shearing between the different tissue types. Magnetic resonance imaging (MRI) has also identified DAI in the brainstem, hippocampus, corpus callosum and at interfaces between the brain and dura mater (Guthrie *et al.*, 1999).

The concept proposed by Strich (1956, 1961) that DAI is an immediate effect of a closed head injury has often been challenged. Jellinger and Seitelberger (1970), although agreeing that one aetiological factor of DAI was mechanical damage to the nerve fibres, suggested that vascular, oedematous and anoxic damage to the cerebral cortex and basal ganglia played a significant role in the pathogenesis of white matter changes. Adams *et al.* (1982), in a study involving a comparison of fatal head trauma cases with and without DAI, failed to find any significant differences between the two groups with respect to the incidence of cerebral oedema or hypoxic brain damage. They concluded that DAI occurs immediately, at the time of impact, and is not secondary to any other form of brain damage. Adams *et al.* (1982) described DAI in terms of a triad of distinctive features: a focal lesion in the corpus callosum; a focal lesion in the dorsolateral quadrants of the rostral brainstem; and microscopic evidence of diffuse damage to axons, such as axonal retraction balls, microglial stars and degeneration of specific fibre tracts in the white matter.

The findings of Adams *et al.* (1982) were supported by those of Gennarelli *et al.* (1982), who induced DAI in the brains of non-human primates by means of imparting angular acceleration. DAI identical to that known to occur in humans subsequent to traumatic head injury was produced and three grades of severity were identified. In the most severe grade, DAI was characterized by focal lesion in the dorsolateral quadrant of the rostral brainstem in addition to a lesion in the corpus callosum and axonal damage in the cerebral white matter. Gennarelli *et al.* (1982) concluded that the degree of DAI was directly related to the duration and severity of coma and the clinical outcome. These findings suggest that there exists a continuum of axonal injury and were later supported by Blumbergs, Jones and North (1989), who described similar grades of DAI in humans. According to Adams *et al.* (1991), even people who have sustained a mild head injury and are rendered unconscious for as little as five minutes after injury have some degree of DAI.

Although DAI is still largely classed as a primary injury, that classification has been further challenged in recent years by Letarte (1999). He argued that, although immediate traumatic axotomy occurs, most of the axonal disruption occurs later. According to Letarte (1999), the majority of axons that will eventually suffer damage remain in continuity immediately after injury, and that it is not until around six hours post-injury that the neurofilaments are destroyed and axotomy occurs (Teasdale and Graham, 1998). The model of axonal injury proposed by Letarte (1999) is different from the immediate, irreversible mechanism described by earlier researchers and implies that the deterioration in patients post-injury may be due to this progressive secondary injury and raises the possibility of developing medical strategies to intervene in this progressive degeneration of axons.

Primary focal lesions

A brain contusion (bruise) consists of an area of brain tissue characterized by multifocal capillary haemorrhages, vascular engorgement and oedema. A linear impact on the skull may result in transient distortion and in-bending of the bone near the point of impact, causing compression of adjacent brain tissue and bruising of the brain in an area directly below the area of impact. Such contusions which occur at the point of impact are termed 'coup' contusions. In addition to causing lesions at this site, the impact may cause the brain to strike the skull at a point opposite to the point of trauma, thereby resulting in additional vascular disruption and bruising at this latter site. Contusions of the latter type are termed 'contre-coup' contusions. Both coup and contre-coup lesions may cause specific and localizable behavioural alterations that accompany closed head injury (Lezak, 1983). The symptoms produced by a brain contusion depend on the size and location of the contusion, and may include speech, language and swallowing disorders. In that intracellular swelling of adjacent structures is frequently associated with contusions, secondary brain damage may develop, leading some authors to suggest that the clinical significance of contusions lies more in the risk of the secondary injuries caused by the mass effects than the focal damage itself (Gennarelli, 1993).

Irrespective of the point of impact, brain contusions are most often found in the orbital and lateral surfaces of the frontal and temporal lobes which occupy the anterior and middle cranial fossae (Auerbach, 1986). The frequent presence of contusions in these sites is due to the brain abrading against the irregular and jagged skull surfaces with which it interfaces (Bigler, 1990). Similarly, the frequent occurrence of contusions on the medial surface of the hemispheres and in the corpus callosum are thought to result from the movement of the brain against the falx cerebri and the tentorium (Gurdjian and Gurdjian, 1976). Previously, contusions were considered to occur in cortical regions only, however, computerized tomography (CT) scans have identified contusions within deep areas of the brain.

When a brain contusion is sufficiently severe to cause a visible breach in the continuity of the brain, it is referred to as a 'laceration'. Lacerations are more typically associated with penetrating head injuries than closed head injuries and tend to be associated with more severe and prolonged neurological sequelae than contusions.

Although intracerebral haematoma associated with closed head injury is usually considered a secondary insult or a primary complication rather than the result of immediate impact injury (Levin, Benton and Grossman, 1982), traumatic basal ganglia haematoma has been reported to be indicative of severe primary brain damage (MacPherson *et al.*, 1986; Coloquhoun and Rawlinson, 1989). A distinct and relatively rare traumatic entity, traumatic basal ganglia haematoma occurs in approximately 3% of severe closed head injuries. Although it can occur in isolation or in association with other intracerebral haematomas and contusions, it is mostly found in patients who have suffered severe diffuse white matter injury (Coloquhoun and Rawlinson, 1989).

A severe closed head injury can cause dysfunction of a variety of cranial nerves, either by damaging the cranial nerve nuclei in the brainstem or disrupting the nerves themselves in either their intracranial or extracranial course (Murdoch, 1990). Contusions of the brainstem can damage the cranial nerve nuclei, leading to flaccid paralysis of the muscles innervated by the affected nerves. In particular, should these affected muscles include the muscles supplied by cranial nerves V, VII, X or XII, speech disorders may result. The most common cause of damage to the cranial nerves in their intracranial course is fracture of the base of the skull. The facial nerve (VII) is most commonly affected by this condition leading to flaccid paralysis of the muscles of facial expression. Branches of the facial (VII) and trigeminal (V) nerves may be damaged extracranially by trauma to the face. In general, traumatic cranial nerve palsies are permanent, the exceptions being those resulting from contusions of extracranial branches of the nerves (Murdoch, 1990).

Secondary neuropathophysiological effects of traumatic brain injury

Primary brain injury can generate a variety of secondary insults to the brain which in turn trigger a pathophysiological cascade of events. Secondary injury has the potential to be limited with appropriate therapeutic interventions (Gjerris, 1986) and includes cerebral oedema, intracranial haemorrhage, ischaemic brain damage, pathological changes associated with increased intracranial pressure (ICP), cerebral atrophy and ventricular enlargement.

Secondary diffuse lesions

According to Bigler (1990), cerebral oedema, which involves an increase in brain volume due to an accumulation of excess water in the brain tissue, is 'the most common secondary effect of brain injury' (p. 32). Adams *et al.* (1980) described three types of brain swelling: localized brain swelling, which occurs around a contusion; unilateral brain swelling, which involves diffuse swelling of one cerebral hemisphere; and brain swelling, which involves diffuse swelling of both cerebral hemispheres. Oedema resulting from TBI is most commonly vasogenic and results from an increase in the permeability of brain capillaries, which allows water and other solutes to exude out into the extracellular spaces within the brain tissue (Levin, Benton and Grossman, 1982; Pang, 1985). Various neuropathological changes may occur as a result of sustained cerebral oedema, including stretching and tearing of axonal fibres; compression of brain tissue, resulting in cell loss; compression of blood vessels, with subsequent infarction of brain tissue; and herniation of the brain (Bigler, 1990).

Elevated ICP occurs when there is an increase in one of the intracranial constituents – blood, brain, cerebrospinal fluid or extracellular fluid – within the non-compliant skull (Pang, 1985). A sudden increase in ICP is a common finding after closed head injury, most frequently due to the development of extradural, subdural or intracerebral haematomas or generalized cerebral swelling. Uncontrolled increases in ICP may cause herniation (a shift of part of the brain to another cranial compartment) and can also impede cerebral blood flow, resulting in ischaemic brain damage (Levin, Benton and Grossman, 1982; Pang, 1985; Murdoch, 1990). Murdoch (1990) described three types of cerebral herniation due to raised ICP following traumatic head injury: transtentorial herniation, in which the medial portions of the temporal lobes are herniated through the tentorial hiatus due to an increase in the ICP above the level of the tentorium cerebelli; tonsillar herniation, where the cerebellar tonsils are displaced down through the foramen magnum; and axial herniation, which occurs when there is a downward displacement of the entire brainstem due to increased ICP. Transtentorial herniation causes compression of the brainstem and interferes with the functioning of the reticular formation, thereby leading to a deterioration in the level of consciousness. At the same time, the third cranial nerve is also compressed, causing pupillary dilation, first on the side of the herniation and later on the other side as well. Eventually, if untreated, compression of the brainstem will lead to death. The level of consciousness and the state of the pupils of the eyes are, therefore, critical factors that require monitoring following closed head injury. The only structure compressed by tonsillar herniation is the medulla and the first sign of its presence is often either respiratory insufficiency or apnea. Although no structures are actually compressed by axial herniation, distortion of the brainstem caused by its downward displacement may cause altered levels of consciousness and changes in respiration.

Ischaemic brain damage is also widely recognized as a common sequela of closed head injury (Graham, Adams and Doyle, 1978; Adams *et al.*, 1980) and ranges from focal necrosis to wide areas of infarction. Although areas of infarction are generally related to the presence of contusions, haematomas, distortion and herniation of the brain and raised ICP, Adams (1975) also defined a specific category of ischaemic brain damage characterized by different patterns of neuronal necrosis and infarction of the brain, which was not directly associated with these factors. Graham and Adams (1971) analysed 100 cases of closed head injury and discovered an unusually high incidence of diffuse neocortical necrosis even after known causes (e.g. cardiac arrest, status epilepticus, contusions, raised ICP, etc.) were eliminated. In a further study of 151 cases, Graham, Adams and Doyle (1978) confirmed a high incidence (91%) of ischaemic brain damage following closed head injury. They also reported that ischaemic brain following traumatic head injury was more frequently found in the hippocam-

pus (81%) and basal ganglia (79%) than in the cerebral cortex (46%).

The development of cerebral atrophy and ventricular enlargement in the brain following a severe closed head injury has been frequently documented (Cullum and Bigler, 1986; Bigler *et al.*, 1993). Cullum and Bigler (1986) were able to demonstrate that the average ventricular enlargement in patients with TBI was twice that of the normal person. They also reported the associated presence of marked cortical atrophy following brain injury, which tended to occur more frequently in the frontal and temporal areas of the brain, as well as in a diffuse pattern throughout the cerebral tissue. Traumatically induced cerebral atrophy and ventricular enlargement have been found to be related to subsequent neuropsychological deficits in complex reasoning and problem-solving, memory, language, intellect and social–emotional functioning (Levin, Benton and Grossman, 1982; Cullum and Bigler, 1986).

Secondary focal lesions

Intracranial haemorrhages are common complications of a closed head injury and may involve bleeding into the extradural, subdural and subarachnoid spaces, into the ventricles or directly into the brain tissues (Adams, 1975). Although these haemorrhages may occur immediately following impact, their effects are usually not evident until they are of sufficient volume to act as intracranial space-occupying lesions.

Extradural haematomas usually result from laceration of the middle meningeal artery by fractured bone and involve bleeding between the skull bones and the dura mater (Figure 4.2). Haematomas of this type usually collect and enlarge fairly rapidly and signs of ICP become evident within a short period post-injury. Typically, although the patient may have been knocked unconscious at the time of head injury, consciousness is quickly recovered and then within 1–2 hours the patient becomes increasingly drowsy and develops paralysis down one side of the body as a result of compression of the ipsilateral cerebral hemisphere by the expanding haematoma. Eventually, the patient demonstrates pupillary dilation and loses consciousness from compression of the third cranial nerve and brainstem,

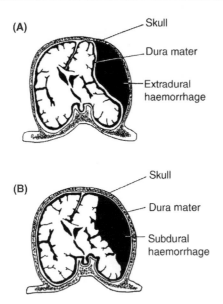

(A)
Skull
Dura mater
Extradural haemorrhage

(B)
Skull
Dura mater
Subdural haemorrhage

Figure 4.2   (A) Extradural haemorrhage. (B) Subdural haemorrhage.

respectively, as a consequence of herniation of the temporal lobe through the tentorial hiatus. Treatment of an extradural haematoma requires an emergency operation which involves the drilling of a burr-hole over the bruise site and evacuating the clot. If left untreated, the patient will die as a result of compression of vital centres (e.g. respiratory centres) in the brainstem. Extradural haemorrhage has been reported to occur in approximately 10% of closed head injured persons (Adams *et al.*, 1980).

Subdural haemorrhage is more common than extradural haemorrhage and is attributed to the rupture of small blood vessels within the subdural space, leading to bleeding between the dura mater and arachnoid (Figure 4.2). Adams *et al.* (1980) recorded an incidence of 45% of subdural haematomas in their series of head injured subjects. Subdural haematomas develop much more slowly than extradural haematomas and, consequently, although the neurological signs and symptoms resulting from associated increased ICP are the same, they appear at a much later time, in some cases days, in others weeks, after the traumatic head injury. If the haematoma develops to the stage of causing transtentorial herniation, as in the case of extradural haematoma,

surgical evacuation of the clot is again required to prevent compression of the brainstem.

Subarachnoid haemorrhage occurs following rupture of the blood vessels that cross the subarachnoid space between the arachnoid and pia mater. Such haemorrhages are common occurrences after closed head injury and can be detected by the presence of blood in the cerebrospinal fluid. Although patients with subarachnoid haemorrhages may experience severe headaches and stiffness of the neck for many days, they normally recover spontaneously.

Intracerebral haemorrhages may present in the brain following closed head injury either singularly or in a multiple format (Adams, 1975). These haematomas are usually directly related to contusions and therefore occur mainly in the subfrontal or temporal regions. Those occurring deep within the brain (e.g. in the basal ganglia) are thought to be due to the effects of shear strains on the small vessels at the moment of impact and are therefore usually regarded as primary injuries. An incidence of 42% of intracerebral haematomas has been reported in a study of closed head injury subjects by Adams *et al.* (1980).

Other complications of traumatic brain injury

In addition to the primary and secondary brain damage outlined above, patients who experience a closed head injury may also suffer from a number of other medical complications that may impact on their post-trauma quality of life. These further complications include: skull fractures, rhinorrhea and otorrhea, and post-traumatic epilepsy and post-traumatic vertigo.

Skull fractures

The various different types of skull fracture associated with traumatic head injury are listed in Table 4.3.

There is no direct relationship between the severity of any damage to the skull and the extent to which the brain is damaged. Although severe fractures of the skull are usually associated with severe cerebral injury, the brain may be

Table 4.3 The different types of skull fracture.

Fracture type	Description
Simple	Cracks or fissures in the skull bone, skin intact
Compound	Cracks in the skull bone, scalp also breached
Comminuted	The damaged skull bone is broken into several pieces
Depressed	A piece of broken skull bone is driven inwards and may cause laceration or compression on the underlying brain tissue

extensively damaged without the skull being fractured. Alternatively, a fracture of the skull may occur without severe damage to the brain. Consequently, the fracture itself is of little importance in relation to the occurrence of persistent neurological deficits following traumatic head injury. Rather, the presence of neurological impairments is dependent on the location and extent of damage to the underlying structures, particularly the brain itself. Overall, depressed skull fractures are the most likely to produce severe and permanent neurological signs due to the possibility of the dislodged piece of bone causing lacerations of the brain tissue.

Rhinorrhea and otorrhea

These terms refer to the leakage of cerebrospinal fluid from the nose (rhinorrhea) and ear (otorrhea) subsequent to traumatic head injury. Rhinorrhea occurs following fracture of the frontal bone with associated tearing of the dura mater and arachnoid. Otorrhea, on the other hand, is caused by injuries to the base of the skull. As injuries in this latter region often damage the brainstem as well, otorrhea is of more serious prognostic importance than rhinorrhea. Infections and meningitis are potential hazards of both conditions.

Post-traumatic epilepsy and post-traumatic vertigo

Although not incapacitating, these two complications of closed head injury may have a profound effect on the lifestyle of the head injured patient. Post-traumatic epilepsy occurs most commonly

after penetrating head injuries, the epilepsy being triggered by the formation of scar tissue as a result of brain laceration. The scar may act as an irritating focus to trigger epileptic fits. In some cases, convulsions may occur very shortly after impact (within 24 hours), especially in children. Where it occurs in adult head injury cases, however, the epilepsy usually develops within the first two years post-injury. Although more common in cases of penetrating head injuries, post-traumatic epilepsy can also occur subsequent to closed head injuries and may be triggered by the development of subdural haematomas.

Some degree of vertigo accompanied by vomiting and unsteadiness is common after head injury. Post-traumatic vertigo may last for days or weeks or may persist in some cases for many months.

Medical management of traumatic brain injury

There are two major components to contemporary treatment of patients with TBI. These include: (1) rapid evacuation of haematomas and control of increasing ICP and (2) prevention of hypotension and hypoxia and maintenance of cerebral perfusion pressure (CPP) (Letarte, 1999). This current approach, however, has only been implemented since the mid-1980s. It evolved as a consequence of a greater understanding of the mechanisms of cerebral oedema and ischaemic brain injury brought about by research at the level of cellular physiology.

Until the mid-1980s, the paradigm for the treatment of patients with TBI was very much focused on prevention of increasing ICP. There is evidence that, even from the earliest of times, an awareness existed of the special importance of brain swelling on the outcome from head injury. Archaeological findings indicate that, in multiple and widespread locations throughout human evolution, trephination was practised. From the early 1900s to the mid-1950s, rapid evacuation of space-occupying lesions, and particularly haematomas, was the principal treatment for head injured patients, with surgery being the only available treatment method. This treatment, however, was only made available to patients deemed to have space-occupying lesions and being, therefore, eligible for surgery. Consequently, many patients who presented as lucid initially went on to deteriorate and often die as the result of untreated space-occupying lesions. Reilly and Adams (1975) reported that many patients with lucid intervals who later died, so-called talk-and-die patients, had space-occupying lesions that were potentially treatable. Fortunately, a means of rapidly identifying patients with space-occupying lesions was provided by the introduction of the CT scanner in the mid-1970s. The introduction of this technology also had the effect of intensifying the surgical focus of the treatment of patients with head injury.

Although still focused on the treatment of elevated ICP, non-surgical therapies for the treatment of TBI were introduced in the mid-1950s. The first effective non-operative treatment for elevated ICP became available with the introduction of urea by Javid and Settlage (1956). Urea was followed by mannitol and in rapid sequence by a series of steroids. Parallel and complementary to these developments was the description of a technique by Lundberg (1960) which allowed continuous monitoring of ICP. Consequently, by the early 1960s a means of quantifying cerebral oedema as well as methods for treating elevated ICP was available.

The catalyst to changing the paradigm for the treatment of patients with head injury from being ICP-centred to one that also recognized the need to maintain cerebral perfusion was a publication by Miller and Sweet (1978) that highlighted ischaemia as a significant threat to patients with head injury. This work culminated in Rosner and co-workers (Rosner and Coley, 1986; Rosner and Daughton, 1990; Rosner, 1995) defining a clinical approach to head injury that recognizes ischaemia as of equal importance to oedema and mass effect in terms of need for treatment.

Letarte (1999) predicted that in addition to these essential components, a third component in the form of pharmacotherapy would be added to the treatment of patients with TBI early in the new millennium. In particular, pharmacotherapy will aim to combat the neurochemical mediations of secondary injury and will be augmented by new techniques for monitoring brain function such as cerebral blood flow (e.g. Xenon CT) brain metabolism (e.g. positron emission tomography (PET)) and global cerebral oxygenation (e.g. jugular bulb monitoring) among others. Using these new techniques, clinicians will not only be able to view the structure of the injured brain but will also be able to map its blood flow and in so doing monitor the adequacy of attempts to maintain CPP. By being able to monitor the metabolism of the brain, clinicians will be able to track markers of neurological injury and thereby better estimate the severity of the patient's injuries.

Language disorders subsequent to traumatic brain injury

Basis of language impairments following traumatic brain injury

Early history – Egyptian papyrus to World War Two

Communication impairments in the form of speech and/or language disorders are commonly reported sequelae of traumatic head injury. Archaeological evidence suggests that the relationship between traumatic head injury and the occurrence of communication disorders was known to a number of ancient civilizations. Papyrus records indicate that the Egyptians were aware of the relationship as early as 3000–2500 BC (Breasted, 1930). A Roman, Valerius Maximus (30 AD), described a learned man of Athens who lost his memory for words after being struck on the head with a stone. Despite the centuries that this relationship has been known, it is only in recent times that detailed descriptions of the speech-language disorders occurring subsequent to head trauma have started to appear in the literature. Many of the early studies only noted the presence of speech-language disorders in patients who had suffered traumatic head injury without providing detailed descriptions of the disorder (e.g. Lichtheim, 1885; Russell, 1932). It was only following the Second World War that detailed descriptions of post-traumatic language disorders subsequent to penetrating (open) head injuries were published (Schiller, 1947; Goldstein, 1948). Similar analyses of language disorders caused by non-penetrating (closed) head injuries have only appeared in the literature in any number since the early 1970s. Even today, our knowledge of the nature and basis of linguistic impairments following closed head injury remains incomplete and controversy remains relating to the terminology applied to language disorders associated with TBI, especially as it relates to the presence or absence of aphasia following TBI. Much of the controversy surrounding the terminology applied to the language impairments observed subsequent to TBI has been due to the inherent variability of the TBI population, the inconsistencies in the methodological parameters used in investigations and the differences in the theoretical perspectives or the nomenclature adopted by the different researchers.

The controversy over terminology

In the 1970s many researchers used nomenclature associated with aphasia to classify the observed linguistic deficits in individuals with TBI (Luria, 1970; Heilman, Safran and Geschwind, 1971; Thomsen, 1975; Levin, Grossman and Kelly, 1976; Groher, 1977). In doing so, the incidence of aphasia was found to be relatively rare when large series of consecutive cases were studied. In one of the most widely noted studies in the literature, Heilman, Safran and Geschwind (1971) examined 750 consecutive acute admissions and diagnosed only 2% (13 cases) as having 'aphasia'. Of these, nine cases were classified as having 'anomic

aphasia', which was defined as fluent speech with relatively intact comprehension and repetition in the presence of verbal paraphasia and impaired object naming. The remaining four cases were found to exhibit fluent paraphasic speech, poor comprehension and impaired repetition characteristic of Wernicke's aphasia. No subjects were classified as either Broca's or global aphasics.

Other studies (Thomsen, 1975; Stone, Lopes and Moody, 1978) yielded similar results to those of Heilman, Safran and Geschwind (1971). Thomsen (1975) examined language disorders in the acute stage of severe closed head injury, and found amnestic (anomic) aphasia and verbal paraphasia to be the most frequent symptoms, with perseveration, dysgraphia and literal paraphasia occurring less frequently. On reassessment between 23 and 50 months later, none had recovered completely; 13 exhibited evidence of a language deficit when tested without showing clinical manifestations of a language disorder (subclinical aphasia); half had persistent deficits of expression (mostly evident on naming tasks); two had resolved from mixed to sensory (Wernicke's) aphasia; and one had resolved from sensory to anomic aphasia. Thomsen (1975) concluded that aphasia following closed head injury is a receptive rather that an expressive disorder contributing to a neuropsychological syndrome often dominated by residual defects of general memory.

Levin, Grossman and Kelly (1976) examined language-disordered patients with mild to severe closed head injuries. They found a trend towards expressive or anomic aphasia in mild–moderate closed head injured patients and mixed deficits in the majority of severe closed head injured cases, the latter group being more prone to linguistic disturbance than the former. It was also noted that closed head injured patients who also had a period of prolonged coma often exhibited a general non-specific linguistic disturbance when consciousness returned.

Language and memory disorders following closed head injury were investigated by Groher (1977), using subjects averaging 17.1 days in coma and excluding cases involving skull fracture. Each patient was assessed as soon as possible after regaining consciousness, using the Porch Index of Communicative Ability (Porch,

1967) and the Wechsler Memory Scale Form I (Wechsler, 1945). Reassessments followed every 30 days for four months. In the acute stages, gestural skills were poorer than graphic skills, which were poorer than verbal skills. All subjects were reported to show marked anomia with literal and nominal paraphasic errors. Reading comprehension was poor, and nine out of the 14 subjects had spastic dysarthria (from which six recovered). Oral apraxia was not observed in any subject. At the final assessment, all subjects could make their needs known and converse readily. However, nine of the 14 subjects used inappropriate language and displayed confused thought content. Groher (1977) proposed that the initial communication problems exhibited by patients following closed head injury comprise both confused language and aphasic disabilities but that the aphasic component resolves leaving the patient with the language of confusion.

In the 1980s the debate over how best to conceptualize and describe the language behaviour following TBI intensified with the publication of a series of studies by Sarno (Sarno, 1980, 1984; Sarno, Buonaguro and Levita, 1986). In her first paper, Sarno reported on the performance of 56 TBI patients on four subtests of the Neurosensory Centre Comprehensive Examination for Aphasia (NCCEA) (Spreen and Benton, 1969). Before testing, the patients had been divided into three groups on the basis of clinical observation: aphasia only (32%), dysarthria with subclinical aphasic disorder (38%) and subclinical aphasic disorder only (30%). The diagnosis of aphasia was limited to patients who 'manifested specific deficits in the processing of information via the speech code' (p. 686), and the type of aphasia was classified according to Geschwind (1971) and Benson (1967). Subclinical aphasia disorder was defined as 'evidence of linguistic processing deficits on testing in the absence of clinical manifestation of linguistic impairments' (p. 687). The results indicated that all TBI patients suffered some degree of linguistic impairment. In contrast to the earlier studies, a larger proportion of patients evidenced classical aphasic syndromes (32%). Of these, the most frequent syndrome was fluent aphasia (39%). Anomia, which was the predom-

inant linguistic disorder found in earlier studies (Heilman, Safran and Geschwind, 1971; Thomsen, 1975; Levin, Grossman and Kelly, 1976; Groher, 1977), occurred in only two (11%) patients in Sarno's group. The subclinical aphasic group was the least impaired and evidenced deficits in the subtests of Visual Naming, Word Fluency and the Token Test.

In 1984, Sarno repeated her original study assessing 69 TBI patients admitted to a rehabilitation centre. In this series, no patient who was assigned to the aphasia group was considered anomic. In the subclinical group, there were deficits in specific linguistic processing tasks (Sentence Repetition, Word Fluency, Token Test) as well as a 'general decrease in richness and complexity' of verbal processing (p. 478). The author concluded that diffuse brain damage, severe enough to cause coma, will result in some form of verbal impairment.

In a later study, Sarno, Buonaguro and Levita (1986) applied a similar but more extensive methodology to a group of 125 TBI patients. Once again, all subject groups displayed compromised verbal functions in the form of aphasia (29.6%), dysarthria (34.4%) and subclinical aphasia (36%). The authors concluded that a severity continuum of verbal impairment was present in TBI, with the subclinical group being the least impaired.

Sarno's (1980, 1984) perspective on linguistic impairment following TBI evoked some criticism by those concerned with the limitations of using the conceptual framework established by classic aphasia theory to explain the verbal deficits in the TBI population. Holland (1982) contested the appropriateness of applying aphasia-related principles and nomenclature to describe individuals who did not demonstrate the focal lesions which underpin the traditional aphasic syndromes. While Holland agreed that aphasia can and does exist following TBI, she argued that most often the language was not disturbed in a typically aphasic way. Rather, she asserted that the language problems in TBI occurred as a manifestation of more general memory and cognitive deficits. Holland (1982) considered that the language deficits observed following TBI could be best described as 'disorders of language use', rather than the disorders of language form typical of true aphasic language. She further proposed that the term 'subclinical aphasia' does nothing to describe the language problems of the head injured patient and argued that, although aphasic patients exist in the head injured population, in the majority of head injury cases the associated language disturbance is not the same disorder as the aphasia associated with vascular lesions. She identified three features that distinguish head injury from the stroke population that might underlie their different language outcomes. The first distinction is that, although aphasiology arose from investigations into the effects of open head injuries caused by fragment penetration in wartime on language, closed head injuries are the most common type of head trauma encountered in civilian life. As indicated previously, closed head injuries generally cause diffuse brain damage rather than focal lesions, as found most often in stroke cases. Consequently, the language disorders found in closed head injury cases are likely to be the outcome of more general and more pervasive memory and cognitive deficits (Holland, 1982). The language deficit in closed head injury patients may, therefore, be superseded by other cognitive and memory deficits which need to be taken into account when treating these cases. Second, Holland (1982) indicated that the difference in language outcome might be explained by the fact that, as a result of the numerous cognitive and memory sequelae, closed head injury rehabilitation is more interdisciplinary than post-stroke aphasia rehabilitation. Third, Holland (1982) pointed out that there is an important demographic difference between the head injury and stroke populations, the occurrence of head injury being highest in the age group from 15 to 24 years of age and stroke being more common in middle to old age. The lower mean age of head injury patients compared with stroke cases could be expected to be associated with a better prognosis for recovery of language function.

Like Holland (1982), consideration of the pathophysiology underlying the neurobehavioural symptoms of TBI also led Hagen (1984) to oppose the use of a traditional, aphasia-related conceptual framework when evaluating and diagnosing the verbal impairments in this population. In his benchmark deliberation on the topic, Hagen argued that an approach to diagnosing and treating language disorders that had been developed from knowledge and experience with other types of neurological impairments could not be successfully applied to TBI. He considered that the observed language disorder in TBI is 'a secondary consequence of an underlying impairment, suppression and/or disorganization of the nonlinguistic cognitive processes that support language processes' (p. 252). Hagen argued that the neuropathology of TBI disrupts cognitive processes such as attention, sequencing, memory, categorization and associative abilities, and as a result the individual with a TBI has difficulty in organizing and integrating incoming information and is impaired in their capacity to interact efficiently and appropriately with the environment. This cognitive disorganization can be reflected in the person's language, which may be disoriented, disorganized, confused, stimulus bound, disinhibited or reduced in initiation. Holland (1982) believed that it is in the area of language pragmatics that post-stroke aphasia and head injured communication contrast most vividly. Aphasic language can be considered a disorder of form while head injured language is better considered a disorder of use. In support of this suggestion, Milton, Prutting and Binder (1984) using the Pragmatic Protocol (Prutting and Kirchner, 1983) reported a mean of 7.6 behaviours demonstrated by the head injured group to be judged inappropriate while a mean of only 0.6 inappropriate behaviours was recorded for a group of normal subjects. The 10 pragmatic behaviours that were most frequently judged to be inappropriate in the head injured group were prosody, affect, topic selection, topic maintenance, turn-taking initiation, turn-taking pause time, turn-taking contingency, quantity/conciseness and fluency. The highest proportion of inappropriate pragmatic behaviours exhibited by the head injured adults was the illocutionary/perlocutionary act, suggesting that breakdown most often occurs in the way the head injured adults function as discourse partners.

Thus, by the mid- to late 1980s, it had become widely accepted that language problems following TBI occurred against a backdrop of cognitive deficits. Indeed, this conceptualization is central to the current thinking that the language deficits which emerge following TBI are either secondary to the cognitive disruptions common following TBI or interdependent on disrupted cognitive processes (Chapman, Levin and Culhane, 1995).

Nature of language disorders following traumatic brain injury

Performance on standardized language assessments

The current conviction that cognitive impairment is the foundation of communication deficits found after TBI has evolved through the realization that most TBI individuals display overall normal performance on conventional aphasia tests in the presence of aberrant functional communicative ability (Thomsen, 1975; Levin, Grossman and Rose, 1979; Holland, 1982; Hagen, 1984; Milton, Prutting and Binder, 1984; Prigatano, Roueche and Fordyce, 1986). While their abilities on specific subtests, namely word finding, verbal fluency and comprehension of complex commands, have consistently been found to be below normal, the overall performances are not usually impaired enough to meet the criteria of aphasia as specified by the tests used (Levin, Grossman and Kelly, 1976, 1979; Sarno, Buonaguro and Levita, 1986). In addition, it has been observed that TBI subjects display qualitative differences in performance to aphasics on standardized test batteries (Levin, Grossman and Rose, 1979; Holland, 1982; Prigatano, Roueche and Fordyce, 1986).

Consistent with the observation that communication problems exist after TBI in the presence of proficiency in tests of primary language function, it has been argued that the communication problems following TBI cannot be adequately measured using traditional clinical test batteries designed to measure comprehension and production of language in aphasics. Such tests focus on specific linguistic processes and are seen as insensitive to the broader communication deficits

in TBI. Most standardized tasks fail to test language skill beyond the level of the sentence and the use of highly structured tasks may disguise the functional difficulties observed in more natural communicative situations (Hagen, 1984; Milton, Prutting and Binder, 1984; Benjamin *et al.*, 1989; Ehrlich and Barry, 1989; Parsons *et al.*, 1989; Coelho, Liles and Duffy, 1991a, b).

While standardized measures of language have been denounced as insensitive to deficits experienced by TBI patients, it is likely that the selected assessments have been insufficient and incomplete. Even in the more recent research, language measures used to determine the presence and severity of linguistic disorders in the TBI populations have often been limited to basic tests for aphasia (Ehrlich and Barry, 1989; Coelho, Liles and Duffy, 1991a; McDonald, 1992; McDonald and van Sommers, 1993; McDonald and Pearce, 1995) or subtests from neuropsychological assessment batteries (Hartley and Jensen, 1991; Chapman *et al.*, 1992). These types of tests are designed to assess primary language skill but fail to examine language comprehensively on more complex tasks. It is not surprising, therefore, that TBI individuals have frequently been found to display facile performances on assessments of primary language function in the presence of poor communicative performances in social contexts.

Communicative competence requires operational language beyond the primary language process or symbolic level, and involves proficiency with metacognitive and metalinguistic operations (Baker, 1982; Wiig, 1984; Wiig and Becker-Caplan, 1984). Metalinguistic skill and the ability to consciously and efficiently access and manipulate the semantic system are linguistically based operations requiring an intricate interplay of primary language processes, cognitive processes and executive processes such as self-monitoring and social judgement. The contribution of linguistic proficiency, where linguistic proficiency includes facility with primary language and higher-level cognitive-linguistic operations, must receive greater emphasis in the systematic and holistic evaluation of communication competence in TBI.

The tendency to limit the assessment of language in subjects with TBI to aphasia batteries fails to systematically investigate the mature and functional linguistic system. As a result, several researchers have concluded on the basis of performance on aphasia batteries or subtests of neuropsychological batteries that language function after TBI is largely intact (Milton, Prutting and Binder, 1984; Mentis and Prutting, 1987; Ehrlich and Barry, 1989; Coelho, Liles and Duffy, 1991a, b; Hartley and Jensen, 1991; McDonald and van Sommers, 1993; McDonald and Pearce, 1995).

In an effort to redress the inadequacy of the standardized language assessments often used in investigating TBI subjects, Hinchcliffe, Murdoch and Chenery (1998) examined 25 people who had suffered a severe TBI on a test battery which allowed assessment of language function across different modalities and along a hierarchy of complexity, structure and predictability. The primary focus of their test battery was on oral language and was based on the Hinchcliffe, Murdoch and Chenery (1998) conceptual model of verbal communicative competence, which is reproduced in Figure 4.3. This model represents schematically the interplay between linguistic and other cognitive processes and emphasizes the contribution of a proficient language system to the achievement of oral communicative competence. In this model, a proficient language system embraces primary and higher-order linguistic functions which, together with input from primary and higher-order cognitive processes, form the substratum of discourse ability and communicative competence. The test battery used by Hinchcliffe, Murdoch and Chenery (1998) therefore included tests which evaluated primary language processes, as well as tests designed to examine the integrity of linguistic skill on complex and linguistically demanding tasks.

The results indicated that, when compared with matched controls, individuals recovering from TBI had minor deficits in primary language function as measured by traditional tests of aphasia, but the differences in performance between the TBI subjects and their matched controls were further pronounced on language tasks which are more demanding on metalinguistics and the lexical semantic system.

Performance on standardized tests of primary language function

The findings of Hinchcliffe, Murdoch and Chenery (1998) supported those of previous investigations which have identified in groups of TBI subjects deficiencies in confrontation naming, verbal associative tasks, auditory comprehension (Levin, Grossman and Kelly, 1976; Sarno, 1980, 1984; Sarno, Buonaguro and Levita, 1986) and reading comprehension (Sarno, 1984). While their results revealed such deficits on rudimentary linguistic tasks, the subjects in the Hinchcliffe, Murdoch and Chenery (1998) sample did not display symptoms typical of the aphasic syndromes demonstrated by head injured persons described in earlier research reports (Heilman, Safran and Geschwind, 1971; Levin, Grossman and Kelly, 1976; Groher, 1977; Sarno, Buonaguro and Levita, 1985). Indeed, in describing the performance by the subject group on tests of naming (the Object Naming subtest of the WAB and the Boston Naming Test), Hinchcliffe, Murdoch and Chenery (1998) concluded that the TBI subjects had linguistic impairments which were qualitatively and quantitatively different from the impairments encountered by sufferers of focal cerebral lesions but they were nonetheless deficient on these tasks when compared to non-brain-damaged controls. In particular, the error behaviour on tests of naming did not reflect symptoms observed in the classic description of anomic aphasia (Geschwind, 1971). Instead, the error behaviour of the TBI subjects resembled that of the normal control subjects with delayed word retrieval and self-cueing of correct responses through semantic association and circumlocution.

Performance on tests of higher-order language

Standardized assessments of linguistic proficiency, which test metalinguistic competence, integrative language skills and the ability to manipulate the lexical semantic system, have been shown to discriminate consistently between TBI subjects and their matched controls (Hinchcliffe, Murdoch and Chenery, 1998). Error analysis of the performance by TBI subjects on subtests of

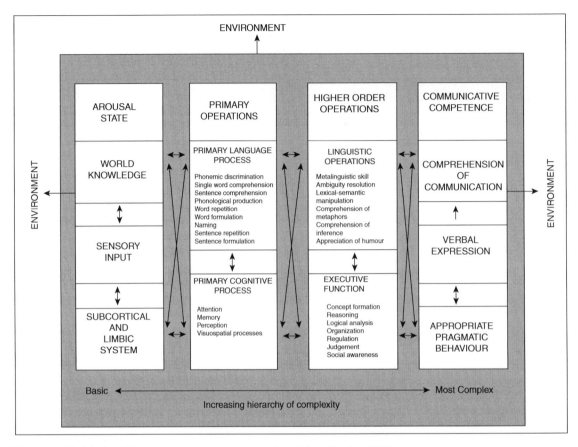

Figure 4.3 Model of verbal communicative competence (adapted from Hartley, 1995).

the Test of Language Competence – Expanded (TLC-E) edition, Level 2 (Wiig and Secord, 1989) by Hinchcliffe, Murdoch and Chenery (1998) revealed key features of higher-order language abilities after TBI.

The TBI subjects had difficulty recognizing and expressing alternative interpretations of ambiguities in sentences, reflecting inefficiency in achieving lexical access and shifting cognitive-linguistic set (Wiig, Alexander and Secord, 1988). Difficulty on the TLC-E listening comprehension tasks revealed reduced ability to attend to salient information and integrate information in order to recognize plausible inferences or draw logical conclusions. The TLC-E was also shown to be a sensitive measure of the verbal planning and monitoring ability of TBI individuals. The Oral Expression subtest of the TLC-E requires cogni-

tive flexibility, conceptual integration, lexical access and choice, as well as synthesis and monitoring of semantic, syntactic and pragmatic variables (Bock, 1982; Wiig, Alexander and Secord, 1988). Performance by the TBI subjects on this subtest was marked by response behaviour suggestive of impulsivity and lack of reflection, evaluation and planning. Because of such task behaviour, the TBI subjects had difficulty in monitoring the linguistic integrity and relevance of the sentence and often produced sentences that were semantically, pragmatically and/or syntactically deviant.

Hinchcliffe, Murdoch and Chenery (1998) also found the TBI subjects in their study to be significantly less competent than matched control subjects in explaining the meaning of metaphorical expressions included in the Figurative Language (FL) subtest of the TLC-E. This task requires the subjects to verbally interpret a metaphoric statement and then to match this statement to another expression denoting the same meaning. Previous investigators (Wiig and Secord, 1985; Towne and Entwistle, 1993) had found TBI subjects who had attained relatively high levels of cognitive functioning, as measured by the Rancho Los Amigos Level of Cognitive Functioning Scale (LOCF) (Hagen, 1984), were able to perform similarly to normal control subjects on this task. In contrast, Hinchcliffe, Murdoch and Chenery (1998) found that despite relatively high LOCF scores, their TBI subjects had difficulty transcending literal meanings in order to interpret the figurative expressions. Difficulty with interpreting figurative language may reflect a reduced appreciation of the denotation of words (Zurif *et al.*, 1974) and a diminished acceptance of connotative language (Gardner and Denes, 1973). The poor performance by the TBI group on this task could also be attributed to poor formulation of verbal explanation as well as failure to utilize contextual cues to determine the non-literal meaning of the sentence.

The Word Test – Revised (Huisingh *et al.*, 1990) was found to be sensitive to disorders of expressive vocabulary and semantic ability following TBI (Hinchcliffe, Murdoch and Chenery, 1998). The TBI group attained significantly lower scores than their matched controls on all the tasks which required them to make semantic associations, recognize and explain semantic incongruity, retrieve semantically similar or opposite words, recognize alternative meanings of words and formulate explanations containing critical semantic elements in order to define nouns and verbs. Poor performances on these tasks reflect impaired verbal planning and reasoning, difficulty recognizing and expressing critical semantic attributes of words, poor organization, categorization and recall of lexical items and depressed mental flexibility.

Although little attention has been given to the impact of right-hemisphere brain damage on the language function of people with TBI, it has been suggested that communicative behaviours seen in TBI patients resemble language disorders associated with right-hemisphere damage (McDonald, 1993). In TBI, the right and left cerebral hemispheres are equally vulnerable to damage and it is well recognized that the right cerebral hemisphere has a significant role in normal language processing (Code, 1987; Bryan, 1988, 1989). Hinchcliffe, Murdoch and Chenery (1998) found four of the six subtests of the Right Hemisphere Language Battery (RHLB) (Bryan, 1989) proved to be difficult for TBI subjects in their study. Performances on the Metaphor Picture Test (MP) revealed that the TBI subjects were significantly less adept at comprehending figurative speech than the normal controls, even when supportive contextual cues were available. The TBI subjects demonstrated a disruption in the comprehension of implicature and appreciation of connotative meaning (Winner and Gardner, 1977). This difficulty is consistent with the performance of the TBI group on the FL subtest of the TLC-E. The TBI subjects made significantly more errors on the Inferential Meaning test (IN) of the RHLB than their matched controls. This finding further attests to the apparent difficulty TBI subjects encounter in appreciating the implicature in messages. It seems that the TBI subjects fail to utilize the information provided in order to draw a conclusion. It is uncertain as to whether the deficit lies in the failure to correctly perceive and attend to salient detail or in the failure to make use of the contextual information in order to make an inference.

The TBI subjects attained a significantly poorer score than the control group on the Humour (HU) subtest of the RHLB. In this task, the subjects heard an unfinished joke and were instructed to select an appropriate punchline to complete the joke. Right-hemisphere-damaged (RHD) patients have been found to perform poorly on this task and display a tendency to select irrelevant endings. This behaviour is said to indicate that the RHD subjects appreciate that the joke must end in surprise, but they cannot determine the ending which is tied coherently with the body of the joke (Brownell *et al.*, 1983). The TBI subjects in the Hinchcliffe, Murdoch and Chenery (1998) study did not favour one type of ending in their erroneous selections. Poor performance on this task provides further evidence of failure by the TBI subjects to integrate across a narrative unit, attend to salient semantic information and appreciate implied meaning.

There is evidence, therefore, that impairments in the language system following TBI can be delineated using standardized and sensitive measures of linguistic function. It is important, however, to use a test battery which appropriately reflects the complexity of the mature language system in order to delineate the nature of the language behaviour of TBI subjects. The use of single language measures, such as naming, or measures of primary language function only, give limited information as to the nature and extent of the language profile of the TBI person and may lead to inappropriate generalizations regarding the entire language system following TBI (Chapman, Levin and Culhane, 1995).

The use of a comprehensive battery of language measures provides a means to reliably assess improvements in language performance over time and a foundation on which to base understanding of the deficits realized in discourse behaviour. Tests which tax the ability to integrate linguistic and non-linguistic components of communication and metalinguistic ability have been shown to consistently discriminate between the present sample of TBI subjects and normal control subjects. These tests have the advantage of isolating linguistic and cognitive-linguistic tasks and of assessing the ability of people with TBI to manipulate the semantic system under varying contextual constraints. As such, they provide the examiner with snapshots of an individual's ability to successfully use the fundamental components of language: language content, form and use. While impairment in cognitive functioning following TBI is unquestionable and pervasive, to date, the data available suggesting an influential association between cognitive processes, such as attention and memory on the one hand and linguistic function on the other, are insufficient to determine whether the relationship between cognitive deficits and linguistic impairments is linear or causative. Based on the evidence available, it can be argued that impairments in the linguistic system following TBI are real, clinically identifiable and should be considered fundamental to breakdown in communicative competence.

The language disorders described above primarily relate to published findings based on the examination of adults who have suffered TBI. For a description of the language impairments associated with childhood TBI see Chapter 12.

Recovery of language function following traumatic brain injury

In general, the prognosis for recovery of language function following head injury appears to be good. Despite this good prognosis, however, the mechanisms of recovery following head injury are still the subject of much controversy. The removal of haematomas and the associated relief of increased intracranial pressure together with the spontaneous recovery of physiological abnormalities account for at least some of the recovery observed during the first 1–3 weeks post-injury. During this period, oedema may subside, blood flow to brain areas not irreversibly damaged may increase and increased intracranial pressure associated with haemorrhage or dynamic alterations of the circulation of the cerebrospinal fluid may return to normal. According to Heilman and Valenstein (1979), recovery continues at a maximal rate for up to three months and then slows. The mechanisms underlying recovery, however, are poorly understood. It is possible that recovery in the acute stage is the result of temporarily inactive but undamaged neural tissue resuming normal activity. This suggestion, however, is based on the assumption that damage to one part of the brain creates a state of shock by depriving other parts of the brain of the normal stimulation thereby causing them to become temporarily inactive. Longer-term recovery (over weeks or months) may involve a process of functional reorganization of neural tissue while factors such as axonal regrowth, collateral sprouting and denervation hypersensitivity of the central nervous system may also contribute to the recovery of function (Fingers, 1978).

Although the severity of the head injury does not have an influence, recovery from head injury appears to follow a set course (Jennett and Teasdale, 1981). Recovery from coma is characterized by opening of the eyes at times (evidence that the brainstem mechanisms concerned with wake-fulness are recovering) and then uttering a few words. Some patients then go through a period of cerebral irritation, which is characterized by noisy, disinhibited behaviour such as swearing, attempting to get out of bed and an aggressive attitude to others. During the subsequent phase, the patient is quiet but confused about temporal, spatial and personal orientation. The end of post-traumatic amnesia marks a crucial stage of the recovery process. The duration of post-traumatic amnesia has been reported to be closely related to the ultimate degree of recovery and to the likelihood of cognitive sequelae (Brooks *et al.*, 1980). Once the patient is out of post-traumatic amnesia, more subtle abnormalities of behaviour may be displayed. At this stage, although the patient may be able to return home, the family is warned that some erratic behaviour can still be expected. Neurological recovery is largely completed by six months post-injury and the patient therefore needs to be encouraged to adapt physically, mentally and socially to any deficit still evident at this time.

Groher (1977) investigated the language and memory abilities of closed head injured patients after regaining consciousness four months post-trauma. He reported that a significant improvement in both language and memory functioning most often occurred within the first month after regaining consciousness. In particular, verbal skills were the first to return and were superior to comprehension capabilities for the first month. After four months, expressive and receptive language skills were grossly functional for conversational purposes. Further, all memory tasks, with the exception of orientation skills, were within normal limits at this time. After four months, comprehension abilities were as good as verbal skills. Writing performance was just becoming functional after four months. At the conclusion of the study, all patients were reported to be able to converse readily and could make their needs known. Despite this, signs of language impairment such as processing delays and word-finding difficulty were still evident and although they scored well on most standardized measurements for aphasia they still displayed problems of relevancy, inhibition of verbal output and with the

sequential organization of ideas into logical outcomes. Although some of the head injured patients examined by Groher (1977) were able to return to work, all reported problems in completing job tasks to their employer's satisfaction. In particular, the patients lacked judgement in the performance of their jobs, lacked initiative, forgot details easily and showed poor concentration. Groher (1983) has proposed that, although head injured patients recover basic language skill within the first six months post-injury, they continue to show deficits in the analysis and synthesis of expressive and receptive language. In a study of 56 head injured patients at a mean injury-test interval of seven months, Sarno (1980) found that seven patients had obvious aphasia but all others displayed only a 'subclinical aphasia', suggesting that, although the prognosis for recovery of language abilities following head injury appears to be good, subtle language impairment may persist long term.

Jennett (1983) summarized the different physiological activities that operate at the different stages of recovery following head injury. He presumed that improvements in the first minutes after injury indicate the resolution of transitory dysfunction that may not have had any structural component. Recovery after several days post-injury, however, is more likely to be due to the resolution of temporary structural abnormalities such as oedema and vascular permeability. The mechanism that underlies recovery after months or years possibly involves the restoration of function in recovering damaged brain structures or the diversion of that function to other normally redundant undamaged areas of the brain. Jennett and Teasdale (1981) concluded that most recovery beyond the first month following trauma is due to the functional use of alternative or redundant neurological pathways.

It has often been suggested that neurobehavioural recovery following brain injury is better in children than in adults. The difference, for example, in the often observed rapid recovery rate of children with acquired aphasia compared to that of adult aphasics was once interpreted as a demonstration of better recovery potential in children (Lenneberg, 1967; Levin and Eisenberg, 1979). It is not clear, however, how the basic mechanisms of injury might differ in children compared to adults to produce the different recovery pattern. Strich (1969) suggested that the shearing strains produced by rotational acceleration in head trauma are less pronounced in smaller brains. If true, this could result in a lesser amount of microscopic neuronal injury in young children than in adults following a comparable closed head injury. Alternatively, it is conceivable that the reported better prognosis for head injured children might be related to the different nature of their head injuries compared to those suffered by adults. Most head injuries suffered by children result from falls or low-speed accidents and, consequently, many paediatric head injuries are associated with less severe rotational acceleration (Levin, Benton and Grossman, 1982). Most head injuries sustained by adults, on the other hand, result from high-speed motor vehicle accidents, which are, by their nature, likely to yield greater diffuse brain injury. Jamison and Kaye (1974) observed that persistent neurological deficits were present only in children injured in road traffic accidents.

Head injury represents an area in which the maxim of better recovery in children has been questioned in recent years (Levin, Ewing-Cobbs and Benton, 1983). Although the rate of spontaneous recovery in children following closed head injury is often striking, persistent long-term language disorders have been reported (Gaidolfi and Vignolo, 1980; Satz and Bullard-Bates, 1981; Jordan, Ozanne and Murdoch, 1988) and even when specific linguistic symptoms resolve, cognitive and academic difficulties often remain. Acquired language disorders in children are covered in greater detail in Chapter 12.

Speech disorders subsequent to traumatic brain injury

Dysarthria constitutes one of the most persistent sequelae of severe TBI, often remaining beyond the resolution of any concomitant language disorder (Najenson *et al.*, 1978; Sarno and Levin, 1985). Despite this recognition, the literature relating to the prevalence and natural course of post-TBI dysarthria is unclear. Depending on factors such as the measures used, the stage post-injury when the measures were taken, the population studied and so on, estimates of the prevalence of dysarthria following TBI vary from 8 to 100% (Rusk, Block and Lowmann, 1969; Dresser *et al.*, 1973; Groher, 1977; Sarno, Buonaguro and Levita, 1986). Rusk, Block and Lowmann (1969) reported that approximately one-third of 96 survivors of severe TBI exhibited dysarthria during the acute phase of their recovery. Sarno, Buonaguro and Levita (1986) observed dysarthria in 34% of their 124 subjects with severe TBI. This was corroborated by Olver, Ponsford and Curran (1996), who also reported that motor speech problems were evident in 34% of their 103 severe TBI subjects five years post-injury. Two separate long-term follow-up studies of children who had suffered severe TBI indicated that 10% of children and 8% of adolescents were unintelligible (Ylvisaker, 1986). In a study of 14 TBI patients, Groher (1977) noted that all demonstrated dysarthria shortly after regaining consciousness.

One frequently observed feature of the dysarthria following TBI is the persistent nature of the disorder. In a follow-up study of 40 severe TBI cases, Thomsen (1984) reported that all 15 subjects who exhibited dysarthria in the acute stage (approximately four months post-injury) continued to demonstrate dysarthria 10–15 years later. Rusk, Block and Lowmann (1969) noted that, of their original 30 TBI subjects diagnosed as dysarthric, half of those subjects remained unimproved 5–15 years later. The remaining 50%, however, had made significant improvements in speech production. Such findings suggest that the prognosis for complete resolution of the dysarthric speech disturbance in individuals with severe TBI is poor (Hartley and Levin, 1990). Despite the often persistent and resilient nature of dysarthria post-TBI, however, the findings of several studies suggest that the restoration of functional verbal communication is possible in TBI cases many years post-injury, and certainly long after the accepted period of neurological recovery has passed (Beukelman and Garrett, 1988; Workinger and Netsell, 1992).

The presence of a persistent dysarthria has important implications for the long-term quality of life of survivors of severe TBI. As pointed out by Beukelman and Yorkston (1991), the presence of such a disorder reduces the individual's ability to function in communication situations that require understandable, efficient and natural-sounding speech (e.g. public speaking, vocational positions that require independent interaction with the public, etc.). In its most severe form, the dysarthria may necessitate the use of alternative and/or augmentative communication systems to bypass the impaired speech production apparatus. Put simply, the presence of a dysarthria may impede the successful return of the affected TBI patient to study, work or general social activities, leading to a loss of vocational standing and social isolation.

Despite the persistent nature of dysarthria in TBI and its potentially devastating social and economic impact on the lives of many survivors of TBI, very little research into its nature and severity has been reported. In particular, until recently there has been a conspicuous lack of research into the physiological bases of the motor breakdown in the various major components of the speech production mechanisms of TBI subjects. Most reports in the literature have included only clinical descriptions of the speech disturbances, single case studies or physiological investigations of small groups of TBI cases. Kent, Netsell and Bauer (1975) in a cinefluorographic study and Lehiste (1965) in an acoustic analysis provided case studies of dysarthria following TBI that detailed deficits in lingual movement, slow rate and incoordination in articulatory activity. Detailed physiological investigations of the functioning of the speech mechanism in survivors of TBI with dysarthria have yet to be reported. Because physiological assessment of the individual motor subsystems of the speech mechanism (i.e. respiratory, laryngeal, velopharyngeal and articulatory subsystems) is crucial in defining the underlying speech motor pathophysiology necessary for the development of optimal treatment programmes (Netsell, 1986; Abbs and De Paul, 1989), further research of this type is necessary. The most comprehensive series of perceptual and physiological studies of dysarthria associated with TBI reported to date was conducted by Theodoros and colleagues (Murdoch *et al.*, 1993; Theodoros and

Murdoch, 1994; Theodoros *et al.*, 1993, 1994; Theodoros, Murdoch and Stokes, 1995).

Severity and type of dysarthria following traumatic brain injury

Examination of the literature reveals wide variability in the severity and type of dysarthria reported to occur in association with TBI, with the severity covering the entire spectrum of dysfunction from mild articulatory imprecision through to total unintelligibility (Sarno, Buonaguro and Levita, 1986). Consistent with the multifocal nature of the brain damage associated with TBI and, depending on the specific site of the lesion, a number of different types of dysarthria have been reported to occur following TBI (Theodoros, Murdoch and Chenery, 1994). As would be expected based on the pathophysiology of TBI, the majority of dysarthric TBI patients exhibit a mixed form of dysarthria reflecting involvement of multiple motor systems, with a preponderance of spastic and ataxic features (Theodoros, Murdoch and Chenery, 1994). In an investigation of the perceptual speech characteristics of 27 TBI subjects with dysarthria, Theodoros, Murdoch and Chenery (1994) identified the presence of four specific types of dysarthria (spastic, hypokinetic, ataxic and flaccid) and four mixed dysarthrias (spastic-ataxic, spastic-hypokinetic, spastic-flaccid and flaccid-ataxic). Marquardt, Stoll and Sussman (1990) suggested that the most frequently occurring form of dysarthria post-TBI is spastic dysarthria, characterized by imprecise articulation, harsh voice quality, reduced stress, monopitch and monoloudness. Spastic dysarthria was also observed by Theodoros, Murdoch and Chenery (1994) to be one of the most frequently occurring components of the mixed dysarthrias exhibited by their TBI patients but only occurring in three (11%) cases in isolation. Spastic dysarthria is generally regarded as resulting from bilateral upper motor neurone lesions (Murdoch, 1990). According to Marquardt, Stoll and Sussman (1990), spastic dysarthria following TBI usually occurs in conjunction with spastic quadriplegia.

Damage to the bulbar cranial nerve nuclei within the brainstem or to the bulbar cranial nerves in their peripheral course (due to either direct insult and/or the shearing effects of acceleration/deceleration in TBI) leads to flaccid dysarthria. Depending on which particular cranial nerves/nuclei are damaged, the characteristics of the flaccid dysarthria will vary; however, nasal emission, hypernasality, breathiness and consonant imprecision are features of flaccid dysarthria frequently reported in TBI cases. Theodoros, Murdoch and Chenery (1994) identified flaccid dysarthria in four (15%) of their TBI cases in isolation and as part of a mixed dysarthria in three other TBI cases.

Some authors have reported the dysarthria evidenced in their TBI cases to be predominantly of the ataxic type (Simmons, 1983), a condition usually associated with generalized damage to the cerebellum or its connections in the brainstem. In support of these findings, Theodoros, Murdoch and Chenery (1994) identified the features of ataxic dysarthria in the speech of approximately 41% of their TBI group. The most frequently occurring form of dysarthria reported by Theodoros, Murdoch and Chenery (1994) was mixed spastic-ataxic, occurring in 30% of their subjects. Excess and equal stress, irregular articulatory breakdown, distorted vowels and a harsh voice quality are commonly reported features of ataxic dysarthria (Darley, Aronson and Brown, 1975).

Although less common, hypokinetic and hyperkinetic dysarthria may also occur in TBI patients, reflecting damage to the extrapyramidal pathways in the region of the basal ganglia and upper brainstem nuclei (Murdoch, 1990). Theodoros, Murdoch and Chenery (1994) reported that four of their 27 dysarthric TBI subjects exhibited hypokinetic dysarthria, with a further three subjects demonstrating mixed spastic-hypokinetic dysarthria.

Perceptual features of dysarthria following traumatic brain injury

The perceptual features of dysarthria following TBI encompass a broad range of abnormal speech features involving all aspects of the speech production process. Abnormal speech features reported to be exhibited by TBI patients include imprecise articulation, phonatory weakness, reduced pitch and loudness variation, hypernasality, a slow or rapid rate of speech and excessively increased or decreased loudness (Ylvisaker, 1992).

The most frequently occurring deviant speech dimensions identified by Theodoros, Murdoch and Chenery (1994) in 27 severe TBI cases included disturbances of prosody, resonance, articulation and respiration, with those deviant speech dimensions pertaining to phonation being less apparent in the speech output of their cases. Abnormal prosodic features noted to be present by Theodoros, Murdoch and Chenery (1994) included impaired rate (70% of TBI subjects exhibited a reduction in rate, while 30% of subjects demonstrated an increased rate of speech), rate fluctuations, short rushes of speech, reduced variation of pitch and loudness, impaired maintenance of loudness, unsteadiness of pitch, excess and equal stress, reduced phrase length and prolonged interword and/or intersyllable intervals. The deviant prosodic features reported by Theodoros, Murdoch and Chenery (1994) are consistent with those observed in the speech of TBI subjects by other researchers (Vogel and von Cramon, 1983; Yorkston *et al.*, 1984; Bellaire, Yorkston and Beukelman, 1986; Ziegler *et al.*, 1988).

Disorders of resonance, in particular hypernasality, have frequently been observed clinically in the speech of individuals following TBI, and the prevalence of this disorder was confirmed by Theodoros, Murdoch and Chenery (1994), who reported that their TBI dysarthric subjects exhibited greater levels of nasality and mixed nasality than non-speech-impaired controls with 26/27 (or 96%) of their subjects exhibiting hypernasality. Resonatory disturbances have also been reported in several case studies of TBI individuals (Workinger and Netsell, 1992; McHenry, Wilson and Minton, 1994).

Articulatory imprecision is another major component of dysarthria following TBI. Theodoros, Murdoch and Chenery (1994) found consonant imprecision to be present in 26 (i.e. 96%) of their

27 TBI cases with dysarthria and was the most discriminating deviant speech feature for differentiating TBI subjects from normal controls. An increase in the length of phonemes and distortion of vowels was also present in the speech output of 75% of these TBI subjects.

Certain perceptual characteristics of the speech output of TBI patients with dysarthria also indicate that the majority of these cases have inadequate respiratory support for speech production. Theodoros, Murdoch and Chenery (1994) reported that 24/27 (89%) of their TBI cases were perceived to exhibit insufficient supply and/or control of expiratory air flow to enable them to phrase correctly and maintain adequate pitch and volume control during speech.

Individual case studies of TBI subjects have indicated the presence of weak, breathy phonation in some subjects (McHenry, Wilson and Minton, 1994), whereas other patients have presented with strained/strangled vocal quality (Workinger and Netsell, 1992). The perceptual analysis of phonation in TBI patients reported by Theodoros, Murdoch and Chenery (1994) indicated that the deviant phonatory features of hoarseness, harshness and intermittent breathiness were more evident in 81, 48 and 46% of the TBI subjects respectively, compared with normal-speaking controls.

Overall, the intelligibility of TBI subjects with dysarthria has been reported to be significantly reduced compared with matched controls in relation to single-word and sentence intelligibility, rate of intelligible speech and communication efficiency (Theodoros, Murdoch and Chenery, 1994). The reduction in intelligibility appears to be the result of the combined effects of deficits in all five aspects of speech, namely prosody, articulation, resonance, respiration and phonation.

Acoustic features of dysarthria following traumatic brain injury

To date, the acoustic characteristics of dysarthria associated with TBI have been poorly defined. By far the majority of studies have only involved single cases, or at best only small groups of TBI patients. Further, in many reported studies, the acoustic features of the speech of TBI patients have been reported in conjunction with acoustic features of other neurologically disordered groups (e.g. cerebrovascular accident cases), making it impossible to identify the specific acoustic anomalies attributable to TBI. Those acoustic studies that have been reported have identified disorders in the areas of articulation, prosody and phonation post-TBI.

Acoustic features indicative of articulatory disorders identified by Ziegler and von Cramon (1983a, b, 1986) included centralization of vowel formants (leading to vowel reduction and distortion), articulatory undershoot on lip rounding and protrusion, lingual undershoot, increased word and syllable durations, inadequate voicing, spirantization (i.e. frication of stop gaps due to incomplete constriction), evidence of tongue retraction and the presence of slow, large amplitude cycles in formant trajectories, indicating slow, exaggerated protrusions and retractions of the tongue. Prosodic disturbances identified by way of acoustic analysis in a single TBI case with ataxic dysarthria by Simmons (1983) included changes in fundamental frequency contour as well as alterations in the temporal aspects of speech and articulatory gestures. Specifically, Simmons (1983) identified the presence of a flat fundamental frequency contour and the lack of high-frequency energy in the vowel formants, consistent with the perceptual qualities of monotonous and unnatural speech. Alterations in the temporal aspects of speech identified by Simmons (1983) using temporal acoustic measures included equal syllable duration with no variation in pause time, consistent with a speech pattern of excess and equal stress. Simmons (1983) also observed syllable durations in this TBI case to be longer than normal.

In an evaluation of the phonatory function of 24 subjects with central dysphonia (18 subjects with TBI), Hartmann and von Cramon (1984) identified specific acoustic features associated with 'breathy', 'rough' and 'tense' vocal qualities. Increase time lag of pre-exhalation and spectral energy about 5 kHz typified 'breathy' vocal quality, while increased fundamental frequency perturbation (jitter), especially in males, was characteristic of 'rough' voice quality. An increase in spectral energy in the 1–5 kHz range as well as increased variance of spectral energy above 5 kHz was associated with 'tense' vocal quality.

Physiological features of dysarthria following traumatic brain injury

Respiratory function following traumatic brain injury

Physiological assessment of the respiratory function of persons following TBI has identified impaired lung volumes and abnormal chest wall movements during speech breathing. McHenry, Wilson and Minton (1994), using respiratory inductance plethysmography, identified reduced inspiratory volume (11% of vital capacity) in a traumatically brain injured woman with flaccid dysarthria. Spirometric and kinematic assessment of the respiratory function of 20 severe TBI subjects conducted by Murdoch *et al.* (1993) using strain-gauge pneumographs revealed the presence of (1) significantly reduced lung capacities (i.e. vital capacity (VC) and forced expiratory volume in one second (FEV_1) compared with those of matched controls and (2) abnormalities in the two-part coordination of the chest wall, involving the rib cage and abdomen, during expiration.

Laryngeal function following traumatic brain injury

Physiological assessments have demonstrated contrasting patterns of laryngeal function in TBI patients with the findings of some studies suggestive of hypofunction and others of hyperfunctional patterns. Netsell and Daniel (1979), in a single case study of a severe TBI person, recorded high glottal air flows consistent with hypoadduction of the vocal folds, compared with normative data (Iwata, von Leden and Williams, 1972). Using a pneumotachometer and differential transducer attached to a face mask, Netsell, Lotz and Barlow (1989) recorded considerably higher laryngeal air flow during vowel production for a TBI subject with dysarthric speech compared with a normal individual. Netsell, Lotz and Barlow (1989) inferred from these results

that the dysarthric speaker demonstrated problems with rapid abduction and adduction of the vocal folds, in addition to inefficient vocal fold adduction in the midline. Similarly, McHenry, Wilson and Minton (1994) recorded laryngeal aerodynamic data consistent with a hypofunctioning larynx in an 18-year-old female following a severe TBI. Specifically, the subject recorded low subglottal pressures and laryngeal resistance values in conjunction with high air flows. In a further study, McHenry (1996) predominantly found hypolaryngeal valving in a group of 26 subjects with severe TBI. Specifically, 61.5% of subjects demonstrated reduced laryngeal airway resistance, 19.2% had resistance values that were within normal limits, while the remaining 19.3% of subjects exhibited increased laryngeal airway resistance values.

In contrast, Theodoros and Murdoch (1994) identified hyperfunctional laryngeal activity as the predominant form of laryngeal dysfunction in a group of TBI subjects, with five different patterns of laryngeal hyperfunction being identified. Hyperfunctional vocal fold vibratory patterns and aerodynamic characteristics – such as increased fundamental frequency, decreased duty cycle and closing time, increased glottal resistance and subglottal pressure and reduced phonatory air flow and ad/abduction rate of the vocal folds – were evident in the instrumental findings, but never altogether in one subject (Theodoros and Murdoch, 1994). Statistical analysis identified five subgroups of TBI subjects with varying degrees and combinations of hyperfunctional laryngeal features. It was suggested by Theodoros and Murdoch (1994) that the hyperfunctional laryngeal activity identified in their subjects could be accounted for by both diffuse cortical and subcortical neuronal damage that is commonly sustained by TBI and that would account for bilateral lesions of the upper motor neurones and corticobulbar fibre tracts resulting in spasticity of the laryngeal musculature. Furthermore, Theodoros and Murdoch (1994) proposed that the different manifestations of hyperfunctional laryngeal activity reflected a combination of the various glottal and respiratory force adjustments deployed by the individual subjects in response to spasticity in the vocal folds and strategies to compensate for impairment in other subsystems of the speech production mechanism.

Velopharyngeal function following traumatic brain injury

Velopharyngeal incompetence is a prominent physiological characteristic of dysarthric speech disturbance associated with TBI. Several individual case studies have identified velopharyngeal dysfunction in TBI persons with dysarthric speech (Netsell and Daniel, 1979; Netsell, Lotz and Barlow, 1989; Workinger and Netsell, 1992; McHenry, Wilson and Minton, 1994). Essentially, these studies identified high nasal air flows and nasalance values, in addition to reduced velopharyngeal resistance and intraoral pressures (Netsell, Lotz and Barlow, 1989; McHenry, Wilson and Minton, 1994). McHenry, Wilson and Minton (1994) reported the findings of an increased nasalance score (50%), reduced velopharyngeal resistance, increased nasal air flow and a reduced intraoral pressure in their severely brain injured case. Similarly, Netsell, Lotz and Barlow (1989) identified the presence of a very high nasal air flow with a concomitant reduction in intraoral pressure in a TBI person during the production of the word 'pamper', indicating that the subject failed to close the velopharynx for the /p/ segment following the nasal /m/.

Confirmation of the frequent occurrence of velopharyngeal dysfunction in the TBI population has been provided by a group study in which an indirect instrumental assessment of velopharyngeal competency was performed on 20 dysarthric TBI subjects and their matched controls (Theodoros *et al.*, 1993). The results of this study revealed significantly increased nasality, based on a nasality index across non-nasalized utterances, in the speech output of TBI subjects compared with the controls. The findings were suggestive of impaired functioning of the velopharyngeal valve.

Articulatory function following traumatic brain injury

Physiological deficits in the articulatory components of the speech mechanism, such as the lips, tongue and jaw have also been reported in brain injured individuals. Kent, Netsell and Bauer (1975), in an early case study of a person with dysarthria following head trauma, identified a reduction in the ranges of lingual mobility, restrictions in the direction of tongue movements and a slow rate of articulation, using cineradiographic techniques. Several aspects of lip force control such as peak force overshoot, force stability during the hold phase of muscle contraction and the rate of force recruitment have also been found to be significantly impaired in TBI subjects (Barlow and Netsell, 1989; Barlow and Burton, 1990). In addition, greater force impairment of the lower lip compared with the upper lip, and a relationship between deficits in lip force control and the magnitude of the target force, have been identified in this population (Barlow and Netsell, 1989). Barlow and Burton (1990), in applying a ramp-and-hold force paradigm in a preliminary investigation to assess the upper and lower lips of four TBI adults with dysarthric speech, identified a degree of force control impairment affecting one or both lips in each subject with considerable individual variation in the manifestation of this impairment. Using a similar ramp-and-hold task, McHenry, Wilson and Minton (1994) identified an impaired ability to rapidly recruit lingual force when attempting to reach a target level in a severely brain injured subject. Furthermore, the subject demonstrated reduced maximum voluntary forces for the upper and lower lips and the tongue. In another single case study of a TBI subject with mild spastic-flaccid dysarthria, Robin, Somodi and Luschei (1991) assessed the tongue strength of the subject on a maximum tongue pressure task and found that the TBI subject produced a weaker maximum tongue pressure compared with a matched control subject. Theodoros, Murdoch and Stokes (1995) also identified significant impairment of lip and tongue function in a group of 18 TBI subjects with dysarthric speech, based on strength, endurance and rate measures. Overall, the study indicated the presence of a slightly greater degree of impairment in tongue function compared with lip function.

The differing degrees of impairment of lip and tongue function are consistent with previous reports of differential subsystem impairment in dysarthric speakers (Hunker, Abbs and Barlow, 1982; Abbs, Hunker and Barlow, 1983). The findings highlight the importance of assessing each functional component of the speech mechanism independently in TBI patients, to accurately define the nature of the underlying pathophysiological deficits of the perceived articulatory disorder.

Summary

Much of our current understanding of the speech-language disorders occurring subsequent to TBI has come from studies reported since the 1980s. It is in the current century, however, that the importance of communication abilities for the long-term quality of life of survivors of TBI has begun to be recognized. Several factors that appear to have minimized the perceived importance of speech-language deficits following TBI to various health professionals include: the failure of researchers to develop terminology to adequately describe the disorders; the lack of empirical data regarding the nature of speech-language disorders post TBI; the failure of researchers to recognize the disorders as unique speech-language symptomatology; the perception that communicative disorders post TBI resolve completely, especially in children; and an opinion that communication disorders in TBI cases need only be treated as an accessory for medical management.

Advances in recent years in our understanding of the basic mechanisms involved in brain damage associated with TBI have enabled the introduction of important improvements in the medical management of TBI cases. This in turn has led to improved survival rates for persons with TBI. The improved survival rate, combined with the increasing incidence of TBI in most Western countries and the now recognized serious economic and social consequence of associated speech-language disorders, has necessitated greater research efforts aimed at a better understanding of the nature of communicative impairments following TBI, which in turn will lead to the development of more effective treatment strategies.

References

Abbs, J.H. and De Paul, R. (1989) Assessment of dysarthria: the critical prerequisite to treatment, in *Disorders of Communication: the Science of Intervention* (ed. M.M. Leahy), Taylor & Francis, London, pp. 206–277.

Abbs, J.H., Hunker, C.J. and Barlow, S.M. (1983) Differential speech motor subsystem impairments with suprabulbar lesions: neurological framework and supporting data, in *Clinical Dysarthria* (ed. W.R. Berry), College Hill Press, San Diego, CA, pp. 21–56.

Adams, J.H. (1975) The neuropathology of head injuries, in *Handbook of Clinical Neurology: Injuries of the Brain and Skull: Part 1*, vol. 23 (eds P.J. Vinken and G.W. Bruyn), North-Holland Publishing Company, Amsterdam, pp. 35–65.

Adams, J.H., Graham, D.I., Gennarelli, T.A. and Maxwell, W.L. (1991) Diffuse axonal injury in nonmissile head injury. *Journal of Neurology, Neurosurgery, and Psychiatry*, **54**, 481–483.

Adams, J.H., Graham, D.I., Murray, L.S. and Scott, G. (1982) Diffuse axonal injury due to non-missile head injury in humans. An analysis of 45 cases. *Annals of Neurology*, **12**, 557–563.

Adams, J.H., Graham, D.I., Scott, G. *et al.* (1980) Brain damage in fatal non-missile head injury. *Journal of Clinical Pathology*, **33**, 1132–1145.

Adams, J.H., Mitchell, D.E., Graham, D.I. and Doyle, D. (1977) Diffuse brain damage of immediate impact type: its relationship to primary brainstem damage in head injury. *Brain*, **100**, 489–502.

Annegers, J.F., Grabow, J.D., Kurland, L.T. and Laws, E.R. (1980) The incidence, causes and secular trends of head trauma in Olmstead County, Minnesota. *Neurology*, **30**, 912–919.

Auerbach, S.H. (1986) Neuroanatomical correlates of attention and memory disorder in traumatic brain injury: an application of neurobehavioral subtypes. *Journal of Head Trauma Rehabilitation*, **3**, 1–12.

Baker, L. (1982) An evaluation of the role of metacognitive deficits in learning disabilities. *Topics in Learning and Learning Disabilities*, **2**, 26–36.

Barlow, S.M. and Burton, M.K. (1990) Ramp-and-hold force control in the upper and lower lips: developing new neuromotor assessment applications in traumatic brain-injured adults. *Journal of Speech and Hearing Research*, **33**, 660–675.

Barlow, S.M. and Netsell, R. (1989) Clinical neurophysiology for individuals with dysarthria, in *Recent*

Advances in Clinical Dysarthria (eds K.M. Yorkston and D.R. Beukelman), College Hill Press, Boston, pp. 53–82.

Bellaire, K., Yorkston, K.M. and Beukelman, D.R. (1986) Modification of breathing patterning to increase naturalness of a mildly dysarthric speaker. *Journal of Communication Disorders*, **19**, 271–280.

Benjamin, L., Debinski, A., Fletcher, D. *et al.* (1989) The use of the Bethesda conversational skills profile in closed head injury, in *Theory and Function: Bridging the Gap* (ed. V. Anderson), Australian Society for the Study of Brain Impairment, Melbourne, pp. 57–64.

Benson, D.F. (1967) Fluency in aphasia: Correlation with radioactive scan localization. *Cortex*, **3**, 373–394.

Beukelman, D.R. and Garrett, K. (1988) Augmentative and alternative communication for adults with acquired severe communication disorders. *Augmentative and Alternative Communication*, **4**, 104–121.

Beukelman, D.R. and Yorkston, K.M. (1991) Traumatic brain injury changes the way we live, in *Communication Disorders Following Traumatic Brain Injury* (eds D.R. Beukelman and K.M. Yorkston), Pro-Ed, Austin, TX, pp. 1–13.

Bigler, E.D. (1990) Neuropathology of traumatic brain injury, in *Traumatic Brain Injury* (ed. E. Bigler), Pro-Ed, Austin, TX, pp. 13–49.

Bigler, E.D., Kurth, S., Blatter, D. and Abildskov, T. (1993) Day-of-injury CT as an index to pre-injury brain morphology: degree of post-injury degenerative changes identified by CT and MR neuroimaging. *Brain Injury*, **7**, 125–134.

Blumbergs, P.C., Jones, N.R. and North, J.B. (1989) Diffuse axonal injury in head trauma. *Journal of Neurology, Neurosurgery and Psychiatry*, **52**, 838–841.

Bock, J.K. (1982) Toward a cognitive psychology of syntax: information processing contributions to sentence formulation. *Psychological Review*, **89**, 1–47.

Breasted, J.H. (1930) *The Edwin Smith Surgical Papyrus*, vol. **1**. University of Chicago Press, Chicago.

Brooks, D.N., Aughton, M.E., Bond, M.R. *et al.* (1980) Cognitive sequelae in relationship to early indices of severity of brain damage after severe blunt head injury. *Journal of Neurology, Neurosurgery and Psychiatry*, **43**, 529–534

Brownell, H.H., Michel, D., Powelson, J. and Gardner, E. (1983) Surprise but not sensitivity to verbal humour in right hemisphere patients. *Brain and Language*, **27**, 20–27.

Bryan, K. (1988) Assessment of language disorders after right hemisphere damage. *British Journal of Disorders of Communication*, **23**, 111–125.

Bryan, K. (1989) *The Right Hemisphere Language Battery*, Far Communications, Southampton.

Chapman, S., Culhane, K., Levin, H. *et al.* (1992) Narrative discourse after closed head injury in children and adolescents. *Brain and Language*, **43**, 2–62.

Chapman, S., Levin, S. and Culhane, K. (1995) Language impairment in closed head injury, in *Handbook of Neurological Speech and Language Disorders* (ed. S. Kirschner), Marcel Decker, New York, pp. 387–429.

Code, C. (1987) *Language, Aphasia and the Right Hemisphere*, John Wiley & Sons Ltd, Chichester.

Coelho, C.A., Liles, B.Z. and Duffy, R.J. (1991a) Discourse analysis with closed head injured adults. Evidence for differing patterns of deficits. *Archives of Physical Medicine and Rehabilitation*, **72**, 465–468.

Coelho, C.A., Liles, B.Z. and Duffy, R.J. (1991b) The use of discourse analyses for the evaluation of higher level traumatically brain-injured adults. *Brain Injury*, **5**, 381–392.

Coloquhoun, I.R. and Rawlinson, J. (1989) The significance of haematomas of the basal ganglia in closed head injury. *Clinical Radiology*, **40**, 619–621.

Cullum, C.M. and Bigler, E.D. (1986) Ventricle size, cortical atrophy, and the relationship with neuropsychological status in closed head injury: a quantitative analysis. *Journal of Clinical Experimental Neuropsychology*, **8**, 437–452.

Darley, F.L. (1982) *Aphasia*, W. B. Saunders, Philadelphia.

Darley, F.L., Aronson, A.E. and Brown, J.R. (1975) *Motor Speech Disorders*, W.B. Saunders Company, Philadelphia.

Dresser, A.C., Meirowsky, A.M., Weiss, G.J. *et al.* (1973) Gainful employment following head injury: prognostic factors. *Archives of Neurology*, **29**, 111–116.

Ehrlich, J. and Barry, P. (1989) Rating communication behaviours in head-injured adults. *Brain Injury*, **3**, 193–198.

Fingers, S. (1978) *Recovery from Brain Damage*, Plenum Press, New York.

Finlayson, M.A.J. and Garner, S.H. (1994) Challenges in rehabilitation of individuals with acquired brain injury, in *Brain Injury Rehabilitation: Clinical Considerations* (eds M.A.J. Finlayson and S.H. Garner), Williams & Wilkins, Baltimore, pp. 3–10.

Friede, R.L. (1973) *Developmental Neuropathology*, Springer, New York.

Gaidolfi, E. and Vignolo, L.A. (1980) Closed head injuries of school aged children: neuropsychological sequelae in early adulthood. *Italian Journal of Neurological Sciences*, **1**, 65–73.

Gardner, K. and Denes, G. (1973) Connotative judgements by aphasic patients on a pictorial adaption of the semantic differential. *Cortex*, **9**, 183–412.

Gennarelli, T.A. (1993) Mechanisms of brain injury. *Journal of Emergency Medicine*, **11**, 5–11.

Gennarelli, T.A., Thibault, L.E., Adams, H.J. *et al.* (1982) Diffuse axonal injury. *Annals of Neurology*, **12**, 212–223.

Geschwind, N. (1971) Current concepts: aphasia. *North England Journal of Medicine*, **284**, 645–656.

Gjerris, F. (1986) Head injuries in children: special features. *Acta Neurochirurgica*, **36** (Suppl.), 155–158.

Goldstein, K. (1948) *Language and Language Disturbances*, Grune & Stratton, New York.

Graham, D.I. and Adams, J.H. (1971) Ischaemic brain damage in fatal head injuries. *Lancet*, **1**, 265–266.

Graham, D.J., Adams, J.H. and Doyle, D. (1978) Ischaemic brain damage in fatal nonmissile head injuries. *Journal of Neurological Science*, **39**, 213–234.

Groher, M. (1977) Language and memory disorders following closed head trauma. *Journal of Speech and Hearing Research*, **20**, 212–222.

Groher, M. (1983) Communication disorders, in *Rehabilitation of the Head Injured Adult* (eds M. Rosenthal, E. Griffith, M. Bond and J.D. Miller), F.A. Davis, Philadelphia.

Gurdjian, E.S. and Gurdjian, E.S. (1976) Cerebral contusions: re-evaluation of the mechanism of their development. *Journal of Trauma*, **16**, 35–51.

Guthrie, E., Mast, J., Richards, P. *et al.* (1999) Traumatic brain injury in children and adolescents. *Child and Adolescent Psychiatric Clinics of North America*, **8**, 807–826.

Hagen, C. (1984) Language disorders in head trauma, in *Language Disorders in Adults: Recent Advances* (ed. A. Holland), College-Hill Press, San Diego, pp. 245–281.

Hagen, C., Malkmus, D. and Burditt, G. (1979) *Intervention Strategies for Language Disorders Secondary to Head Trauma: Short Course*, American Speech-Language and Hearing Association, Atlanta.

Hartley, L. (1995) *Cognitive-Communicative Abilities Following Brain Injury: a Functional Approach*, Singular Publishing Group Inc., San Diego.

Hartley, L. and Jensen, P.J. (1991) Narrative and procedural discourse after closed head injury. *Brain Injury*, **6**, 271–281.

Hartley, L.L. and Levin, H.S. (1990) Linguistic deficits after closed head injury: a current appraisal. *Aphasiology*, **4**, 353–370.

Hartmann, E. and von Cramon, D. (1984) Acoustic measurement of voice quality in central dysphonia. *Journal of Communication Disorders*, **17**, 425–440.

Heilman, K.M., Safran, A. and Geschwind, N. (1971) Closed head trauma and aphasia. *Journal of Neurology, Neurosurgery and Psychiatry*, **34**, 265–269.

Heilman, K.M. and Valenstein, C. (1979) *Clinical Neuropsychology*, Oxford University Press, New York.

Hendrick, E.B., Hardwood-Nash, D. and Hudson, A.R. (1964) Head injuries in children: a survey of 4465 consecutive cases at the Hospital for Sick Children, Toronto, Canada. *Clinical Neurosurgery*, **11**, 45–65.

Hillbom, E. (1959) Delayed effects of traumatic brain injuries: neurological remarks. *Acta Psychiatrica Scandinavica*, **137**, 7.

Hinchcliffe, F.J., Murdoch, B.E. and Chenery, H.J. (1998) Towards a conceptualization of language and cognitive impairment in a closed head-injury: use of clinical measures. *Brain Injury*, **12**, 109–132.

Holbourn, A.H.S. (1943) Mechanics of head injuries. *Lancet*, **2**, 438–441.

Holland, A.L. (1982) When is aphasia aphasia? The problem of closed head injury, in *Clinical Aphasiology*, vol. 12 (ed. R. Brookshire), BRK Publishers, Minneapolis, pp. 345–349.

Huisingh, R., Barrett, M., Bachman, L. *et al.* (1990) *The Word Test – Revised*, LinguiSystems, East Moline, IL.

Hunker, C., Abbs, J. and Barlow, S.M. (1982) The relationship between parkinsonian rigidity and hypokinesia of the orofacial system: a quantitative analysis. *Neurology*, **32**, 755–761.

Iwata, S., von Leden, H. and Williams, D. (1972) Air flow measurement during phonation. *Journal of Communication Disorders*, **5**, 67–69.

Jamison, D.L. and Kaye, H.H. (1974) Accidental head injury in children. *Archives of Diseases of Childhood*, **49**, 376–381.

Javid, M. and Settlage, P. (1956) Effect of urea on cerebrospinal fluid pressure in human subjects: preliminary report. *Journal of the American Medical Association*, **160**, 943–949.

Jellinger, K. (1983) The neuropathology of pediatric head injuries, in *Pediatric Head Trauma* (ed.

K. Shapiro), Futura, Mount Kisco, NY, pp. 87–115.

Jellinger, K. and Seitelberger, F. (1970) Protracted post-traumatic encephalopathy: pathology, pathogenesis, and clinical implications. *Journal of Neurological Sciences*, **10**, 51–94.

Jennett, B. (1983) Scope and scale of the problem, in *Rehabilitation of the Head Injured Adult* (ed. J.D. Miller), F.A. Davis, Philadelphia, pp. 61–75.

Jennett, B. (1986) Head trauma, in *Diseases of the Nervous System* (eds A.K. Asbury, G.M. McKann and W.I. McDonald), W.B. Saunders, Philadelphia, pp. 1282–1297.

Jennett, B. and Teasdale, G. (1981) *Management of Head Injuries*, F.A. Davis, Philadelphia.

Jordan, F.M., Ozanne, A.E. and Murdoch, B.E. (1988) Long-term speech and language disorders subsequent to closed head injury in children. *Brain Injury*, **2**, 179–185.

Katz, M.D. (1992) Neuropathology and neurobehavioural recovery from closed head injury. *Journal of Head Trauma Rehabilitation*, **7**, 1–15.

Kent, R.D., Netsell, R. and Bauer, L. (1975) Cineradiographic assessment of articulatory mobility in the dysarthrias. *Journal of Speech and Hearing Disorders*, **40**, 467–480.

Klauber, M.R., Barrett-Connor, E., Marshall, L.F. and Bowers, S.A. (1981) The epidemiology of head injury: a prospective study of an entire community – San Diego County, California, 1978. *American Journal of Epidemiology*, **113**, 500–509.

Kraus, J.F., Black, M.A., Hessal, N. *et al.* (1984) The incidence of acute brain injury and serious impairment in a defined population. *American Journal of Epidemiology*, **119**, 186–201.

Lehiste, I. (1965) Some acoustic characteristics of dysarthric speech. *Biblotheca Phonetica*, **2**, 1–124.

Lenneberg, E. (1967) *Biological Foundations of Language*, John Wiley & Sons, Inc., New York.

Letarte, P.B. (1999) Neurotrauma care in the new millennium. *Surgical Clinics of North America*, **79**, 1449–1470.

Levin, H.S., Benton, A.L. and Grossman, M.D. (1982) *Neurobehavioural Consequences of Closed Head Injury*, Oxford University Press, New York.

Levin, H.S. and Eisenberg, G.M. (1979) Neuropsychological outcome of closed head injury in children and adolescents. *Child's Brain*, **5**, 281–292.

Levin, H.S., Ewing-Cobbs, L. and Benton, A.L. (1983) Age and recovery from brain damage, in *Aging and the Recovery of Function in the Central Nervous System* (ed. S.W. Scheff), Plenum Publishing, New York, pp. 233–240.

Levin, H.S., Grossman, R.G. and Kelly, P.J. (1976) Aphasia disorder in patients with closed head injury. *Journal of Neurology, Neurosurgery, and Psychiatry*, **39**, 1062–1070.

Levin, H.S., Grossman, R.G. and Rose, S.E. (1979) Long term neuropsychological outcome of closed head injury. *Journal of Neurosurgery*, **50**, 412–422.

Lezak, M. (1983) *Neuropsychological Assessment*, 2nd edn, Oxford University Press, New York.

Lichtheim, L. (1885) On aphasia. *Brain*, **7**, 433–484.

Lindenberg, R. and Freytag, E. (1969) Morphology of brain lesions from blunt trauma in early infancy. *Archives of Pathology (Chicago)*, **87**, 298–305.

Lundberg, N. (1960) Continuous recording and control of ventricular fluid pressure in neurosurgical practice. *Acta Psychiatrica Scandinavica*, **36** (Suppl.), 1–193.

Luria, A.R. (1970) *Traumatic Aphasia*, Mouton, The Hague.

Marquardt, T.P., Stoll, J. and Sussman, H. (1990) Disorders of communication in traumatic brain injury, in *Traumatic Brain Injury: Mechanisms of Damage, Assessment, Intervention and Outcome* (ed. E.D. Bigler), Pro-Ed, Austin, TX, pp. 181–205.

MacPherson, P., Teasdale, E., Dhaker, S. *et al.* (1986) The significance of traumatic haematoma in the region of the basal ganglia. *Journal of Neurology, Neurosurgery and Psychiatry*, **49**, 29–34.

McDonald, S. (1992) Communication disorders following closed head injury: new approaches to assessment and rehabilitation. *Brain Injury*, **6**, 283–292.

McDonald, S. (1993) Viewing the brain sideways: frontal versus right hemisphere explanations of non-aphasic language disorders. *Aphasiology*, **7**, 535–549.

McDonald, S. and Pearce, S. (1995) 'The Dice Game' a new test of pragmatic language skills after closed head injury. *Brain Injury*, **9**, 255–271.

McDonald, S., Togher, L. and Code, C. (1999) The nature of traumatic brain injury: basic features and neuropsychological consequences, in *Communication Disorders Following Traumatic Brain Injury* (eds S. McDonald, L. Togher and C. Code), Psychology Press, Hove, pp. 19–54.

McDonald, S. and van Sommers, P. (1993) Pragmatic language skills after closed head injury: ability to negotiate requests. *Cognitive Neuropsychology*, **10**, 297–315.

McHenry, M.A. (1996) Laryngeal airway resistance following traumatic brain injury, in *Disorders of Motor Speech: Assessment, Treatment and Clinical Characterization* (eds D.A. Robin, K.M. Yorkston and D.R. Beukelman), Paul H. Brooks Publishing Co., Baltimore, pp. 229–240.

McHenry, M., Wilson, R.L. and Minton, J.T. (1994) Management of multiple physiologic system deficits following traumatic brain injury. *Journal of Medical Speech-Language Pathology*, **2**, 59–74.

Menkes, J.H. and Till, K. (1995) Postnatal trauma and injuries by physical agents, in *Textbook of Child Neurology* (ed. J.H. Menkes), Williams & Wilkins, Baltimore, pp. 557–597.

Mentis, M. and Prutting, C. (1987) Cohesion in the discourse of normal and head injured adults. *Journal of Speech and Hearing Research*, **30**, 88–89.

Miller, J.D. and Sweet, R.C. (1978) Early insults to the injured brain. *Journal of the American Medical Association*, **240**, 439–442.

Milton, S., Prutting, C. and Binder, G. (1984) Appraisal of communication competence in head injured adults, in *Clinical Aphasiology*, vol. **14** (ed. R. Brookshire), BRK Publishers, Minneapolis, pp. 114–123.

Murdoch, B.E. (1990) *Acquired Speech and Language Disorders: A Neuroanatomical and Functional Neurological Approach*, Chapman and Hall, London.

Murdoch, B.E., Theodoros, D.G., Stokes, P.D. and Chenery, H.J. (1993) Abnormal patterns of speech breathing in dysarthria following severe closed head injury. *Brain Injury*, **7**, 295–308.

National Head Injury Foundation. (1985) *An Educator's Manual: What Educators Need to Know About Students with Traumatic Brain Injury*. National Head Injury Foundation, Framingham, MA.

Najenson, T., Sazbon, L., Fiselzon, J. *et al.* (1978) Recovery of communicative functions after prolonged traumatic coma. *Scandinavian Journal of Rehabilitation Medicine*, **10**, 15–21.

Naugle, R.I. (1990) Epidemiology of traumatic brain injury in adults, in *Traumatic Brain Injury: Mechanisms of Damage, Assessment, Intervention, and Outcome* (ed. E.D. Bigler), Pro-Ed, Austin, TX, pp. 69–103.

Netsell, R. (1986) *A Neurobiological View of Speech Production and the Dysarthrias*, College Hill Press, San Diego.

Netsell, R. and Daniel, B. (1979) Dysarthria in adults: Physiologic approach in rehabilitation. *Archives of Physical Medicine and Rehabilitation*, **60**, 502–508.

Netsell, R., Lotz, W.K. and Barlow, S.M. (1989) A speech physiology examination for individuals with dysarthria, in *Recent Advances in Clinical Dysarthria* (eds K.M. Yorkston and D.R. Beukelman), College Hill Press, Boston, pp. 4–37.

Olver, J.H., Ponsford, J.L. and Curran, C.A. (1996) Outcome following traumatic brain injury: a comparison between 2 and 5 years after injury. *Brain Injury*, **10**, 841–848.

Pang, D. (1985) Pathophysiologic correlates of neurobehavioural syndromes following closed head injury, in *Head Injury Rehabilitation: Children and Adolescents* (ed. M. Ylvisaker), Pro-Ed, Austin, TX, pp. 3–70.

Parsons, C.L., Lambier, J., Snow, P. *et al.* (1989) Conversational skills in closed head injury: Part 1. *Australian Journal of Human Communication Disorders*, **17**, 37–46.

Porch, B.E. (1967) *Porch Index of Communicative Ability*, Consulting Psychologists Press, Palo Alto, CA.

Prigatano, G., Roueche, J. and Fordyce, D. (1986) Nonaphasic language disturbances after brain injury, in *Neuropsychological Rehabilitation after Brain Injury* (ed. G.P. Prigatano), John Hopkins University Press, Baltimore, pp. 18–28.

Prutting, C. and Kirchner, D. (1983) Applied pragmatics, in *Pragmatic Assessment and Intervention Issues in Language* (eds T. Gallagher and C. Prutting), College Hill Press, San Diego.

Reilly, P.L. and Adams, J.H. (1975) Patients with head injury who talk and die. *Lancet*, **2**, 375–377.

Robin, D.A., Somodi, L.B. and Luschei, E.S. (1991) Measurement of strength and endurance in normal and articulation disordered subjects, in *Dysarthria and Apraxia of Speech: Perspectives on Management* (eds C.A. Moore, K.M. Yorkston and D.R. Beukelman) Paul Brookes Publishing Co., Baltimore, pp. 173–184.

Rosner, M.J. (1995) Introduction to cerebral perfusion pressure management. *Neurosurgical Clinics of North America*, **6**, 761–773.

Rosner, M.J. and Coley, I.B. (1986) Cerebral perfusion pressure, intracranial pressure and elevation. *Journal of Neurosurgery*, **65**, 636–641.

Rosner, M.J. and Daughton, S. (1990) Cerebral perfusion pressure management in head trauma. *Journal of Trauma*, **30**, 933–940.

Rusk, H., Block, J. and Lowmann, E. (1969) Rehabilitation of the brain-injured patient: a report of 157 cases with long-term follow-up of 118, in *The Late*

Effects of Head Injury (eds E. Walker, W. Caveness and M. Critchley), Charles C. Thomas, Springfield, MA, pp. 327–332.

Russell, W.R. (1932) Cerebral involvement in head injury: a study based on the examination of two hundred cases. *Brain*, **55**, 549–603.

Russell, W.R. and Espir, M.L.E. (1961) *Traumatic Aphasia*, Oxford University Press, London.

Sarno, M. (1980) The nature of verbal impairment after closed head injury. *Journal of Nervous and Mental Disease*, **168** (11), 685–692.

Sarno, M. (1984) Verbal impairment after closed head injury: report of a replication study. *Journal of Nervous and Mental Disease*, **172** (8), 475–479.

Sarno, M.T., Buonaguro, A. and Levita, E. (1986) Characteristics of verbal impairment in closed head injured patients. *Archives of Physical Medicine and Rehabilitation*, **67**, 400–405.

Sarno, M.T. and Levin, H.S. (1985) Speech and language disorders after closed head injury, in *Speech and Language Evaluation in Neurology: Adult Disorders* (ed. J.K. Darby), Grune & Stratton, New York, pp. 323–339.

Satz, P. and Bullard-Bates, C. (1981) Acquired aphasia in children, in *Acquired Aphasia* (ed. M.T. Sarno), Academic Press, New York, pp. 23–74.

Schiller, F. (1947) Aphasia studied in patients with missile wounds. *Journal of Neurology, Neurosurgery and Psychiatry*, **10**, 183–197.

Simmons, N. (1983) Acoustic analysis of ataxic dysarthria: an approach to monitoring treatment, in *Clinical Dysarthria* (ed. W. Berry), College Hill Press, San Diego, pp. 283–294.

Spreen, O. and Benton, A.L. (1969) *Neurosensory Centre Comprehensive Examination for Aphasia: Manual for Directions*, University of Victoria, Victoria, BC.

Stone, J.L., Lopes, J.R. and Moody, R.A. (1978) Fluent aphasia after closed head injury. *Surgical Neurology*, **9**, 27–29.

Strich, S.J. (1956) Diffuse degeneration of the cerebral white matter in severe dementia following head injury. *Journal of Neurology, Neurosurgery and Psychiatry*, **19**, 163–185.

Strich, S.J. (1961) Shearing of nerve fibres as a cause of brain damage due to head injury. *Lancet*, **2**, 443–448.

Strich, S.J. (1969) The pathology of brain damage due to blunt head injuries, in *The Late Effects of Head Injury* (eds A.E. Walker, W.F. Caveness and M.

Critchley), Charles C. Thomas, Springfield, IL, pp. 501–524.

Tate, R.L., McDonald, S. and Lulham, J.L. (1998) Traumatic brain injury: severity of injury and outcome in an Australian population. *Journal of Australia and New Zealand Public Health*, **22**, 11–15.

Teasdale, G.M. and Graham, D.I. (1998) Craniocerebral trauma: protection and retrieval of the neuronal population after injury. *Neurosurgery*, **43**, 723–738.

Teasdale, G. and Jennett, B. (1974) Assessment of coma and impaired consciousness: a practical scale. *Lancet*, **2**, 81–84.

Teasdale, G.M. and Jennett, B. (1976) Assessment and prognosis of coma after head injury. *Acta Neurochirurgica*, **34**, 45–55.

Teuber, H.L. (1975) Recovery of function after brain injury in man, in *Outcome of Severe Damage to the Central Nervous System* (eds R. Porter and D.W. Fitzsimons), CIBA Foundation Symposium No. 34, Elsevier/Excerpta Medica, Amsterdam.

Theodoros, D.G. and Murdoch, B.E. (1994) Laryngeal dysfunction in dysarthric speakers following severe closed head injury. *Brain Injury*, **8**, 667–684.

Theodoros, D.G., Murdoch, B.E. and Chenery, H.J. (1994) Perceptual speech characteristics of dysarthric speakers following severe closed head injury. *Brain Injury*, **8**, 101–124.

Theodoros, D.G., Murdoch, B.E. and Stokes, P.D. (1995) A physiological analysis of articulatory dysfunction in dysarthric speakers following severe closed head injury. *Brain Injury*, **9**, 237–254.

Theodoros, D.G., Murdoch, B.E., Stokes, P.D. and Chenery, H.J. (1993) Hypernasality in dysarthric speakers following severe closed head injury: a perceptual and instrumental analysis. *Brain Injury*, **7**, 59–69.

Thomsen, I.V. (1975) Evaluation and outcome of aphasia in patients with severe closed head trauma. *Journal of Neurology, Neurosurgery and Psychiatry*, **38**, 713–718.

Thomsen, I.V. (1984) Late outcome of very severe blunt head injury: a 10–15 year second follow-up. *Journal of Neurology, Neurosurgery and Psychiatry*, **47**, 260–268.

Towne, R. and Entwistle, L. (1993) Metaphoric comprehension in adolescents with traumatic brain injury and adolescents with language learning disability. *Language, Speech and Hearing Sciences in Schools*, **24**, 100–107.

Vernon-Levett, P. (1991) Head injuries in children. *Critical Care Nursing Clinics of North America*, **3**, 411–421.

Vogel, M. and von Cramon, D. (1983) Articulatory recovery after traumatic midbrain damage: a follow-up study. *Folia Phoniatrica et Logopaedica*, **35**, 294–309.

Wechsler, D. (1945) *Wechsler Memory Scale Form 1*, Psychological Corporation, New York.

Wiig, E. (1984) Language disabilities in adolescents: a question of cognitive strategies. *Topics in Language Disorders*, **4**, 41–58.

Wiig, E., Alexander, E. and Secord, W. (1988) Linguistic competence and level of cognitive functioning in adults with traumatic closed head injury, in *Neuropsychological Studies of Nonfocal Brain Injury: Trauma and Dementia* (ed. H. Whitaker), Springer-Verlag, New York, pp. 186–199.

Wiig, E. and Becker-Caplan, L. (1984) Linguistic retrieval strategies and word-finding difficulties among children with language disabilities. *Topics in Language Disorders*, **4**, 1–18.

Wiig, E. and Secord, E. (1985) *Test of Language Competence*, Charles E. Merrill, Columbus, OH.

Wiig, E. and Secord, E. (1989) *Test of Language Competence – Expanded*, Charles E. Merrill, Columbus, OH.

Winner, E. and Gardner, H. (1977) The comprehension of metaphor in brain damaged patients. *Brain*, **100**, 717–729.

Workinger, M. and Netsell, R. (1992) Restoration of intelligible speech 13 years post-head injury. *Brain Injury*, **6**, 183–187.

Ylvisaker, M. (1986) Language and communication disorders following pediatric head injury. *Journal of Head Trauma Rehabilitation*, **1**, 48–56.

Ylvisaker, M. (1992) Communication outcome following traumatic brain injury. *Seminars in Speech and Language*, **13**, 239–250.

Yorkston, K.M. and Beukelman, D.R. (1991) Motor speech disorders, in *Communication Disorders Following Traumatic Brain Injury* (eds D.R. Beukelman and K.M. Yorkston), Pro-Ed, Austin, TX, pp. 251–315.

Yorkston, K.M., Beukelman, D.R. and Bell, K.R. (1988) *Clinical Management of Dysarthric Speakers*, Little Brown, Boston.

Yorkston, K.M., Beukelman, D.R., Minifie, F. and Sapir, S. (1984) Assessment of stress patterning in dysarthric speakers, in *The Dysarthrias: Physiology, Acoustics, Perception, Management* (eds M. McNeil, A. Aronson and J. Rosenbek), College Hill Press, San Diego, pp. 131–162.

Ziegler, W., Hoole, P., Hartmann, E. and von Cramon, D. (1988) Accelerated speech in dysarthria after acquired brain injury: acoustic correlates. *British Journal of Disorders of Communication*, **23**, 215–228.

Ziegler, W. and von Cramon, D. (1983a) Vowel distortion in traumatic dysarthria: a formant study. *Phonetica*, **40**, 63–78.

Ziegler, W. and von Cramon, D. (1983b) Vowel distortion in traumatic dysarthria: lip rounding versus tongue advancement. *Phonetica*, **40**, 312–322.

Ziegler, W. and von Cramon, D. (1986) Spastic dysarthria after acquired brain injury: an acoustic study. *British Journal of Disorders of Communication*, **21**, 173–187.

Zurif, E.B., Caramazza, A., Myerson, R. and Galvin, J. (1974) Semantic feature representation of normal and aphasic language. *Brain and Language*, **1**, 167–187.

Language disorders subsequent to right-hemisphere lesions

5

Introduction

The extent to which language is represented in the right hemisphere has been a topic of controversy since the late nineteenth century, when the British neurologist John Hughlings Jackson (1874) was the first to propose that the right cerebral hemisphere contributes to language processing. Although since the work of Broca (1861, 1865) the left hemisphere has been traditionally viewed as being dominant for language, in recent years there has been an accumulation of evidence suggesting that the right hemisphere of dextrals does play an important role in normal linguistic functioning (Searleman, 1977; Lesser, 1978; Delis *et al.*, 1983; Tompkins, 1995; Myers, 1999; Côté *et al.*, 2007). Importantly, not all individuals with right-hemisphere damage present with communication disorders and those that do exhibit a variety of symptoms which vary according to the nature of the communicative event, the relative fatigue of the patient and the extent of their neuropathology. Perusal of the relevant literature reveals that a diversity of language and language-related perceptual and cognitive disturbances have been reported in association with damage to the right cerebral hemisphere, the most frequent of which include: cognitive and subtle communicative deficits, affective and emotional deficits, and neglect of visual half space. Reviews of the role of the right hemisphere have concluded that this hemisphere may have a unique role in the processing of non-literal, context-bound, complex features of language such as understanding figurative language, stories, jokes and other forms of discourse, integrating complex linguistic information with the context and appreciating indirect speech acts (Code, 1987; Joanette, Goulet and Hannequin, 1990).

Lateralization of language function

Historically, hemispheric specialization for language was unanticipated until the reports of Broca (1861, 1865). Broca is generally regarded as being the first to ascribe speech dominance to the cerebral hemisphere contralateral to the preferred hand. Broca (1861) reported that the centre for speech was located in the third frontal convolution of the left cerebral hemisphere. In a later publication (Broca, 1865), he indicated that only the left hemisphere appeared to be involved in patients with impaired language function. Broca believed that the speech dominant hemisphere in right-handed persons was the left hemisphere, while in left-handers the dominant hemisphere was the right hemisphere.

Broca's correlation of aphasia with focal brain damage in the left hemisphere was subsequently corroborated and the importance of the left hemisphere for language became widely accepted. Terms such as 'dominant' and 'non-dominant', and 'major' and 'minor' were applied to the left and right cerebral hemispheres respectively. Reports of language impairments following right-hemisphere damage in left-handers added tentative support for Broca's idea (Zangwill, 1964). More recent reports, however, have provided convincing evidence that Broca's presumed one-to-one correlation between handedness and hemispheric dominance for language is overly simplistic (Schuell, Jenkins and Jiminez-Pabon, 1964; Zangwill, 1964; Penfield and Roberts, 1966; Rossi and Rosandini, 1967).

Currently, it is believed that most people (approximately 96%) are left-hemispheric dominant for language, which is related to handedness in the following way: approximately 93% of the population is right-handed and it is commonly estimated that 90–99% of all right-handers have their language functions predominantly subserved by the left hemisphere (Penfield and Roberts, 1959; Zangwill, 1960; Pratt and Warrington, 1972); the remaining 7% of the population are thought to be left-handed, with approximately 50–70% of these non-right-handers having their language functions localized primarily within the left hemisphere (Goodglass and Quadfasel, 1954; Zangwill, 1967; Hecaen and Sauguet, 1971; Warrington and Pratt, 1973). There is, therefore, a higher proportion of right-hemisphere language representation in non-right-handers than in right-handers (Strauss, Wada and Kosaka, 1983).

It has been suggested by some authors that most non-right-handers have considerable language function in both hemispheres (bilateral language dominance) (Luria, 1970; Gloning, 1977). The bilaterality of language function in non-right-handers is readily apparent from two observations, the greater frequency of aphasia

following brain injury in non-right-handers (Gloning *et al.*, 1969) and their better recovery rate (Luria, 1970). Beaumont (1974) formulated a general model for cerebral organization which also accounted for the fact that language abilities are less clearly lateralized in non-right-handers by simply suggesting that more diffuse cerebral representation is a general characteristic of these individuals.

Linguistic functions of the right hemisphere

Experimental approaches and techniques

Research relating to the linguistic functions of the right hemisphere has involved a variety of experimental approaches which have utilized subjects of varying levels of neurological integrity including: neurologically normal subjects, hemispherectomized subjects, commissurotomized subjects, aphasic individuals with left-hemisphere lesions and patients with acquired right-hemisphere lesions.

In addition to the diversity of subjects, a variety of techniques have been used to study the language abilities of the right hemisphere. The techniques employed have included dichotic listening (Johnson, Sommers and Weidner, 1977; Pettit and Noll, 1979; Caldas and Botelho, 1980), visual half-field tachistoscopic presentation (Moore and Weidner, 1974), intracarotid amobarbital injection (Kinsbourne, 1971), regional cortical blood flow (Meyer *et al.*, 1980) and electroencephalography (Tikofsky, Kooi and Thomas, 1960). More recently, functional neuroimaging studies based on either positron emission tomography (PET) (Posner and Raichle, 1994) or functional magnetic resonance imaging (fMRI) (Lehericy *et al.*, 2000) have demonstrated bilateral hemisphere activation in individuals performing language-related tasks such as word generation, passive listening and silent sentence repetition, thereby suggestive of a role for the right cerebral hemisphere in language processing.

Studies based on normal subjects

Studies involving neurologically normal subjects have contributed to both the current knowledge of language lateralization and the knowledge of the linguistic functions of the right hemisphere. In normal human subjects, while morbidity and trauma are presumed absent, it cannot be said that the cerebral hemispheres operate truly independently. Laterality differences, however, can be demonstrated in normal subjects and the findings generally complement those obtained from studies of clinical populations (Bradshaw and Nettleton, 1983). One of the richest sources of information on right-hemisphere linguistic function comes from studies of normal individuals who have suffered right-hemisphere damage secondary to stroke or trauma. In addition, researchers have also learnt a great deal about language lateralization by studying the effects of various surgical procedures in the brain on language abilities.

Language symptoms of right-hemisphere damage

Adults with right-hemisphere damage may appear to be communicatively competent upon initial or superficial contact, with language problems only becoming evident with more in-depth conversational exchange and social interaction (Tompkins, 1995; Myers, 1999). By using the more traditional aphasia test batteries therefore, clinicians may find it difficult to determine the presence of a language disturbance in a right-handed patient who has suffered either a vascular or traumatic lesion in the right cerebral hemisphere. Despite this, the majority of speech pathologists know from clinical experience that many right-handed patients with right-hemisphere damage do not communicate normally. Even though on the surface these patients appear to retain the basics of language, closer examination often reveals that they lack a complete understanding of the context of an utterance, the pre-suppositions entailed in the utterance or the tone of a conversational exchange.

The speech of persons with damaged right hemispheres has been described as excessive and rambling, inappropriate, confabulatory, irrelevant, literal and sometimes bizarre (Gardner, 1975; Collins, 1975; Gardner *et al.*, 1975; Tompkins, 1995; Myers, 1999). Some authors have highlighted that the comments made by patients with right-hemisphere damage are often off-colour (e.g. production of socially inappropriate comments) and many exhibit inappropriate humour (e.g. disproportionate response to slapstick humorous situations that depict someone either endangered or injured – so-called gallows humour) (Gardner *et al.*, 1975). In addition, these patients have often been observed to focus on insignificant details in conversation or make tangential remarks and the usual range of intonation is frequently observed to be lacking (Gardner, 1975; Ross and Mesulam, 1979). Myers (1979, 1986) reported that the speech of these patients is characterized by difficulty in extracting critical pieces of information, in seeing the relationships among them and in reading conclusions or drawing inferences based on those relationships. In other words, right-hemisphere-damaged patients appear to have a basic problem integrating and organizing information and an inability to form an overall gestalt of information given (Wapner, Hamby and Gardner, 1981; Myers, 1986).

It is well documented in the literature that severe disturbances in the linguistic components of language (i.e. phonology, syntax, lexical semantic) are often seen in association with lesions of the left cerebral hemisphere. In contrast, lesions of the right hemisphere of dextrals rarely impair the semantic or grammatical components of language. Consequently, the role of the right hemisphere in language has been considered rudimentary by some researchers. It must be remembered, however, that language comprises other components in addition to the aforementioned linguistic components. Benson (1986) identified four major divisions of language: syntactic (relational) language, semantic (definitional) language, prosodic (vocal) language and gestural (motor) language. While semantics and syntax belong to the linguistic facet of language, the latter two components, gestural and prosodic language, have been referred to as belonging to the extra- or paralinguistic facets of language. Evidence from research carried out in recent years suggests that although the traditional linguistic components of language are largely the concern of the dominant left hemisphere, the right hemisphere appears vital for the processing of the extralinguistic aspects of language which contemporary students of language would include as part of pragmatics or the discourse function of language. We will now examine in further detail the effects of right-hemisphere damage on both the linguistic and extralinguistic components of language.

Linguistic deficits following right-hemisphere damage

The findings of several studies have suggested that the traditional linguistic components of language are lateralized primarily to the left cerebral hemisphere in dextrals. In particular, of all the components of language, the syntactic component appears to be the most clearly lateralized, being almost totally an activity of the left hemisphere (Zaidel and Peters, 1981; Zaidel, 1985). On the other hand, although the left hemisphere is also primarily responsible for the semantic component of language, the available evidence from split-brain and hemispherectomy studies (see below) suggests that the non-dominant right hemisphere also possesses some semantic linguistic functions. Lesser (1974) found that right-hemisphere-damaged patients were not impaired in their use of syntax or phonological discrimination but had marked difficulty on a semantic test of language comprehension. Gainotti *et al.* (1981) also concluded that right-hemisphere lesions consistently impair semantic lexical discrimination but do not hamper phoneme discrimination.

Mild syntactic and semantic deficits were found by Hier and Kaplan (1980) to occur in only some right-hemisphere-damaged patients. They did, however, report a high level of correlation between the occurrence of verbal deficits and hemianopia which led Millar and Whitaker (1983) to the conclusion that verbal deficits in these patients are likely to occur only in association with other deficits of the impaired right hemisphere. Myers (1986) argued that deficits in straightforward expressive and receptive tasks (e.g. nam-

ing, word discrimination, following simple commands, word and sentence reading and writing) should not be considered a major source of right-hemisphere communication impairment. In agreement with Millar and Whitaker (1983), she concluded that deficits evident on various language tests may be attributed to deficits in other processing functions of the right hemisphere. Further, Myers (1986) also highlighted that linguistic deficits, when evident in right-hemisphere-damaged patients, tend to be mild. Millar and Whitaker (1983) indicated that there is good evidence that the right hemisphere contributes to many factors of human behaviour that play a role in communication. Consequently, they suggested that right-hemisphere-damaged patients exhibit a cognitive affective disorder rather than a linguistic disorder.

Adults with right-hemisphere damage usually have no difficulty with basic comprehension and expression, although linguistic tasks such as complex auditory comprehension (Hier and Kaplan, 1980), word fluency (Adamovich and Henderson, 1983) and naming (Gainotti *et al.*, 1981) have been demonstrated to be difficult for right-hemisphere-damaged subjects; when they are present, these deficits are mild and do not significantly affect communicative competence (Myers, 1984, 1999). Rather, it is linguistic deficits at a higher level, where integration and organization of information is necessary, that disturbs the communicative abilities of patients with right-hemisphere damage. Consequently, deficits are often more apparent on tasks with increased demands on cognitive resources. Thus, an individual with right-hemisphere damage may have little difficulty on straightforward tasks (e.g. basic comprehension task) but may breakdown when the task becomes more cognitively demanding (e.g. complex comprehension task involving several steps or instructions). The difficulty level increase may involve factors such as adding time constraints, inferences or metalinguistic/metacognitive demands (e.g. requiring consideration of another person's point of view). Further, communicative problems such as deficits in comprehension in persons with right-hemisphere damage are often evidenced on tasks where multiple interpretations are possible, and where the patient is required to select the most appropriate meaning.

The comprehension deficits exhibited by right-hemisphere-damaged subjects has been described by Diggs and Basili (1987) as diminishing the ability of these patients to appreciate antonymic contrasts, interpret proverbs and figures of speech, solve incongruent statements and understand logico-grammatical and other linguistically complex sentences. They observed that comprehension problems in these patients increased with memory load and linguistic complexity. Hier and Kaplan (1980) also found the comprehension of logico-grammatical sentences and abstract interpretation of proverbs to be impaired in right-hemisphere-damaged subjects.

Yet another feature of the comprehension abilities of right-hemisphere-damaged patients reported in the literature is that they tend to interpret figurative/non-literal language literally. Individuals with right-hemisphere damage do not appear to fully appreciate the abstract meanings of words and phrases (Myers and Linebaugh, 1981; Kempler *et al.*, 1999), with responses reflecting a literal interpretation. More specifically, they appear to have difficulty in generating alternative meanings and interpret figurative language such as idioms, proverbs and metaphors literally. Further, they may also have a problem comprehending some aspects of humour, irony and sarcasm (Myers and Linebaugh, 1981; Bihrle, Brownell and Powelson, 1986; Van Lanker and Kempler, 1987). The results of a study carried out by Foldi, Cicone and Gardner (1983) in which right-hemisphere-damaged patients were required to interpret both direct and indirect speech indicate that they interpret indirect speech literally, without taking contextual information into account. Similarly, Myers and Linebaugh (1981) observed that right-hemisphere-damaged adults tend to relate more readily to denovative rather than connotative aspects of language, a tendency which could possibly prevent them from grasping intended or implied meaning embedded in an utterance. Myers and Linebaugh (1981) also reported that their subjects with right-hemisphere damage responded literally to idiomatic expressions more frequently than control subjects and had difficulty determining the correct context of utterances. Further, their right-hemisphere-damaged subjects tended to interpret an idiom analytically, breaking it down into its constituent elements rather than processing it as a whole using context to aid interpretation. According to Weylman *et al.* (1989), individuals with right-hemisphere damage may interpret requests such as 'Can you close the door?' literally, and thereby respond with a verbal response ('yes') rather than performing the action indirectly suggested by the speaker. Vanhalle *et al.* (2000), however, have reported that requests of this type are more often interpreted correctly if the request is set in a natural context rather than taken out of context such as in experimental or clinical settings.

The discourse of individuals with right-hemisphere damage has been described as factual but off-target, disjointed and poorly organized. The verbal output often resembles a list of details or sentences rather than a coherent story (Benowitz, Moya and Levine, 1990; Beeman, 1993). In particular, persons with right-hemisphere damage may have problems in identifying main ideas or themes in self-generated stories or descriptions of pictured scenes or videos (e.g. Cookie Theft picture) (Joanette *et al.*, 1986; Cherney, Drimmer and Halper, 1997). They may see the individual elements but fail to deduce the overall theme or message. Further, they exhibit reduced cohesion of discourse production, do not efficiently use themes as clues to organize sentences into coherent stories (Schneiderman, Murasugi and Saddy, 1992) and may find difficulty identifying main ideas from written or spoken texts (Hough, 1990). Therefore, despite being aware of the individual elements depicted in a pictured scene and the individual sentences conveyed in verbal output, individuals with right-hemisphere damage may be unable to extract what Myers (1997) called 'the macrostructure' of verbal discourse or visual events. For example, when describing the Cookie Theft picture from the Boston Diagnostic Aphasia Examination (Goodglass and Kaplan, 1983), individuals with right-hemisphere damage may be able to identify individual elements such as the cookie jar, the woman washing dishes, the water running over the sink and so on without being able to deduce the core concept being depicted.

Several authors have investigated the ability of right-hemisphere-damaged adults to interpret and process narratives (e.g. Wapner, Hamby and Gardner, 1981; Gardner *et al.*, 1983). These studies have shown that, as in the case of idioms, right-hemisphere-damaged patients tend to use a logical analytical style to infer directly information leading to literal and abnormal interpretation of emotional, moral and humorous content. When asked to retell the narrative, these patients were generally able to recall isolated details but had difficulty inhibiting tangential and confabulatory responses. They were reported to constantly violate the story boundary allowing personal experiences and opinions to intrude. The right-hemisphere-damaged patients also displayed problems in ordering and integrating specific information and were unable to judge the appropriateness of facts, situations and characterizations to the story. It has been suggested by Wapner, Hamby and Gardner (1981) that these results indicate a poor integration of language elements and a diminished appreciation of narrative form. Wapner, Hamby and Gardner (1981) have proposed that these deficits in right-hemisphere-damaged adults are due to an underlying problem acquiring a sense of the overall gestalt of linguistic entities. If Wapner and co-workers are correct, this problem would lead to a disturbance of the basic schema of language and would make the appreciation of the relationships between language elements difficult. Wapner, Hamby and Gardner (1981) summarized the effect of these deficits by suggesting that without this organizing principle right-hemisphere-damaged adults are consigned to an undirected rambling discourse and are unable to judge which details matter and what overall points they yield. This suggestion is supported by the findings of studies which have shown that patients with right-hemisphere damage provide less information using an equal or greater number of words when compared to normal subjects (Myers, 1979; Rivers and Love, 1980; Diggs and Basili, 1987). The factual but disorganized verbal output of persons with right-hemisphere damage may also be the outcome of problems these individuals have with the generation and interpretation of inferences. Although individuals with right-hemisphere damage have few if any problems with basic inferences, such as those required to link two sentences together, they do often experience difficulties with elaborative inferences (i.e. those that add information to a passage such as predictions and character emotions) (Lehman and Tompkins, 2000).

Overall, right-hemisphere-damaged patients primarily have difficulty in the interpretation, integration and organization of linguistic elements and context. They fail to appraise information holistically or to form an overall structure as a reference base to aid their interpretation and production of complex language.

Extralinguistic deficits following right-hemisphere damage

Although in the past most studies have examined the effects of right-hemisphere damage on the more traditional linguistic components of language, an increasing amount of research in recent years has focused on the contribution of the right hemisphere to the pragmatic, prosodic and emotional aspects of communication. In fact, Myers (1986, 1997) considered the most important part of the communication deficit exhibited by right-hemisphere-damaged patients to be the impairment in these so-called extralinguistic components of language.

Categories of extralinguistic deficits. Myers (1986) distinguished between two different categories of extralinguistic deficits: affective-prosodic disturbances and pragmatic disorders. Affective-prosodic disturbances relate to the comprehension and expression of emotional tone (affect) conveyed through mechanisms such as facial expression, gesture (body language) and prosodic features of oral speech (intonation contour, volume, rate and rhythm), These intonation patterns convey both linguistic and emotional information. 'Pragmatics' refers to the use of language in linguistic and situational context. According to Code (1987), 'pragmatics represents an interface between language and other aspects of behaviour and is concerned not with linguistic entities themselves but with the total behavioural-social context in which communication takes place and the actual intentions behind an utterance message' (p. 88). Put more simply, pragmatics involves the relationship between language and social contexts, including the intent of the communication exchange.

Affective-prosodic disturbances. Reports in the literature have indicated that patients with right-hemisphere lesions have difficulties with both the production and comprehension of prosody. In particular, they have a disturbance in the affective (emotional) component of prosody (Tucker, Watson and Heilman, 1977; Ross and Mesulam, 1979; Brownell and Martino, 1998; Borod *et al.*, 2000). In particular, right-hemisphere-damaged patients have been described as having 'flat-affect' and monotonous speech (Ross and Mesulam, 1979). Subjects sustaining right-hemisphere damage have also been reported to be impaired in their ability to evaluate emotional situations presented through non-verbal means, particularly those presented through facial expressions (Benowitz *et al.*, 1983). Affective gestural impairment was also reported by Lundgren, Moya and Benowitz (1983), who found impaired ability in right-hemisphere-damaged patients to perceive affect from facial expression and to interpret body language. An inability to express emotion through either vocal melody or gesture, a condition referred to by Ross (1981) as 'aprosodia', has been reported to be associated with damage to the right posterior inferior frontal area (the analogue of Broca's area in the left hemisphere). Further, Ross (1981) also suggested that the emotional quality of speech cannot be comprehended if there is damage in the posterior temporal parietal area of the right hemisphere. These findings have led some authors to conclude that the right hemisphere is dominant for processing affective-prosody (Ross and Mesulam, 1979; Ross, 1981; Emmorey, 1987).

Based on his observations of the effects of right-hemisphere damage on prosody, Ross (1981) proposed a theory that the functional anatomic organization of affective prosody in the right hemisphere mirrors that of propositional language in the left hemisphere. He proposed a method of assessment and classification of 'prosodic disorders' (aprosodias) similar to that used for aphasic language disorders based on prosodic comprehension, repetition and expression. Ross hypothesized that after damage to the anterior right hemisphere, prosodic expression and repetition would be impaired but prosodic comprehension would remain intact and that damage to the posterior right hemisphere would result in impaired prosodic comprehension and repetition with fluent expression. Ross (1981) also forecast the existence of transcortical aprosodic syndromes in which prosodic repetition is basically intact.

Ross's theory of aprosodia extends beyond his results and was based on the case histories of 10 patients only. Within his limited subject group, Ross was unable to demonstrate all of the aprosodias that he proposed. Although his own research does not provide conclusive support for Ross's theory, the basic premise of differential localization in affective prosody in the right hemisphere gains support from the work of Roberts, Kinsella and Wales (1982). In agreement with the differential anterior/posterior damage profile advanced by Ross (1981), these latter authors found that patients with posterior right-hemisphere damage performed significantly worse on prosodic discrimination tasks than patients with anterior right-hemisphere damage.

It could be argued that these reported affective-prosody deficits described in the research relating to the effects of right-hemisphere damage on language might be related to the global problem that right-hemisphere-damaged adults have in integrating and processing information. The inability to discriminate and produce affective and prosodic information may be due to inefficient and inaccurate integration of affect and prosody with language leading to deficits in the interpretation and production of messages.

Clinically, one other important finding of research in this area is that after right-hemisphere damage, affect may not match mood (Ross, 1985). Hence, 'flat-affect' displayed by right-hemisphere-damaged patients need not reflect an underlying depressed mood but rather a specific affective-prosody deficit. Roberts, Kinsella and Wales (1982), after comparing performance on tasks discriminating linguistic prosody and affective prosody, found right-hemisphere-damaged adults to have differential difficulty with certain emotional tones of voice. Their results suggested that it is not emotion itself that is difficult for patients with right-hemisphere lesions, but rather the prosodic element of emotional (affective) speech. These findings were supported to some extent by Kinsella (1986), who demonstrated similar deficits of prosodic discrimination in right-hemisphere-damaged subjects when required to judge sentence type by prosodic cues alone.

Pragmatic deficits. Pragmatic deficits associated with damage to the right hemisphere are interrelated with the deficiencies in affective-prosody and linguistic-cognitive processing described above (Myers, 1986). Some authors have suggested that pragmatic difficulties form the crux of right-hemisphere disorders (Joanette and Ansaldo, 1999; Myers, 2001). Clinical observation of the conversational abilities of right-hemisphere-damaged patients shows that these individuals are unable to appreciate the context and tone of a conversation or the presuppositions entailed. Studies that have investigated conversational behaviour in persons with lesions in the right hemisphere have indicated that these individuals take fewer turns in conversation and talk more about themselves than non-neurologically impaired controls. Further, they tend to prolong conversations rather than terminating them in response to cues from their conversational partners (Kennedy *et al.*, 1994; Kennedy, 2000). Their discourse often focuses on insignificant and tangential details and includes inappropriate humour and comments, giving their language an excessive and rambling nature. Myers (1986) suggested that the reason why right-hemisphere-damaged patients are unable to use contextual clues results from their difficulty in 'evaluating the significance of sensory input, in associating it with prior knowledge and integrating multiple features of experience into a meaningful pattern or context' (p. 456). Further, she suggested that the inability of these patients to use contextual cues occurring in conjunction with an essentially intact linguistic system is the reason why patients with right-hemisphere damage react to literal rather than metaphorical, humorous or idiomatic speech forms and why they confabulate, miss the point and include tangential detail in their con-

versation. Myers (1986) has suggested that it is these two deficits (i.e. the tendency to interpret words and events on a literal, superficial basis and the failure to establish an adequate organizational framework) that constitute the two major pragmatic deficits in patients with right-hemisphere damage.

The inability of right-hemisphere-damaged patients to interpret contextual information and organize their response was well illustrated in a study carried out by Myers (1979). Eight right-hemisphere-damaged patients and eight matched non-brain-damaged control patients were asked to describe the Cookie Theft picture from the Boston Diagnostic Aphasia Examination. Using the list of concepts normally used in describing the picture, Myers classified the concepts as either literal (e.g. reaching up; has finger to mouth) or interpretive (e.g. asking for cookie; saying 'shhh') and then compared the frequency of these two types of concepts in both the right-hemisphere-damaged and control groups. The results indicated that patients with right-hemisphere damage used significantly fewer interpretive concepts compared to the control group. Myers (1979) also noted that the right-hemisphere-damaged group produced a large number of irrelevant comments. She concluded that right-hemisphere-damaged patients have difficulty integrating information both on a perceptual and on a more formal level and that this deficit is manifest in their verbal output of irrelevant and often excessive information and a literal treatment of questions and events.

Prutting and Kirchner (1987) analysed the pragmatic abilities of right-hemisphere-damaged adults in conversation. They reported that these patients were similar to aphasic adults when comparing the mean percentage of appropriate pragmatic behaviours (84% compared with 82%). However, the right-hemisphere-damaged adults manifested a distinctive cluster of inappropriate behaviours. The pragmatic behaviours most frequently judged to be inappropriate in this group included eye gaze, prosody, adjacency, contingency, quantity and conciseness. Adjacency and contingency are turn-taking behaviours that relate to the ability to continue conversation and share a topic.

A number of authors have proposed that the pragmatic disorder exhibited by individuals with right-hemisphere damage represents a disruption of 'theory of mind' (Brownell and Martino, 1998; Winner *et al.*, 1998). Theory of mind has been characterized as the ability to infer the mental states of others, such as their beliefs, knowledge and desires and may represent the central cognitive ability that underlies our ability to engage in social interaction (Happe, Brownell and Winner, 1999). Happe, Brownell and Winner (1999) defined theory of mind as 'the ability to attribute thoughts and feelings to self and others' (p. 211). It involves seeing another person's point of view, and understanding how much another person knows, particularly if it is different from what you know. Individuals with right-hemisphere damage do not appear to take into account another person's perspective, interpreting information based on their own viewpoint. This may account for problems these individuals have attributing emotions to characters in stories, and the overpersonalization observed in their conversation.

The observation that left-hemisphere-damaged aphasic patients communicate better than they talk (Holland, 1977) and right-hemisphere-damaged patients perhaps talk better than they communicate has led to the hypothesis that the right hemisphere is responsible for simultaneously organizing and integrating different elements of conversation while the left hemisphere is critical for literal language (phonology, syntax and low-level semantics) (Foldi, Cicone and Gardner, 1983).

Other neuropsychological sequelae of right-hemisphere damage

In addition to the language disorders outlined above, damage to the right hemisphere is also associated with a number of other neuropsychological deficits. The primary information-processing functions of the right hemisphere are those of attention and perception. Consequently, the deficits that occur following right-hemisphere damage fall primarily in the areas of neglect, denial, visual and spatial perceptual disorders as well as constructional disturbances.

Myers (1999) reported that between 30 and 60% of patients with right-hemisphere damage exhibit visuospatial neglect. Unilateral neglect is a condition in which the patient fails to attend and respond to stimuli on one side of the body. It occurs more commonly and with greater severity following right-hemisphere lesions than left-hemisphere lesions. Neglect typically affects the side of space contralateral to the brain lesion. Consequently, individuals with right-hemisphere damage usually exhibit neglect in the left side of space. Visual neglect is the most common type and it frequently affects communication, particularly reading and writing. If an object referred to by a conversational partner is located in the left visual field, verbal communication can also be involved. Individuals with visual neglect may not read words or letters (neglect dyslexia) placed in the left side of space. Likewise when writing, persons with visual neglect often commence writing in the middle of the page rather than at the left margin. Once considered a unitary disorder, the neglect syndrome has been classified by Myers (1986) into two distinct types: parietal and frontal neglect. The symptoms of parietal neglect range from a failure to respond to simultaneous bilateral stimulation to a failure to report any incoming stimuli from an area to the left of the patient's midline. When specifically directed to left-sided stimuli, patients may report what is there, but on their own, without constant reminders, they will attend to the right side only. The symptoms of frontal neglect include impaired performance on cancellation and scanning tasks as well as on tests of block design, copying and spontaneous drawing, indicating impaired constructional abilities. Although neglect is far more prevalent on the left, it can occur also on the right. Further, although most common in vision, neglect can also involve olfaction, audition and sensation. Anosognosia (denial of illness) often is present in conjunction with visual neglect and has been reported to occur in up to 40% of individuals with right-hemisphere damage (Blake *et al.*, 2002).

Other neuropsychological disorders that are the observed effect of impaired attention and perception following right-hemisphere damage include impaired facial recognition (prosopagnosia) and impaired geographic and topological orientation. Prosopagnosia (face blindness) is generally accepted as a deficit in visual integration and, along with topological disorientation, can lead to the wrong conclusion that the patient is suffering from a psychiatric condition. The condition results in social, pragmatic and identity problems. Even the faces of close friends or relatives may not be recognized. The fusiform gyrus, an area of the brain important for visual functions, has been linked with dissociation of the neural centres that link emotionality and visual pattern recognition and is a suggested site of brain damage associated with prosopagnosia. Myers (1986) described 'topological disorientation' as being the failure to assimilate visual cues. Patients with this problem have difficulty reading a map, remembering familiar routes and learning new ones, a factor that explains why many individuals with right-hemisphere damage easily get lost, can't find their way home or may be found wandering hospital wards. Reduplicative paramnesia has also been reported in association with lesions of the right hemisphere. This disorientation is specific to location such that patients may know that they are in a specific ward in a hospital but may be convinced that the hospital itself is far away in another city.

Lesions in either the left or the right parietal lobes are often associated with constructional disturbances. As in the case of neglect, right-hemisphere lesions tend to be associated with more frequent and severe constructional deficits than left-hemisphere lesions.

Development of language lateralization: evidence from focal brain lesions and hemispherectomy

The surgical removal of a total cerebral hemisphere (hemispherectomy) has occasionally been performed as a treatment for various diseases of the brain (Basser, 1962; Smith and Burklund, 1966; Smith and Sugar, 1975). Two predominant types of hemispherectomy are performed: anatomical removal and functional removal. Anatomical removal involves complete removal of the hemisphere with the exception of the basal ganglia, while functional removal involves removal of the temporal and/or parietal lobes with disconnection of the white matter tracts between the frontal and occipital lobes (Rassmussen, 1983; Villemure and Mascott, 1993). Functional removal is performed more often than anatomical removal, because the latter is associated with significant side effects such as increased risk of bleeding, subdural haematomas, increased intracranial pressure, hemosiderosis, hemiparesis and visual field defects. The most striking aspect of the literature on hemispherectomy, as pointed out by Searleman (1977), concerns the enormous difference between children and adults, particularly in relation to post-operative speech-language functioning. Brain lesions incurred early in childhood have been reported to have relatively mild consequences on language development, especially in comparison to lesions acquired later in adult life (Vargha-Khadem *et al.*, 1992; Muter, Taylor and Vargha-Khadem, 1997; Reilly, Bates and Marchman, 1998). These findings have been interpreted in relation to the 'plasticity' and 'equipotentiality' of the immature brain. What Zangwill (1960) called the 'equipotentiality' of the two cerebral hemispheres refers to their analogous capacity to subserve language functions subsequent to unilateral brain damage (Lenneberg, 1967) so that a shift of language competency from one hemisphere to the other is easily accomplished at a young age. 'Plasticity', on the other hand, refers to the compensatory mechanisms that may underlay lesion-induced neurofunctional and behavioural reorganization following brain injury. The theory of equipotentiality, however, has been challenged by the findings of studies that suggest the presence of early specialization of the left hemisphere for language acquisition (Bates *et al.*, 1997). More recently, it has been suggested that equipotentiality and left-hemisphere specialization represent the two extreme ends of a continuum whereby, although the left hemisphere may be innately predisposed to language learning and processing, this predisposition may remain sufficiently plastic for the right hemisphere to acquire and mediate language in circumstances where the left hemisphere is damaged by focal brain injury (Satz, Strauss and Whitaker, 1990; Vicari *et al.*, 2000; Chilosi *et al.*, 2001).

Recently, several neuroimaging studies have provided evidence to support the concept of equipotentiality and plasticity of the immature brain by identifying the presence of right-hemisphere specialization for language subsequent to early damage to the left language areas (Müller *et al.*, 1999; Lazar *et al.*, 2000). According to Staudt *et al.* (2002), the reorganization of language in the right hemisphere involving regions which are mostly homotopic to the language areas in the left hemisphere of healthy right-handers, thereby suggesting a 'near equipotentiality of the two hemispheres at a topological level' (p. 964).

Several authors have hypothesized that both cerebral hemispheres possess equal potential for language until at least four or five years of age (Lenneberg, 1967; Osgood and Miron, 1963). Further, it is believed by several researchers that the non-dominant hemisphere retains an ability to assume responsibility for language through the first 10 or 12 years of life and possibly beyond (Smith, 1966; Lenneberg, 1967; Cummings *et al.*, 1979). For this reason, although children who have begun to develop language may exhibit a language disturbance following cerebral damage, the resulting language disorder is usually only temporary and mild. It appears, therefore, that the cerebral dominance for language develops with age and consequently the younger the child at the onset of acquired aphasia is, the less complete the dominance for language in one hemisphere is and the better the other hemisphere can assume language function.

Hemispherectomies, when performed in childhood, are primarily for the treatment of intractable epilepsy arising from brain damage. It has been reported that the presence of epilepsy alone may change the pattern of lateralization (Piccirilli *et al.*, 1988; Riva *et al.*, 1993). For example, children with benign focal epilepsy with no documented brain lesion have been reported to have a bilateral representation of language processing (Piccirilli *et al.*, 1988). It would appear that left frontal or parietal brain injury may

displace language functions partially or totally to the right hemisphere (Rassmussen and Milner, 1977), and early left temporal lobe epilepsy may displace language with the left hemisphere (Devinsky and Vazquez, 1993) or to the right hemisphere (Helmstaedter *et al.*, 1994). In those cases where hemispherectomy has involved removal of the right hemisphere, aphasia, at least in the classic sense, has not been recorded.

In contrast to the minimal effects of hemispherectomies in children on speech-language function, hemispherectomy in late childhood or adult life has been reported to have a serious effect on cognition as well as speech-language function (Whitaker and Ojemann, 1977). Although hemispherectomies involving the removal of the dominant left hemisphere in adults are performed infrequently, they produce quite a different language outcome from the equivalent operation in children (Basser, 1962; Smith, 1966; Smith and Sugar, 1975). Removal of the left hemisphere in this situation, usually for the treatment of glioma, results in a permanent aphasia of a type similar to that seen in cases of global aphasia (Basser, 1962; Smith, 1966). Right hemispherectomy in adults, on the other hand, is usually characterized by impaired visuospatial functioning and intact speech and language (Basser, 1962; Searleman, 1977). Where there is evidence that the left hemisphere has been diseased since childhood, later removal of that hemisphere has also been reported to result in little or no language impairment, suggesting that the right hemisphere is able to assume responsibility for language function in these cases (Smith and Sugar, 1975).

Language functions of the right hemisphere: evidence from commissurotomy

The corpus callosum is the major commissure connecting the two cerebral hemispheres. Occasionally, the corpus callosum is severed in a surgical operation (split-brain surgery or commissurotomy) primarily to control the spread of intractable epilepsy from one hemisphere to the other (Searleman, 1977). Transection of the anterior two-thirds of the corpus callosum as well as complete transection have been used, with the latter procedure generally being more effective (Black, Holmes and Lombroso, 1992). A variety of techniques have been developed to investigate the language abilities of the isolated right hemisphere following section of the corpus callosum (Sperry and Gazzaniga, 1967; Gazzaniga, 1970; Zaidel, 1976). Overall, these techniques have demonstrated that the isolated right hemisphere is capable of considerable language function. Gazzaniga and Sperry found in a series of studies in commissurotomized patients that each hemisphere, when structurally isolated from the other, functions autonomously (Gazzaniga and Sperry, 1967; Sperry and Gazzaniga, 1967). For example, Gazzaniga and Sperry (1967) found that linguistic information (words) presented visually to the right hemisphere could not be communicated in writing or speech, but had to be expressed through non-verbal responses. If, for instance, the word 'spoon' was flashed to the subject's left visual field, he or she would subsequently be able to point to a picture of a spoon with his or her left hand, although he or she would be able to name it. Through the use of non-verbal responses such as this, Sperry and Gazzaniga (1967) were able to show that the right (non-dominant) hemisphere is not 'word-blind' or 'word-deaf', as first suggested by Geschwind (1965a,b), who proposed that the right hemisphere is completely incapable of utilizing or comprehending verbal stimuli. Nebes and Sperry (1971) further showed that the right hemisphere is not limited to just matching single words to objects but rather that it can pick out from a group of hidden objects the one that is verbally described.

The work of Sperry and colleagues with commissurotomized patients suggests that the comprehension of both spoken and written language is represented in both the left and right cerebral hemispheres, although the degree of representation in the right is unknown. Levy (1970) was able to demonstrate that the right hemisphere can comprehend verbal stimuli and carry out spoken commands. In a further series of experiments with commissurotomized patients, Levy, Trevarthen and Sperry (1972) demonstrated what appears to be an upper limit for right-hemisphere linguis-

tic abilities. They found that although the right hemisphere can usually comprehend verbal stimuli it is totally unable to make phonological transformations. For example, the right hemisphere may comprehend the meaning of the words 'ache' and 'lake', but it would never know that they rhyme (Levy, 1974). Zaidel (1983) claimed, in direct contrast to the earlier findings of Gazzaniga and Hillyard (1971), that the right hemisphere of commissurotomized patients possesses considerable syntactic capabilities.

Zaidel (1976), from his study of both hemispherectomized and commissurotomized subjects, noted that his data, in conjunction with the data of other authors, suggested a complex model of development of language laterality of the brain. He felt that some, but not all, auditory language functions continue to develop in the right hemisphere past what is generally regarded as the critical period of language acquisition. From the results of a series of further studies in this area, Zaidel (1978a,b) concluded that the right hemisphere represents the limited linguistic competence that can be acquired by a more general purpose, non-linguistic cognitive apparatus through repeated exposure to experience and through the formation of associations. He attributed the following characteristics to the right hemisphere: no speech, little writing; surprisingly rich auditory lexicons; substantial visual vocabularies; a good grasp of pictorial semantics in terms of everyday social experience; poor ability to evoke the sound image of a word; a rudimentary level of syntax; practically no ability to read sentences; no grapheme-to-phoneme-correspondence rules; and better auditory comprehension than comprehension of written words or phrases. Gazzaniga *et al.* (1984) also reported that the right hemisphere of split-brain subjects has a rich lexicon, although not as rich as that of the left hemisphere as well as a limited control of syntax.

Based on a review of split-brain subjects, Gazzaniga (1983) concluded that language and speech in the right hemisphere can exist at either a rudimentary or a sophisticated level. He determined that, among the small subset of his subjects who possessed a well-developed level of language in the right hemisphere, in almost every case it was attributable to brain pathology occurring prior to commissurotomy. Levy (1983) critically reviewed Gazzaniga's (1983) paper and, while agreeing that the normal right hemisphere is non-linguistic, contested some of Gazzaniga's other findings. Levy claimed, for example, that the results provided by Gazzaniga did not imply that early brain damage produces any reorganization and bilateralization of language. Further, Zaidel (1983) opposed the claim of Gazzaniga (1983) that when right-hemisphere language does occur it does not show a consistent and unique form of organization but varies widely as a function of the extent of pre-surgical left-hemisphere damage. Zaidel (1983) felt that this latter claim implied that right-hemisphere language carried no special theoretical linguistic significance.

Overall, therefore, the results from split-brain studies suggest that the right hemisphere has a considerable capacity to comprehend verbal stimuli. Gazzaniga (1970), however, has warned that it is often possible to overestimate the linguistic abilities of the right hemisphere of split-brain subjects, owing to what he termed 'cross-cueing' strategies. In the process of cross-cueing, one hemisphere may learn how to transmit information extracallosally to the other by initiating gestures, orienting responses or even verbalizations that can be picked up and acted upon by the other hemisphere. In addition to cross-cueing, other methodological and theoretical problems also arise when interpreting the results of human commissurotomy studies and when generalizing these results to the normal population. It must be remembered that the surgery is rather traumatic, involving manipulation of the brain as well as the disruption of its blood supply, factors which could possibly affect the patient's later performance on particular linguistic tasks. Commissurotomy subjects may also be prone to bilateral language representation as a result of early cerebral damage from epileptic seizures. Functional reorganization of the brain may occur in patients who have had long-standing epilepsy, and a higher percentage of bilateral language representation in these subjects could account for the relatively high degree of linguistic skills observed in several of the reported studies (Searleman, 1977). One additional problem is the pos-

sibility of interhemispheric transmission by other midbrain commissures. Finally, the disconnected right hemisphere is not subject to the mutual facilitation and inhibition of the normal brain, with the result that its functioning must in some sense inevitably be abnormal. These shortcomings need to be taken into account when interpreting the results obtained from studies involving commissurotomized subjects.

As a consequence of the above problems reported to be associated with commissurotomy and owing to the undesirability of dividing the optic chiasma in humans, a number of techniques have been developed by various researchers to present language material to the right hemisphere only of both commissurotomized and normal subjects. These techniques include methods such as the use of a scleral contact lens system (Zaidel, 1976; 1978a,b), tachistoscopy (Zurif and Bryden, 1969) and a key-tapping method (Tsunoda, 1975). In general, these studies have tended to confirm the findings of the reported split-brain investigations. Overall, the results of these latter investigations suggest that the right hemisphere of commissurotomized subjects is capable of some language function. In particular, the right hemisphere appears to be able to recognize (comprehend) some printed and spoken words. Its ability to express language material, however, is extremely limited.

Anatomical differences between the left and right hemispheres

A number of researchers have provided evidence that the speech-language centres of the left hemisphere are anatomically better developed than equivalent regions in the right hemisphere. Geschwind and Levitsky (1968) reported that the planum temporale (that part of the auditory association cortex posterior to Heschl's gyrus on the superior lateral surface of the temporal lobe (Brodmann areas 22 and 42) and which includes the speech reception area of Wernicke) was larger on the left in 65% and larger on the right in 11% of the 100 brains they studied. Their findings have since been confirmed by other researchers

(Wada, Clarke and Hamm, 1975; Rubens, Mahowald and Hutton, 1976).

In general, studies of the morphological asymmetries between the two cerebral hemispheres have indicated the presence of a complex and interrelated set of differences in the anatomy of the posterior sylvian region. These include differences in the position of the Fissure of Sylvius and size of the parietal operculum as well as the development of the planum temporale. Although it is possible that these differences in the structure of the posterior sylvian region of the two hemispheres may in some way provide a neuroanatomical substrate for left-hemisphere dominance for speech-language (Geschwind and Levitsky, 1968; LeMay and Culebras, 1972; Wada, Clarke and Hamm, 1975; Galaburda *et al.*, 1978), most authors have advised caution in applying a functional importance to these asymmetries. Despite this cautionary advice, however, a number of factors highlight the possible link between hemisphere asymmetry and cerebral dominance for language. First, the posterior sylvian region of the dominant hemisphere coincides with Wernicke's area and is known to be involved in language processing. Second, the greater development of the planum temporale in the left hemisphere has been demonstrated in infant and foetal brains (Witelson and Pallie, 1973; Wada, Clarke and Hamm, 1975) as well as adults, thereby suggesting that physical asymmetry may precede functional asymmetry. Third, the asymmetry of the parietal opercula has been found to be absent in the majority of left-handers (LeMay and Culebras, 1972). Finally, Ratcliff *et al.* (1980) reported asymmetries of the posterior sylvian branches of the middle cerebral artery in favour of the dominant hemisphere in 59 patients for whom lateralization was known from Wada testing. The asymmetry, however, was significantly reduced in patients with atypical cerebral dominance.

The role of the right hemisphere in recovery from aphasia

As early as the middle of the nineteenth century, Broca (1861) postulated that the minor hemisphere possessed an inherent ability to mediate speech following major hemisphere damage. Since that time, a number of researchers have implicated the right hemisphere in the recovery of language function following a left-hemisphere lesion. Luria (1963) offered three possible explanations for the recovery of language function in these cases: (a) the injury is of a transitory nature, (b) reorganization within the left hemisphere allows compensatory functioning of adjacent undamaged structures or (c) there is a complete transfer of language to corresponding areas in the right hemisphere (dominance shift). Klingman and Sussman (1983) further suggested that the observed recovery may be a product of the right hemisphere working in conjunction with the damaged left hemisphere to mediate language function.

Experimental techniques

A variety of experimental techniques have been used to assess the relative involvement of the left and right hemispheres in the recovery from aphasia. The techniques employed have included dichotic listening (Sparks, Goodglass and Nickel, 1970; Johnson, Sommers and Weidner, 1977; Pettit and Noll, 1979; Caldas and Botelho, 1980), visual half-field tachistoscopic presentation (Moore and Weidner, 1974), intracarotid amobarbital injection (Kinsbourne, 1971), regional cortical blood flow (Meyer *et al.*, 1980) and electroencephalography (Tikofsky, Kooi and Thomas, 1960).

Dichotic listening tests

The most commonly used method to study hemispheric language lateralization in aphasia has been the dichotic listening test. Studies using this method have generally demonstrated either an emerging left-ear preference during the course of language recovery (Johnson, Sommers and Weidner, 1977; Pettit and Noll, 1979; Caldas and Botelho, 1980) or no ear advantage (Schulhoff and Goodglass, 1969). The emergence of a left-ear preference parallel to language recovery has been taken to suggest that the right hemisphere may participate in some way in language processing. However, development of a left-ear preference does not appear to occur uniformly across different aphasic groups. Caldas and Botelho (1980) administered three different dichotic listening tests to a group of aphasic subjects at various stages of the recovery process. Interestingly, the non-fluent aphasics demonstrated a tendency to increase left-ear preference, while fluent aphasics in direct contrast demonstrated an increase of right-ear preference in a verbal dichotic test. Caldas and Botelho (1980) suggested that these findings indicate a compensatory function of the right hemisphere in cases of non-fluent aphasia (due to a pre-rolandic lesion), but not in cases of fluent aphasia of post-rolandic origin.

The importance placed upon such results obtained from dichotic listening studies has been questioned (Berlin and McNeil, 1976; Linebaugh, 1978). Many researchers have failed to recognize the vulnerability of the dichotic listening technique to both the acoustic and phonetic variables of the dichotic (simultaneous) stimuli. Acoustic parameters such as voice onset timing, signal intensity, frequency range and length of stimuli have been shown to alter the right-ear advantage, which, it is claimed, is typically displayed by normal subjects (Berlin and McNeil, 1976). A significant phonetic variable has also been discovered in that it has been noted in dichotic listening experiments, performed with consonant–vowel syllables, that voiceless stop consonants are more intelligible than voiced consonants (Lowe *et al.*, 1970; Berlin *et al.*, 1973). This effect is so powerful that, if voiceless consonants were presented to the left ear and voiced consonants to the right ear as a dichotic listening task, the results could be expected to show a left-ear advantage (Berlin and McNeil, 1976). Ideally, dichotic stimuli should be truly simultaneous, with maximum phonetic and acoustic competition. Unfortunately, however, the necessary methodological processes for accurate stimulus matching have not been widely used to date since they depend on computerized simulated speech.

Interpretation of the left-ear advantage as an indication of right-hemisphere involvement in language functioning has been criticized to the extent that the dichotic paradigm is considered merely to illustrate a 'lesion effect' (Linebaugh, 1978). That is, the lesion of the left auditory cortex causes degradation of the contralateral right-ear signal. The existence of a lesion effect is supported by the fact that the presence of pathology in the left hemisphere has been demonstrated to variably produce extinction of stimuli presented to the left ear, to the right ear or to neither after dichotic stimulation (Sparks, Goodglass and Nickel, 1970). The observed variability can be attributed to the anatomical locus of the pathology (Benson, 1979).

Visual half-field tachistoscopic presentation

A right-hemisphere superiority in visual linguistic decoding has been demonstrated in aphasic subjects with the technique of visual half-field tachistoscopic presentation (Moore and Weidner, 1974). Normal subjects typically exhibit a left-hemisphere superiority. The reversal of hemisphere dominance for the decoding of visual language in aphasics supports the 'dominance shift' hypothesis in the recovery of language following left-hemisphere pathology. However, several studies reviewed by Searleman (1977) suggested that both the dichotic and tachistoscopic techniques may be measuring factors unrelated to language lateralization and may vary considerably in terms of reliability. In addition, both techniques only measure low-level speech perception and comprehension abilities (Searleman, 1977; Klingman and Sussman, 1983). Research in both audition and vision has provided evidence that hemispheric asymmetries are found primarily at later higher-order stages of information processing than those stages investigated by dichotic and tachistoscopic paradigms (Berlin and McNeil, 1976; Madden and Nebes, 1980).

Intracarotid amobarbital injection (Wada Test)

The technique of intracarotid amobarbital injection, developed by Wada and Rasmussen (1960), has been used to investigate the source of residual aphasic speech. Kinsbourne (1971) reported three right-handed aphasic subjects in which speech production continued during anaesthetization of the left hemisphere. In two of those cases, a subsequent contralateral injection arrested speech production demonstrating that dominance for residual speech production had shifted to the right hemisphere. Unfortunately, other aphasic subjects tested failed to support the 'hemispheric shift' hypothesis, leading Kinsbourne to conclude that the right hemisphere is not always the source of aphasic speech.

Regional cortical blood flow measurement

Regional cortical blood flow measurements, obtained during the period of aphasic language recovery from left hemisphere infarction, have yielded interesting results. A failure of regional cerebral blood flow to increase in Broca's area during behavioural activation in eight right-handed aphasic subjects who had demonstrated good speech recovery within three months post-onset of aphasia was reported by Meyer *et al.* (1980). In contrast, these subjects showed a significant increase in regional cerebral blood flow in the corresponding posterior frontal and peri-sylvian regions of the right hemisphere, thereby indicating right-hemisphere participation in the recovery from aphasia. Unfortunately, regional cerebral blood flow measurements cannot be performed without some risk to the subject, which poses limitations for its use as an experimental technique (Kertesz, 1979).

Electroencephalography

Further evidence to support a role for the right hemisphere in language recovery in aphasia has come from electroencephalographic studies. Tikofsky, Kooi and Thomas (1960) established a relationship between electroencephalogram readings and recovery of speech in aphasic subjects. They found that abnormal electroencephalogram recordings over the right hemisphere significantly lessened the prognosis for speech recovery, whereas abnormal readings over the left hemisphere had no observable relationship to speech recovery.

Linguistic-manual time-sharing paradigm

Klingman and Sussman (1983) adapted the linguistic-manual time-sharing paradigm initially developed by Kinsbourne and Cook (1971) as a speech output based lateralization measure. The paradigm involves the concurrent performance of a linguistic and uni-manual task (e.g. separate left or right index finger tapping). When normal, right-handed subjects perform simultaneous right index finger tapping and verbalization tasks (both programmed by the left hemisphere), disruption in finger tapping rate is evident in comparison to tapping in silence. Left finger tapping and verbalization (programmed by the right and left hemispheres respectively) produces non-significant disruption in manual performance compared to the control condition. Performance impairments of the right hand indicate left hemisphere lateralization of speech production in normal subjects (Kinsbourne and Cook, 1971). Theoretically, the basis for the laterality effect, revealed by the concurrent performance paradigm, relies upon the notion of 'functional cerebral space' (Kinsbourne and Hicks, 1978). Hypothetically, the cerebral programmes which control the two performances share the same intrahemispheric functional space, such that, concurrent task performance overtaxes the capacity of the processing centre and one task must necessarily suffer.

The linguistic-manual paradigm was administered by Klingman and Sussman (1983) to eight non-fluent aphasics and a matched normal control group. As expected, the normal subjects only displayed disruption in right index finger tapping rates during concurrent linguistic and manual tasks. Collectively, the aphasic subjects displayed symmetrical manual disruption indicative of bilateral language representation. Three aphasic subjects revealed consistent right-hemisphere lateralization.

Clinic observation of recovered aphasics

Perhaps the most salient evidence for right-hemisphere mediation in aphasic language recovery has come from the accumulated case reports documenting the effect of right-hemisphere lesions in recovered aphasic patients subsequent to original left-hemisphere pathology (Russell and Espir, 1961; Levine and Mohr, 1979; Cambier *et al.*, 1983). These studies have tended to show that the language abilities of recovered aphasics are impaired following damage to the right hemisphere to a greater extent than would normally be expected subsequent to a right-hemisphere lesion, thereby suggesting that there has been a shift of language function in these patients, at least in part, from the left to the right hemisphere. Although there appears to be a considerable corpus of evidence available to support a role for the right hemisphere in the processes of recovery from aphasia, the exact nature of this role remains uncertain.

Summary

Ever since the late nineteenth century, controversy has surrounded the role of the right cerebral hemisphere in language function. Paul Broca was the first to introduce the concept of cerebral dominance for language when in 1861 he ascribed speech dominance to the cerebral hemisphere contralateral to the preferred hand. Hughlings Jackson in 1874 was the first to propose that the right cerebral hemisphere contributes to language processing. Subsequently, a variety of experimental approaches and techniques have been utilized in an attempt to further clarify the contribution of the right cerebral hemisphere to language, including: dichotic listening tasks, visual half-field tachistoscopic presentation, intracarotid amobarbital injection and electroencephalography. In addition, research in this field has employed a variety of different subjects of varying levels of neurological integrity, including: neurologically normal persons, hemispherectomized patients, commissurotomized patients, aphasic individuals with left-hemisphere lesions and secondary right-hemisphere lesions, and patients with right-hemisphere lesions.

Overall, the findings of these studies suggest that people with right-hemisphere damage have difficulty in the interpretation, integration and organization of linguistic elements and context. They fail to fully appraise information holistically and to form an overall structure as a reference base to aid their interpretation and production of complex language. In addition, they also have problems in the pragmatic, prosodic and emotional aspects of communication (the so-called extralinguistic components of language). Although some evidence is available to suggest a role for the right cerebral hemisphere in the recovery from aphasia, the precise nature of that role has yet to be fully defined.

References

Adamovich, B. and Henderson, J. (1983) Can we learn more from word fluency measures with aphasic right brain injured and closed head trauma patients?, in *Clinical Aphasiology Conference Proceedings* (ed. R.H. Brookshire), BRK Publishers, Minneapolis, pp. 124–131.

Basser, L. (1962) Hemiplegia of early onset and the faculty of speech with special reference to the effects of hemispherectomy. *Brain*, **85**, 427–460.

Bates, E., Thal, D., Trauner, D. *et al.* (1997) From first words to grammar in children with focal brain injury. *Developmental Neuropsychology*, **13**, 275–343.

Beaumont, J.G. (1974) Handedness and hemisphere function, in *Hemisphere Function in the Human Brain* (eds S.J. Diamond and J.G. Beaumont), Paul Elek, London, pp. 78–91.

Beeman, M. (1993) Semantic processing in the right hemisphere may contribute to drawing inferences from discourse. *Brain and Language*, **44**, 80–120.

Benowitz, L.I., Bear, D.M., Rosenthal, R. *et al.* (1983) Hemispheric specialization in non-verbal communication. *Cortex*, **19**, 5–12.

Benowitz, L.I., Moya, K.L. and Levine, D.N. (1990) Impaired verbal reasoning and constructional apraxia in subjects with right hemisphere damage. *Neuropsychologia*, **28**, 231–241.

Benson, D.F. (1979) *Aphasia, Alexia and Agraphia*, Churchill Livingstone, New York.

Benson, D.F. (1986) Aphasia and lateralization of language. *Cortex*, **22**, 71–86.

Berlin, C.I., Lowe-Bell, S.S., Cullen, J.K. *et al.* (1973) Dichotic speech perception: an interpretation of right ear advantage and temporal offset effects. *Journal of the Acoustical Society of America*, **53**, 699–709.

Berlin, C.I. and McNeil, M.R. (1976) Dichotic listening, in *Contemporary Issues in Experimental Phonetics* (ed. N.J. Lass), Academic Press, New York, pp. 75–87.

Bihrle, A.M., Brownell, H.H. and Powelson, J. (1986) Comprehension of humorous and nonhumorous materials by left and right brain-damaged patients. *Brain and Cognition*, **5**, 399–411.

Black, M.P., Holmes, G. and Lombroso, C. (1992) Corpus callosum section for intractable epilepsy in children. *Pediatric Neurosurgery*, **18**, 298–304.

Blake, M., Duffy, J.R., Myers, P.S. and Tompkins, C.A. (2002) Prevalence and patterns of right hemisphere cognitive/communicative deficits: retrospective data from an inpatient rehabilitation unit. *Aphasiology*, **16**, 537–548.

Borod, J.C., Pick, L.H., Andelman, E. *et al.* (2000) Verbal pragmatics following unilateral stroke: emotional content and valence. *Neuropsychology*, **14**, 112–124.

Bradshaw, J.L. and Nettleton, N.C. (1983) *Human Cerebral Asymmetry*, Prentice-Hall, Englewood Cliffs, NJ.

Broca, P. (1861) Portée de la parole. Ramollissement chronique et destruction partielle du lobe antérieur gauche du cerveau. *Bulletins de la Société d'anthropologie de Paris*, **2**, 219.

Broca, P. (1865) Sur le siége de la faculté du langage articulé. *Bulletins de la Société d'anthropologie de Paris*, **36**, 337–393.

Brownell, H. and Martino, G. (1998) Deficits in inference and social cognition: the effects of right hemisphere brain damage on discourse, in *Right Hemisphere Language Comprehension: Perspectives from Cognitive Neuroscience* (eds M. Beeman and C. Chiarello), Lawrence Erlbaum, Mahwah, NJ, pp. 309–328.

Caldas, A.C. and Botelho, M.A.S. (1980) Dichotic listening in the recovery of aphasia after stroke. *Brain and Language*, **10**, 145–151.

Cambier, J., Elghozi, D., Signaret, J.L. and Henin, D. (1983) Contribution of the right hemisphere to language in aphasic patients: disappearance of this language after a right-sided lesion. *Paris Review Neurologique*, **139**, 55–63.

Cherney, L.R., Drimmer, D.P. and Halper, A.S. (1997) Informational content and unilateral neglect: a longitudinal investigation of five subjects with right hemisphere damage. *Aphasiology*, **11**, 351–364.

Chilosi, A.M., Cipriani, P.P., Bertuccelli, B. *et al.* (2001) Early cognitive and communication development in children with focal brain lesions. *Journal of Child Neurology*, **16**, 309–316.

Code, C. (1987) *Language, Aphasia and the Right Hemisphere*, John Wiley & Sons, Ltd, Chichester.

Collins, M. (1975) The minor hemisphere, in *Clinical Aphasiology Conference Proceedings* (ed. R. Brookshire), BRK Publishers, Minneapolis, pp. 49–65.

Côté, H., Payer, M., Giroux, F. and Joanette, Y. (2007) Towards a description of clinical communication impairment profiles following right-hemisphere damage. *Aphasiology*, **21**, 739–749.

Cummings, J.L., Benson, D.F., Walsh, M.J. and Levine, H.L. (1979) Left-to-right transfer of language dominance: a case study. *Neurology*, **29**, 1547–1549.

Delis, D.C., Wapner, W., Gardner, H. and Moses, J.A. (1983) The contribution of the right hemisphere to the organization of paragraphs. *Cortex*, **19**, 43–50.

Devinsky, O. and Vazquez, B. (1993) Behavioral changes associated with epilepsy. *Neurology Clinics*, **11**, 127–149.

Diggs, C. and Basili, A.G. (1987) Verbal expression of right cerebrovascular accident patients: convergent and divergent language. *Brain and Language*, **30**, 130–146.

Emmorey, K.D. (1987) The neurological substrates for prosodic aspects of speech. *Brain and Language*, **30**, 305–321.

Foldi, N.S., Cicone, M. and Gardner, H. (1983) Pragmatic aspects of communication in brain-damaged patients, in *Language Functions in Brain Organization* (ed. S.J. Segalowitz), Academic Press, New York, pp. 123–137.

Gainotti, G., Caltagirone, C., Miceli, G. and Masullo, C. (1981) Selective semantic-lexical impairment of language comprehension in right brain damaged patients. *Brain and Language*, **13**, 201–211.

Galaburda, A.M., Le May, M., Kemper, T. and Geschwind, N. (1978) Right–left asymmetries in the brain. *Science*, **199**, 852–856.

Gardner, H. (1975) *The Shattered Mind*, Knopf, New York.

Gardner, H., Brownell, H.H., Wapner, W. and Michelow, D. (1983) Missing the point: the role of the right hemisphere in the processing of complex linguistic materials, in *Cognitive Processing in the Right Hemisphere* (ed. E. Perecman), Academic Press, New York, pp. 201–223.

Gardner, H., King, P., Flamm, L. and Silverman, J. (1975) Comprehension and appreciation of humorous material following brain damage. *Brain*, **98**, 399–412.

Gazzaniga, M.S. (1970) *The Bisected Brain*, Appleton-Century-Crofts, New York.

Gazzaniga, M.S. (1983) Right hemisphere following brain bisection: a 20-year perspective. *American Psychologist*, **38**, 525–537.

Gazzaniga, M.S., Charlotte, S., Smylie, S. *et al.* (1984) Profiles of right hemisphere language and speech following brain bisection. *Brain and Language*, **22**, 206–220.

Gazzaniga, M.S. and Hillyard, S. (1971) Language and speech capacity of the right hemisphere. *Neuropsychologia*, **9**, 273–280.

Gazzaniga, M.S. and Sperry, R.W. (1967) Language after sectioning of the cerebral commissures. *Brain*, **90**, 131–148.

Geschwind, N. (1965a) Disconnection syndromes in animals and man. Part 1. *Brain*, **88**, 237–294.

Geschwind, N. (1965b) Disconnection syndromes in animals and man. Part 2. *Brain*, **88**, 585–644.

Geschwind, N. and Levitsky, W. (1968) Human brain: left–right asymmetries in temporal speech region. *Science*, **161**, 186–187.

Gloning, I., Gloning, K., Haub, C. and Quatember, R. (1969) Comparison of verbal behaviour in right-handed and non-right-handed patients with anatomically verified lesion of one hemisphere. *Cortex*, **5**, 43–52.

Gloning, K. (1977) Handedness and aphasia. *Neuropsychologia*, **15**, 353–358.

Goodglass, H. and Kaplan, E. (1983) *The Boston Diagnostic Aphasia Examination*, Lea & Febiger, Philadelphia.

Goodglass, H. and Quadfasel, F.A. (1954) Language laterality in left-handed aphasics. *Brain*, **77**, 510–548.

Happe, F., Brownell, H. and Winner, E. (1999) Acquired 'theory of mind' impairments following stroke. *Cognition*, **70**, 211–240.

Hecaen, H. and Sauguet, J. (1971) Cerebral dominance in left-handed subjects. *Cortex*, **7**, 19–48.

Helmstaedter, C., Kurthen, M., Linke, D. and Elger, C. (1994) Right hemisphere restitution of language and memory functions in right hemisphere language-dominant patients with left temporal lobe epilepsy. *Brain*, **117**, 729–737.

Hier, D.B. and Kaplan, J. (1980) Verbal comprehension deficits after right hemisphere damage. *Applied Psycholinguistics*, **1**, 279–294.

Holland, A. (1977) Some practical considerations in aphasic rehabilitation, in *Rationale for Adult Aphasia Therapy* (eds M. Sullivan and M.S. Kommers), University of Nebraska Press, Nebraska, pp. 37–45.

Hough, M.S. (1990) Narrative comprehension in adults with right and left hemisphere brain damage: theme organization. Brain and Language, **38**, 253–277.

Jackson, J.H. (1874) On the nature of the duality of the brain. Reprinted in J. Taylor (ed.), *Selected Writings of John Hughlings Jackson*, Vol. 2 (pp. 129–145), Hodder & Stoughton, London.

Joanette, Y. and Ansaldo, A.I. (1999) Clinical note: acquired pragmatic impairments and aphasia. *Brain and Language*, **68**, 529–534.

Joanette, Y., Goulet, P. and Hannequin, D. (1990) *Right Hemisphere and Verbal Communication*, Springer-Verlag, New York.

Joanette, Y., Goulet, P., Ska, B. and Nespoulous, J.-L. (1986) Informative content of narrative discourse in right-brain-damaged right-handers. *Brain and Language*, **29**, 81–105.

Johnson, J., Sommers, R. and Weidner, W. (1977) Dichotic ear preference in aphasia. *Journal of Speech and Hearing Research*, **20**, 116–129.

Kempler, D., Van Lancker, D., Marchman, V. and Bates, E. (1999) Idiom comprehension in children and adults with unilateral brain damage. *Developmental Neuropsychology*, **15**, 327–349.

Kennedy, M.R.T. (2000) Topic scenes in conversations with adults with right hemisphere brain damage. *American Journal of Speech-Language Pathology*, **9**, 72–86.

Kennedy, M., Strand, E., Burton, W. and Petersen, C. (1994) Analysis of first-encounter conversations of right-hemisphere damaged participants. *Clinical Aphasiology*, **22**, 67–80.

Kertesz, A. (1979) *Aphasia and Associated Disorders: Taxonomy, Localization and Recovery*, Grune & Stratton, New York.

Kinsbourne, M. (1971) The minor cerebral hemisphere as a source of aphasic speech. *Archives of Neurology*, **25**, 303–306.

Kinsbourne, M. and Cook, J. (1971) Generalized and lateralized effects on concurrent verbalization on a unimanual skill. *Quarterly Journal of Experimental Psychology*, **23**, 341–345.

Kinsbourne, M. and Hicks, R.E. (1978) Functional cerebral space: a model for overflow transfer and interference effects in human performance, in *Attention and Performance VII* (ed. J. Requin), Erlbaum, Hillsdale, NJ, pp. 71–79.

Kinsella, G. (1986) Rehabilitation of prosodic impairment following right hemisphere lesions, in *Proceedings of the Tenth Annual Brain Impairment*

Conference (eds V. Anderson, J. Ponsford and P. Snow), Australian Society for the Study of Brain Impairment, Melbourne, pp. 52–65.

Klingman, K.C. and Sussman, H.M. (1983) Hemisphericity in aphasic language recovery. *Journal of Speech and Hearing Research*, **26**, 248–256.

Lazar, R., Marshall, R., Pile-Spellman, J. *et al.* (2000) Interhemispheric transfer of language in patients with left frontal cerebral arteriovenous malformation. *Neuropsychologia*, **38**, 1325–1332.

Lehericy, S., Cohen, L., Bazin, B. *et al.* (2000) Functional MR evaluation of temporal and frontal language dominance compared with Wada test. *Neurology*, **54**, 1625–1633.

Lehman, M.T. and Tompkins, C.A. (2000) Inferencing in adults with right hemisphere brain damage: an analysis of conflicting results. *Aphasiology*, **14**, 485–499.

LeMay, M. and Culebras, A. (1972) Human brain: morphologic differences in the hemispheres demonstrable by carotid arteriography. *New England Journal of Medicine*, **287**, 168–170.

Lenneberg, E. (1967) *Biological Foundations of Language*, John Wiley & Sons, Inc., New York.

Lesser, R. (1974) Verbal comprehension in aphasia: an English version of three Italian tests. *Cortex*, **10**, 247–263.

Lesser, R. (1978) *Linguistic Investigations of Aphasia: Studies in Language Disability and Remediation*, Elsevier, New York.

Levine, D.N. and Mohr, J.P. (1979) Language after bilateral cerebral infarctions: role of the minor hemisphere in speech. *Neurology*, **29**, 927–938.

Levy, J. (1970) Information processing and higher psychological functions in the disconnected hemispheres of commissurotomy patients. Doctoral Dissertation: California Institute of Technology.

Levy, J. (1974) Cerebral asymmetries as manifested in split brain man, in *Hemispheric Disconnection and Cerebral Function* (eds M. Kinsbourne and W.D. Smith), Charles C. Thomas, Springfield, IL, pp. 34–47.

Levy, J. (1983) Language, cognition and the right hemisphere: a response to Gazzaniga. *American Psychologist*, **38**, 538–541.

Levy, J., Trevarthen, C. and Sperry, R.W. (1972) Perception of bilateral chimeric figures following hemispheric disconnection. *Brain*, **95**, 61–78.

Linebaugh, C.W. (1978) Dichotic ear preference in aphasia: another view. *Journal of Speech and Hearing Research*, **21**, 598–600.

Lowe, S.S., Cullen, J.K., Berlin, C.I. *et al.* (1970) Perception of simultaneous dichotic and monotic monosyllables. *Journal of Speech and Hearing Research*, **13**, 812–822.

Lundgren, K., Moya, K. and Benowitz, L. (1983) Perception of nonverbal cues after right brain damage, in *Clinical Aphasiology Conference Proceedings* (ed. R.H. Brookshire), BRK Publishers, Minneapolis, pp. 74–83.

Luria, A.R. (1963) *Restoration of Function after Brain Injury*, Pergamon Press, London.

Luria, A.R. (1970) *Traumatic Aphasia*, Mouton, The Hague.

Madden, D.J. and Nebes, R.D. (1980) Visual perception and memory, in *The Brain and Psychology* (ed. M.C. Wittrock), Academic Press, New York, pp. 26–38.

Meyer, J.A., Sakai, F., Yamaguchi, F. *et al.* (1980) Regional changes in cerebral blood flow during standard behavioural activation in patients with disorders of speech and mentation compared to normal volunteers. *Brain and Language*, **9**, 61–77.

Millar, J.M. and Whitaker, H.A. (1983) The right hemisphere's contribution to language: a review of the evidence from brain-damaged subjects, in *Language Functions and Brain Organization* (ed. S.J. Segalowitz), Academic Press, New York, pp. 121–139.

Moore, W. and Weidner, W. (1974) Bilateral tachistoscopic word perception in aphasic and normal subjects. *Perceptual and Motor Skills*, **39**, 1003–1011.

Müller, R., Rothermel, R.D., Behen, M.E. *et al.* (1999) Language organization in patients with early and late left-hemisphere lesion: a PET study. *Neuropsychologia*, **37**, 545–547.

Muter, V., Taylor, S. and Vargha-Khadem, F. (1997) A longitudinal study of early intellectual development in hemiplegic children. *Neuropsychologia*, **35**, 289–298.

Myers, P.S. (1979) Profiles of communication deficits in patients with right cerebral hemisphere damage: implications for diagnosis and treatment, in *Clinical Aphasiology Conference Proceedings* (ed. R.H. Brookshire), BRK Publishers, Minneapolis, pp. 27–36.

Myers, P.S. (1984) Right hemisphere impairment, in *Language Disorders in Adults* (ed. A. Holland), College-Hill Press, San Diego, pp. 85–97.

Myers, P.S. (1986) Right hemisphere communication impairment, in *Language Intervention Strategies in*

Adult Aphasia (ed. R. Chapey), Williams & Wilkins, Baltimore, pp. 105–118.

Myers, P.S. (1997) Right hemisphere syndrome, in *Aphasia and Related Neurogenic Language Disorders* (ed. L.L. LaPointe), Thieme, New York, pp. 201–225.

Myers, P.S. (1999) *Right Hemisphere Damage: Disorders of Communication and Cognition*, Singular Publishing Group, San Diego.

Myers, P.S. (2001) Towards a definition of RHD syndrome. *Aphasiology*, **15**, 913–918.

Myers, P.S. and Linebaugh, C.W. (1981) Comprehension of idiomatic expressions by right-hemisphere-damaged adults, in *Clinical Aphasiology Conference Proceedings* (ed. R.H. Brookshire), BRK Publishers, Minneapolis, pp. 254–261.

Nebes, R.D. and Sperry, R.W. (1971) Hemisphere disconnection syndrome with cerebral birth injury in the dominant arm area. *Neuropsychologia*, **9**, 247–259.

Osgood, C. and Miron, M. (1963) *Approaches to the Study of Aphasia*, University of Illinois Press, Chicago.

Penfield, W. and Roberts, L. (1959) *Speech and Brain Mechanisms*, Princeton University Press, Princeton.

Penfield, W. and Roberts, L. (1966) *Speech and Brain Mechanisms*, Atheneum, New York.

Pettit, J.M. and Noll, J.D. (1979) Cerebral dominance in aphasia recovery. *Brain and Language*, **7**, 191–200.

Piccirilli, M., D'Alessandro, P., Tiacci, C. and Ferroni, A. (1988) Language lateralization in children with benign partial epilepsy. *Epilepsia*, **29**, 19–25.

Posner, M.I. and Raichle, M. (1994) *Images of Mind*, Scientific American Library, New York.

Pratt, R.T.C. and Warrington, E.K. (1972) The assessment of cerebral dominance in unilateral ECT. *British Journal of Psychiatry*, **121**, 327–328.

Prutting, C. and Kirchner, D. (1987) A clinical appraisal of the pragmatic aspects of language. *Journal of Speech and Hearing Disorders*, **52**, 105–119.

Rassmussen, T. (1983) Hemispherectomy for seizures revisited. *Canadian Journal of Neuroscience*, **10**, 71–78.

Rassmussen, T. and Milner, B. (1977) The role of early left-brain injury in determining lateralization of cerebral speech functions. *Annals of the New York Academy of Science*, **299**, 355–369.

Ratcliff, G., Dila, C., Taylor, L. and Milner, B. (1980) The morphological asymmetry of the hemispheres and cerebral dominance for speech: a possible relationship. *Brain and Language*, **11**, 87–98.

Reilly, J.S., Bates, E. and Marchman, V.A. (1998) Narrative discourse in children with early focal brain injury. *Brain and Language*, **61**, 335–375.

Riva, D., Panteleoni, C., Milani, N. and Giorgi, C. (1993) Hemispheric specialization in children with unilateral epileptic focus with and without computed tomography demonstrated lesion. *Epilepsia*, **34**, 69–73.

Rivers, D.L. and Love, F.J. (1980) Language performance on visual processing tasks in right hemisphere lesion cases. *Brain and Language*, **10**, 348–366.

Roberts, C., Kinsella, G. and Wales, R. (1982) Disturbances in processing prosodic features of language following right hemisphere lesions, in *Proceedings of the 1982 Brain Impairment Workshop* (eds G.V. Stanley and K.W. Walsh), Australian Society for the Study of Brain Impairment, Melbourne, pp. 73–81.

Ross, E.D. (1981) The aprosodias: functional anatomic organization of the affective components of language in the right hemisphere. *Archives of Neurology*, **38**, 561–569.

Ross, E.D. (1985) Modulation of affect and nonverbal communication by the right hemisphere, in *Principles of Behavioural Neurology* (ed. M.M. Mesulan), F.A. Davis, Philadelphia, pp. 154–163.

Ross, E.D. and Mesulam, M.M. (1979) Dominant language functions of the right hemisphere: prosody and emotional gesturing. *Archives of Neurology*, **36**, 144–148.

Rossi, G. and Rosandini, G. (1967) Experimental analysis of cerebral dominance in man, in *Brain Mechanisms Underlying Speech and Language* (eds C.H. Millikan and F. Darley), Grune & Stratton, New York, pp. 169–176.

Rubens, A.B., Mahowald, M.W. and Hutton, J.T. (1976) Asymmetry of the lateral (sylvian) fissures in man. *Neurology*, **26**, 620–624.

Russell, W.R. and Espir, M.L.E. (1961) *Traumatic Aphasia: a Study of Aphasia in War Wounds of the Brain*, Oxford University Press, Oxford.

Satz, P., Strauss, E. and Whitaker, H. (1990) The ontogeny of hemispheric specialization: some old hypotheses revisited. *Brain and Language*, **38**, 596–614.

Schneiderman, E.I., Murasugi, K.G. and Saddy, J.D. (1992) Story arrangement ability in right-brain-damaged patients. *Brain and Language*, **43**, 107–120.

Schuell, H., Jenkins, J. and Jiminez-Pabon, E. (1964) *Aphasia in Adults*, Harper and Row, New York.

Schulhoff, C. and Goodglass, H. (1969) Dichotic listening, side of brain injury and cerebral dominance. *Neuropsychologia*, 7, 148–160.

Searleman, A. (1977) A review of right hemisphere linguistic capabilities. *Psychological Bulletin*, **84**, 503–528.

Smith, A. (1966) Speech and other functions after left dominant hemispherectomy. *Journal of Neurology, Neurosurgery and Psychiatry*, **29**, 467–471.

Smith, A. and Burklund, C.W. (1966) Dominant hemispherectomy. *Science*, **153**, 1280.

Smith, A. and Sugar, O. (1975) Development of above normal language intelligence 21 years after left hemispherectomy. *Neurology*, **25**, 813–818.

Sparks, R., Goodglass, H. and Nickel, B. (1970) Ipsilateral versus contralateral extinction in dichotic listening resulting from hemispheric lesions. *Cortex*, **6**, 249–260.

Sperry, R.W. and Gazzaniga, M.S. (1967) Language following surgical disconnection of the hemispheres, in *Brain Mechanisms Underlying Speech and Language* (eds C.H. Milikan and F. Darley), Grune & Stratton, New York, pp. 185–195.

Staudt, M., Lidzba, K., Grodd, W. *et al.* (2002) Right-hemispheric organization of language following early left-sided brain lesions: functional MRI topography. *Neuroimage*, **16**, 954–967.

Strauss, E., Wada, J. and Kosaka, B. (1983) Writing hand posture and cerebral dominance for speech. *Cortex*, **20**, 143–147.

Tikofsky, R.S., Kooi, K.A. and Thomas, M.H. (1960) Electroencephalographic findings and recovery from aphasia. *Neurology*, **10**, 154–156.

Tompkins, C.A. (1995) *Right Hemisphere Communication Disorders: Theory and Management*, Singular Publishing Group, San Diego.

Tsunoda, T. (1975) Functional differences between right and left cerebral hemispheres detected by the key tapping method. *Brain and Language*, **2**, 152–170.

Tucker, D.M., Watson, R.T. and Heilman, K.M. (1977) Discrimination and evocation of affectively intoned speech in patients with right parietal disease. *Neurology*, **27**, 947–950.

Vanhalle, C., Lemieux, S., Joubert, S. *et al.* (2000) Processing of speech acts by right hemisphere brain-damaged patients: an ecological approach. *Aphasiology*, **14**, 1127–1142.

Van Lanker, D.R. and Kempler, D. (1987) Comprehension of familiar phrases by left- but not by right-hemisphere damaged patients. *Brain and Language*, **35**, 265–277.

Vargha-Khadem, F., Isaacs, E., Van Der Werf, S. *et al.* (1992) Development of intelligence and memory in children with hemiplegic cerebral palsy. *Brain*, **115**, 315–329.

Vicari, S., Albertoni, A., Chilosi, M. *et al.* (2000) Plasticity and reorganization during language development in children with early brain injury. *Cortex*, **36**, 31–36.

Villemure, J.G. and Mascott, C. (1993) Hemispherectomy: the peri-insular approach: technical aspects. *Epilepsia*, **34** (Suppl. 6), 48.

Wada, J., Clarke, R. and Hamm, A. (1975) Cerebral hemispheric asymmetry in humans. *Archives of Neurology*, **32**, 239–246.

Wada, J. and Rasmussen, T. (1960) Intracarotid injection of sodium amytal for the lateralization of cerebral speech dominance: experimental and clinical observations. *Journal of Neurosurgery*, **17**, 266–282.

Wapner, W., Hamby, S. and Gardner, H. (1981) The role of the right hemisphere in the apprehension of complex linguistic materials. *Brain and Language*, **14**, 15–33.

Warrington, W.K. and Pratt, R.T.C. (1973) Language laterality in left handers assessed by unilateral ECT. *Neuropsychologia*, **11**, 423–428.

Weylman, S., Brownell, H.H., Roman, M. and Gardner, H. (1989) Appreciation of indirect requests by left and right brain damaged patients: the effects of verbal context and conventionality of wording. *Brain and Language*, **62**, 89–106.

Whitaker, H. and Ojemann, G.A. (1977) Lateralization of higher cortical functions: a critique. *Annals of the New York Academy of Sciences*, **229**, 459–473.

Winner, E., Brownell, H., Happe, F. *et al.* (1998) Distinguishing lies from jokes: theory of mind deficits and discourse interpretation in right hemisphere brain-damaged patients. *Brain and Language*, **62**, 89–106.

Witelson, S.F. and Pallie, W. (1973) Left hemisphere specialization for language in the newborn: neuroanatomical evidence of asymmetry. *Brain*, **96**, 641–646.

Zaidel, E. (1976) Auditory vocabulary of the right hemisphere following brain bisection or hemidecortication. *Cortex*, **12**, 191–211.

Zaidel, E. (1978a) Concepts of cerebral dominance in the split brain, in *Cerebral Correlates of Conscious Experience* (eds P.A. Buser and A. Rougeul-Buser), Elsevier North Holland Biomedical Press, Amsterdam, pp. 273–281.

Zaidel, E. (1978b) Auditory language comprehension in the right hemisphere following cerebral commissurotomy and hemispherectomy: a comparison with child language and aphasia, in *Language, Acquisition and Language Breakdown: Parallels and Divergencies* (eds A. Caramazza and E.B. Zurif), Johns Hopkins University Press, Baltimore, pp. 98–112.

Zaidel, E. (1983) A response to Gazzaniga: language in the right hemisphere, convergent perspectives. *American Psychologist*, **38**, 542–546.

Zaidel, E. (1985) Right hemisphere language, in *The Dual Brain: Hemispheric Specialization In Humans* (eds D.F. Benson and E. Zaidel), The Guilford Press, New York, pp. 58–65.

Zaidel, E. and Peters, A.M. (1981) Phonological encoding and ideographic reading by the disconnected right hemisphere: two case studies. *Brain and Language*, **14**, 205–234.

Zangwill, O.L. (1960) *Cerebral Dominance and its Relation to Psychological Function*, Charles C. Thomas, Springfield, IL.

Zangwill, O.L. (1964) Intelligence in aphasia, in *Disorders of Language* (eds A.V.S. De Ruek and M. O'Connor) Little, Brown and Company, Boston, pp. 86–97.

Zangwill, O.L. (1967) Speech and the minor hemisphere. *Acta Neuropsychologica*, **67**, 1013–1020.

Zurif, E.B. and Bryden, M.P. (1969) Familial handedness and left–right differences in auditory and visual perception. *Neuropsychologia*, 7, 179–187.

Language disturbances in dementia syndromes

6

Introduction

Dementia is a clinical syndrome in which there is a persistent impairment in intellectual function as a consequence of acquired brain disease with compromise in at least three of the following spheres of mental activity: language, memory, visuospatial skills, emotion or personality and cognition (abstraction, calculation, judgement, etc.) (Cummings, Benson and LoVerme, 1980; Cummings and Benson, 1983). According to the text revision of the fourth edition *Diagnostic and Statistical Manual of Mental Disorders* (DSM-IV-TR) (American Psychiatric Association, 2000), dementia is defined as an impairment in short- and long-term memory with related changes in abstract thinking, judgement, other higher-cortical functions or personality that causes significant social and occupational impairments. Importantly, in order to make a diagnosis of dementia according to DSM-IV-TR criteria, evidence of an organic cause of the memory and intellectual impairments is also required. Although most definitions of dementia indicate that language impairment may be present, research is now available to suggest that disturbed language function may be present at all stages of some dementia syndromes (Irigaray, 1973; Obler and Albert, 1981; Bayles, 1982; Murdoch *et al.*, 1987, 1988; Smith, Murdoch and Chenery, 1989; Chenery and Murdoch, 1994).

Dementia is a disorder which affects the adult and geriatric population, being most common in people over the age of 65 years. Up to 20% of persons in this age group have been reported to have some degree of dementia (Reifler, Larson and Hanley, 1982; Graves and Kukull, 1994). Currently, the size of the geriatric population in most Western countries is increasing, both in terms of absolute numbers and as a percentage of the overall population. Estimates taken in the United States suggest that by the year 2030 approximately 20% of the US population will be over 65 years of age; this figure represents in excess of 50 million persons (Plum, 1979; Wells, 1981). If, as suggested in the literature, language impairment is a common feature of dementia, the rapidly increasing incidence of the disorder has important implications for the future caseloads of those speech-language pathologists involved in the treatment of adult neurologically disordered clients. As we move further into the twenty-first century, we can expect that demented persons will form an ever-increasing proportion of the clients requiring speech pathology services.

During the past two decades, a greater level of interest in dementia and its effects on language function has been reflected in a rise in the number of studies reported in the literature devoted to the investigation of the language abilities of demented patients. It is now evident that different patterns of language impairment may accompany the different types of dementia. For this reason, prior to reviewing the findings of studies which have investigated the language abilities of demented patients, the major dementia-producing diseases will be discussed in terms of their characteristics and underlying neuropathologies.

Types of dementia

Dementia can be the product of a number of different conditions and diseases and, depending on the aetiology, the impairment in mental abilities can be either reversible or irreversible. The major types of dementia are listed in Table 6.1.

In the region of 70 different diseases and conditions have been identified as potential causes of dementia. They include chronic cortical degenerative diseases (e.g. Alzheimer's disease, Pick's disease, dementia with Lewy bodies), cerebrovascular diseases (e.g. vascular dementia, Binswanger's disease), endocrine disorders (e.g. thyroid disease, diabetes, Cushing's disease), nutritional deficiencies (e.g. vitamin B_{12}, thiamine), systemic diseases (e.g. respiratory diseases, anaemia), extrapyramidal syndromes (e.g. Parkinson's disease, Huntington's disease), infectious disorders (e.g. encephalitis, Creutzfeldt–Jakob disease) and various other neurological conditions (e.g. traumatic brain injury, tumours, normal pressure hydrocephalus). By far the most common cause of dementia is Alzheimer's disease, accounting for some 50–60% of all persons with dementia (Tomlinson, Blessed and Roth, 1970). Vascular dementias (e.g. those caused by multi-infarcts or ischaemia) account for approximately 20% of cases. According to Eastley and Wilcock (2000), approximately 13% of individuals with dementia have a potentially reversible form of the disorder. This 13% includes those with conditions such as drug toxicity, thyroid disease, vitamin deficiency and normal pressure hydrocephalus.

Although dementia is more commonly associated with neurological disorders that involve cortical structures (e.g. Alzheimer's disease), it is now also widely recognized that dementia may also accompany neurological disorders that primarily involve subcortical structures such as the basal ganglia, thalamus and brainstem (e.g. Parkinson's disease and Huntington's disease). A number of important differences recognized clinically serve to distinguish cortical dementia from subcortical dementia. In particular, subcortical dementing illnesses affect the motor system and are therefore associated with movement disorders such as the rigidity and bradykinesia of Parkinson's disease, whereas motor impairments are not evident in cortical dementias until late in their clinical course.

The dementia-producing diseases most commonly seen by a speech pathologist include: Alzheimer's disease, dementia with Lewy bodies, Pick's disease, vascular dementia, dementia associated with extrapyramidal syndromes and Korsakoff's syndrome.

Alzheimer's disease

Alzheimer's disease is a progressive, degenerative disorder of uncertain aetiology that represents the single, most frequently diagnosed cause of dementia (Terry and Katzman, 1983; Brookmeyer, Gray and Kawas, 1998) accounting for approximately one-half of all cases of irreversible dementia (Reifler, Larson and Hanley, 1982). The condition is reported to afflict in the region of 6–10% of all persons over the age of 65 years, with the figure rising to 33% at age 90. It has been estimated that this represents a prevalence of 10–20 million cases worldwide (Brookmeyer, Gray and Kawas, 1998; Ballard, 2000). For this reason, it has received the greatest amount of attention in the literature relating to language disturbances in dementia.

Although originally described as 'pre-senile dementia', Alzheimer's disease is now considered essentially the same as senile dementia of the Alzheimer-type. The neuropathological findings

Table 6.1   Major causes of dementia.

Cortical dementias
Alzheimer's disease
Pick's disease

Extra pyramidal syndromes (subcortical dementias)
Parkinson's disease
Hepatolenticular degeneration (Wilson's disease)
Huntington's disease
Progressive supranuclear palsy
Idiopathic basal ganglia calcification

Hydrocephalus

Metabolic and toxic encephalopathies
Nutritional deficiencies, for example vitamin B_{12} deficiency
Endocrine disturbances, for example hypothyroidism, hyperthyroidism, Cushing's disease, Addison's disease, diabetes
Drug toxicity
Heavy-metal exposure
Alcohol abuse (Korsakoff's syndrome)

Cardiovascular disease
Vascular dementia, for example large-vessel vascular dementia, Binswanger's disease

Infectious diseases
Human immunodeficiency virus (HIV)
Neurosyphilis
Herpes simplex encephalitis
Creutzfeldt–Jakob disease

Miscellaneous dementia syndromes
Neoplastic
Post-traumatic
Post-anoxic

and the behavioural alterations in these diseases are essentially indistinguishable (Haase, 1977) and the age of onset has been eliminated as a criterion for the diagnosis of Alzheimer's disease. The term 'Alzheimer's disease' is now used for all age groups.

Diagnosis of Alzheimer's disease is usually made between 70 and 79 years of age and the condition is associated with a marked decrease in life expectancy.

Characteristics of Alzheimer's disease

The symptomatology of Alzheimer's disease includes: intellectual dysfunctions sufficient to interfere with social behaviour, absence of the characteristics of delirium, memory impairment, indication of brain damage and at least one of either personality change, impairment in abstract thinking, poor judgement or other disturbance of higher-cortical function (e.g. aphasia, apraxia, agnosia or constructional difficulty). Memory loss is the most marked feature of cognitive decline in Alzheimer's disease and often appears as the first symptom of the condition (Hyman, Van Hoesen and Damasio, 1990). The behavioural symptoms exhibited by the majority of patients with Alzheimer's disease include personality changes (e.g. disinhibition, disengagement, apathy); delusions (e.g. persecution, theft, infidelity, abandonment, etc.); hallucinations (e.g. visual, auditory, gustatory, olfactory); mood disorders (e.g. depression, anxiety, mania); sleep, eating and sexual disorders; and restlessness, pacing, wandering, repetitive behaviours (Teri and Logsdon, 1991).

Alzheimer's disease is known to pass through a series of stages as the condition progresses (Kertesz and Kertesz, 1988). The first stage, termed 'forgetfulness', may last for 2–4 years and is initially signalled by impairment of recent memory (often noticed only by family members). In addition to memory impairment for recent events, this early stage is also characterized by spatial and temporal disorientation and a lack of spontaneity; social competence at this time is preserved and, although an overt language disorder may not be present, sensitive assessment can identify some degree of language impairment. The

second stage, termed the 'confusional stage', is accompanied by progressive cortical involvement with the appearance of more frank symptoms of language impairment. There is increased intellectual deterioration, and personality changes become more prominent. Depression, which may be apparent in the earlier stage of the disorder, may give way to an agitated restless state. A frontal lobe gait disorder may become apparent, with short, slow, shuffling steps, flexed posture, wide base and difficulty initiating walking. The third and final stage, termed the 'terminal stage', is characterized by rigidity and bradykinesia. Previously preserved social graces are lost and psychiatric symptoms, including psychosis, paranoia, hallucinations or delusions, may be prominent. Primitive reflexes are commonly found. Other late features may include myoclonus, incontinence, spasticity, extensor plantar responses and hemiparesis. Mutism, incontinence and a bed-ridden state are terminal manifestations.

Epidemiological studies have identified several potential risk factors for Alzheimer's disease, including advanced age, a positive family history (especially in first-degree relatives) and apolipoprotein E (ApoE) genotype. The single most consistently identified risk factor for Alzheimer's disease across numerous studies is advanced age, with the incidence and prevalence of Alzheimer's disease increasing with age. Although a positive family history is another risk factor, the most common form of Alzheimer's disease occurs sporadically. Rare, early-onset, pre-senile forms of Alzheimer's disease do occur with an autosomal-dominant pattern of inheritance but account for less than 5% of cases globally. The genetic basis of most hereditary forms of Alzheimer's disease involves genes that encode amyloid precursor protein leading to the increased deposition of amyloid in the neurones of affected individuals (see pathology section below). High deposition of β-amyloid also occurs in individuals with Down syndrome (Trisomy 21), many of whom develop Alzheimer's disease by their mid-30s. The ApoE gene is located on chromosome 19. The presence of the E4 allele form of this gene is associated with increased risk of Alzheimer's disease and a younger age at onset. In addition to the above, lower education levels and head injury with loss of consciousness also increase the risk of Alzheimer's disease (Jorm, 2000). In contrast, high educational attainment, the use of anti-inflammatory medications and replacement oestrogen for postmenopausal women are associated with reduced risk of Alzheimer's disease (Jorm, 2000).

Pathological changes in the brain in Alzheimer's disease

Pathological changes reported to occur in the brains of Alzheimer patients include both morphological and neurochemical alterations. The brains of Alzheimer patients have been found to be underweight (usually less than 1 kg) (Corsellis, 1976; Tomlinson, 1977) and characterized by diffuse ventricular dilation, atrophy and neuronal loss in both grey and white matter. The morphological changes, however, are not spread diffusely throughout the cerebral cortex. On gross examination the areas of brain damage, although widespread, can be seen to primarily involve the temporal and frontal lobes, the hippocampus, parahippocampus and hippocampal gyrus (Tomlinson, 1977). At the same time, areas of cortex subserving primary motor, somatosensory and visual functions are relatively spared (Jervis, 1937; McMenemy, 1940). Motor abnormalities do not usually appear until the late stages of the disorder and subcortical structures do not become involved until after the dementia is well established (Cummings and Benson, 1983).

A number of characteristic histological changes are evident in the neurones of the cerebral cortex in Alzheimer's disease. These changes include senile (neuritic) plaques and neurofibrillary tangles. Senile (or neuritic) plaques are small spherical areas of tissue degeneration consisting of granular deposits and remnants of neuronal processes. These plaques develop as a result of inappropriate accumulation of the protein β-amyloid in the brain. Beta-amyloid is formed during the processing of amyloid precursor protein, a compound that is thought to help regulate synaptic function, possibly by regulating excitotoxic activity of glutamate. In Alzheimer's disease, amyloid precursor protein is processed abnormally leading to β-amyloid being slowly deposited in the extracellular spaces within the brain. Beta-amyloid, especially in its aggregated form is known to be toxic to surrounding synapses and neurones, causing synaptic membrane destruction and eventually cell death.

Senile plaques have a three-layered structure with an outer zone of degenerating neuritic processes, a middle zone of swollen axons and dendrites and a central core of β-amyloid. In Alzheimer's disease, these plaques are distributed diffusely in the cerebral cortex. Typically, senile plaques initially develop in the hippocampus and the basal forebrain, and from there gradually spread to involve the neocortical and subcortical grey matter of the temporal, parietal, frontal and, eventually, occipital cortex. Subcortical nuclei only become involved relatively late in the process. The formation of these plaques correlates with the increasing loss of synapses, the formation of senile plaques in the hippocampus corresponding to the onset of the earliest clinical sign, namely short-term memory loss.

Neurofibrillary tangles represent one of the most characteristic morphological changes in Alzheimer's disease. These lesions form within the neurones and comprise a microtubule-associated protein, tau, that has a vital role in the maintenance of neuronal cytoskeletal structure and function. In Alzheimer's disease, tau becomes dissociated from the cytoskeleton, forming neurofibrils that become twisted and contorted into a helical shape within the neuronal cytoplasm (Jervis, 1937). As a consequence, the cytoskeletal structure of the neurone collapses, interfering with the transport of intracellular elements within the neurone. Neurofibrillary tangles develop and conform to an anatomical pattern that correlates with the clinical syndrome, with the number and distribution of tangles being directly related to the severity of the dementia. Together with senile plaques, the presence of neurofibrillary tangles represents the most important diagnostic criteria for Alzheimer's disease.

Neuropathologies such as senile plaques and neurofibrillary tangles can only be definitely identified via direct histological examination of the brain tissue. Consequently, confirmation of Alzheimer's disease in most cases is currently dependent on autopsy, with the occasional rare case being verified by biopsy (Shore, Overman and Wyatt, 1983; Martin *et al.*, 1985). Such limitations emphasize the need to make ante-mortem diagnoses on the basis of some other identifiable symptom complex. Berg (1985) reported that the term 'Dementia of the Alzheimer's type' is used to refer to the disorder diagnosed by clinical criteria, but not histologically verified as Alzheimer's disease. However, the terms 'dementias of the Alzheimer's type' and 'Alzheimer's disease' are used interchangeably by different authors.

As indicated above, the histological changes in Alzheimer's disease are not spread diffusely throughout the cerebral cortex but rather occur in specific topographic patterns. The neurofibrillary tangles and senile plaques are most evident in the temporal–parietal–occipital junction area with the frontal lobe being affected to a lesser degree. Significant involvement also occurs in the temporal–limbic cortex and the posterior cingulated gyrus. In the limbic cortex the hippocampus, entorhinal area (the anterior part of the parahippocampal gyrus) and the amygdala are affected. Additional histological changes evident in the affected cortical areas in Alzheimer's disease include a loss of neurones, accumulation of neuronal lipofuscin and astrocyte hyperplasia (Corsellis, 1976; Terry *et al.*, 1981; Dowson, 1982). Although the cerebral cortex is the primary region affected in Alzheimer's disease, histological changes including senile plaques and neurofibrillary tangles have also been reported in subcortical structures such as the thalamus, hypothalamus and mammillary bodies (McDuff and Sumi, 1985).

The importance of the histological changes outlined above is that they interfere with nerve transmission at the cellular level, and consequently the changes in cognitive function observed in Alzheimer's disease can largely be related to the predominant brain areas affected by the histological alterations. For instance, the memory impairment seen in Alzheimer's disease is believed to be associated with the damage to the limbic system, especially the hippocampus. Although the causes of the morphological changes are unknown, in recent years it has been suggested that they may be the by-products of a malfunction in the cholinergic system (a neuronal network that transmits

nerve impulses through acetylcholine) (Whitehouse *et al.*, 1981; Gottfries *et al.*, 1983). Levels of enzymes such as choline acetyltransferase involved in the manufacture of acetylcholine have been found to be reduced by 80% in the cerebral cortex and hippocampus of patients with Alzheimer's disease (Davies, 1983). The distribution of this biochemical reduction closely parallels the topography of the histological alterations, the reduction in enzyme activity being most marked in those brain areas with the greatest concentration of senile plaques and neurofibrillary tangles.

It is possible that the cholinergic deficit in Alzheimer's disease is related to histological changes in the nucleus basalis of Meynert located beneath the globus pallidus in the basal forebrain (Coyle, Price and de Long, 1983). In the region of 70% of the cholinergic activity in the cerebral cortex appears to reside in axon terminals with cell bodies located in this nucleus making it the principal origin of cortical cholinergic innervation. In Alzheimer's disease, the extensive reduction of cholinergic neurones occurs within the nucleus basalis along with histological changes, suggesting that the lack of cortical cholinergic input and the development of senile plaques and neurofibrillary tangles are related. The cholinergic deficiency in Alzheimer's disease has led to the therapeutic use of acetylcholinesterase inhibitors, which enhance cholinergic neurotransmission by inhibiting acetylcholine breakdown.

In addition to the cholinergic hypothesis outlined above, other alternative causes of Alzheimer's disease proposed in the literature include aluminium intoxication (Crapper, Krishnan and Quittkart, 1976), disordered immune function (Behan and Behan, 1979; Mitler *et al.*, 1981), viral infection (de Boni and Crapper, 1978) and dysfunction of cellular microtubules (Heston *et al.*, 1981). As mentioned previously, a hereditary factor has also been suggested. Larrson, Sjörgren and Jacobson (1963) reported that first-order relatives of persons suffering from Alzheimer's disease have a four times greater chance of having the disease than individuals without such familial relationship. Further evidence for a genetic factor comes from the finding that individuals with Down syndrome develop the neuropathological changes typical of Alzheimer's disease if they survive to middle life (Reisberg, 1981). Like Down syndrome, therefore, Alzheimer's disease, at least in some forms, may be the consequence of chromosomal abnormality (Reisberg, 1981). An increased incidence of Down syndrome has been found in families of persons with Alzheimer's disease. Alternatively, the disease may represent an exaggeration of normal ageing, since the associated histological changes are also found in brains from normal, older individuals, but to a lesser extent.

Differential diagnosis and medical treatment of Alzheimer's disease

The differential diagnosis of Alzheimer's disease is problematic, with confirmation dependent on histological evidence at post-mortem. Currently, there are no specific diagnostic tests for Alzheimer's disease that can be applied to living patients, nor are there any specific biological markers of Alzheimer's disease. Magnetic resonance imaging (MRI) may be helpful in arriving at a tentative diagnosis by revealing the presence of generalized atrophy of the brain, enlargement of the ventricles and widening of the cortical sulci and atrophy of the hippocampi and amygdala. Further, the absence of motor deficits, especially in the early to middle stages, helps to differentiate Alzheimer's disease from many other forms of dementia (e.g. dementia associated with Parkinson's disease, vitamin B_{12} deficiency, tertiary neurosyphilis). However, at various stages, Alzheimer's disease may resemble other dementia syndromes without motor signs such as Korsakoff's syndrome, Pick's disease and HIV dementia complex. In the early stages, Alzheimer's disease may resemble depression or pure memory disorders such as the Korsakoff's amnestic syndrome. More advanced Alzheimer's disease needs to be distinguished from conditions such as Pick's disease, vascular dementia and Creutzfeldt–Jakob disease among others. As Alzheimer's disease progresses, symptoms typical of Parkinsonism (e.g. rigidity, bradykinesia, short, slow shuffling steps) become evident, making clinical differentiation from dementia with Lewy bodies and other Parkinsonian diseases more difficult.

Currently, there is no treatment available that has been unequivocally shown to reverse existing deficits associated with Alzheimer's disease or to arrest disease progression. Pharmacological treatment of Alzheimer's disease is, therefore, only symptomatic. Because cholinergic neuronal pathways degenerate and choline acetyltransferase is depleted in the brains of individuals with Alzheimer's disease, cholinergic replacement therapy has been used in an effort at the symptomatic treatment of cognitive dysfunction. Acetylcholinesterase inhibitors such as donepezil, rivastigmine, galantamine and tacrine among others have been shown to mildly reduce the decline in cognitive function based on performance on standardized tests of cognitive function. However, once these medications are stopped, individuals often show a precipitous decline to severity levels that would have been reached without the medication. Other experimental treatments under investigation include vaccines directed against β-amyloid and the metal chelator, clioquinol. Behavioural disturbances (e.g. insomnia, agitation, hallucinations, delusions) associated with Alzheimer's disease may require treatment with antipsychotic drugs, antidepressants and anxiolytic drugs.

Dementia with Lewy bodies

Lewy bodies are spherical, eosinophilic staining, intracytoplasmic inclusion bodies that hallmark histopathological lesions of Parkinson's disease. In individuals with Parkinson's disease, these bodies occur within the neurones of the substantia nigra and other brainstem nuclei. Up to 25% of older demented patients who come to autopsy are identified as having Lewy bodies in the cerebral cortex and brainstem, making dementia with Lewy bodies the second-most-common form of dementia. A synaptic protein called α-synuclein is the major component of Lewy bodies found in both dementia with Lewy bodies and Parkinson's disease. These bodies also contain tau, a protein also known to be present in the neurones of individuals with Alzheimer's disease and Pick's disease.

Clinical manifestations of dementia with Lewy bodies include cognitive decline, behavioural change and motor dysfunction. In contrast to Alzheimer's disease, dementia with Lewy bodies is characterized clinically by cognitive decline without prominent early-memory impairment. Another distinctive feature is a fluctuating mental status which may be dramatic, ranging from relatively lucid to severe confusion. Episode duration and frequency vary greatly, lasting minutes, days or weeks. These patients also experience well-formed visual hallucinations and usually exhibit motor signs of Parkinson's disease (especially bradykinesia and rigidity) within 1–2 years of dementia.

Although memory loss in dementia with Lewy bodies is less severe than in Alzheimer's disease, these patients have a greater problem retrieving previously learnt information than encoding new information and consequently show a greater benefit with cueing than do patients with Alzheimer's disease. In Alzheimer's disease, encoding difficulty predominates and therefore patients do not benefit as much from practice or from cueing. Visuospatial and constructional skills tend to be impaired earlier in dementia with Lewy bodies than in Alzheimer's disease so that these patients may show geographical disorientation in familiar surroundings (e.g. their own home) while their memory is only mildly impaired. Executive function is also impaired significantly earlier in dementia with Lewy bodies than in Alzheimer's disease. Based on neuropsychological testing, patients with dementia with Lewy bodies are often more impaired than those with Alzheimer's disease on verbal fluency, psychomotor speed, executive function (problem solving, abstract reasoning, ability to complete tasks) and visuospatial/constructional ability but are similarly impaired on episode memory and language (Galasko *et al.*, 1998).

Cholinergic central nervous system deficits occur in dementia with Lewy bodies in the same way they do in Alzheimer's disease. Consequently, these patients may respond well to anticholinesterase drugs such as donepezil or tacrine. Indeed, some small clinical trials have produced some evidence to suggest that these drugs do have a favourable effect on cognitive outcome measures in dementia with Lewy bodies.

Pick's disease (frontal temporal dementia)

Pick's disease is a primary degenerative dementia that bears some clinical resemblance to Alzheimer's disease. The condition accounts for approximately 15–20% of all degenerative dementias. The aetiology is unknown and the condition is mostly regarded as an idiopathic degenerative process affecting the neuronal cell body. Typically, the age of onset is broad, ranging from 21 to 75 years, with onset most commonly occurring between the ages of 40 and 60 years (Haase, 1977). Death usually occurs within 2–15 years (Slaby and Wyatt, 1974). Men and women are equally affected. Pick's disease is characterized by a progressive intellectual deterioration marked by a diminished sense of responsibility and loss of social graces manifested by a disinhibited personality. In particular, at least in the early stages, these behavioural disturbances are more prominent than cognitive dysfunction. Importantly, memory is less impaired, especially in the early stages, than in Alzheimer's disease. The relative sparing of memory may be due to the fact that the hippocampal formation is less affected in Pick's patients than in persons with Alzheimer's disease. Language abnormalities and a wide variety of personality changes are among the earliest intellectual alterations to occur in Pick's disease (Wechsler *et al.*, 1982). The changes in personality may include irritability, depression, socially inappropriate activity, hypersexuality, loss of personal propriety and other behavioural disinhibitions. Abnormalities of motor and sensory systems are conspicuously absent during most of the course of the disease, but as it advances a Parkinsonian-type of extrapyramidal syndrome often develops and pyramidal system abnormalities may also appear. In the late stages of Pick's disease, intellectual deterioration may affect all areas of intellectual function and terminally these patients are mute and immobile with both urinary and faecal incontinence.

Pathologically, the brains of patients with Pick's disease are reduced in size. The atrophy, as evident on computerized tomographic (CT) and MRI scans and at autopsy, selectively involves either the frontal or temporal lobes, or both (Corsellis, 1976). In particular, the anterior and medial temporal areas and the orbitofrontal cortex show the most severe atrophic changes while the parietal lobe, the pre-central gyrus (primary motor cortex) and the posterior one-third of the superior temporal gyrus tend to be spared (Corsellis, 1976; Cummings and Duchen, 1981).

In most cases of Pick's disease, two characteristic histopathological features are evident in the neurones within the affected areas of the cerebral cortex. These features include intracytoplasmic Pick bodies and 'inflated' neurones. Pick bodies are dense intracellular structures about the same size as the nucleus which occur in the neuronal cytoplasm. These bodies are characteristic of Pick's disease in that they do not occur in normal ageing and are rare in diseases other than Pick's disease. Inflated neurones (also referred to as Pick cells) are enlarged nerve cells in which the nuclei are displaced to one side even though no body is evident in the cytoplasm to cause the displacement. Other histopathological changes including loss of neurones, astrocyte hyperplasia (gliosis) and microglial cell proliferation are also evident in the affected cortical areas of Pick's disease.

Neurone loss and astrocytic gliosis also occur to a variable extent in the basal ganglia, thalamus and subthalamic nucleus. Pick bodies, however, tend to be confined to the cerebral cortex and are not found in subcortical structures (Corsellis, 1976; Cummings and Duchen, 1981). There is no apparent selective involvement of one transmitter system in Pick's disease as occurs in the cholinergic system of Alzheimer patients.

A definitive differential diagnosis of Pick's disease is not possible during life and relies instead on identification of the histological features of the condition outlined above at post-mortem. These include the distinctively circumscribed pattern of lobular atrophy preferentially involving the frontal and anterior lobes, the presence of Pick inclusion bodies and Pick cells, the absence of amyloid plaques and neurofibrillary tangles characteristic of Alzheimer's disease. During

life, although not definitive, Pick's disease and Alzheimer's can sometimes be separated by the generally earlier onset in the case of Pick's disease and the more prominent behavioural than cognitive impairment at presentation. In addition, an MRI scan may help eliminate other potential mechanisms of frontal lobe pathology such as tumour or infection and can demonstrate the presence of atrophy predominantly involving the frontal and temporal lobes.

Currently, there is no effective treatment for Pick's disease. There appears to be no basis for the use of acetylcholinesterase inhibitors as used in Alzheimer's disease and, although sedatives may be administered to combat behavioural problems, in some cases (e.g. benzodiazepines) they may actually exacerbate undesirable behaviours such as agitation. Drugs such as atypical neuroleptics, mood stabilizers and atypical anxiolytics (e.g. trazodone, buspirone) may be of some help with reducing problematic behaviours.

Vascular dementia

Vascular dementia is the third-most-common form of dementia after Alzheimer's disease and dementia with Lewy bodies (Jorm and Jolley, 1998). The condition is defined clinically by sudden onset of cognitive decline, stepwise deterioration and focal neurological findings (Erkinjuntti and Rockwood, 2003). Although historically vascular dementia was termed multi-infarct dementia, more recently the concept of vascular dementia has been extended beyond the original concept of multi-infarct dementia as introduced by Hachinski, Lassen and Marshall (1974) to include all forms of cognitive loss due to cerebrovascular disease. Consequently, vascular dementia now encompasses a group of clinical syndromes related to different vascular mechanisms and changes in the brain, with different causes and clinical manifestations.

Vascular dementia is predominantly a disease of older people. According to Herbert and Brayne (1995), the prevalence of vascular dementia ranges from 1–2 to 4.2% of persons aged 65 years and older with the incidence increasing with increasing age. Men and women are affected equally. The condition results from ischaemic, hypoperfusive or haemorrhagic brain lesions that are associated with numerous clinical syndromes. The major subcategories of ischaemic vascular dementia include large-vessel vascular dementia and subcortical ischaemic vascular dementia. Large-vessel vascular dementia includes multi-infarct vascular dementia and strategic single-infarct dementia. The former is associated with multiple large complete infarcts occurring secondary to diseases of the extracranial arteries that can involve both cortical and subcortical structures, usually with perifocal incomplete infarction involving the cerebral white matter. Strategic single-infarct dementia, in contrast, involves a single infarct in functionally critical areas of the brain, such as the angular gyrus, thalamus, territory of the anterior cerebral artery and others.

Subcortical ischaemic vascular dementia involves small-vessel disease as the chief vascular aetiology in which lacunar infarction and ischaemic white matter lesions, particularly involving the periventricular white matter and frontal region, are the primary types of brain lesions and the primary location of lesions is subcortical. Two clinical syndromes related to subcortical ischaemic vascular dementia are lacunar state and subcortical arteriosclerotic encephalopathy (Binswanger's disease). The clinical manifestations of subcortical ischaemic vascular dementia result from interruption of parallel circuits from the pre-frontal cortex to the basal ganglia and corresponding thalamocortical connections by ischaemic lesions.

Although hypertension is the most common aetiological factor, vascular dementia may be caused by a large number of different disease entities (e.g. atherosclerosis, diabetes, Binswanger's disease, cardiac disease, etc.). Features identified by Hachinski *et al.* (1975) which serve to differentiate vascular dementia from other dementias include: abrupt onset, stepwise deterioration in intellectual function, fluctuating course, nocturnal confusion, relative preservation of personality, depression, somatic complaints, emotional lability, a history of hypertension, a history of strokes, evidence of associated atherosclerosis and focal neurological signs and symptoms. If a number of these features are present, then vascular

dementia should be suspected. However, a diagnosis of vascular dementia can rarely be reached in the absence of vascular lesions (e.g. territorial infarctions, lacunas and white matter changes) as demonstrated by neuroimaging.

Most of the patients also exhibit pseudobulbar-like bilateral abnormalities including rigidity, spasticity, hyper-reflexia, gait abnormalities and dysarthria. Because the exact nature of the cognitive and language deficits depends on the site, location and extent of the cerebral infarctions, speech-language deficits in the form of an aphasia, apraxia of speech and/or dysarthria may form components of the overall symptom complex in vascular dementia. Although overt aphasia is an uncommon clinical sign of vascular dementia, individual cases may exhibit a range of aphasic deficits, including word-finding difficulties, word fluency deficits and high-level language dysfunction (Murdoch and Lethlean, 1996). These latter deficits may include problems with verbal explanation, verbal reasoning, reconstruction of sentences, the formation of inferences and the interpretation of absurdities, ambiguities and metaphors (Murdoch and Lethlean, 1996).

Currently, there is no approved symptomatic pharmacological treatment for vascular dementia despite numerous compounds having been purported to be useful in the symptomatic treatment of vascular dementia, including antithrombotics, ergot alkaloids, nootropics, thyrotropin-releasing hormone analogue, ginkgo biloba extracts, plasma viscosity drugs, hyperbaric oxygen, antioxidants and serotonin, among others. Other drugs that have been the subject of controlled clinical trials include central acetylcholinesterase inhibitors such as donepezil and galanthamine.

Dementia in extrapyramidal syndromes

Extrapyramidal syndromes are disorders in which the major pathological changes occur in the basal ganglia, thalamus and upper brainstem while the cerebral cortex is relatively spared. The principal extrapyramidal syndromes in which dementia may be present include Parkinson's disease, Huntington's disease, progressive supranuclear palsy, Wilson's disease and idiopathic basal ganglia calcification. The characteristics and neuropathology of each of these disorders is described in Chapters 10 and 11 in relation to hypokinetic, hyperkinetic and mixed dysarthrias.

The dementia syndromes associated with the various extrapyramidal disorders have similar characteristics and are collectively referred to as 'subcortical dementia'. The features of subcortical dementia include: mental slowness, inertia and lack of initiative, memory impairment that profits from structure and cues, slowness of cognitive processing and disturbances of mood (including depression).

Subcortical dementias differ from cortical dementias in two important ways. First, subcortical dementias in general lack the language disturbance (at least in the early stages), agnosia, apraxia and alexia that are characteristic of the cortical dementia syndromes such as seen in Alzheimer's and Pick's disease. Second, the subcortical dementias are different in that each of the extrapyramidal syndromes is associated with a prominent movement disorder (e.g. bradykinesia, tremor, rigidity, chorea, myoclonus, dystonia, etc.) as part of their clinical symptomatology. Consequently, the majority of patients with extrapyramidal disorders exhibit a dysarthria (see Chapters 10 and 11).

Dementia has been reported to affect approximately 10–15% of individuals with Parkinson's disease, the prevalence increasing with age (Velakoulis and Lloyd, 2000). Typically, the classic motor symptoms such as tremor, hypokinesia and rigidity associated with Parkinson's disease precede the development of cognitive and language impairments (see Chapter 3). It has been suggested that symptoms such as depression, anxiety, loss of self-esteem, suicidal thoughts, delusions, visual hallucinations, delirium, fatigue and sleep disturbances may be related to treatment with dopaminergic drugs (e.g. levodopa) (Liberman, 1998).

Huntington's disease, an autosomal dominant heredo-degenerative condition is also characterized by a movement disorder, psychiatric symptoms and dementia. The signs of dementia usually become apparent after chorea and psychiatric symptoms have been present for some years. A memory disorder affecting all aspects of memory is usually an early and prominent feature. Language, however, is usually relatively intact until the later stages of the disorder (see Chapter 3). According to Chua and Chiu (2000), personality alterations, mood disorders (e.g. depression), psychosis, aggressive behaviour, apathy, irritability, emotional lability, impulsivity, disinhibition and suicide are common in Huntington's disease. (The clinical features and neuropathological bases of both Parkinson's disease and Huntington's disease are discussed more fully in Chapters 3 and 10.)

Korsakoff's syndrome

Korsakoff's syndrome (formerly known as 'Korsakoff's psychosis') has been defined as an isolated loss of recent memory in a fully awake, alert and cooperative patient who has normal immediate recall, remote memory and manipulation of old knowledge (Ross, 1980). The condition may be encountered in a variety of disorders (e.g. closed head injury, vascular infarction of the left or both medial temporal lobe(s), herpes simplex encephalitis, anoxia, tuberculous meningitis, etc.) and may be either permanent or transient (Ross, 1980). Traditionally, however, it is linked to alcoholism and Wernicke's encephalopathy.

Wernicke's encephalopathy and Korsakoff's syndrome represent two clinical aspects of the same pathological process that occurs in response to chronic alcohol abuse. Wernicke's encephalopathy represents the acute stage of this process and Korsakoff's syndrome the chronic residual mental deficit that usually occurs in the latter stages of Wernicke's encephalopathy. Excessive alcohol intake over a long period causes changes in the stomach that interfere with the absorption of vitamins, especially thiamine (vitamin B_1). The resultant deficiency of vitamin B_1 causes damage to several regions of the brain including the brainstem, thalamus, mammillary bodies (which receive strong hippocampal input), hypothalamus and the frontal and associative areas of the neocortex. These morphological changes are associated with a triad of symptoms which characterize Wernicke's encephalopathy. These include mental changes, paralysis of eye movements and an ataxic gait.

The most striking mental change in Korsakoff's syndrome is an amnesia for recent events (recent-memory disturbance) coupled with an inability to acquire new memories. Long-term memory is also frequently affected, although to a lesser extent. Although lesions of the mammillary bodies were long believed to be the anatomic basis of the distinctive memory deficit, the results of more recent clinicopathological studies have suggested that lesions of the medial thalamus, especially those involving the dorsomedial nucleus and the medial pulvinar (see Chapter 3) correlate best with the amnestic symptoms (Haller, 1980). With thiamine supplementation and a balanced diet, patients with Wernicke–Korsakoff syndrome may become more alert but the memory problems persist.

It should be noted that in addition to Wernicke–Korsakoff syndrome, there is now evidence to suggest that an alcoholic dementia also exists. In contrast to Wernicke–Korsakoff syndrome, in which difficulties in learning new information represent the predominant mental disability (Cutting, 1978), alcoholic dementia is characterized by neuropsychological deficits which include poor memory, poor abstraction, impaired planning and poor constructions (Ron, 1977; Lishman, 1981).

Korsakoff's syndrome can be prevented or its severity reduced by the prompt administration of thiamine to patients with Wernicke's encephalopathy. Patients with established Korsakoff's syndrome should also receive thiamine to prevent the progression of deficits, although existing deficits are unlikely to be reversed.

Language disorders in cortical dementias

Language disorders in Alzheimer's disease

A language deficit is a significant component of the symptomatology of Alzheimer's disease (Bayles and Kaszniak, 1987), with the most obvious manifestation of such a deficit being a conver-sational word-finding problem. While the grammatical structure is mostly retained, the speech of individuals with Alzheimer's disease tends to be vague, repetitive and circumlocutory. The ability to formulate complex syntactic structures appears to be almost unaffected; however, the speech of persons with Alzheimer's disease has a paucity of meaningful content words, instead consisting mostly of empty, meaningless words (e.g. thing, stuff), pronouns without antecedents (e.g. it) and vague circumlocutions (e.g. 'Oh that's that one that you put on there when you have to go') (Hier, Hagenlocker and Shindler, 1985; Nicholas *et al.*, 1985; Kempler, Curtiss and Jackson, 1987).

Although the recognized diagnostic criteria do not specify that the presence of a language impairment is mandatory in order to make a diagnosis of Alzheimer's disease, the results of a number of studies utilizing sensitive indicators of language functioning such as detailed aphasia batteries or conversational analysis have indicated that a language deficit, in a more or less severe form, is present at all stages of the disorder (Appell, Kertesz and Fisman, 1982; Bayles 1982; Cummings *et al.*, 1985; Murdoch *et al.*, 1987; Bayles, Tomoeda and Trosset, 1992; Bayles, Tomoeda and Trosset, 1993). In fact, a language disorder was noted by Alzheimer in 1907 (Alzheimer, 1969) as part of the clinical findings in the first description of Alzheimer's disease. Based on their performance on the Western Aphasia Battery (Kertesz, 1980), Appell, Kertesz and Fisman (1982) found all 25 subjects in their sample of Alzheimer patients to be aphasic. Both Cummings *et al.* (1985) and Murdoch *et al.* (1987) concluded that the presence of a language impairment is an important diagnostic criterion of Alzheimer's disease.

Patterns of language decline in Alzheimer's disease

Patients with Alzheimer's disease exhibit a progressive decline in communicative ability with different language abilities being affected at different stages of the disorder. Early reports such as that by Bayles (1982) suggested that the semantic and pragmatic systems are the most vulnerable throughout the course of the disease while phonological and syntactic aspects of language are relatively preserved until the later stages of the disease. A number of authors have suggested that the patterns of language impairment evidenced at certain stages correspond to specific aphasia syndromes. During the early stages of dementia, speech output is fluent, well articulated and syntactically preserved and auditory comprehension abilities for conversational material and reading aloud are intact. Hier, Hagenlocker and Shindler (1985) reported that the language deficit exhibited by early-stage Alzheimer patients shows considerable similarity to anomic or semantic aphasia with respect to mean length of utterance, number of subordinate clauses, anomic index, empty word and conciseness index on a picture description task. A number of other authors have also reported anomic aphasia as a prominent feature of early-stage Alzheimer's disease (Constantinidis, Richards and de Ajuriaguerra, 1978; Kertesz, 1979; Sandson, Obler and Albert, 1987). In order to attain the correct name of an object on a naming task, early-stage Alzheimer patients may circumlocute in a similar manner to healthy older persons. However, they require more time on average than normal older people to retrieve the target word and are less able to utilize phonemic cues to facilitate retrieval (Obler and Albert, 1981). Although verbal paraphasias may be present in the spontaneous speech of Alzheimer patients, in the early stage of the disorder these, where they occur, tend to be self-corrected.

During the mid-stage of Alzheimer's disease, language becomes increasingly paraphasic. Moderately affected Alzheimer patients demonstrate an increasing number of uncorrected verbal and literal paraphasic errors in discourse and in their responses to naming tasks. Neologisms also become more frequent and auditory comprehension ranges from mild to moderately impaired. Overall, the language abilities in the midstage resembles either a transcortical sensory aphasia (in the absence of a repetition deficit) or a Wernicke's aphasia (in the presence of a repetition deficit). Murdoch *et al.* (1987) found that the language of patients with moderate to moderately severe dementia of the Alzheimer type resembled that of transcortical sensory aphasia. Cummings *et al.* (1985) also reported that the language disorder in

Alzheimer's disease throughout most of its course resembles a transcortical sensory aphasia. However, these latter authors reported that as the disease progresses repetition abilities deteriorate and the language disorder then resembles a Wernicke's aphasia.

In the late stage of Alzheimer's disease, breakdown in pragmatic function is the primary alteration in language abilities. Sandson, Obler and Albert (1987) described late-stage Alzheimer patients as non-fluent, echolalic, palilalic and perseverative. At the terminal, or end, stage, the patient may be mute or restricted to echolalia or palilalia, and auditory comprehension for spoken language is severely impaired. The severe language impairments at this time is reminiscent of global aphasia.

Components of language affected by Alzheimer's disease

Patients with Alzheimer's disease do not show an equal degree of impairment across the different types of linguistic knowledge but rather show greater impairment on those components of language more highly dependent on cognition. Language tasks that are performed with minimal demands upon attentional and memory processes (e.g. oral reading, repetition, automatic speech) are less vulnerable to the effects of a dementing illness such as Alzheimer's disease than are tasks (e.g. story retelling, discourse production, sentence comprehension) that are heavily dependent for their successful performance on higher-order cognitive processing. The semantic and pragmatic language systems appear to be more impaired in dementia than do syntactic and phonological systems (Irigaray, 1973; de Ajuriaguerra and Tissot, 1975; Whitaker, 1976; Schwartz, Marin and Saffran, 1979; Bayles and Boone, 1982; Murdoch *et al.*, 1987) possibly as a consequence of their greater reliance on conscious processing (Bayles, 1985).

Pragmatic language abilities in Alzheimer's disease. The term 'pragmatic language abilities' refers to an individual's ability to use language effectively and represents a speaker's ability to judge contextual effects, perceive and express emotions and use conversational conventions. Pragmatics appears to be the area of linguistic knowledge most dependent upon cognition, which may explain why pragmatic deficits are more apparent than phonologic or syntactic difficulties in persons with Alzheimer's disease (Bayles, Tomoeda and Caffrey, 1982). Although pragmatics is a difficult aspect of language to quantify, a number of researchers have investigated language functions thought to have a pragmatic focus, such as testing the ability of Alzheimer patients to describe, their ability to provide a narrative and their ability to relate context and meaning. Hier, Hagenlocker and Shindler (1985) suggested that the most obvious linguistic deficit in Alzheimer patients is their failure to use language to convey information. Irigaray (1967) and Obler and Albert (1981) reported that patients with Alzheimer's disease exhibit a difficulty with sentence construction and narrative (description) tasks. Such difficulty is manifested by a paucity of commands, questions, indirect requests, second-person pronouns and terms inferring speaker awareness of the truth value of a statement (e.g. perhaps). These findings reflect a breakdown in the use of language as a tool for communication, information conveyance, direction of action and generation of concepts and propositions (Appell, Kertesz and Fisman, 1982).

As a test of their functional communicative abilities, Murdoch *et al.* (1988) compared the performance of a group of Alzheimer subjects on the Communicative Abilities in Daily Living (CADL) (Holland, 1980) with that of an appropriately constituted control group. They found that the Alzheimer patients were impaired in all areas of functional communication compared to the control group except humour/metaphor/absurdity with the poorest performance being observed in those categories of the CADL more highly dependent on cognition.

Syntactic language abilities in Alzheimer's disease.
On the basis of a large-scale study, Irigaray (1973) concluded that phonological and syntactic linguistic codes are comparatively preserved in Alzheimer's disease compared with lexical semantic abilities. Although his observation has been supported by many researchers (including Whitaker, 1976; Schwartz, Marin and Saffran, 1979; Appell, Kertesz and Fisman, 1982), it is now evident that Irigaray's findings may not

represent the true extent of the alterations in syntactic abilities that occur in dementia. De Ajuriaguerra and Tissot (1975) concluded that the intellectual regression which occurs in dementia has implications for language, extending beyond the lexical semantic domain. Schwartz, Marin and Saffran (1979) further suggested that it is not uncommon to find reports of syntactic disturbances in the late stages of deteriorating dementia. To the extent that syntax maps logical relations which are beyond the limited competence of the dementia patient, syntactic ability will also be affected.

Similarly, Constantinidis, Richards and de Ajuriaguerra (1978) reported that close examination reveals, in many instances, that syntax does not escape the general disorganization of language production present in Alzheimer patients. Breakdown may occur in the use of phrase markers and grammatical agreement, and sentences and phrases are often left unfinished (aposiopesis). Critchley (1984) noted that aposiopesis is a conversation trait manifested by the memory deficits of the aged and, hence, is not unique to patients with Alzheimer' disease. In agreement, Hier, Hagenlocker and Shindler (1985) found no significant difference between the number of sentence fragments provided by persons with Alzheimer's disease and matched control subjects. Furthermore, Obler and Albert (1981) reported that the ability of patients to repeat long and short syntactic sequences depended upon the frequency of occurrence of the semantic (lexical) components included in those sequences.

A more recent study by Tomoeda, Bayles and Boone (1990) confirmed that patients with probable Alzheimer's disease have more difficulty with increasing syntactic complexity than do age-matched controls. Rochon, Waters and Caplan (1994) investigated sentence comprehension in 23 early-stage patients with probable Alzheimer's disease. Although they were able to achieve equivalent scores to control subjects on sentences of complex syntax, the patients with probable Alzheimer's disease had greater difficulty comprehending sentences with two semantic propositions. Overall, therefore, it would appear that there is some evidence for some dissolution in complex levels of syntactic functioning in Alzheimer's disease even though syntactic skills remain relatively spared compared to the semantic component of language.

Semantic language abilities in Alzheimer's disease. Performance on various naming tasks is frequently used to determine the status of a patient's semantic language abilities. Although naming impairment is one of the most commonly reported language deficits associated with Alzheimer's disease (Bayles, 1982; Bayles and Boone, 1982; Bayles and Tomoeda, 1983; Blackburn and Tyrer, 1985; Chui *et al.*, 1985; Hier, Hagenlocker and Shindler, 1985; Bayles, Tomoeda and Trosset, 1993; Chenery and Murdoch, 1994; Chenery, Murdoch and Ingram, 1994), the cause of the naming deficit is still disputed. Some investigators hypothesize that misnaming in Alzheimer's disease results from a misperception of the stimuli, while others attribute failure to linguistic factors such as the erosion of referential boundaries of semantic classes (Schwartz, Marin and Saffran, 1979; Bayles and Tomoeda, 1983). Bayles, Tomoeda and Caffrey (1982) and de Ajuriaguerra and Tissot (1975) suggested that word-finding difficulties and a decrease in functional vocabulary are responsible for the poor performance of Alzheimer patients on naming tasks.

The finding that naming is facilitated in Alzheimer patients when the function of an object is demonstrated led to the hypothesis that dementia patients are perceptually impaired (Lawson and Barker, 1968). In agreement with this hypothesis, it was found by Rochford (1971) that the types of naming error produced by demented patients are consistent with an impairment of visual recognition and relatively unimpaired verbal ability. The naming performance of the demented patients was described by Rochford as verbally fluent but perceptually off course.

Several studies, however, have failed to support the suggestion that visuoperceptual problems may be responsible for the naming difficulty exhibited (Schwartz, Marin and Saffran, 1979; Bayles, 1982; Martin and Fedio, 1983; Kirshner, Webb and Kelly, 1984; Smith, Murdoch and Chenery, 1989). Bayles and Tomoeda (1983) found that, when misnaming occurred, it was most likely to be semantically associated to the target (e.g. 'truck' for 'bus'), many of the error responses provided by Alzheimer patients being both semantically and visually similar to the stimulus (e.g. a watch is semantically and visually similar to a clock). These authors suggested that the proportion of error responses related only visually to the target was smaller than would be expected if perceptual impairment caused misnaming, as Rochford (1971) and Lawson and Barker (1968) suggested.

Smith, Murdoch and Chenery (1989) investigated the lexical semantic abilities of a group of Alzheimer subjects using both visual and tactile naming tasks. The results of their study support a semantic network disruption rather than a visuoperceptual deficit as the basis of the naming disturbance observed in Alzheimer patients. Based on the pattern of error responses provided in the naming tasks, they concluded that patients with Alzheimer's disease are able to identify the semantic class to which the target in the naming task belongs, but cannot provide the lexeme corresponding to the correct individual class member.

The ability of Alzheimer patients to demonstrate, through gesture, the recognition of objects they cannot name is further evidence against the interpretation of a perceptual impairment as the basis of the naming impairment (Schwartz, Marin and Saffran, 1979). Further, the observation that naming errors become more semantically unrelated as the dementia worsens does not support Rochford's interpretation. Rather, it seems reasonable to predict that, if the visual signal was degraded, as would occur in a perceptual disorder, the naming errors would be more random and only related semantically to the stimulus by chance.

Martin *et al.* (1985) believe that patients with Alzheimer's disease display either a loss of or an inability to utilize those attributes which serve to distinguish semantically related words. Similarly, Grober *et al.* (1985) suggested that the saliency of essential attributes might be reduced in Alzheimer's disease so that the more important, referent-defining attributes are considered by these patients to be no more important than other less essential attributes. The reduced importance given to the essential attributes in turn changes the organization of semantic information from a set of ordered attributes (ordered with respect to the importance of the concept) to a set of more equally weighted attributes, such that the patient may not appreciate the relative importance of the attribute in delineating meaning or for lexical mapping. Such a change in the semantic organization can consequently affect the encoding of new information into both the semantic memory and episodic memory (Grober *et al.*, 1985). Further, any cognitive process into which the disorganized knowledge enters could be profoundly affected. Hence, the naming difficulties exhibited by individuals with Alzheimer's disease may represent semantic deficits causing memory defects rather than the reverse condition.

The loss of semantic information in Alzheimer's disease may represent an extreme case where the weight assigned to specific attributes has become so reduced that they are at a level below that needed for correct identification. Disorganization of the patient's semantic knowledge may result in deficits of lexical access (Bayles and Tomoeda, 1983; Martin and Fedio, 1983; Martin *et al.*, 1985). Such difficulties may be manifested as circumlocutions, semantic paraphasias or the use of indefinite anaphoric reference (the use of empty words, use of vague superordinate or generic words as replacements for words identifying specific meanings or entities) (de Ajuriaguerra and Tissot, 1975; Obler and Albert, 1981). Jargon, extremely laconic speech or mutism may also present as manifestations of more profound lexical disturbances (Obler and Albert, 1981).

Schwartz, Marin and Saffran (1979) suggested that, as a result of semantic reorganization in dementia, names no longer specify a unique referent (or class of referents) but rather a population of referents representing a more global extension of the word's application. Similarly, Martin and Fedio (1983) found that patients with Alzheimer's disease often substitute either a more general, high-order (superordinate category) name or the name of an object from the same semantic category. That is, Alzheimer patients tend to produce semantic field errors involving either a hierarchical relationship or a linear, within category, relationship.

Schwartz, Marin and Saffran (1979) suggested that the lexical loss in Alzheimer's disease is characterized by a systematic and progressive loss of semantic attributes that define referents – the more specific distinguishing attributes being lost before the more general ones. Warrington (1975) provided similar reasoning. Bayles and Tomoeda (1983) concluded that the referential boundaries of items in the mental lexicon appear to erode concurrently with the demise in the patient's ability to abstract and generalize. These latter authors further noted that the more abstract sets of semantic features and intellect appear to deteriorate concurrently and they argued that linguistic impairment, rather than perceptual impairment, better explains the majority of naming errors produced by demented patients.

Theories of semantic impairment in Alzheimer's disease

As outlined above, a deficit in the cognitive processing of word meanings, termed a 'semantic memory deficit', is a hallmark feature of the disease process in Alzheimer's disease. Indeed, the significance of the naming deficits is such that Hodges and Patterson (1995) have termed these difficulties 'semantic dementia', in which there is a progressive yet selective loss of semantic memory with relative preservation of other linguistic (phonological and syntactic) and non-verbal cognitive abilities (e.g. complex perceptual and visuospatial skills). While a large corpus of research has provided unequivocal evidence for the existence of such a deficit, there is continuing disagreement as to its precise nature. At issue is the question of whether the semantic deficit seen in Alzheimer's disease reflects specific disruption of the structural components of the semantic memory system (Martin, 1992a,b; Salmon and Chan, 1994). Alternatively, semantic memory impairments may be more closely linked to deficits in other cognitive domains which mediate the access and retrieval of information contained in an otherwise intact semantic network (Nebes, 1992; McGlinchey-Berroth and Milberg, 1993). Consequently, a large body of literature has grown around the investigation of language and communication difficulties that arise from the unavailability of semantic information in Alzheimer's disease, with the major focus of this work directed at determining the processes underlying the unavailability of this information. Two major hypotheses have been proposed to account for the semantic memory deficits that occur in Alzheimer's disease, namely the degraded stores hypothesis and the impaired access hypothesis (Glosser and Friedman, 1991; Salmon and Chan, 1994).

Degraded stores hypothesis. The 'degraded stores' hypothesis suggests a breakdown in the organization and structure of semantic knowledge in Alzheimer's disease. According to this view, the representation of semantic knowledge is lost as a consequence of neuronal death in specific regions of the temporal and parietal lobes (Harasty *et al.*, 1999). Degradation of semantic knowledge results in concepts becoming less clearly defined as their characteristic attributes are eliminated. In addition, formerly strong associations between related concepts are weakened as they become less specified.

The majority of evidence in support of degraded semantic representations in Alzheimer's disease has come from studies that have employed off-line measures of semantic memory, such as verbal fluency, picture naming and tasks which assess knowledge of concept meanings. For example, some studies have used these tasks to compare the performances of patients with Alzheimer's disease to the performances of patients with other dementing illnesses, such as Huntington's disease. Butters *et al.* (1987) administered category- and letter-fluency tasks to both patients with Alzheimer's disease and patients with Huntington's disease who were matched in terms of dementia severity. The patients with Huntington's disease were equally impaired on both category- and letter-fluency tasks, whereas patients with Alzheimer's disease demonstrated impaired performance only on the category-fluency task. These results were interpreted as evidence for a specific impairment to the structure of the semantic network in Alzheimer's disease.

Studies of picture naming have also provided evidence for structural degradation of the semantic network in Alzheimer's disease. For example, some authors have demonstrated a predominance of semantic errors in tests of picture naming, early in the course of dementia (LaBarge *et al.*, 1992; Chenery, Murdoch and Ingram, 1996). As the disease progresses, semantic errors appear to give way to less related errors, suggesting a gradual loss of semantic information in Alzheimer's disease. In addition, many studies of semantic attribute knowledge in Alzheimer's disease have demonstrated good knowledge of superordinate category information, with impairment in the knowledge of more specific, defining semantic features (Warrington, 1975; Martin and Fedio, 1983). The results of these studies have been taken as evidence for a bottom-up deterioration of semantic knowledge in Alzheimer's disease with lower-order attributes lost first, while superordinate knowledge is retained into the later stages of the disease.

Impaired access hypothesis. In contrast to the degraded stores hypothesis, the 'impaired access' hypothesis proposes that patients with Alzheimer's disease have difficulty accessing and retrieving information from an otherwise intact semantic network. According to this theory, patients with Alzheimer's disease retain normal semantic structure with fully specified semantic representations, but are unable to efficiently access this information when required. A number of authors have suggested that impairments in other cognitive domains, such as working memory and attention, subserve the semantic retrieval deficits observed in patients with Alzheimer's disease (Spinnler, 1991; Gainotti, 1993). Presumably then, normal semantic knowledge should be exhibited when the operation of consciously controlled retrieval mechanisms is eliminated or reduced.

Evidence for the impaired access hypothesis has come from a number of studies that have reported intact semantic attribute knowledge in Alzheimer's disease. For example, patients with Alzheimer's disease have been shown to be unable to provide lengthy functional descriptions of given objects, but have demonstrated accurate attribute knowledge when asked to choose related items from an array (Grober *et al.*, 1985; Flicker *et al.*, 1987). In addition, the results of a reaction time, relatedness judgement task showed that patients with Alzheimer's disease were just as fast to recognize semantic relationships based on specific functional or physical attributes as those based on superordinate category membership (Nebes and Brady, 1990). The results of these studies have provided evidence to suggest that patients with Alzheimer's disease retain an intact semantic knowledge base, but have difficulty accessing this knowledge as a consequence of impairment to attention-mediated retrieval mechanisms.

Impaired access to degraded stores hypothesis. A third, more moderate, hypothesis has also been proposed to account for the semantic memory deficits observed in patients with Alzheimer's disease (Gainotti, 1993; McGlinchey-Berroth and Milberg, 1993). This third hypothesis combines the major features of the degraded stores and impaired access hypotheses, and suggests that semantic memory deficits are a result of both degraded or disorganized (Grober *et al.*, 1985) semantic representations and failed retrieval mechanisms. As Gainotti stated, 'because of the diffuse and bilateral distribution of cortical lesions, Alzheimer's disease can simultaneously disrupt both specific and general cognitive mechanisms' (p. 290). An account of semantic memory deficits in Alzheimer's disease that combines aspects of both major hypotheses may assist in providing some resolution for the equivocal results of previous studies of semantic memory in this population.

The majority of studies that have attempted to provide support for either the degraded stores or impaired access hypotheses have employed off-line tests of semantic memory. The major problem in interpreting the results of these studies rests with the fact that off-line tasks, such as verbal fluency and picture naming, often involve the operation of extralinguistic cognitive processes that may also be impaired in Alzheimer's disease. For example, the verbal-fluency task requires not only intact semantic memory representations but also unimpaired attention-based search and retrieval strategies, episodic memory monitoring to avoid repetition and an intact phonological lexicon (Ober, Shenaut and Reed, 1995). Likewise, the picture-naming task requires the use of non-semantic cognitive processes, including an intact visuoperceptual system and intact mapping procedures from structural visual description

to semantic representation and from semantic representation to the phonological lexicon (Funnell and Hodges, 1996). While off-line tasks have been useful in identifying and quantifying the semantic memory deficits that occur in Alzheimer's disease, they have been less useful in characterizing the precise nature of these deficits. For example, a deficit in verbal fluency may be primarily associated with failed retrieval mechanisms, rather than degraded concepts.

One experimental paradigm that has been employed extensively in differentiating semantic memory disorders due to disturbed structure from those due to impaired access and retrieval mechanisms is the semantic-priming task. The semantic-priming task may be manipulated methodologically, so that automatic access of semantic representations is assessed independently of controlled, strategic retrieval mechanisms. In addition, semantic priming may be brought about via controlled retrieval processes that are heavily dependent on the operation of other cognitive functions, including working memory and attention (Neely, 1991). The results of studies that have investigated semantic priming effects in Alzheimer's disease have been equivocal, with some studies demonstrating normal semantic priming, while others have reported either reduced or increased priming in Alzheimer's disease (Chenery, 1996). These equivocal findings have been linked to a failure to account for methodological factors in the semantic priming task (Ober and Shenaut, 1995). Reports that priming improves semantic performance in some patients with Alzheimer's disease suggests that, at least in these cases, the ability to recall concepts has not been completely abraded (Chenery, Ingram and Murdoch, 1990; Chenery, Murdoch and Ingram, 1994). Consensus has not yet been reached on whether the semantic difficulties are attributable to the loss of conceptual knowledge, the loss of access to such knowledge or both.

Language disorders in Pick's disease

A diagnosis of Pick's disease can only be made with certainty following the histological examination of the brain tissue at autopsy. Consequently, few reports have appeared in the literature which document the language abilities of patients with Pick's disease. Although in a number of ways Pick's disease and Alzheimer's disease are similar, it appears that the two conditions do differ in the pattern of their associated language impairment.

In some cases of Pick's disease, a language abnormality is the earliest disturbance in intellectual function to appear (Wechsler *et al.*, 1982). Certainly, a disturbance in language function appears early in the course of disease and is a prominent feature of the condition by mid-stage (Cummings and Benson, 1983). Speech, in the initial stage of Pick's disease has been described as slow and deliberate with verbal paraphasias (Holland *et al.*, 1985). By mid-stage, typical language disturbances include anomia, auditory agnosia, excessive use of verbal stereotypes, circumlocutions and echolalia (Cummings and Duchen, 1981; Cummings, 1982; Wechsler *et al.*, 1982; Holland *et al.*, 1985). Speech output at this time is non-fluent (Morris *et al.*, 1984; Holland *et al.*, 1985). As the condition progresses, impaired auditory comprehension abilities also become evident and in the terminal stage of the disorder many patients become completely mute (Cummings and Duchen, 1981).

Although the language disturbance observed in patients with Pick's disease is similar to that evidenced in Alzheimer patients in terms of their word-finding difficulties and naming impairments, the speech output of the two groups differs markedly in relation to fluency. Non-fluent speech is a feature of Pick's disease at a relatively early stage. In patients with Alzheimer's disease, however, it is not until the late stage of the disorder that speech becomes non-fluent. These similarities and differences in speech-language abilities are easily explained by reference to the neuroanatomical involvement in each condition. As described earlier, in Pick's disease the brain areas which show the greatest histological changes are the pre-frontal areas of the cortex and the superior temporal gyrus. Particularly in the early stages, there is relative sparing of the occipital and parietal region. Consequently, Pick patients exhibit impaired speech output in the form of non-fluent speech while their auditory comprehension abilities remain relatively intact until the

later stages. In contrast, the cortical areas most affected in early to mid-stage Alzheimer's disease include the temporal and parietal temporal association areas. Damage in the frontal areas tends to be less severe and temporal lobe involvement is usually greater than parietal (Kemper, 1984). Therefore, the neuropathological changes that occur in Alzheimer's disease in particular involve the posterior language area and posterior borderzone region. The transcortical sensory-like and/or Wernicke's-like aphasia observed in Alzheimer patients by a number of authors (Cummings *et al.*, 1985; Murdoch *et al.*, 1987), therefore, could be expected. Loss of fluent speech in late-stage Alzheimer's disease corresponds to further involvement of the frontal lobe at that time. At the terminal stage of the disorder, extensive atrophy to all cortical association areas parallels the cortical damage found in global aphasia (i.e. a large perisylvian lesion involving the frontal, temporal and parietal lobes).

Relationship between the language of dementia and aphasia

The use of the term 'aphasia' to describe the language deficit occurring in dementia has been questioned by a number of authors (Critchley, 1964; Bayles, 1984). To these authors, aphasia implies the presence of a language deficit in association with a focal brain lesion, the loss in ability to interpret and formulate language being disproportionate to impairment in other cognitive functions. Darley (1982) suggested that the term be applied only in those cases where the aetiology is known and where the patient has a focal and not a diffuse lesion. Further, Bayles, Tomoeda and Caffrey (1982) believed the term should be used for conditions with an abrupt onset and for non-progressive diseases. Clearly, these criteria would be inconsistent with the use of the term 'aphasia' to describe the language disorder in dementia. It is interesting to ask, however, that if the term were applied with rigid adherence to these criteria, how then would one refer to the language disability manifested, for example, by head injury patients with multiple contusions or by patients with neural abscess or progressive cerebral tumours that have spread to involve the patient's language area?

Although not universally accepted, most definitions of aphasia suggest that language impairment can exist in the absence of other cognitive dysfunction. Kitselman (1981) suggested that the primary difference between language impairment in aphasia and dementia is the degree to which the language impairment occurs in isolation. For most people then, language disturbance in dementia cannot be defined as aphasia because in dementia the language disturbance is embedded within a variety of other cognitive deficits, including memory impairment. In aphasia, however, the language disturbance is the primary problem.

Support for considering language disorders in dementia as aphasia syndromes comes from a number of sources. As noted by Joynt (1984), the first descriptions of Alzheimer's disease (1907) and Pick's disease (1892) emphasized the presence of a language disturbance as part of the clinical findings. Since these early reports, a number of other studies have also documented the occurrence of a language deficit in association with dementia (Irigaray, 1973; Obler and Albert, 1981; Appell, Kertesz and Fisman, 1982; Bayles, 1982, 1985; Shore, Overman and Wyatt, 1983; Cummings *et al.*, 1985; Murdoch *et al.*, 1987; Bayles, Tomoeda and Trosset, 1993; Chenery, Murdoch and Ingram, 1996). Nicolosi, Harryman and Krescheck (1983) defined aphasia as 'the inability to speak or to comprehend words arranged in phrases' (p. 11). Hence, they did not suggest any restriction of usage based on characteristics such as onset or lesion site. Based on their definition, it would be appropriate to refer to the language difficulties of demented patients observed in the above studies as aphasia. It is obvious, therefore, that much of the controversy regarding the relationship between language disturbance in aphasia and dementia is related to terminology.

Many authors have compared language deficits in dementia to aphasia syndromes. Based on the lack of a direct parallel between the degree of dementia and the extent of the language disturbance, Seltzer and Sherwin (1983) reported that the language dysfunction demonstrated by

their demented patients reflected a specific language disorder (aphasic disturbance) rather than a non-specific feature of general intellectual deterioration. During the early stages of dementia, it has been reported that the language deficit exhibited by patients with dementia of the Alzheimer type shows considerable similarity to anomic or semantic aphasia (Hier, Hagenlocker and Shindler, 1985). In the later stages of dementia, expressive language and comprehension abilities decline and there is a progressive increase in the emptiness of speech. On a picture description task, the number of prepositional phrases and conciseness of expression decrease while the anomia and number of empty words provided increase. Many researchers have likened these language abilities to Wernicke's aphasia based on the combined presence of comprehension deficit and incoherent but fluent output (Whitaker, 1976; Obler and Albert, 1981).

In contrast to these authors, Hier, Hagenlocker and Shindler (1985) and Whitaker (1976) suggested that, if demented patients' repetition abilities were considered in these comparisons, their language abilities would more closely parallel the characteristics of a transcortical (sensory or mixed) rather than Wernicke's aphasia. Therefore, the importance of considering all available data when attempting to categorize, label or compare patients is emphasized. It is suggested that many such comparisons based on minimal behavioural information complicate and distort the relationship between aphasia and dementia syndromes. Finally, in the terminal stage of dementia, researchers have reported a poverty of output, jargon and comprehension abilities reminiscent of global aphasia.

Schwartz, Marin and Saffran (1979) drew attention to the similarities between the overall language pattern exhibited by Alzheimer patients (preserved syntactic and phonologic capacities in the face of marked semantic loss) and transcortical aphasic patients' language abilities, especially those with the mixed sensorimotor type of transcortical aphasia. Similarly, Cummings *et al.* (1985) reported that Alzheimer patients had fluent paraphasic output and impaired auditory comprehension with relative preservation of the ability to repeat which are characteristics of the transcortical sensory aphasic. They noted that Alzheimer patients performed poorly when executing over-learnt speech sequences – which is also evident in many transcortical sensory aphasics – but, in contrast to transcortical sensory aphasics, showed less paraphasia and echolalia. Murdoch *et al.* (1987) also noted that although the language deficits observed in their subjects with Alzheimer's disease were indicative of transcortical aphasia they showed less neologistic paraphasias of echolalia than expected in transcortical aphasias. Cummings *et al.* (1985) also found that their subjects did not exhibit the completion phenomenon reported to feature in transcortical aphasia. Consequently, Cummings *et al.* (1985) concluded, in agreement with the above researchers, that the language abilities of Alzheimer patients in the later stages more closely resembles the characteristics of Wernicke's aphasia. Whitaker (1976) noted a similar relationship between these two syndromes. However, Schwartz, Marin and Saffran (1979) pointed out that the nature of the semantic loss in transcortical sensory aphasia has not been clearly defined and, therefore, they suggest that Alzheimer patients demonstrate a unique pattern of language alteration which is similar, but not identical, to transcortical sensory aphasia. That is, the comparison does not necessarily infer the similarity of underlying primary deficits, only of clinical manifestations.

The relationship of the language deficits of the early and late stages of Alzheimer's disease to specific aphasic syndromes, however, is not as neat as it may first appear. Early Alzheimer patients have been shown to use fewer total words and prepositional phrases than anomic aphasics do, being more comparable to Wernicke's aphasics in this respect (Hier, Hagenlocker and Shindler, 1985). Similarly, late Alzheimer patients have shown values for mean length of utterance, total words and subordinate clauses which are within the range of the anomic aphasic (Hier, Hagenlocker and Shindler, 1985).

The comparison is further complicated by the clinical observation of a significant increase in fluent aphasia (compared with Broca's non-fluent aphasia) in older adults. Obler *et al.* (1978) demonstrated that different aphasia types distribute differently across older adulthood. Broca's aphasia is more prevalent among patients in their early 50s (mean age 51 years), while Wernicke's aphasia is most prevalent in patients in their early 60s (mean age 63 years). Hence, the similarity between demented patients' language abilities and Wernicke's aphasia may be influenced by the normal ageing effects of these patients' language abilities independent of, or in addition to, the aphasia or dementia syndrome.

It is obvious, though, that much of the controversy regarding the relationship between the language disturbance of aphasia and dementia is related to terminology. Murdoch (1988) stated that, when it comes to the treatment of subjects with Alzheimer's disease, determining whether the language impairment in subjects with Alzheimer's disease is a result of deficits in other cognitive functions is more important than whether this language deficit is called aphasia. As the whole classification debate has resulted from the proposed relationship between cognition and language in dementia, it is, therefore, important that research efforts first try to understand exactly how, and to what degree, cognition and language are related in dementia in contrast to aphasia. Only once this relationship is understood can the debate as to whether the observed deficit represent aphasia be finalized.

Summary

Dementia primarily affects the adult and geriatric populations and is characterized by persistent impairment in intellectual function as an outcome of brain disease with concomitant impairments in three of the following: language, memory, visuospatial skills, emotion or personality and cognition. Given the increasing incidence of dementia, recent decades have seen a growth in research into the effect of various dementia syndromes on language. Most interest has been focused on language function in Alzheimer's disease with a lesser number of studies investigating language skills in Pick's disease, vascular dementia, dementia in extrapyramidal syndromes and Korsakoff's syndrome. In general, patients with cortical dementia (e.g. Alzheimer's disease) tend to show greater impairment on those components of language more highly dependent on cognition with the semantic and pragmatic language systems being the most vulnerable throughout the course of the disease. In contrast, the phonological and syntactic aspects of language are relatively preserved until the later stages of the disease. Although a deficit in the cognitive processing of word meanings, termed a 'semantic memory deficit', is the hallmark feature of Alzheimer's disease, the precise nature of the deficit is unknown. Two theories proposed to account for the semantic memory deficit in dementia include the 'degraded stores' hypothesis and the 'impaired access' hypothesis. Although some authors have utilized terminology derived from aphasia classifications to describe the language impairment observed in individuals with various forms of dementia, the use of such terminology has been questioned.

References

Alzheimer, A. (1969) Alzheimer's disease. *Archives of Neurology*, **21**, 109–110.

American Psychiatric Association (2000) *Diagnostic and Statistical Manual of Mental Disorders, Tex Revision (DSM-IV-TR)*, 4th edn, APA, Washington DC.

Appell, J., Kertesz, A. and Fisman, M. (1982) A study of language functioning in Alzheimer's patients. *Brain and Language*, **17**, 73–91.

Ballard, C. (2000) Criteria for the diagnosis of dementia, in *Dementia* (eds J. O'Brien, D. Ames and A. Burns), Arnold, London, pp. 29–40.

Bayles, K.A. (1982) Language function in senile dementia. *Brain and Language*, **16**, 265–280.

Bayles, K.A. (1984) Language and dementia, in *Language Disorders in Adults: Recent Advances* (ed. A.L. Holland), College Hill Press, San Diego, pp. 85–101.

Bayles, K.A. (1985) Communication in dementia, in *The Aging Brain: Communication in the Elderly* (ed. H.K. Ulatowska), Taylor & Francis, London, pp. 43–57.

Bayles, K.A. and Boone, D.R. (1982) The potential of language tasks for identifying senile dementia. *Journal of Speech and Hearing Disorders*, **47**, 210–217.

Bayles, K.A. and Kaszniak, A.W. (1987) *Communication and Cognition in Normal Aging and Dementia*, College Hill Press, Boston.

Bayles, K.A. and Tomoeda, C. (1983) Confrontation naming impairment in dementia. *Brain and Language*, **19**, 98–114.

Bayles, K.A., Tomoeda, C. and Caffrey, T. (1982) Language and dementia producing diseases. *Communicative Disorders*, 7, 131–146.

Bayles, K.A., Tomoeda, C.K. and Trosset, M.W. (1992) Relation of linguistic communication abilities of Alzheimer's patients to stage of disease. *Brain and Language*, **42**, 454–472.

Bayles, K.A., Tomoeda, C.K. and Trosset, M.W. (1993) Alzheimer's disease: effects on language. *Developmental Neuropsychology*, **9**, 131–160.

Behan, P.O. and Behan, W.M.H. (1979) *Possible Immunological Factors in Alzheimer's Disease: Early Recognition of Potentially Reversible Deficits*, Churchill Livingstone, London, pp. 104–118.

Berg, L. (1985) Does Alzheimer's disease represent an exaggeration of normal aging? *Archives of Neurology*, **42**, 737–739.

Blackburn, I.M. and Tyrer, G.M.B. (1985) The value of Luria's neuropsychological investigation for the assessment of cognitive dysfunction in Alzheimer-type dementia. *British Journal of Clinical Psychology*, **24**, 171–179.

Brookmeyer, R., Gray, S. and Kawas, C. (1998) Projections of Alzheimer's disease in the United States and the public health impact of delaying disease onset. *American Journal of Public Health*, **88**, 1337–1342.

Butters, N., Granholm, E., Salmon, D.P. *et al.* (1987) Episodic and semantic memory: a comparison of amnesic and demented patients. *Journal of Clinical and Experimental Neuropsychology*, **9**, 479–497.

Chenery, H.J. (1996) Semantic priming in Alzheimer's dementia. *Aphasiology*, **10**, 1–20.

Chenery, H.J., Ingram, J. and Murdoch, B.E. (1990) Automatic and volitional processing in aphasia. *Brain and Language*, **38**, 215–232.

Chenery, H.J. and Murdoch, B.E. (1994) The production of narrative discourse in response to animations in persons with dementia of the Alzheimer's type. *Aphasiology*, **8**, 159–171.

Chenery, H.J., Murdoch, B.E. and Ingram, J. (1994) An investigation of confrontation naming performance in Alzheimer's dementia as a function of disease severity. *International Journal of Neuroscience*, **74**, 140.

Chenery, H.J., Murdoch, B.E. and Ingram, J. (1996) An investigation of confrontation naming performance in Alzheimer's dementia as a function of disease severity. *Aphasiology*, **10**, 423–441.

Chua, P. and Chiu, E. (2000) Huntington's disease, in *Dementia* (eds J. O'Brien, D. Ames and A. Burns), Arnold, London, pp. 827–843.

Chui, H., Teng, E.L., Henderson, V.W. and May, A.C. (1985) Clinical subtypes of dementia of the Alzheimer's type. *Neurology*, **35**, 1544–1550.

Constantinidis, J., Richards, J. and de Ajuriaguerra, J. (1978) Dementias with senile plaques and neurofibrillary changes, in *Studies in Geriatric Psychiatry* (eds A.D. Isaacs and F. Post), John Wiley & Sons, Inc., Brisbane, pp. 55–69.

Corsellis, J.A.N. (1976) Ageing and the dementias, in *Greenfield's Neuropathology* (eds W. Blackwood and J.A.N. Corsellis), Year Book Publishers, Chicago, pp. 125–136.

Coyle, J.T., Price, D.L. and de Long, M.R. (1983) Alzheimer's disease: a disorder of cortical cholinergic innervation. *Science*, **219**, 1194–1219.

Crapper, D.R., Krishnan, S.S. and Quittkart, S. (1976) Aluminium neurofibrillary degeneration and Alzheimer's disease. *Brain*, **99**, 67–80.

Critchley, M. (1964) The neurology of psychotic speech. *British Journal of Psychiatry*, **110**, 353–364.

Critchley, M. (1984) And all the daughters of musick shall be brought low: language function in the elderly. *Archives of Neurology*, **41**, 1135–1139.

Cummings, J.L. (1982) Cortical dementias, in *Psychiatric Aspects of Neurologic Disease*, vol. **2** (eds D.F. Benson and D. Blumer), Grune & Stratton, New York, pp. 47–59.

Cummings, J.L. and Benson, D.F. (1983) *Dementia: a Clinical Approach*, Butterworths, Boston.

Cummings, J.L. and Duchen, L.W. (1981) The Klüver–Bucy syndrome in Pick's disease: Clinical and pathologic correlations. *Neurology*, **31**, 1415–1422.

Cummings, J.L., Benson, D.F. and LoVerme, S. (1980) Reversible dementia. *Journal of the American Medical Association*, **243**, 2434–2439.

Cummings, J.L., Benson, D.F., Hill, M.A. and Read, S. (1985) Aphasia in dementia of the Alzheimer's type. *Neurology*, **35**, 394–397.

Cutting, J. (1978) The relationship between Korsakoff's syndrome and alcoholic dementia. *British Journal of Psychiatry*, **132**, 240–251.

Darley, F.L. (1982) *Aphasia*, W.B. Saunders, Philadelphia.

Davies, P. (1983) An update on the neurochemistry of Alzheimer's disease, in *The Dementias* (eds R. Mayeux and W.G. Rosen), Raven Press, New York, pp. 151–170.

de Ajuriaguerra, J. and Tissot, R. (1975) Some aspects of language in various forms of senile dementia (comparisons with language in childhood), in *Foundations of Language Development* (eds E.H. Lenneberg and E. Lenneberg), Academic Press, New York, pp. 323–339.

de Boni, U. and Crapper, D.R. (1978) Paired helical filaments of the Alzheimer type in cultured neurons. *Nature*, **271**, 566–568.

Dowson, J.H. (1982) Neuronal lipofuscin accumulation in ageing and Alzheimer dementia: a pathogenic mechanism? *British Journal of Psychiatry*, **140**, 142–148.

Eastley, R. and Wilcock, G. (2000) Assessment and differential diagnosis of dementia, in *Dementia* (eds J. O'Brien, D. Ames and A. Burns), Arnold, London, pp. 41–47.

Erkinjuntti, T. and Rockwood, K. (2003) Vascular dementia. *Seminars in Clinical Neuropsychiatry*, **8**, 37–45.

Flicker, C., Ferris, S.H., Crook, T., and Bartus, R.T. (1987) Implications of memory and language dysfunction in the naming deficit of senile dementia. *Brain and Language*, **31**, 187–200.

Funnell, E. and Hodges, J.R. (1996) Deficits in semantic memory and executive control: evidence for differing effects upon naming in dementia. *Aphasiology*, **10**, 687–709.

Gainotti, G. (1993) Mechanisms underlying semantic-lexical disorders in Alzheimer's disease, in *Handbook of Neuropsychology*, vol. **8** (eds F. Boller and J. Grafman), Elsevier, Amsterdam, pp. 283–294.

Galasko, D., Salmon, D.P., Lineweaver, T. *et al.* (1998) Neuropsychological measures distinguish patients with Lewy body variant from those with Alzheimer's disease. *Neurology*, **50**, A181.

Glosser, G. and Friedman, R.B. (1991) Lexical but not semantic priming in Alzheimer's disease. *Psychology and Aging*, **6**, 522–527.

Gottfries, C., Adolfsson, R., Aquilonius, S. *et al.* (1983) Biochemical changes in dementia disorders of Alzheimer type. *Neurobiology of Aging*, **4**, 261–271.

Graves, A.B. and Kukull, W.A. (1994) The epidemiology of dementia, in *Handbook of Dementing Illnesses* (ed. J.C. Morris), Marcel Dekker Inc., New York, pp. 23–69.

Grober, E., Buschke, H., Kawas, C. and Fuld, P. (1985) Impaired ranking of semantic attributes in dementia. *Brain and Language*, **26**, 276–287.

Haase, G. (1977) Diseases presenting as dementia, in *Dementia: Contemporary Neurology Series* (ed. C.E. Wells), E.A. Davis, Philadelphia, pp. 231–245.

Hachinski, V.C., Lassen, N.A. and Marshall, J. (1974) Multi-infarct dementia: a cause of mental deterioration in the elderly. *Lancet*, **2**, 207–209.

Hachinski, V.C., Iliff, L.P., Zilkha, E. *et al.* (1975) Cerebral blood flow in dementia. *Archives of Neurology*, **32**, 632–637.

Haller, R.G. (1980) Alcoholism and neurologic disorders, in *Neurology*, vol. 5 (ed. R.N. Rosenberg), Grune & Stratton, New York, pp. 569–588.

Harasty, J.A., Halliday, G.M., Kril, J. and Code, C. (1999) Specific temporoparietal gyral atrophy reflects the pattern of language dissolution in Alzheimer's disease. *Brain*, **122**, 675–686.

Herbert, R. and Brayne, C. (1995) Epidemiology of vascular dementia. *Neuroepidemiology*, **14**, 240–257.

Heston, L.L., Mastrik, A.R., Anderson, E. and White, J. (1981) Dementia of the Alzheimer type. *Archives of General Psychiatry*, **38**, 1085–1090.

Hier, D.B., Hagenlocker, K. and Shindler, A.G. (1985) Language disintegration in dementia: effects of etiology and severity. *Brain and Language*, **25**, 117–133.

Hodges, J.R. and Patterson, K. (1995) Is semantic memory consistently impaired early in the course of Alzheimer's disease? Neuroanatomical and diagnostic implications. *Neuropsychologia*, **33**, 441–459.

Holland, A.L. (1980) *Communicative Abilities in Daily Living*, University Park Press, Baltimore.

Holland, A.L., McBurney, D.H., Moossy, J. and Reinmuth, O.M. (1985) The dissolution of language in Pick's disease with neurofibrillary tangles: a case study. *Brain and Language*, **24**, 36–38.

Hyman, B.T., Van Hoesen, G.W. and Damasio, A.R. (1990) Memory related neural systems in Alzheimer's disease: an anatomic study. *Neurology*, **40**, 1721–1730.

Irigaray, L. (1967) Approche psycholinguistique du langage des déments. *Neuropsychologia*, **5**, 25–52.

Irigaray, L. (1973) *Le Langage des Déments*, Mouton, The Hague.

Jervis, G.A. (1937) Alzheimer's disease. *Psychiatry Quarterly*, **11**, 5–18.

Jorm, A.F. (2000) Risk factors for Alzheimer's disease, in *Dementia* (eds J. O'Brien, D. Ames and A. Burns), Arnold, London, pp. 383–390.

Jorm, A.F. and Jolley, D. (1998) The incidence of dementia: a meta-analysis. *Neurology*, **51**, 728–733.

Joynt, R.J. (1984) The language of dementia, in *Advances in Neurology*, vol. **42** (ed. F.C. Rose), Raven Press, New York, pp. 63–75.

Kemper, T. (1984) Neuroanatomical and neuropathological changes in normal aging and in dementia, in *Clinical Neurology of Aging* (ed. M.L. Albert), Oxford University Press, New York, pp. 9–52.

Kempler, D., Curtiss, S. and Jackson, C. (1987) Syntactic preservation in Alzheimer's disease. *Journal of Speech and Hearing Research*, **30**, 343–350.

Kertesz, A. (1979) *Aphasia and Associated Disorders: Taxonomy, Localization and Recovery*, Grune & Stratton, New York.

Kertesz, A. (1980) *Western Aphasia Battery*, University of Western Ontario, London, Canada.

Kertesz, A. and Kertesz, M. (1988) Memory deficit and language dissolution in Alzheimer's disease. *Journal of Neurolinguistics*, **3**, 103–114.

Kirshner, H.S., Webb, W.G. and Kelly, M.P. (1984) The naming disorder of dementia. *Neuropsychologia*, **22**, 23–30.

Kitselman, K. (1981) Language impairment in aphasia, delirium, dementia and schizophrenia, in *Speech Evaluation in Medicine* (ed. J.E. Darby), Grune & Stratton, New York, pp. 163–181.

Larrson, T., Sjörgren, T. and Jacobson, G. (1963) Senile dementia. *Acta Psychiatrica Scandinavica*, **167** (Suppl.), 1–259.

Lawson, J.S. and Barker, M.G. (1968) The assessment of nominal dysphasia in dementia: the use of reaction time measures. *British Journal of Medical Psychology*, **41**, 411–414.

LaBarge, E., Balota, D.A., Storandt, M. and Smith, D.S. (1992) An analysis of confrontation naming errors in senile dementia of the Alzheimer's type. *Neuropsychology*, **6**, 77–95.

Liberman, A. (1998) Managing the neuropsychiatric symptoms of Parkinson's disease. *Neurology*, **50**, S33–S38.

Lishman, W.A. (1981) Cerebral disorder in alcoholism: syndromes of impairment. *Brain*, **104**, 1–20.

Martin, A. (1992a) Degraded knowledge representations in patients with Alzheimer's disease: implications for models of semantic and repetition priming, in *Neuropsychology of Memory* (eds L.R. Squire and N. Butters), Guilford Press, New York, pp. 220–232.

Martin, A. (1992b) Semantic knowledge in patients with Alzheimer's disease: evidence for degraded representations, in *Memory Function in Dementia* (ed. L. Blackman), Elsevier, Amsterdam, pp. 119–134.

Martin, A. and Fedio, P. (1983) Word production and comprehension in Alzheimer's disease: the breakdown of semantic knowledge. *Brain and Language*, **19**, 124–141.

Martin, A., Brouwers, P., Cox, C. and Fedio, P. (1985) On the nature of the verbal memory deficit in Alzheimer's disease. *Brain and Language*, **25**, 323–341.

McDuff, T. and Sumi, S.M. (1985) Subcortical degeneration in Alzheimer's disease. *Neurology*, **35**, 123–126.

McGlinchey-Berroth, R. and Milberg, W.P. (1993) Preserved semantic memory structure in Alzheimer's disease, in *Adult Information Processing: Limits on Loss* (ed. J. Cerella), Academic Press, San Diego, pp. 407–422.

McMenemy, W.H. (1940) Alzheimer's disease. *Journal of Neurology and Psychiatry*, **3**, 211–240.

Mitler, A.E., Neighbor, A., Katzman, R. *et al.* (1981) Immunological studies in senile dementia of the Alzheimer type: evidence for enhanced suppressor cell activity. *Annals of Neurology*, **10**, 506–510.

Morris, J.C., Cole, M., Banker, B.O. and Wright, D. (1984) Hereditary dysphasic dementias and the Pick-Alzheimer spectrum. *Annals of Neurology*, **16**, 455–466.

Murdoch, B.E. (1988) Language disorders in dementia as aphasia syndromes. *Aphasiology*, **2**, 181–185.

Murdoch, B.E., Chenery, H.J., Boyle, R. and Wilks, V. (1988) Functional communicative abilities in dementia of the Alzheimer type. *Australian Journal of Human Communication Disorders*, **16**, 11–21.

Murdoch, B.E., Chenery, H.J., Wilks, V. and Boyle, R. (1987) Language disorders in dementia of the Alzheimer type. *Brain and Language*, **31**, 122–137.

Murdoch, B.E. and Lethlean, J.B. (1996) Language dysfunction in subcortical arteriosclerotic encephalopathy (Binswanger disease). *Journal of Medical Speech-Language Pathology*, **4**, 275–288.

Nebes, R.D. (1992) Semantic memory function in Alzheimer's disease. *Psychological Bulletin*, **106**, 377–394.

Nebes, R.D. and Brady, C.B. (1990) Preserved organization of semantic attributes in Alzheimer's disease. *Psychology and Aging*, **5**, 574–579.

Neely, J.H. (1991) Semantic priming effects in visual word recognition: a selective review of current findings and theories, in *Basic Processes in Reading: Visual Word Recognition* (eds D. Besner and G.W. Humphreys), Erlbaum, Hillsdale, NJ, pp. 264–336.

Nicholas, M., Obler, L.K., Albert, M.L. and Helm-Estabrooks, N. (1985) Empty speech in Alzheimer's disease and fluent aphasia. *Journal of Speech and Hearing Research*, **28**, 405–410.

Nicolosi, L., Harryman, E. and Krescheck, J. (1983) *Terminology of Communication Disorders*, 2nd edn, Williams & Wilkins, Baltimore.

Ober, B.A. and Shenaut, G.K. (1995) Semantic priming in Alzheimer's disease: meta-analysis and theoretical review, in *Age Differences in Word and Language Processing* (eds P. Allen and T.R. Bashore), Elsevier, Amsterdam, pp. 247–271.

Ober, B.A., Shenaut, G.K. and Reed, B.R. (1995) Assessment of associative relations in Alzheimer's disease: evidence for preservation of semantic memory. *Aging and Cognition*, **2**, 254–267.

Obler, L.K. and Albert, M.L. (1981) Language in the elderly aphasic and in the dementing patient, in *Acquired Aphasia* (ed. M.T. Sarno), Academic Press, New York, pp. 385–398.

Obler, L.K., Albert, M.L., Goodglass, H. and Benson, D.F. (1978) Aging and aphasia types. *Brain and Language*, **6**, 318–322.

Pick, A. (1892) On the relation between aphasia and senile atrophy of the brain, in *Neurological Classics in Modern Translation* (eds D.A. Rottenberg and F.H. Hochberg), Hafner, New York, pp. 221–242.

Plum, F. (1979) Dementia: An approaching epidemic. *Nature*, **279**, 372–373.

Reifler, B.V., Larson, E. and Hanley, R. (1982) Coexistence of cognitive impairment and depression in geriatric outpatients. *American Journal of Psychiatry*, **139**, 623–629.

Reisberg, B. (1981) *Brain Failure*. The Free Press, New York.

Rochford, G. (1971) A study of naming errors in dysphasic and in demented patients. *Neuropsychologia*, **9**, 437–443.

Rochon, E., Waters, G.S. and Caplan, D. (1994) Sentence comprehension in patients with Alzheimer's disease. *Brain and Language*, **46**, 329–349.

Ron, M.A. (1977) Brain damage in chronic alcoholism: a neuropathological, neuroradiological and psychological view. *Psychological Medicine*, 7, 103–112.

Ross, E.D. (1980) Disorders of higher cortical functions: diagnosis and treatment, in *Neurology*, vol. 5 (ed. R.N. Rosenberg), Grune & Stratton, New York, pp. 589–602.

Salmon, D.P. and Chan, A.S. (1994) Semantic memory deficits associated with Alzheimer's disease, in *Neuropsychological Exploration of Memory and Cognition: Essays in Honor of Nelson Butters* (ed. L.S. Cermak), Plenum Press, New York, pp. 61–76.

Sandson, J., Obler, L.K. and Albert, M.L. (1987) Language changes in healthy aging and dementia, in *Advances in Applied Psycholinguistics* (ed. S. Rosenberg), Cambridge University Press, Cambridge, Mass, pp. 272–291.

Schwartz, M.F., Marin, O.S.M. and Saffran, E.M. (1979) Dissociations of language function in dementia: a case study. *Brain and Language*, 7, 277–306.

Seltzer, B. and Sherwin, I. (1983) A comparison of clinical features in early and later onset primary degenerative dementia. *Archives of Neurology*, **40**, 143–146.

Shore, D., Overman, C.A. and Wyatt, R.J. (1983) Improving accuracy in the diagnosis of Alzheimer's disease. *Journal of Clinical Psychiatry*, **44**, 207–212.

Slaby, A.E. and Wyatt, R.J. (1974) *Dementia in the Presenium*, Charles C. Thomas, Springfield, IL.

Smith, S.R., Murdoch, B.E. and Chenery, H.J. (1989) Semantic abilities in dementia of the Alzheimer type. 1: lexical semantics. *Brain and Language*, **36**, 314–324.

Spinnler, H. (1991) The role of attention disorders in the cognitive deficits of dementia, in *Handbook of Neuropsychology*, vol. 5 (eds F. Boller and J. Grafman), Elsevier, Amsterdam, pp. 79–122.

Teri, L. and Logsdon, R.G. (1991) Identifying pleasant activities for Alzheimer's disease patients: the pleasant events schedule A–D. *The Gerontologist*, **31**, 124–127.

Terry, R.D. and Katzman, R. (1983) Senile dementia of the Alzheimer type. *Annals of Neurology*, **14**, 497–506.

Terry, R.D., Peck, A., de Teresa, R. *et al.* (1981) Some morphometric aspects of the brain in senile dementia of the Alzheimer type. *Annals of Neurology*, **10**, 184–192.

Tomlinson, B.E. (1977) The pathology of dementia, in *Dementia: Contemporary Neurology Series* (ed. C.E. Wells), E.A. Davis, Philadelphia, pp. 75–89.

Tomlinson, B.E., Blessed, G. and Roth, M. (1970) Observations on the brains of demented old people. *Journal of Neurological Sciences*, **11**, 205–242.

Tomoeda, C.K., Bayles, K.A. and Boone, D.R. (1990) Speech rate and syntactic complexity effects on the auditory comprehension of Alzheimer patients. *Journal of Communication Disorders*, **23**, 151–161.

Velakoulis, D. and Lloyd, J. (2000) Parkinson's disease and dementia: prevalence and incidence, in *Dementia* (eds J. O'Brien, D. Ames and A. Burns), Arnold, London, pp. 845–852.

Warrington, E.K. (1975) The selective impairment of semantic memory. *Quarterly Journal of Experimental Psychology*, **27**, 635–657.

Wechsler, A.F., Verity, M., Rosenschein, S. *et al.* (1982) Pick's disease. *Archives of Neurology*, **39**, 287–290.

Wells, C.E. (1981) A deluge of dementia. *Psychosomatics*, **22**, 837–838.

Whitaker, H. (1976) A case of isolation of language functions, in *Studies in Neurolinguistics*, vol. 2 (eds H. Whitaker and H.A. Whitaker), Academic Press, New York, pp. 1–58.

Whitehouse, P.J., Price, D.L., Clark, A.W. *et al.* (1981) Alzheimer disease: evidence for the selective loss of cholinergic neurons in the nucleus basalis. *Annals of Neurology*, **10**, 122–126.

Language disorders associated with diseases of the cerebral white matter

7

Introduction

A number of researchers have suggested that the disruption of the cerebral white matter, as may occur in conditions such as subcortical strokes or as a result of demyelinating disorders (e.g. multiple sclerosis), may cause language problems by disconnecting deep brain structures (e.g. the basal ganglia) from the language areas of the cerebral cortex (Damasio *et al.*, 1982; Alexander, Naeser and Palumbo, 1987). Further, as discussed in Chapter 3, models describing the roles of subcortical structures in language have frequently considered the importance of white matter pathways or connections that enable communication not only between the language centres of the cerebral cortex but also between subcortical brain structures and the cerebral cortex (Crosson, 1985; Alexander, Naeser and Palumbo, 1987; Wallesch and Papagno, 1988). Consequently, it would appear that not only are cortical-cortical connections (e.g. arcuate fasciculus) important in language processing but also cortical-subcortical and subcortical-subcortical white matter pathways are also critical for normal language functioning (Wallesch and Papagno, 1988). A schematic

diagram of the major white matter connections is presented in Figure 7.1.

Although contemporary models of subcortical participation in language (see Chapter 3) have proposed roles for structures such as the basal ganglia, thalamus and subthalamic nucleus, emphasis has also been placed on the communication of these structures with the cerebral cortex via critical white matter pathways. Indeed, indirect effects of subcortical dysfunction on the language areas of the cortex have been proposed as possible explanations for language deficits following subcortical vascular lesions. Mechanisms of distance effects, including the influences of mass effect and oedema (Alexander and LoVerme, 1980), cortical ischaemia (Megens *et al.*, 1992) and cortical hypometabolism (Metter *et al.*, 1988; Levasseur *et al.*, 1992) have been proposed which inactivate the cortical language areas causing a disconnection effect and consequent language impairment. It has been suggested that this disconnection effect may have a direct influence on cortical function or interrupt the flow of information from different structures participating in language processing (Robin and Schienberg, 1990). Put more simply, it is suggested that in order for information to be

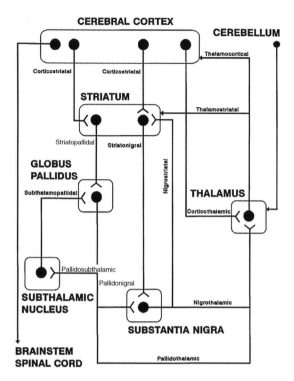

Figure 7.1   Schematic diagram of the major white matter connections in the cortical-subcortical system

transmitted for language processing, critical white matter pathways must be available between the subcortical structures and the cortex (e.g. thalamocortical connections), between different cortical regions (e.g. connections between Wernicke's area and Broca's area via the arcuate fasciculus) and between the subcortical structures themselves (e.g. pallidothalamic connections) (Figure 7.1). Rather than proposing a single cortical or subcortical structure as exclusively responsible for a particular language process, researchers have suggested that the white matter pathways are critical for enabling cortical and subcortical structures to work together in a linked communicative system (Lieberman, Ellenberg and Restum, 1986; Wallesch and Papagno, 1988; Robin and Schienberg, 1990). Therefore, damage anywhere in the circuitry of pathways may result in abnormal balances of inhibitory and excitatory influences and in this way impairs language processing (Crosson, 1985; Robin and Schienberg, 1990). In support of this suggestion,

lesions in the corona radiata (containing bundles of corticoprojectional and thalamocortical fibres subadjacent to the cortex), and the internal capsule (containing projection fibres which connect auditory, parietal and occipital areas and subcortical nuclei) have been reported to be associated with language deficits similar to those located in a pathway endpoint, that is the cortex (Hyman and Tranel, 1989).

Assuming, as outlined above, subcortical white matter pathways do play an important role in language processing, it could be predicted that damage to subcortical white matter pathways in neurological diseases with purely white matter damage, such as occurs in multiple sclerosis, Binswanger's disease and progressive multifocal leukoencephalopathy would result in language impairment. In support of this prediction, individuals with multiple sclerosis (FitzGerald, Murdoch and Chenery, 1987; Lethlean and Murdoch, 1993a, 1997), Binswanger's disease (Leifer, Buonanno and Richardson, 1990; Murdoch and Lethlean, 1996) and progressive multifocal leukoencephalopathy (Berger *et al.*, 1987; Lethlean and Murdoch 1993b) have been reported to exhibit speech-language problems associated with demyelination of the white matter of the central nervous system. The nature of the language disorders reported in association with each of these three conditions is reported below:

Language disorders in multiple sclerosis

Until recently, research into communication problems in multiple sclerosis tended to concentrate on the motor aspects of speech rather than on the possible language problems resulting from subcortical white matter demyelination. Traditionally, cognitive-linguistic abilities were thought to be a function of the cerebral cortex and consequently it was assumed that disruption to these abilities in diseases of the white matter was unlikely. However, it is becoming increasingly evident that the part played by white matter pathways and subcortical structures in both cognitive and language functions may have been underestimated. Researchers now propose that disruption of subcortical and brainstem influence on the cerebral cortex in multiple sclerosis can be responsible for cortical dysfunction, leading to cognitive and linguistic disorders in this population (Crosson, 1985; Alexander, Naeser and Palumbo, 1987; Wallesch and Papagno, 1988; Lethlean and Murdoch, 1994a,b). In particular neural white matter pathways connecting subcortical structures such as the basal ganglia and thalamus to the cortical language areas have been considered important in language function (Alexander, Naeser and Palumbo, 1987). Cognitive impairments subsequent to multiple sclerosis are known to span the entire spectrum and include deficits in memory, intelligence, information processing, abstract and conceptual reasoning and attention (Beatty and Monson, 1989; Blackwood *et al.*, 1991; Rao *et al.*, 1993; Ruchkin *et al.*, 1994). Likewise, in studies where appropriate and sufficiently sensitive language tests have been used, individuals with multiple sclerosis have been shown to exhibit language deficits in the areas of naming, comprehension of logic or grammatical constructions, word fluency, verbal reasoning, word definitions and the interpretation of absurdities, ambiguities and metaphors (Lethlean and Murdoch, 1993a, 1994a,b).

General characteristics of multiple sclerosis

Multiple sclerosis is one of the most common aetiologies for chronic neurological dysfunction in young and middle-aged adults and has been defined as 'an acquired primary demyelinating disease of the central nervous system in which myelin is the target of an autoimmune inflammatory process(es)' (Whitaker and Mitchell, 1997 p. 4).

Neuropathophysiology of multiple sclerosis

Multiple sclerosis is a disease of the white matter of the central nervous system characterized by disseminated demyelination of neuronal axons within the central nervous system with relative preservation of axon integrity (Raine, 1977). Myelin is an insulative lipid that encircles neuronal axons throughout the nervous system, in a sheath-like fashion (Sherwood, 1993). The myelin is manufactured by independent central and peripheral nervous system myelin-producing cells, oligodendrocytes in the central nervous system and Schwann cells in the peripheral nervous system, and provides a high-resistance, low-capacitance insulation for the axon. In the unimpaired nervous system, the myelin produced is characteristically segmented into discrete units along each axon, separated by nodes of Ranvier (Hashimoto and Paty, 1986). Myelinated axons conduct nerve impulses from node to node in a saltatory, rather than a continuous, manner, which allows a reduction in conduction time and an increased metabolic efficiency. It is not surprising, therefore, that demyelination, as occurs in multiple sclerosis, is accompanied by significant conduction abnormalities (Kocsis and Waxman, 1985). Eisen (1983) stated that the pathophysiological hallmark of demyelination is slow conduction, attributed to a reduction in ionic shift propagations along bare axonal segments.

Demyelination of normally myelinated tracts within the central nervous system occurs in a periaxial fashion in multiple sclerosis with little or no axonal degeneration (van Oosten *et al.*, 1995). Irregular grey islands known as plaques are often seen at autopsy in regions where demyelination has occurred, particularly in the optic nerves, pons, medulla oblongata, spinal cord, cerebellum, the superior surface of the corpus callosum and the periventricular regions of the cerebral hemispheres (De Souza, 1990; Matthews *et al.*, 1991). Although multiple sclerosis appears to have a predilection for certain sites within the central nervous system, no myelinated tract within the brain or spinal cord is exempt from attack, (Hallpike, Adams and Tourtellotte, 1983). The anatomical distribution of lesions is highly variable between individuals, and within any one case plaques may vary considerably in size, shape and age (Matthews *et al.*, 1991).

The demyelination process has been described as 'phasic', involving the progression of an acute lesion to a chronic plaque (Hashimoto and Paty, 1986). It has been hypothesized that the acute lesion is the result of an inflammatory reaction involving the infiltration of inflammatory cells (primarily lymphocytes, plasma cells and macrophages) through the blood–brain barrier. These cells accumulate at the site of demyelination and engulf the degenerating myelin (van Oosten *et al.*, 1995). As the lesion becomes chronic, reactive gliosis (formation of scar tissue as a result of astrocyte proliferation) occurs and inflammatory activity becomes less marked resulting in the formation of the typical 'sclerotic plaque'. Accompanying the formation of these plaques, the myelin sheaths and oligodendrocytes are lost and axonal loss also tends to occur, especially in severe, long-standing cases of multiple sclerosis (van Oosten *et al.*, 1995).

It is now generally accepted that remyelination (i.e. the process in which demyelinated axons are reinvested with new myelin sheaths) does occur in the central nervous system and may contribute to lasting recovery from acute relapse in some cases of multiple sclerosis (Scolding and Franklin, 1998). However, in multiple sclerosis this remyelination process is far from complete and myelin repair ultimately fails during progression of the disease, as disability and handicap accumulate. As yet, however, the factors which limit the oligodendritic remyelination process are not understood (Allen, 1991).

Epidemiology and aetiology of multiple sclerosis

The aetiology of multiple sclerosis is unknown. Currently, multiple sclerosis is classified as a T-cell-mediated organ-specific autoimmune disease (Martin and McFarland, 1995). Although evidence acquired from multiple sclerosis patients has supported the autoimmune theory, current thinking regarding the possible aetiology of multiple sclerosis has largely been shaped by studies based on experimental models of central nervous system inflammation, especially experimental allergic encephalomyelitis. Characteristically, the onset of symptoms of multiple sclerosis occurs post-pubescently, with peak incidence rates occurring between 30 and 40 years of age (De Souza, 1990). Onset of symptoms after 60 years of age is rare (Acheson, 1985). There is general agreement that multiple sclerosis is slightly more common in females than males, with female to male ratios reported to be in the order of 1.5 : 1

(Hartelius, Nord and Buder, 1995). Acheson (1985) attributed this female predilection to a possible hormonal interaction. Furthermore, the global distribution of multiple sclerosis illustrates characteristic latitudinal and racial profiles which have provided impetus for the development of numerous environmental and genetic theories of causation (Hashimoto and Paty, 1986).

Environmental and genetic theories of causation
Influence of latitude. It is generally accepted that multiple sclerosis is more common in countries further from the equator, both in the northern and southern hemispheres, with the peak prevalence rates having been documented in Caucasian populations residing at latitudes between 40° and 60° (Rivera, 1986). Specific regions of peak prevalence (i.e. ≥ 50 cases per 100 000 population) include: northern and central Europe, northern North America, New Zealand and parts of Southern Australia (Hashimoto and Paty, 1986). Multiple sclerosis prevalence rates in Australia comply with the latitudinal patterns of the northern hemisphere, with prevalence increasing with distance from the equator. Multiple sclerosis has been reported to be four times more common in Tasmania (the most southern state of Australia) (75.6 cases per 100 000) than in Queensland (a northern state of Australia) (18.6 cases per 100 000) (McLeod, Hammond and Hallpike, 1994).

According to Compston (1994), the uneven geographical distribution associated with multiple sclerosis may indirectly reflect underlying environmental factors of causation. Postulated environmental influences have included nutrition, diet, agricultural production, sanitation, geological environment (e.g. presence/absence of trace elements) (Bauer and Hanefeld, 1993), infectious agents (e.g. viruses, spirochetes, mycoplasma) (Dick, 1976), as well as climate and social customs (Hutter, 1993). The strongest evidence to support an environmental pathogenesis has come from the results of migration studies which have shown that living at greater latitudes during childhood and adolescence increases a person's susceptibility to multiple sclerosis in adult life (Hutter, 1993). Further, documented trends indicate that migration prior to the age of

15 promotes the acquisition of the risk rate of the individual's new environment; however, birthplace risk levels are maintained if migration occurs after 15 years of age (Kurtzke, 1983). Based on these observations, many researchers investigating the possible cause of multiple sclerosis have hypothesized that an environmental agent (possibly a slow virus endemic to temperate climates) present prior to the age of 15 may be responsible for the subsequent manifestation of this disease (Tienari, 1994).

In a recent review, however, Poser (1994) questioned the viability of the often-cited interrelation between prevalence and latitude, in that prevalence of multiple sclerosis varies enormously in populations living on the same latitude. Poser (1994) concluded that genetic susceptibility plays a much more significant part than geography in determining the prevalence of multiple sclerosis in a particular location, although the degree and complexity of genetic control remains largely undefined (Sadovnick, 1994). Currently, there is growing support among multiple sclerosis researchers for the hypothesis that one or more environmental agents trigger the disease in a genetically susceptible host resulting in immune-mediated tissue injury within the central nervous system (Cook *et al.*, 1995). Although the potency of various environmental factors in influencing the expression of multiple sclerosis is unknown, a non-specific infectious agent or agents, socio-economic factors and diet are thought to contribute (Hutter, 1993; Poser, 1994).

Viral conditions. A number of viruses have been reported to cause demyelination in both humans (e.g. subacute sclerosing panencephalitis) and animals (e.g. canine distemper demyelinating encephalomyelitis) (Meulen and Stephenson, 1983). As such, viral-driven aetiological hypotheses have been applied to manifestations of multiple sclerosis (Meulen and Stephenson, 1983). Serological studies of blood serum and cerebrospinal fluid in multiple sclerosis patients have revealed characteristically high antibody titres for measles and, less commonly, elevated titres for rubella, mumps, varicella, herpes, paramyxovirus and human T-cell leukaemia virus 1, among others

(Bauer and Hanefeld, 1993). A distinctive cerebrospinal fluid antibody triad of elevated measles, rubella and zoster antigens was documented in up to 80% of a multiple sclerosis subject sample studied by Felgenhauer *et al.* (1985). Dick (1976) hypothesized that the multiple sclerosis initiating viral agent, most probably acquired during childhood, lies dormant within the central nervous system until adolescence. Post-pubescently the virus is 'awakened' by unidentified stimuli, to precipitate a demyelinating rampage. Hashimoto and Paty (1986) suggested that this post-viral demyelination is immune-mediated.

A viral aetiopathogenesis is supported by habitually elevated levels of specific immunoglobulins in the cerebrospinal fluid of multiple sclerosis patients (Dick, 1976). Hashimoto and Paty (1986) stated that the immune system operates on the premise of an antigen-specific control response to foreign agents. Numerous abnormalities of immune regulation have been identified in multiple sclerosis patients including: virus-specific, antibody-producing plasma cells surrounding areas of demyelination; production of high levels of cerebrospinal fluid immunoglobulins, specifically IgG; and, most strikingly, the loss of suppressor T-lymphocyte cells from the blood, prior to relapse (Rivera, 1986). This characteristic immunological profile may be indicative of a viral reaction, delayed hypersensitivity to viral antigens or an autoimmune response (Leibowitz, 1983). The manifestation of multiple sclerosis in selective hosts subsequent to various viral infections may be attributed to a genetic susceptibility (Tienari, 1994). Ebers (1992) remarked that multiple sclerosis might be feasibly accepted as an autoimmune disease, under genetic influences.

Racial and genetic factors. Although multiple sclerosis occurs in all three of the principal racial groups of the world comprising Caucasoid (white), Mongoloid (Oriental) and Negroid (black) populations, not all racial groups appear to be equally susceptible to the disease. In general it appears that multiple sclerosis is most common in Caucasian populations but rare in Oriental, black African (Tienari, 1994), Australian Aboriginal and Torres Strait Islander populations

(McLeod, Hammond and Hallpike, 1994). Even when residing in high-risk locations, these latter ethnic groups manifest lower-than-expected prevalence rates for multiple sclerosis, suggesting that they may be protected against the disease by some racially determined genetic factor (Hashimoto and Paty, 1986). Further evidence of a genetic influence in the occurrence of multiple sclerosis comes from studies that have shown that first-degree relatives of affected individuals are 25–50 times more likely to develop multiple sclerosis than the general population is. (Wikstrom, Kinnunen and Porras, 1984; Sadovnick *et al.*, 1992). In addition, twin studies have documented concordance rates in monozygotic and dizygotic twins of 25 and 3% respectively, highly suggestive of a genetic influence (Ebers *et al.*, 1986).

The human leukocyte antigen gene complex on chromosome 6 is associated with immune functions (Tienari, 1994). Representations of certain loci on this gene complex have been characteristically linked to autoimmune diseases, including multiple sclerosis (Hauser *et al.*, 1989). Of note, dissimilarities in human leukocyte antigen associations have been identified between different racial groups (Acheson, 1985), and as such the isolation of a universal multiple sclerosis susceptibility gene cannot be substantiated. Despite these variable findings, however, histocompatibility antigen studies have given indisputable validity to the genetic theory of causation (Batchelor, 1985).

In essence, it appears that we cannot sequester the aetiological agents responsible for the manifestation of multiple sclerosis. The combined effects of genetic and environmental influences provide us with the most viable interpretation of neuropathology associated with multiple sclerosis (Poser, 1994). It has been postulated that a genetic susceptibility predisposes the individual to disease acquisition; however, environmental elements of unknown origin are thought to be responsible for activating the onset of clinical symptoms (Poser, 1994).

Clinical signs and symptoms of multiple sclerosis

The clinical signs and symptoms associated with multiple sclerosis vary tremendously from case to case as a consequence of the variability in the anatomic distribution and age of the central nervous system lesions. Despite the fact that demyelination may occur virtually anywhere within the central nervous system, the majority of patients with multiple sclerosis have their initial symptoms in a relatively limited distribution. McAlpine (1972) documented limb weakness, optic neuritis, paraesthesia in the extremities, diplopia, vertigo and impaired micturition to be the most common primary clinical manifestations of multiple sclerosis. Dysarthria, dysphagia, nystagmus, auditory dysfunction, weakness, ataxia, intention tremor, spasticity, sphincter disturbances and altered emotional responses are symptoms that manifest more commonly in patients with long-standing or advanced multiple sclerosis. Pain is not usually a presenting symptom of multiple sclerosis but frequently develops during the course of the illness in such forms as trigeminal neuralgia and pseudoradicular pain. Generalized fatigue subsequent to increases in body temperature or episodes of physical exertion is also frequently seen in multiple sclerosis, and may be persistent or transient in nature (Bauer and Hanefeld, 1993). Fatigue has been noted to result in reduced motivation levels and decreased work performance.

Transient symptoms known as 'paroxysmal attacks' are commonly experienced in multiple sclerosis, especially in the early stages of the disease (Mitchell, 1993). These attacks are usually brief and intense, lasting seconds to minutes and have a tendency to recur in a stereotypic manner for each individual (Matthews *et al.*, 1991). Paroxysmal dysarthria and ataxia have both been frequently reported as the most common type of paroxysmal attacks. Other paroxysmal disorders associated with multiple sclerosis include trigeminal neuralgia, tonic seizures and spasms, and unpleasant quivering sensations (Mitchell, 1993).

The general course of multiple sclerosis is variable and may take several forms including: relapsing–remitting, progressive–relapsing and chronic progressive. Approximately 65% of individuals with multiple sclerosis experience a relapsing–remitting form of the disease at onset, with symptoms usually developing subacutely and resolving over weeks to months, with periods between disease relapses being characterized by a lack of disease progression (Mitchell, 1993). After a varying number of exacerbations, a majority of the individuals with relapsing–remitting multiple sclerosis also enter a secondary progressive phase where symptoms gradually evolve without remission. Progressive–relapsing multiple sclerosis occurs in about 15% of patients and represents a progressive disease from outset, with clear acute relapses, with or without full recovery, with periods between relapses characterized by continuing progression. The chronic progressive form of multiple sclerosis exists in approximately 20% of patients and is characterized by disease progression from outset with only occasional plateaus and temporary minor improvements.

Diagnosis of multiple sclerosis

Diagnosis of multiple sclerosis is difficult and typically made by exclusion, with heavy reliance on clinical history and neurological symptoms using the criteria specified by Poser *et al.* (1983). These criteria are based on dissemination in time and space and the diagnostic categories include 'definite', 'probable' and 'possible' multiple sclerosis. For a definite diagnosis, clinical evidence that two different regions of the central white matter have been affected at different times is needed (Poser *et al.*, 1983). Confirmatory evidence can also be gained by the use of magnetic resonance imaging (MRI) cerebrospinal fluid analysis and multisensory evoked potentials (Rao, 1986). Probable multiple sclerosis is specified in cases where relapse–remitting symptoms are present with only one neurological sign commonly associated with multiple sclerosis. A diagnosis of possible multiple sclerosis is made where relapse–remitting symptoms are present without documented signs or objective signs are insufficient to establish more than one site of central nervous system involvement. Although the diagnosis of multiple sclerosis is far easier and more certain with the availability of cranial MRI, a determination of disease activity and the disease progression remains difficult.

Medical treatment of multiple sclerosis

Effective curative therapy for multiple sclerosis is as yet unavailable. Consequently, medical man-

agement of multiple sclerosis continues to focus on the treatment of acute exacerbations, prevention of relapse and progression and alleviation of the chronic symptoms of the disease (Noseworthy, 1991; Francis, 1993; van Oosten *et al.*, 1995). Acute exacerbations are principally treated with drugs such as corticosteroids that possess properties which accelerate the recovery that usually follows each attack (Rudick and Goodkin, 1992; Ebers, 1994). Most neurologists limit the use of these drugs to only the most serious or disabling episodes (Francis, 1993) since long-term administration does not alter the natural history of the disease significantly and, moreover, steroid side effects outweigh this limited benefit (Ebers, 1994). The corticosteroids, corticotrophin (adrenocorticotrophic hormone, ACTH) and methylprednisolone have been reported to accelerate recovery from relapse in multiple sclerosis equally well (Thompson *et al.*, 1989), although their effects are probably only short-lived (Barkhof *et al.*, 1994). Methylprednisolone is usually the preferred treatment option because it has the convenience of a shorter treatment course (Mitchell, 1993; van Oosten *et al.*, 1995). Another treatment sometimes used in cases of acute exacerbation, especially in pregnant patients (Mitchell, 1993), is plasma exchange. This treatment produces only minimal benefits, which fail to justify the cost (Weiner *et al.*, 1989).

As a result of current thoughts on multiple sclerosis, the drugs used to prevent relapse and slow progression of the disease are typically immunosuppressive agents (Francis, 1993). Immunosuppressive drugs such as azathioprine, cyclophosphamide and cyclosporin may slow the progression of multiple sclerosis to some degree; however, potentially serious adverse side effects including hypertension, anaemia and gastrointestinal complications have limited their use.

Interferon beta (IFN-B) has recently been demonstrated to be of value in reducing relapses and preventing the accumulation of brain lesions over time in multiple sclerosis, without producing serious adverse side effects (Jacobs *et al.*, 1994; Jacobs and Johnson, 1994; Polman and Uitdehaag, 2003). Generally, the interferons act to stimulate the immune system, activating macrophages, enhancing natural killer cells and inhibiting virus replication (Francis, 1993). IFN-B has not yet been observed to have an effect on the accumulation of disability over time (Jacobs *et al.*, 1994). Another recently investigated treatment involving glatiramer acetate (formerly copolymer 1, a mixture of random polymers simulating the amino acid sequence of myelin basic protein) administered daily to patients via subcutaneous injections has shown modest benefits in slowing the progression of both the relapsing/remitting and progressive forms of multiple sclerosis (Francis, 1993; Jacobs *et al.*, 1994).

The symptomatic treatment of multiple sclerosis involves a wide variety of pharmacological agents. Spasticity is experienced frequently in established multiple sclerosis and is most commonly treated with antispastic agents such as baclofen, tizanidine, diazepam and dantrolene carefully titrated to provide relief of spasticity without either producing or exacerbating muscular weakness (van Oosten *et al.*, 1995). Unfortunately, specific treatment is unavailable to combat the disabling effects of muscle weakness (van Oosten *et al.*, 1995).

Ataxia is also a relatively frequent and disabling symptom of multiple sclerosis that is difficult to treat (van Oosten *et al.*, 1995). Most agents used for the problem of ataxia have only a damping effect on incapacitating tremor, with the likelihood of tolerance to the drug(s) developing, as well as the production of unacceptable side effects (Francis, 1993). Fatigue has the potential to impact profoundly on daily living in patients with multiple sclerosis. Amantadine and pemoline are often used to lessen the physiological component of fatigue but the psychological component requires counselling and sometimes the administration of antidepressant drugs (Francis, 1993). Urinary tract symptoms, such as detrusor hyperreflexia and abnormally high post-micturitional volumes, are generally treated using oral anticholinergic medication and intermittent self-catheterization (van Oosten *et al.*, 1995).

Much controversy surrounds the efficacy of currently used multiple sclerosis therapies owing to difficulties in determining whether a patient's condition has stabilized spontaneously or as a response to therapy. Although many therapies have been reported to be effective based on limited trials or following initial application, many have been found later to provide no benefit on the basis of larger trials or after the passage of time (Mitchell, 1993).

Individuals with multiple sclerosis have complex problems and the potential for significant and sometimes severe disability despite the currently used treatments. In view of this, many authors (Noseworthy, 1991; Mitchell, 1993) advocate a multidisciplinary approach to the treatment of multiple sclerosis to provide patients with optimal care. Physical, occupational, speech and recreational therapy are all important in assisting multiple sclerosis patients to experience a good quality of life. Communicative impairment, resulting from the presence of a significant dysarthria, may be an important contributor to a reduction in the quality of life for some individuals with multiple sclerosis. Ultimately, both medical and rehabilitative therapies should be tailored to suit each patient's individual needs (Mitchell, 1993).

Language disorders in multiple sclerosis: evidence from case studies

Despite the recognition at a theoretical level of the importance of connectivity between the cortical and subcortical structures implicated in various neuroanatomical models of language processing (see Chapter 3), documentation of the presence of language deficits in the multiple sclerosis population has consisted primarily of descriptions of individual multiple sclerosis cases with severe communication difficulties supported by a relatively small number of group studies.

Single case studies of subjects with multiple sclerosis have provided evidence for the presence of a language disorder which may be associated with this disease (Friedman, Brem and Mayeaux, 1983; Day, Fisher and Mastaglia, 1987; Achiron *et al.*, 1992). In fact, a variety of language problems have been documented in multiple sclerosis subjects, probably reflecting the variable nature of the disease. Individuals with multiple sclerosis have been reported to present with motor aphasia

(Olmos-Lau, Ginsberg and Geller, 1977), global aphasia (Friedman, Brem and Mayeaux, 1983) and a 'fluent' language disorder with alexia and agraphia (Day, Fisher and Mastaglia, 1987).

Olmos-Lau, Ginsberg and Geller (1977) documented a case of a 17-year-old woman's development of motor aphasia during a second episode of multiple sclerosis. Her speech was characterized by absent spontaneous speech, paraphasias in naming and repetition, intact auditory comprehension, preservation of written language and orofacial apraxia. Friedman, Brem and Mayeaux (1983) described a case of global aphasia in a 32-year-old woman with multiple sclerosis. The case's speech profile revealed non-fluent language production, severely impaired repetition, naming, reading and writing and poor comprehension of simple commands. A computerized tomography (CT) scan at this time revealed white matter plaques in the left periventricular region large enough to interrupt all language pathways including connections from Broca's and Wernicke's areas as well as the arcuate fasciculus. A few months later, the subject improved and a year later presented with mild anomia and intact comprehension. However, repetition for long sentences remained slightly affected and her handwriting was poor and agrammatical.

A case report of alexia with agraphia in multiple sclerosis has been described in the literature (Day, Fisher and Mastaglia, 1987). This 34-year-old woman presented with a jargonic fluent aphasia, which resolved to the presence of mild language deficits including dysnomia, mildly impaired comprehension and repetition and persistent alexia and agraphia. According to Day, Fisher and Mastaglia (1987), the white matter lesion on the CT scan responsible for the aphasic deficits, alexia and agraphia, was appropriately placed to cause a disconnection of the visual cortex from Wernicke's area and the angular gyrus.

Achiron *et al.* (1992) described two subjects with a relapse–remitting disease course who presented with acute onset of severe non-fluent aphasia correlating respectively with large plaques in the left frontal region and the left centrum semiovale as identified by MRI. It was suggested that the plaques were sufficiently large enough to disrupt commissural, association and projection fibres in the dominant frontal temporal region and thus cause motor aphasia.

Language disorders in multiple sclerosis: evidence from group studies

Neuropsychological test batteries

Research into the language abilities of groups of multiple sclerosis subjects has primarily been limited to studies that have utilized neuropsychological assessments rather than tests designed specifically to determine linguistic abilities. This has resulted in varied reports concerning the presence or absence of linguistic deficits in multiple sclerosis, with both intact and impaired language abilities having been identified by researchers using language subtests of neuropsychological batteries (Table 7.1). Language subtests incorporated into neuropsychological assessment batteries are designed to access only basic, functional language abilities but may fail to identify complex linguistic performances of individuals with multiple sclerosis. In fact, performance by multiple sclerosis subjects on restricted language assessments may mask the presence of high-level language difficulties, which may be identified on more complex linguistic tasks. Consequently, studies suggesting linguistic integrity in multiple sclerosis have been based on limited language assessment regimens. Discrepancies in the literature as to whether subjects with multiple sclerosis present with linguistic disturbances may therefore be attributed, in part, to the use of insufficiently sensitive language assessments, which may fail to detect 'high level' language problems. Neuropsychologists primarily interested in cognition and memory in multiple sclerosis have included language subtests such as naming, verbal fluency, spelling, reading and writing in their investigations. A list of these studies appears in Table 7.1. A number of researchers have documented word-finding difficulties in both chronic progressive and relapse–remitting multiple sclerosis groups on naming tasks including the Boston Naming Test (BNT), the abbreviated BNT, the Graded Naming Test and other unspecified tests of naming (Jambor, 1969; Caine *et al.*, 1986; Beatty *et al.*, 1990). Other studies, however, have

Table 7.1 The results of group studies investigating language abilities in subjects with multiple sclerosis.

Task	Researchers	n(*)	Findings
WAIS Verbal Subtests	Callanan *et al.* (1989)	48 (unspec)	intact
	Ivnik (1978)	14 (unspec)	intact
	Jambor (1969)	43 (unspec)	impaired
	Klonoff *et al.* (1991)	86 (RR)	intact
	Lyon-Caen *et al.* (1986)	30 (RR)	intact
	Peyser *et al.* (1980)	55 (unspec)	55% impaired
	Rao *et al.* (1985)	47 (CP)	impaired
	Rao *et al.* (1991)	19 (CP) 30 (RR) 42 (CS)	impaired
	van den Burg *et al.* (1987)	19 (RR)	intact
Comprehension	Anzola *et al.* (1990)	41 (RR)	intact
	Huber *et al.* (1987)	32 (unspec)	intact
Reading	Jambor (1969)	43 (unspec)	intact
	Rao *et al.* (1991)	19 (CP) 39 (RR) 42 (CS)	intact
	Jambor (1969)	43 (unspec)	impaired
	Callanan *et al.* (1989)	48 (unspec)	intact
Writing	Jennekens-Schinkel *et al.* (1990a)	20 (CP) 13 (RR)	intact
	Jennekens-Schinkel *et al.* (1990b)	19 (CP) 20 (RR)	intact
	Jennekens-Schinkel *et al.* (1990a)	20 (CP) 13 (RR)	intact
Spelling	Jennekens-Schinkel *et al.* (1990b)	19 (CP) 20 (RR)	intact
	Jambor (1969)	43 (unspec)	intact

Note: n = number of subjects; * = disease course; WAIS = Wechsler Adult Intelligence Scale; CP = chronic progressive; RR = relapsing–remitting; unspec = unspecified; CS = chronic stable.

reported intact naming abilities in multiple sclerosis groups (Pozzilli *et al.*, 1991; Ron, Callanan and Warrington, 1991). Reduced speed of lexical access is another linguistic deficit which has been inconsistently identified in multiple sclerosis. This finding is indicated by the reported varied performances of individuals with multiple sclerosis on word-fluency tasks (Heaton *et al.*, 1985; FitzGerald, Murdoch and Chenery, 1987; Anzola *et al.*, 1990) and on verbal subtests of the Wechsler Adult Intelligence Scale (WAIS) (Jambor, 1969; Callanan *et al.*, 1989). A majority of studies have reported competent reading, writing and spelling skills and relatively intact comprehension abilities in multiple sclerosis groups (Table 7.1).

Aphasia test batteries

Language assessments designed to test individuals with aphasia following a cerebrovascular accident have also been employed in multiple scle-

rosis group studies (Heaton *et al.*, 1985; FitzGerald, Murdoch and Chenery, 1987; Franklin *et al.*, 1988; Wallace and Holmes, 1993). Heaton *et al.* (1985) used the Aphasia Screening Test (AST) to compare 57 relapse–remitting and 43 chronic progressive multiple sclerosis subjects with a control group. The chronic progressive multiple sclerosis subjects were found to make significantly more errors on the AST than both the relapse–remitting and control groups, whereas the relapse–remitting subjects and the control group performed similarly.

Franklin *et al.* (1988) assessed 60 subjects with chronic progressive multiple sclerosis using the Multilingual Aphasia Examination and the subtest of commands with auditory sequencing from the Western Aphasia Battery. The authors found that, as a group, the multiple sclerosis subjects' receptive and expressive language skills were not significantly different from the control group's.

Further examination of the data revealed that 20% of the multiple sclerosis subjects were impaired on visual naming, 23% on tests of oral comprehension of words and phrases and 18% on tests of verbal fluency.

FitzGerald, Murdoch and Chenery (1987) assessed 20 multiple sclerosis subjects using subtests of the Neurosensory Center Comprehensive Examination for Aphasia (NCCEA; Spreen and Benton, 1969) and the Wiig–Semel Test of Linguistic Concepts (Wiig and Semel, 1974). More than 50% of the subjects performed at a lower than normal level of functioning on subtests of tactile naming, word fluency, sentence construction, writing to dictation and articulation. Poor comprehension of logico-grammatical constructions was also documented. Subtests other than word fluency and sentence construction were regarded as influenced by sensory and motor problems. Although no typical aphasic syndrome was identified in the multiple sclerosis group, the group's language profile appeared to reflect semantic or lexical impairments.

Subsequently, Wallace and Holmes (1993) identified a multiple sclerosis group's cognitive/linguistic deficits on the Arizona Battery for Communication Disorders. When compared to a control group, the multiple sclerosis subjects attained relatively lower scores on the linguistic subtests assessing object description, generative naming, concept definition, generative writing and picture description abilities. Further research using a larger sample of multiple sclerosis subjects was recommended by Wallace and Holmes (1993) because their multiple sclerosis group only consisted of four individuals with a chronic progressive disease course.

High-level language batteries

Despite the documentation of studies hinting at the presence of linguistic impairment in multiple sclerosis, the majority of researchers have provided inadequate information to enable valid description of a characteristic pattern of language breakdown associated with the disease. As indicated earlier, in the majority of studies, language tests which have been used are not sufficiently sensitive to detect potential high-level lan-

guage problems and may be confounded by multiple sclerosis subjects' sensory and motor deficits. Neuropsychological assessments, including tests of naming, verbal fluency and verbal subtests of the WAIS, fail to incorporate measures of high-level language requiring comprehension of complex commands, interpretation of figurative language, inferential reasoning and high-level verbal explanation abilities. While standardized aphasia assessments may assess the gross language abilities of multiple sclerosis groups, they fail to detect more subtle linguistic impairment. Therefore, the need existed for more specific assessment of high-level language abilities in the multiple sclerosis population using tests specifically developed for that purpose so as to describe fully the proposed language disorder.

The most extensive study of the high-level language abilities of persons with multiple sclerosis conducted to date is that reported by Lethlean and Murdoch (1997). The test battery administered by Lethlean and Murdoch included the Test of Language Competence (TLC) (Wiig and Secord, 1985) and the Word Test (TWT; Jorgensen *et al.*, 1981). Their findings indicated that, as a group, the subjects with multiple sclerosis presented with difficulties in understanding ambiguous sentences and metaphoric expressions, making inferences, recreating sentences and exhibited relatively poor performance on voluntary and semantic tasks compared to the controls. Further, Lethlean and Murdoch (1997) reported that individuals with either a chronic progressive or relapse–remitting disease course both had significant high-level language problems. In particular, the division of the multiple sclerosis subjects into groups according to disease course revealed that individuals with both a chronic progressive and a relapse–remitting course experienced significantly more difficulties than the control groups when interpreting ambiguities and metaphors, recreating sentences and forming inferences. Irrespective of disease course, the multiple sclerosis subjects also performed more poorly than the controls on the vocabulary and semantic tasks of TWT including making associations, explaining absurdities, identifying antonyms and defining words. The occurrence of high-level language difficulties in multiple sclerosis was not specifically determined by disease course, as has been previously suggested by some authors (Feinstein *et al.*, 1992). The findings of Lethlean and Murdoch's (1997) investigation did, however, indicate that individuals with a chronic progressive disease course might present with more severe high-level language difficulties when compared to a relapse–remitting group. Further examination of the results revealed that only the chronic progressive group performed more poorly than the control group on the Synonym subtest of the TWT. Overall, the chronic progressive group was more severely impaired on the Recreating Sentences and Understanding Ambiguous Sentences subtests of the TLC and on the Associations, Synonyms and Multiple Definition subtests of TWT.

Although the differences between the performance of the chronic progressive and relapse–remitting subjects and the control group on subtests of TWT were statistically significant, the magnitude of the differences and the clinical meaningfulness of some of the observed differences were questioned by Lethlean and Murdoch (1997). For example, differences in the means of the subjects' identification of synonyms and antonyms in all three groups were less than two points out of a ceiling score of 16 and 14, respectively. Lethlean and Murdoch proposed that the TLC revealed more clinically relevant high-level language deficits in their chronic progressive and relapse–remitting multiple sclerosis groups; therefore, consideration of the multiple sclerosis subjects' performances on the TLC will form the basis of the following theoretical discussion.

According to Bernstein (1987), the use of non-literal language such as ambiguity, metaphorical expressions and so on acts to add a depth and richness to language and allows subtle indirect communication of information. The way in which people process figurative language is a complex procedure, which has been discussed and debated at length in the literature (Baldwin, Luce and Readence, 1982; Bernstein, 1987; Frazier and Rayner, 1987; Simpson and Krueger, 1991), and results so far have been inconclusive.

Understanding ambiguous sentences. Lethlean and Murdoch (1997) noted that both the relapse–remitting and the chronic progressive multiple sclerosis subjects had difficulty identifying two meanings for ambiguous sentences in the TLC. Illustrative examples of the test items include 'And then the man wiped the glasses carefully' (lexical ambiguity), 'Bob did not blame the girl as much as her mother' (surface structure ambiguity) and 'I have always known that flying planes can be dangerous' (deep structure ambiguity). For each of these items, the subjects were required to produce two possible meanings for the sentences with contextual cues. For example, the sentence 'And then the man wiped the glasses carefully' is ambiguous because there is no contextual information to suggest whether the lexically ambiguous word 'glasses' refers to reading glasses or drinking glasses. Some of the multiple sclerosis subjects were able to identify one correct meaning but, even with prompting, failed to evaluate, plan and process a second interpretation of the sentence. Other multiple sclerosis subjects provided two responses but with similar meanings.

Researchers have attempted to explain the normal process of individuals' understanding of lexically ambiguous language (Simpson, 1984; Burgess and Simpson, 1988). Indeed, there is considerable debate in the literature as to whether the comprehension of ambiguity is interactive (i.e. dependent on context) or modular. A review completed by Simpson (1984) has outlined the three major models for ambiguous processing. The first model is the context-dependent, or selective access, model, which is an interactive model proposing that the meanings of ambiguous words are stimulated by the context of the sentence in which they occur (Glucksberg, Kreuz and Rho, 1986). In this context-dependent model, only the contextually appropriate meaning of the ambiguous word is accessed (Simpson, 1981; Simpson *et al.*, 1989). Another model is the single access model, which suggests that the meanings of an ambiguous word are retrieved serially according to their frequency (Hogaboam and Perfetti, 1975). That is, the most frequent meaning is accessed first and if the meaning is appropriate in context the search is discontinued. If, however, the retrieved meaning is not appropriate in context, the search continues to another meaning. In the absence of contextual information, the most frequent meaning is activated first.

The modular-based multiple access model for ambiguous processing proposed by Onifer and Swinney (1981), however, seems to be the one best applied to the model of language processing, outlined by Wallesch and Papagno (1988) (see Chapter 3), which incorporates cortical and subcortical structures and their connections. In turn, Lethlean and Murdoch (1997) suggested that Wallesch and Papagno's (1988) model helped to explain the poor performance by their multiple sclerosis subjects on the Understanding Ambiguous Sentences subtest of the TLC. According to Onifer and Swinney's (1981) model of ambiguous processing, all meanings are simultaneously activated upon presentation of an ambiguous word. Once the meanings of the word have been accessed, the context influences the selection of the appropriate meaning.

In Wallesch and Papagno's (1988) model of language processing, parallel neuroanatomical modules provide alternatives (e.g. different meanings for an ambiguous sentence) which are transmitted to the thalamus via the globus pallidus. Only one response, however, is released by the thalamus to be produced by the cortex. The parallel modules originating in the cortex form cortico-striato-pallido-thalamo-cortical loops, which enable the production of alternative interpretations of ambiguous items. Lethlean and Murdoch (1997) proposed that interruptions of the cortical-subcortical pathways within a modular system might have resulted in the multiple sclerosis subjects' failure to provide alternative meanings for the ambiguous sentences.

The interpretation of syntactically ambiguous sentences has been found to be heavily influenced by the prosodic patterns used by the speaker (Beach, 1991). The subtest of the TLC requiring the interpretation of syntactically ambiguous sentences, however, did not provide the intonation or phrasing cues for the subjects examined by Lethlean and Murdoch (1997). Indeed, both their chronic progressive and relapse–remitting multiple sclerosis subjects had difficulty identifying two meanings for ambiguous sentences with deep and surface structure ambiguities. In the absence of prosodic information, it is possible that the syntactically ambiguous sentences are processed in a modular way, similar to lexically ambiguous

sentences, where the two potential meanings are determined based on the information given by the cortex and integrated and organized by the subcortical structures according to Wallesch and Papagno's (1988) model of language processing. It is recognized, however, that within each module it is likely that different processes will be carried out on lexical versus syntactic ambiguities.

Explanation of metaphorical expressions. The chronic progressive and relapse–remitting multiple sclerosis subjects tested by Lethlean and Murdoch (1997) experienced more difficulty than control subjects when explaining metaphorical expressions in the TLC. For example, when one subject was asked to interpret the metaphor 'There is rough sailing ahead for us' in the situation 'Two students moving into a new town', she responded, 'There is a rough area ahead for them.' According to Bernstein (1987), the term 'metaphor' means to carry over meaning and the comprehension of a metaphor requires the individual to convey aspects of one object over to another object so that it is spoken of as the first object. Gentner (1983) described three types of metaphors, namely attribute, relational and double metaphors. The metaphorical expressions in the TLC consist of relational metaphors in which the topic and vehicle share a relationship. In the example 'There is rough sailing ahead for us', the relationship between the topic 'moving to a new town' and the vehicle 'going in a sailing boat in rough weather' is that both express the notions of 'the future' and 'of difficulties'. Lethlean and Murdoch (1997) suggested that their multiple sclerosis subjects' difficulty in the figurative language tasks may not necessarily reflect an inability to understand these metaphorical relationships but rather that their difficulty is a reflection of poor verbal explanation abilities. Indeed, the subjects' performances improved when they were required to match metaphorical expressions such as 'There is rough sailing ahead for us' with similar underlying meanings from a choice of four items: one a correct match (e.g. 'We will be facing a hard road') and three distracters representing an opposite metaphor (e.g. 'The rough times are behind us now'), a literal interpretation (e.g. 'The waves are going to make it hard to sail') and a non-related metaphor (e.g. 'It took the wind out of our sails'). Children have also been found to perform better on a multiple choice task of understanding metaphors than verbally explaining metaphors (Bernstein, 1987).

Recreating sentences. Lethlean and Murdoch (1997) suggested that organizational linguistic difficulties were reflected in their chronic progressive and relapse–remitting multiple sclerosis group's significantly poor performance on the Recreating Sentence subtest of the TLC. Some of their multiple sclerosis subjects had difficulty integrating and organizing three words that had to be incorporated into a sentence in a given context. For example, each subject had to formulate a sentence with the words 'difficult', 'nonetheless' and 'now' in the context of 'moving house'. A picture of the scenario 'moving house' was provided for the subjects with the words printed above the picture. In addition, the context and the words were read aloud by the examiner. Certain multiple sclerosis subjects were found to have difficulty including all three words in the construction of their sentences and so produced an intact sentence with one or two of the words. For example, one subject constructed the sentence: 'It was difficult job packing up nonetheless it will be for the better'. Other subjects attempted to include all three words but produced sentences which were awkward, incomplete and/or semantically, pragmatically and syntactically inconsistent. For example, one subject produced the non-sentence: 'Nonetheless the last furniture had to go now being difficult'. The findings of sentence construction difficulties in multiple sclerosis subjects by Lethlean and Murdoch (1997) support previous findings (e.g. FitzGerald, Murdoch and Chenery, 1987). Indeed, Bock (1982) has suggested that recreating sentences demands the conceptual integration and synthesis of semantic, pragmatic and syntactic variables. Lethlean and Murdoch (1997) proposed that their multiple sclerosis subjects' poor performance on the recreating sentence items of the TLC may reflect inefficient strategies used to complete the task (with a possible cognitive origin) and/or difficulties in integrating and monitoring linguistic information.

One of the roles of the basal ganglia in language processing outlined in Wallesch and

Papagno's (1988) model is one of integrating and monitoring linguistic information. It is suggested that with the potential disconnection of the cortical structures from subcortical input, owing to demyelination of subcortical white matter pathways in multiple sclerosis, the cortex would have difficulty organizing and integrating the three words into a syntactically, semantically and pragmatically appropriate sentence. Lethlean and Murdoch (1997) speculated that the compromised performance of their multiple sclerosis subjects on the Sentence Construction subtest of the TLC, which required the application of internalized morphologic and syntactic rules (Wiig and Semel, 1974), may have been related to poor intentional self-monitoring abilities. Indeed, a goal-directed intentional role of the deep subcortical nuclei has been proposed by Wallesch (1985), where the will of an individual must be integrated when formulating language.

Making inferences. The chronic progressive and relapse–remitting multiple sclerosis subjects studied by Lethlean and Murdoch (1997) also performed significantly below the control group on the TLC subtests of Making Inferences. The subjects were required to read two statements relating a story and then complete the story by choosing from four inferences which best explained what could have happened. The statements and inferential choices were read out by the examiner to ensure that the items were read accurately. According to Wiig and Secord (1985), reduced scores on this inferential subtest of the TLC, as demonstrated by Lethlean and Murdoch's (1997) multiple sclerosis group represent inactive processing and an ability to generate hypotheses.

Summary: high-level language abilities. Lethlean and Murdoch (1997) concluded that the high-level language dysfunction identified in their multiple sclerosis groups appears to be representative of a more diffuse brain impairment associated with white matter demyelination in multiple sclerosis. Although the diffuse and variable involvement of the cerebral white matter tracts in multiple sclerosis (Rao *et al.*, 1985) make it difficult to provide precise statements concerning the anatomical substrate that influences high-level language processing in this disease, it would appear that Wallesch and Papagno's (1988) model of language processing is useful for explaining, in part, the high-level language dysfunction in multiple sclerosis observed by Lethlean and Murdoch (1997). Certainly, the findings of Lethlean and Murdoch (1997) support the suggestion that individuals with interruptions in subcortical white matter pathways, such as occurs in multiple sclerosis, may experience high-level language problems.

Discourse assessments

Only two reported studies have attempted to document the spoken narrative abilities of individuals with multiple sclerosis (Wallace and Holmes, 1993; Arnott *et al.*, 1997). Wallace and Holmes (1993) administered a picture description subtest, as part of the Arizona Battery for Communication Disorders of Dementia (ABCD) (Bayles and Tomoeda, 1991), to a group of persons with multiple sclerosis. Similar to the reported findings in closed head injury and right hemisphere damage groups (Ehrlich, 1988; Parsons *et al.*, 1989; Joanette and Goulet, 1990), the multiple sclerosis subjects produced fewer utterances per minute, less complete syntactically correct utterances per minute and a smaller number of information units per utterance than matched controls did. However, this was a pilot study involving only four subjects, all with a chronic progressive disease course. The study was also designed to test the sensitivity of the ABCD to cognitive/linguistic deficits in multiple sclerosis, and not to document narrative abilities. Nevertheless, by highlighting deficits of informative content and communicative efficiency in narrative discourse, the results of the Wallace and Holmes (1993) study signified that discourse skills in multiple sclerosis warranted further investigation.

In a larger study, Arnott *et al.* (1997) elicited discourse samples from 47 persons with multiple sclerosis and 47 matched controls in response to computer-generated, animated sequences. In particular, the information conveyed during narrative discourse was analysed by these authors to ascertain whether multiple sclerosis affects a person's ability to effectively plan message content. Within the conceptual level of discourse processing, data were analysed for story schema

and informative content. Arnott *et al.* (1997) reported that the two groups, multiple sclerosis and control, could not be distinguished by measures of the quantity of information conveyed. However, there was a difference in the nature of the information produced by the two groups. The persons with multiple sclerosis produced less essential story information than control subjects, while a tendency for the individuals with multiple sclerosis to produce more incorrect and ambiguous information than controls was also noted. Arnott *et al.* (1997) postulated that both pragmatic and cognitive skills impact on performance in the narrative genre, hence deficits in these areas might have contributed to the observed performance deficits. They considered the nature of the discourse deficits observed to be consistent with subcortical plaque damage affecting fibre tracts between and within the cerebral hemispheres. It was concluded by Arnott *et al.* (1997) that discourse analysis may be sensitive to subtle communication impairments subsequent to multiple sclerosis, which prompted further investigation of discourse abilities in this population.

Language disorders in multiple sclerosis: clinical implications

An awareness of the presence of high-level language deficits in individuals with multiple sclerosis is important for speech-language pathologists involved in the rehabilitation of those people who have this disease. The findings of various studies are indicative of the need for researchers and clinicians to use more sensitive language assessments to accurately quantify and describe the linguistic abilities of individuals with multiple sclerosis. The presence of disturbed language abilities in multiple sclerosis has important implications for the rehabilitation and management of patients with multiple sclerosis in that language disorders may have a considerable negative impact on an individual's daily life. It is essential, therefore, that clinicians take into account when planning their management of clients with multiple sclerosis the impact of possible high-level language impairments on such activities as work, self-care, interpersonal relationships and other aspects of social life beyond the physical disability associated with multiple sclerosis. Further recognition of those people with multiple sclerosis who present with high-level language difficulties will then enable clinicians to develop and make available rehabilitation strategies aimed at maximizing language skills.

Language disorders in Binswanger's disease

Binswanger's disease, also referred to as 'subcortical arteriosclerotic encephalopathy', usually affects older individuals and is characterized by progressive demyelination of subcortical white matter pathways in combination with atherosclerosis of the long penetrating arteries of the deep cerebral white matter. Characteristically, affected individuals are aged between 50 and 70 years with more than 80% having a history of hypertension, diabetes or both. According to neuroanatomical and neuroradiological findings, those areas of the brain most often involved in Binswanger's disease include the white matter in the periventricular (Libon *et al.*, 1990) and frontal areas (Bennett *et al.*, 1990; Forstl, Howard and Levy, 1991).

The clinical features of Binswanger's disease are varied and may include a history of persistent severe hypertension and systemic vascular disease, acute strokes and progressive dementia (Babikian and Ropper, 1987; Caplan, 1988; Yao *et al.*, 1990). Motor disturbances such as pseudobulbar palsy (Caplan, 1988; Ferrer *et al.*, 1990), psychiatric signs and symptoms (Venna *et al.*, 1988) and a gradual accumulation of focal neurological signs including gait disturbance, hemiplegia, hemianopia, sensory disturbances and aphasia (Babikian and Ropper, 1987; Bennett *et al.*, 1990) have also been associated with Binswanger's disease. The course of Binswanger's disease is intermittently progressive with a step-wise decline in intellectual function typically over 3–10 years. Primary treatment is aimed at reducing the risk of dementia and involves treating arterial hypertension, cardiac disease, lipid abnormality and diabetes. In cases

where cerebrovascular disease is identified, secondary treatment involves acute management of stroke and its complications. Prevention of stroke recurrence by appropriate antiplatelet or anticoagulant therapy and addressing primary risk factors are also important. In cases where dementia has developed, cholinesterase inhibitors may be of some benefit.

Although researchers have suggested that overt aphasia is an uncommon clinical sign of the disease (Babikian and Ropper, 1987; Sacquegna *et al.*, 1989; Summergrad and Peterson, 1989), individual cases of Binswanger's disease may exhibit a range of 'aphasic' deficits (DeReuck *et al.*, 1980; Garcia-Albea, Cabello and Franch, 1987; Kertesz, Polk and Carr, 1990; Libon *et al.*, 1990). Subjects with Binswanger's disease have been found to present with language profiles reflecting a non-fluent motor type of aphasia (Huang, Wu and Luo, 1985), fluent Wernicke's aphasia (Leifer, Buonanno and Richardson, 1990) and a mixed aphasia (Garcia-Albea, Cabello and Franch, 1987). More specifically, word-finding difficulties (Kinkel *et al.*, 1985; Libon *et al.*, 1990) and word-fluency deficits (Kinkel *et al.*, 1985; Roman, 1987; Gallassi *et al.*, 1991) have also been identified in Binswanger's disease.

In their study, Sacquegna *et al.* (1989) described subjects with Binswanger's disease who presented without cortical signs of aphasia, apraxia or agnosia and suggested that the dementia of Binswanger's disease is compatible with a so-called subcortical dementia. Traditionally, one of the differential characteristics of cortical dementia (e.g. Alzheimer's disease) and subcortical dementia (e.g. Parkinson's disease and progressive supranuclear palsy) is the presence of language deficits in the clinical profile of individuals with cortical dementia but a relatively rare occurrence of language problems in those with subcortical dementia (Cummings and Benson, 1984; Huber and Paulson, 1985). Murdoch (1990), however, has suggested that individuals with multi-infarct vascular dementia, such as has been reported to occur in Binswanger's disease, may exhibit both subcortical and cortical clinical signs. Similarly, multiple sclerosis subjects with demyelination of subcortical white pathways have been found to present with signs of both cortical and subcortical dementia (Beatty and Monson, 1989).

Although overt aphasia is an uncommon clinical sign of Binswanger's disease, in addition to word-finding difficulties and word-fluency deficits, the presence of subtle, high-level language deficits have been reported to occur in this population (Murdoch and Lethlean, 1996). These latter deficits may include problems with verbal explanation, verbal reasoning, the reconstruction of sentences, the formation of inferences and the interpretation of absurdities, ambiguities and metaphors (Murdoch and Lethlean, 1996). Given that the diffuse subcortical white matter lesions associated with Binswanger's disease appear to be well placed to disrupt ascending and descending connections between cortical and subcortical structures, it was suggested by Murdoch and Lethlean (1996) that the language deficits in Binswanger's disease may reflect a frontal lobe system deficit resulting from multiple disconnections of cortico-striato-pallido-thalamo-cortical loops responsible for language processing (Wallesch and Papagno, 1988). The progression of intellectual deficits which has been identified in Binswanger's disease has also been reported to result from cortical disconnection, most likely caused by hypoperfusion (DeReuck *et al.*, 1980; Roman, 1987) and ischaemic damage (Yao *et al.*, 1990).

The findings of Murdoch and Lethlean (1996) highlight the need for clinicians and researchers to be aware that individuals with Binswanger's disease may develop language problems as their intellectual abilities deteriorate. The importance of this need is made even greater considering that the use of high-level language assessment may assist in the early diagnosis of this potentially treatable disease.

Language disorder in progressive multifocal leukoencephalopathy

Progressive multifocal leukoencephalopathy is a fatal demyelinating disease of the central nervous system caused by a polyomavirus (Koralnik, 2004). The disease tends to occur in immunocompromised individuals secondary to immunosuppressive therapy (Hseuh and Reyes, 1988), autoimmune disorders such as acquired immunodeficiency syndrome (AIDS) (Hseuh and Reyes, 1988; Major *et al.*, 1992), lymphoproliferative diseases (Hseuh and Reyes, 1988) and Hodgkin's disease (Pansky and Allen, 1980). Progressive multifocal leukoencephalopathy has been reported to occur in AIDS at a much higher frequency than in other conditions associated with disorders of the immune system (Krupp *et al.*, 1985), with AIDS accounting for up to 85% of cases (Major *et al.*, 1992). A male-to-female ratio of 7.6 : 1.0 has been reported with the highest incidence of occurrence between the ages of 25 and 50 years (Berger *et al.*, 1998). No effective therapy is currently available, although affected individuals on highly active antiretroviral therapy may experience a prolonged clinical course.

Progressive multifocal leukoencephalopathy has been described as a multiple sclerosis-like disease, typically involving either a relapse–remitting course or, more commonly, fatal progression (Corral *et al.*, 2004). The virus primarily infects oligodendrocytes, resulting in demyelination of the central nervous system. Those parts of the central nervous system most often involved are the cerebral white matter, deep layers of the cortex and corticomedullary junction. Lesions may be of varying size and are most marked in the cerebral subcortical white matter and less frequently affect the cerebellum, optic nerves and spinal cord. The clinical features of progressive multifocal leukoencephalopathy may include focal neurological signs including hemiparesis, ataxia, speech-language disturbances, visual defects, sensory impairments and sometimes seizures (Berger *et al.*, 1987; Hseuh and Reyes, 1988). Deterioration of mental performance (Berger *et al.*, 1987) and presence of dementia (Sutherland, 1981) have also been described.

Although language disturbances have been reported to occur in progressive multifocal leukoencephalopathy (Berger *et al.*, 1987; Hseuh and Reyes, 1988; Llewelyn *et al.*, 1990), assessments of the language utilized in the reported studies have largely been restricted to subjective observations of language abilities. In most cases, the authors have also been non-specific regarding the type of language disorder exhibited by their patients with progressive multifocal leukoencephalopathy. The most detailed and comprehensive language evaluation of a person with progressive multifocal leukoencephalopathy documented to date was that reported by Lethlean and Murdoch (1993b). The major features of the language abilities of the 33-year-old female case they examined included intact auditory comprehension, repetition, reading and writing associated with poor initiation of speech and marked reduction of spontaneous speech in conversation. Naming deficits and impaired performance on high-level language tasks, including verbal reasoning, reconstruction of sentences, formulation of inferences and interpretation of absurdities, ambiguities and metaphors were identified. The findings of Lethlean and Murdoch (1993b) highlight the need for clinicians to be aware that persons with progressive multifocal leukoencephalopathy are at risk of developing language impairments, this need being made even greater given the increasing incidence of AIDS in the general population.

Summary

Although several models describing the role of subcortical structures in language have highlighted the importance of white matter pathways, only in recent times have reports appeared in the literature of language disorders associated with diseases of the cerebral white matter such as multiple sclerosis, Binswanger's disease and progressive multifocal leukoencephalopathy. Individuals with multiple sclerosis have been reported to exhibit a variety of language problems including motor aphasia, global aphasia and a fluent-language disorder with alexia and agraphia. This variation is thought to result from the variable nature of multiple sclerosis with the specific parts of the central nervous system affected varying from one individual to another. Reports also vary concerning the presence or absence of linguistic deficits in multiple sclerosis with both intact and impaired language abilities being reported. Unfortunately, much of the reported research into language function in multiple sclerosis has been based on the use of neuropsychological assessments rather than tests specifically designed to determine linguistic abilities, and consequently the tests employed might not have been sufficiently sensitive to detect high-level linguistic deficits. Those studies that have utilized high-level language test batteries have identified several areas of deficit in high-level language function in multiple sclerosis, including difficulties understanding ambiguous sentences and metaphoric expressions, difficulties making inferences and recreating sentences and poor performance on voluntary and semantic tasks.

Although overt aphasia is an uncommon clinical sign, patients with Binswanger's disease have also been reported to exhibit a range of language profiles, including a non-fluent motor type of aphasia, Wernicke's type aphasia and mixed aphasia as well as high-level language deficits. Naming deficits and impaired performance on high-level language tests have also been documented in progressive multifocal leukoencephalopathy. Overall, these findings suggest that white matter pathways are critical for enabling cortical and subcortical structures to work together in a linked neural network to facilitate normal language processing.

References

Acheson, E.D. (1985) The epidemiology of multiple sclerosis, in *McAlpine's Multiple Sclerosis* (ed. W.B. Matthews), Churchill Livingstone, Edinburgh, pp. 3–27.

Achiron, A., Ziu, I., Djaldetti, R. *et al.* (1992) Aphasia in multiple sclerosis: clinical and radiographic correlations. *Neurology*, **42**, 2195–2197.

Alexander, M.P. and LoVerme, S.R. (1980) Aphasia after left hemisphere intracerebral haemorrhage. *Neurology*, **30**, 1193–1202.

Alexander, M.P., Naeser, M.A. and Palumbo, C.L. (1987) Correlations of subcortical CT lesion sites and aphasia profiles. *Brain*, **110**, 961–991.

Allen, I.V. (1991) Pathology of multiple sclerosis, in *McAlpine's Multiple Sclerosis*, 2nd edn (eds W.B. Matthews, A. Compston, I.V. Allen and C.N. Martyn), Churchill Livingstone, Edinburgh, pp. 341–378.

Anzola, G.P., Bevilaqual, L., Cappa, S.F. *et al.* (1990) Neuropsychological assessment in patients with relapsing–remitting multiple sclerosis and mild functional impairment: correlation with magnetic resonance imaging. *Journal of Neurology, Neurosurgery and Psychiatry*, **53**, 142–145.

Arnott, W.L., Jordan, F.M., Murdoch, B.E. and Lethlean, J.B. (1997) Narrative discourse in multiple sclerosis: an investigation of conceptual structure. *Aphasiology*, **11**, 969–991.

Babikian, V. and Ropper, A.H. (1987) Binswanger's disease: a review. *Stroke*, **18**, 2–12.

Baldwin, R., Luce, T. and Readence, O. (1982) The impact of subschema on metaphorical processing. *Reading Research Quarterly*, **4**, 528–543.

Barkhof, F., Tas, M.W., Frequin, S.T. *et al.* (1994) Limited duration of the effect of methylprednisolone on changes on MRI in multiple sclerosis. *Neuroradiology*, **36**, 382–387.

Batchelor, J.R. (1985) Immunological and pathological aspects, in *McAlpine's Multiple Sclerosis* (ed. W.B. Matthews), Churchill Livingstone, Edinburgh, pp. 281–300.

Bauer, H.J. and Hanefeld, F.A. (1993) *Multiple Sclerosis: its Impact from Childhood to Old Age*, W.B. Saunders, London.

Bayles, K.A. and Tomoeda, C.K. (1991) *Arizona Battery for Communication Disorders of Dementia Test Manual*, Canyonlands, Tucson, AZ.

Beach, C.M. (1991) The interpretation of prosodic patterns at points of syntactic structure ambiguity: evidence for cue trading relations. *Journal of Memory and Language*, **30**, 644–663.

Beatty, W.W., Goodkin, D.E., Hertsgaard, D. and Monson, N. (1990) Clinical and demographic predictors of cognitive performance in multiple sclerosis: do diagnostic type, disease, duration and disability matter? *Archives of Neurology*, **47**, 305–308.

Beatty, W.W. and Monson, N. (1989) Lexical processing in Parkinson's disease and multiple sclerosis. *Journal of Geriatric Psychiatry and Neurology*, **2**, 145–152.

Bennett, D.A., Wilson, R.S., Gilley, D.W. and Fox, J.H. (1990) Clinical diagnosis of Binswanger's disease. *Journal of Neurology, Neurosurgery and Psychiatry*, **53**, 961–965.

Berger, J.R., Kaszovitz, B., Donovan-Post, J.D. and Dickinson, G. (1987) Progressive multifocal leukoencephalopathy associated with human immunodeficiency virus infection. *Annals of Internal Medicine*, **107**, 78–87.

Berger, J.R., Pall, L., Lanska, D. and Whiteman, M. (1998) Progressive multifocal leukoencephalopathy in patients with HIV infection. *Journal of Neurovirology*, **4**, 59–68.

Bernstein, D.K. (1987) Figurative language: assessment strategies and implications for intervention. *Folia Phoniatrica et Logopaedica*, **39**, 130–144.

Blackwood, H.D., LaPointe, L.L., Holtzapple, P. *et al.* (1991) Lexical semantic abilities of individuals with multiple sclerosis and aphasia, in *Clinical Aphasiology* (ed. R.E. Prescott), Pro Ed, Austin, TX, pp. 121–127.

Bock, T.K. (1982) Toward a cognitive psychology of syntax: information processing contributions to sentence formulation. *Psychological Review*, **89**, 1–47.

Burgess, C. and Simpson, G.B. (1988) Cerebral hemispheric mechanisms in the retrieval of ambiguous word meanings. *Brain and Language*, **33**, 86–103.

van den Burg, W., van Zomeren, A.H., Minderhoud, J.M. *et al.* (1987) Cognitive impairment in patients with multiple sclerosis and mild physical disability. *Archives of Neurology*, **44**, 494–501.

Caine, E.D., Bamford, K.A., Schiffer, R.B. *et al.* (1986) A controlled neuropsychological comparison of Huntington's disease and multiple sclerosis. *Archives of Neurology*, **43**, 249–254.

Callanan, M.M., Logsdail, S.J., Ron, M.A. and Warrington, E.K. (1989) Cognitive impairment in patients with clinically isolated lesions of the type seen in multiple sclerosis: a psychometric and MRI study. *Brain*, **112**, 361–374.

Caplan, L.R. (1988) Binswanger's disease. *Current Opinion in Neurology and Neurosurgery*, **1**, 57–62.

Compston, A. (1994) The epidemiology of multiple sclerosis: principles, achievements and recommendations. *Annals of Neurology*, **36** (Suppl. 2), 211–217.

Cook, S.D., Rohowsky-Kochan, C., Bansil, S. and Dowling, P.C. (1995) Evidence for multiple sclerosis as an infectious disease. *Acta Neurologica Scandinavica*, **161**, 34–42.

Corral, I., Quereda, C., Garcia-Villenueva, M. *et al.* (2004) Focal monophasic demyelinating leukoencephalopathy in advanced HIV infection. *European Neurology*, **52**, 36–41.

Crosson, B. (1985) Subcortical functions in language: a working model. *Brain and Language*, **25**, 257–292.

Cummings, J.L. and Benson, D.F. (1984) Subcortical dementia: review of an emerging concept. *Archives of Neurology*, **41**, 874–879.

Damasio, A.R., Damasio, H., Rizzo, M. *et al.* (1982) Aphasia with nonhaemorrhagic lesions in the basal ganglia and internal capsule. *Archives of Neurology,* **39**, 15–20.

Day, T.J., Fisher, A.G. and Mastaglia, F.L. (1987) Alexia with agraphia in multiple sclerosis. *Journal of the Neurological Sciences,* **78**, 343–348.

DeReuck, J., Crevits, L., DeCoster, W. *et al.* (1980) Pathogenesis of Binswanger chronic progressive subcortical encephalopathy. *Neurology,* **30**, 920–928.

De Souza, L. (1990) *Multiple Sclerosis: Approaches to Management,* Chapman and Hall, London.

Dick, G. (1976) The etiology of multiple sclerosis. *Central African Journal of Medicine,* **23**, 129–130.

Ebers, G.C. (1992) Infections and demyelinating disease: editorial overview. *Current Opinions in Neurology and Neurosurgery,* **5**, 173–174.

Ebers, G.C. (1994) Treatment of multiple sclerosis. *The Lancet,* **343**, 275–279.

Ebers, G.C., Bulman, D.E., Sadovnick, A.D. *et al.* (1986) A population-based study of multiple sclerosis in twins. *New England Journal of Medicine,* **315**, 1638–1642.

Ehrlich, J.S. (1988) Selective characteristics of narrative discourse in head-injured and normal adults. *Journal of Communication Disorders,* **21**, 1–9.

Eisen, A. (1983) Neurophysiology in multiple sclerosis. *Neurologic Clinics,* **1**, 615.

Feinstein, A., Kartsounis, L.D., Miller, D.H. *et al.* (1992) Clinically isolated lesions of the type seen in multiple sclerosis: a cognitive, psychiatric and MRI follow up study. *Journal of Neurology, Neurosurgery and Psychiatry,* **55**, 869–876.

Felgenhauer, K., Schadlich, H.J., Nekic, M. and Ackermann, R. (1985) Cerebrospinal fluid antibodies: a diagnostic indicator for multiple sclerosis. *Journal of Neurological Sciences,* **71**, 291–299.

Ferrer, I., Bella, R., Serrano, M.T. *et al.* (1990) Arteriosclerotic leukoencephalopathy in the elderly and its relation to white matter lesions in Binswanger's disease, multi-infarct encephalopathy and Alzheimer's disease. *Journal of Neurological Sciences,* **98**, 37–50.

FitzGerald, F.J., Murdoch, B.E. and Chenery, H.J. (1987) Multiple sclerosis: associated speech and language disorders. *Australian Journal of Human Communication Disorders,* **15**, 15–33.

Forstl, H., Howard, R. and Levy, R. (1991) Binswanger's clinical and neuropathological criteria for 'Binswanger's disease'. *Journal of Neurology, Neurosurgery and Psychiatry,* **54**, 1122–1123.

Francis, D.A. (1993) The current therapy of multiple sclerosis. *Journal of Clinical Pharmacy and Therapeutics,* **18**, 77–84.

Franklin, G.M., Heaton, R.K., Nelson, L.M. *et al.* (1988) Correlation of neuropsychological and MRI findings in chronic progressive multiple sclerosis. *Neurology,* **38**, 1826–1829.

Frazier, L. and Rayner, K. (1987) Resolution of syntactic category ambiguities: eye movements in parsing lexically ambiguous sentences. *Journal of Memory and Language,* **26**, 505–526.

Friedman, J.H., Brem, H. and Mayeaux, R. (1983) Global aphasia in multiple sclerosis. *Annals of Neurology,* **13**, 222–223.

Gallassi, R., Morreale, A., Montagna, P. *et al.* (1991) Binswanger's disease and normal pressure hydrocephalus: clinical and neuropsychological comparison. *Archives of Neurology,* **48**, 1156–1159.

Garcia-Albea, E., Cabello, A. and Franch, O. (1987) Subcortical arteriosclerotic encephalopathy (Binswanger's disease): a report of five cases. *Acta Neurologica Scandinavica,* **75**, 295–303.

Gentner, D. (1983) Structure mapping: a theoretic framework for analogy. *Cognitive Science,* **7**, 155–170.

Glucksberg, S., Kreuz, R.J. and Rho, S. (1986) Context can constrain lexical access: implications for models of language comprehension. *Journal of Experimental Psychology: Learning, Memory and Cognition,* **12**, 323–335.

Hallpike, J.F., Adams, W.M. and Tourtellotte, W.N. (1983) *Multiple Sclerosis,* Chapman and Hall, London.

Hartelius, L., Nord, L. and Buder, E. (1995) Acoustic analysis of dysarthria associated with multiple sclerosis. *Clinical Linguistics and Phonetics,* **9**, 95–120.

Hashimoto, S.A. and Paty, D.W. (1986) Multiple sclerosis. *Disease-a-Month,* **32**, 517–589.

Hauser, S.L., Fleischnick, E., Weiner, H.L. *et al.* (1989) Extended major histocompatibility complex haplotypes in patients with multiple sclerosis. *Neurology,* **39**, 275–277.

Heaton, R.K., Nelson, L.M., Thompson, D.S. *et al.* (1985) Neurological findings in relapsing–remitting and chronic progressive multiple sclerosis. *Journal of Consulting and Clinical Psychology,* **53**, 103–110.

Hogaboam, T.W. and Perfetti, C.A. (1975) Lexical ambiguity and sentence comprehension. *Journal of Verbal Learning and Verbal Behavior,* **14**, 265–274.

Hseuh, C. and Reyes, C.V. (1988) Progressive multifocal leukoencephalopathy. *American Family Physician*, **37**, 129–132.

Huang, K., Wu, L. and Luo, Y. (1985) Binswanger's disease: progressive subcortical encephalopathy or multi-infarct dementia. *Canadian Journal of Neurological Sciences*, **12**, 88–94.

Huber, S.J. and Paulson, G.W. (1985) The concept of subcortical dementia. *American Journal of Psychiatry*, **142**, 1312–1317.

Huber, S.J., Paulson, G.W., Shuttleworth, E.C. *et al.* (1987) Magnetic resonance imaging correlates of dementia in multiple sclerosis. *Archives of Neurology*, **44**, 732–736.

Hutter, C. (1993) On the causes of multiple sclerosis. *Medical Hypotheses*, **41**, 93–96.

Hyman, B.T. and Tranel, D. (1989) Hemianesthesia and aphasia: an anatomical and behavioral study. *Archives of Neurology*, **46**, 816–819.

Ivnik, R.J. (1978) Neuropsychological stability in multiple sclerosis. *Journal of Consulting and Clinical Psychology*, **46**, 913–923.

Jacobs, L., Goodkin, D.E., Rudick, R.A. and Herndon, R. (1994) Advances in specific therapy for multiple sclerosis. *Current Opinions in Neurology*, **7**, 250–254.

Jacobs, L. and Johnson, K.P. (1994) A brief history of the age of interferons as treatment of multiple sclerosis. *Archives of Neurology*, **51**, 1245–1252.

Jambor, K.L. (1969) Cognitive functioning in multiple sclerosis. *British Journal of Psychiatry*, **115**, 765–775.

Jennekens-Schinkel, A., Laboyrie, P.M., Lanser, J.B. and Van Der Velde, E.A. (1990a) Cognition in patients with multiple sclerosis: after four years. *Journal of Neurological Sciences*, **99**, 229–247.

Jennekens-Schinkel, A., Lanser, J.B., Van Der Velde, E.A. and Sanders, E.A. (1990b) Performances of multiple sclerosis patients in tasks requiring language and visuoconstruction: assessment of outpatients in quiescent disease stages. *Journal of the Neurological Sciences*, **95**, 89–105.

Joanette, Y. and Goulet, P. (1990) Narrative discourse in right-brain-damaged right-handers, in *Discourse Ability in Brain Damage* (eds Y. Joanette and H.H. Brownell), Springer-Verlag, New York, pp. 131–153.

Jorgensen, C., Barrett, M., Huisingh, R. and Sachman, L. (1981) *The Word Test: a Test of Expressive Vocabulary and Semantics*, LinguiSystems, Moline, IL.

Kertesz, A., Polk, M. and Carr, T. (1990) Cognition and white matter changes on MRI in dementia. *Archives of Neurology*, **47**, 387–391.

Kinkel, W.R., Jacobs, L., Polachini, I. *et al.* (1985) Subcortical arteriosclerotic encephalopathy (Binswanger's disease): computed tomographic, nuclear magnetic resonance and clinical correlations. *Archives of Neurology*, **42**, 951–959.

Klonoff, H., Clark, C., Oger, J. *et al.* (1991) Neuropsychological performance in patients with mild multiple sclerosis. *Journal of Nervous and Mental Disease*, **179**, 127–131.

Kocsis, J.D. and Waxman, S.G. (1985) Demyelination: causes and mechanisms of clinical abnormality and functional recovery, in *Handbook of Clinical Neurology*, vol. 47 (eds P.J. Vinken, G.W. Bruyn, H.L. Klawans and J.C. Koetsier), Elsevier Science, New York, pp. 29–47.

Koralnik, I.J. (2004) New insights into progressive multifocal leukoencephalopathy. *Current Opinion in Neurology*, **17**, 365–370.

Krupp, L.B., Lipton, R.B., Swerdlow, M.L. *et al.* (1985) Progressive multifocal leukoencephalopathy: clinical and radiographic features. *Annals of Neurology*, **17**, 344–349.

Kurtzke, J.F. (1983) Epidemiology of multiple sclerosis, in *Multiple Sclerosis* (eds J.F. Hallpike, C.W.M. Adams and W.W. Tourtellotte), Williams and Wilkins, Baltimore, pp. 47–96.

Leibowitz, S. (1983) The immunology of multiple sclerosis, in *Multiple Sclerosis* (eds J.F. Hallpike, C.W.M. Adams and W.W. Tourtellotte), Williams and Wilkins, Baltimore, pp. 379–412.

Leifer, D., Buonanno, F.S. and Richardson, E.P. (1990) Clinicopathologic correlations of cranial MRI of periventricular white matter. *Neurology*, **40**, 911–918.

Lethlean, J.B. and Murdoch, B.E. (1993a) Language problems in multiple sclerosis. *Journal of Medical Speech-Language Pathology*, **1**, 47–57.

Lethlean, J.B. and Murdoch, B.E. (1993b) Language function in progressive multifocal leukoencephalopathy: a case study. *Journal of Medical Speech-Language Pathology*, **1**, 27–34.

Lethlean, J.B. and Murdoch, B.E. (1994a) Naming in multiple sclerosis: effects of disease course, duration, age, and education level. *Journal of Medical Speech-Language Pathology*, **2**, 43–56.

Lethlean, J.B. and Murdoch, B.E. (1994b) Naming errors in multiple sclerosis: support for a combined semantic/perceptual deficit. *Journal of Neurolinguistics*, **8**, 207–223.

Lethlean, J.B. and Murdoch, B.E. (1997) Performance of subjects with multiple sclerosis on tests of high level language. *Aphasiology*, **11**, 39–57.

Levasseur, M., Baron, J.C., Sette, G. *et al.* (1992) Brain energy metabolism in bilateral paramedian thalamic infarcts: a PET study. *Brain*, **115**, 795–807.

Libon, D.J., Scanlon, M., Swenson, R. and Coslet, H.B. (1990) Binswanger's disease: some neuropsychological considerations. *Journal of Geriatric Psychiatry and Neurology*, **3**, 31–40.

Lieberman, R.R., Ellenberg, M. and Restum, W.H. (1986) Aphasia associated with verified subcortical lesions: three case reports. *Archives of Physical Medicine and Rehabilitation*, **67**, 410–414.

Llewelyn, J.G., Valentine, A.R., Bradley, C. *et al.* (1990) Multifocal central nervous system lesions and retropharyngeal lymphadenopathy on magnetic resonance imaging: an association that suggested progressive multifocal leukoencephalopathy in a patient with acute aphasia. *British Journal of Radiology*, **63**, 897–899.

Lyon-Caen, O., Jouvent, R., Hauser, S. *et al.* (1986) Cognitive function in recent onset demyelinating diseases. *Archives of Neurology*, **43**, 1138–1141.

Major, E.O., Amemiya, K., Tornatore, C.S. *et al.* (1992) Pathogenesis and molecular biology of progressive multifocal leukoencephalopathy, the JV virus-induced demyelinating disease of the human brain. *Clinical Microbiological Reviews*, **5**, 49–73.

Martin, R. and McFarland, J.F. (1995) Immunological aspects of experimental allergic encephalomyelitis and multiple sclerosis. *Critical Reviews in Clinical Laboratory Science*, **32**, 121–182.

Matthews, W.B., Compston, A., Allen, I.V. and Martyn, C.N. (1991) *McAlpine's Multiple Sclerosis*, Churchill Livingstone, Edinburgh.

McAlpine, D. (1972) *Multiple Sclerosis: a Reappraisal*, Churchill Livingstone, Edinburgh.

McLeod, J.G., Hammond, S.R. and Hallpike, J.F. (1994) Epidemiology of multiple sclerosis in Australia. *Medical Journal of Australia*, **160**, 117–122.

Megens, J., Van Loon J., Goffin, J. and Gybels, J. (1992) Subcortical aphasia from thalamic abscess. *Journal of Neurology, Neurosurgery and Psychiatry*, **55**, 319–321.

Metter, E.J., Riege, W.R., Hanson, W.R. *et al.* (1988) Subcortical structure in aphasia: analysis based on (F18) – fluorodeoxyglucose positron emission to-

mography and computed tomography. *Archives of Neurology*, **45**, 1229–1234.

Meulen, V. and Stephenson, J.R. (1983) The possible role of viral infections in multiple sclerosis and other related demyelinating diseases, in *Multiple Sclerosis* (eds J.F. Hallpike, C.W.M. Adams and W.W. Tourtellotte), Williams and Wilkins, Baltimore, pp. 241–274.

Mitchell, G. (1993) Update on multiple sclerosis therapy. *Medical Clinics of North America*, **77**, 231–249.

Murdoch, B.E. (1990) *Acquired Speech and Language Disorders: a Neuroanatomical and Functional Neurological Approach*, Chapman & Hall, London.

Murdoch, B.E. and Lethlean, J.B. (1996) Language dysfunction in subcortical arteriosclerotic encephalopathy (Binswanger's disease). *Journal of Medical Speech-Language Pathology*, **4**, 275–288.

Noseworthy, J.H. (1991) Therapeutics of multiple sclerosis. *Clinical Neuropharmacology*, **14**, 49–61.

Olmos-Lau, B.N., Ginsberg, M.D. and Geller, J.B. (1977) Aphasia in multiple sclerosis. *Neurology*, **27**, 623–626.

Onifer, W. and Swinney, D.A. (1981) Accessing lexical ambiguities during sentence comprehension: effects of frequency of meaning and contextual bias. *Memory and Cognition*, **9**, 225–236.

van Oosten, B.W., Truyen, L., Barkhof, F. and Polman, C.H. (1995) Multiple sclerosis therapy. *Drugs*, **49**, 200–212.

Pansky, B. and Allen, D.J. (1980) *Review of Neuroscience*, Macmillan, New York.

Parsons, C.L., Lambier, J., Snow, P. *et al.* (1989) Conversational skills in closed head injury: part 1. *Australian Journal of Human Communication Disorders*, **17**, 37–46.

Peyser, J.M., Edwards, K.R., Poser, C.M. and Filskov, S.B. (1980) Cognitive function in patients with multiple sclerosis. *Archives of Neurology*, **37**, 577–579.

Polman, C.H. and Uitdehaag, B.M. (2003) New and emerging treatment options for multiple sclerosis. *Lancet Neurology*, **2**, 563–566.

Poser, C.M. (1994) The epidemiology of multiple sclerosis: a general overview. *Annals of Neurology*, **36** (Suppl. 2), 180–193.

Poser, C.M., Paty, D.W., Scheinberg, L. *et al.* (1983) New diagnostic criteria for multiple sclerosis. *Annals of Neurology*, **13**, 227–231.

Pozzilli, C., Passafiume, D., Bernardi, S. *et al.* (1991) SPECT, MRI and cognitive functions in multiple sclerosis. *Journal of Neurology, Neurosurgery and Psychiatry*, **54**, 110–115.

Raine, C.S. (1977) The etiology and pathogenesis of multiple sclerosis: recent developments. *Pathobiology Annual*, **7**, 347–384.

Rao, S.M. (1986) Neuropsychology of multiple sclerosis: a critical review. *Journal of Clinical and Experimental Neuropsychology*, **8**, 502–542.

Rao, S.M., Glatt, S., Hammeke, T.A. *et al.* (1985) Chronic progressive multiple sclerosis: relationship between cerebral ventricular size and neuropsychological impairment. *Archives of Neurology*, **42**, 678–682.

Rao, S.M., Grafman, J., DiGiulo, D. *et al.* (1993) Memory dysfunction in multiple sclerosis: its relation to working memory, semantic encoding and implicit learning. *Neuropsychology*, **7**, 364–374.

Rao, S.M., Leo, G.J., Bernardin, L. and Unverzagt, F. (1991) Cognitive dysfunction in multiple sclerosis: 1. frequency, patterns and predictions. *Neurology*, **41**, 658–691.

Rivera, V.M. (1986) Multiple sclerosis: is the mystery beginning to unfold? *Postgraduate Medicine*, **79**, 217–232.

Robin, D.A. and Schienberg, S. (1990) Subcortical lesions and aphasia. *Journal of Speech and Hearing Disorders*, **55**, 90–100.

Roman, G.C. (1987) Senile dementia of the Binswanger type: a vascular form of dementia in the elderly. *Journal of the American Medical Association*, **258**, 1782–1788.

Ron, M.A., Callanan, M.M. and Warrington, E.K. (1991) Cognitive abnormalities in multiple sclerosis: a psychometric and MRI study. *Psychological Medicine*, **21**, 59–68.

Ruchkin, D.S., Grafman, J., Krauss, G.L. *et al.* (1994) Event-related brain potential evidence for verbal memory deficit in multiple sclerosis. *Brain*, **117**, 289–305.

Rudick, R. and Goodkin D. (1992) *Treatment of Multiple Sclerosis*, Springer-Verlag, Berlin.

Sacquegna, T., Guttmann, S., Giuliani, S. *et al.* (1989) Binswanger's disease: a review of the literature and a personal contribution. *European Neurology*, **29**, 20–22.

Sadovnick, A.D. (1994) Genetic epidemiology of multiple sclerosis: a survey. *Annals of Neurology*, **36**, S194–S203.

Sadovnick, A.D., Ebers, G.C., Wilson, R.W. and Paty, D.W. (1992) Life expectancy in patients with multiple sclerosis. *Neurology*, **42**, 991–994.

Scolding, N.J. and Franklin, R.J.M. (1998) Axon loss in multiple sclerosis. *Lancet*, **352**, 340–341.

Sherwood, L. (1993) *Human Physiology: from Cells to Systems*, 2nd edn, West Publishing Co., New York.

Simpson, G.B. (1981) Meaning dominance and semantic context in the processing of lexical ambiguity. *Journal of Verbal Learning and Verbal Behavior*, **20**, 120–136.

Simpson, G.B. (1984) Lexical ambiguity and its role in models of word recognition. *Psychological Bulletin*, **96**, 316–340.

Simpson, G.B. and Krueger, M.A. (1991) Selective access of homograph meanings in sentence context. *Journal of Memory and Language*, **30**, 627–643.

Simpson, G.B., Peterson, R.R., Casteel, M.A. and Burgess, C. (1989) Lexical and sentence context effects in word recognition. *Journal of Experimental Psychology: Learning, Memory, and Cognition*, **15**, 88–97.

Spreen, O. and Benton, A.L. (1969) *Neurosensory Center Comprehensive Examination for Aphasia*, University of Victoria, Victoria.

Summergrad, P. and Peterson, B. (1989) Binswanger's disease (part II): pathogenesis of subcortical arteriosclerotic encephalopathy and its relation to other dementing processes. *Journal of Geriatric Psychiatry and Neurology*, **2**, 171–181.

Sutherland, J.M. (1981) *Fundamentals of Neurology*, Griffin Press, Adelaide.

Thompson, A.F., Kennard, C., Swash, M. *et al.* (1989) Relative efficacy of intravenous methylprednisolone and ACTH in the treatment of acute relapse in MS. *Neurology*, **39**, 969–971.

Tienari, P.J. (1994) Multiple sclerosis: multiple etiologies, multiple genes? *Annals of Medicine*, **26**, 259–269.

Venna, N., Mogocsi, S., Jay, M. *et al.* (1988) Reversible depression in Binswanger's disease. *Journal of Clinical Psychiatry*, **49**, 23–26.

Wallace, G.L. and Holmes, S. (1993) Cognitive-linguistic assessment of individuals with multiple sclerosis. *Archives of Physical Medicine and Rehabilitation*, **74**, 637–643.

Wallesch, C.W. (1985) Two syndromes of aphasia occurring with ischaemic lesions involving the left basal ganglia. *Brain and Language*, **25**, 357–361.

Wallesch, C.W. and Papagno, C. (1988) Subcortical aphasia, in *Aphasia* (eds F.C. Rose, R. Whurr and M.A. Wyke), Whurr Publishers, London, pp. 256–287.

Weiner, H.L., Dau, P.C., Khatri, B.O. *et al.* (1989) Double-blind study of true vs sham plasma exchange in patients treated with immunosuppression for acute attacks of multiple sclerosis. *Neurology*, **39**, 1143–1149.

Whitaker, J.N. and Mitchell, G.W. (1997) Clinical features of multiple sclerosis, in *Multiple Sclerosis: Clinical and Pathogenic Basis* (eds C.S. Raine, H.F. McFarland and W.W. Tourtellotte), Chapman and Hall, London, pp. 3–19.

Wiig, E.R. and Secord, W. (1985) *Test of Language Competence*, Merril, Columbus.

Wiig, E.R. and Semel, E.M. (1974) Development of comprehension of logico-grammatical sentences by grade school children. *Perceptual and Motor Skills*, **38**, 175–176.

Wikstrom, M. Kinnunen, E. and Porras, J. (1984) The age-specific prevalence ratio of familial multiple sclerosis. *Neuroepidemiology*, **3**, 74–82.

Yao, H., Sadoshima, S., Kuwabara, Y. *et al.* (1990) Cerebral blood flow and oxygen metabolism in patients with vascular dementia of the Binswanger type. *Stroke*, **21**, 1694–1699.

Neurological disturbances associated with aphasia 8

Introduction

A number of neurological disturbances are commonly encountered in patients with aphasia. These associated neurological disturbances include apraxia, agnosia, alexia, agraphia and Gerstmann syndrome. Although each of these disturbances may occur in isolation, they are most often observed as part of an aphasic disturbance. Where they do occur as part of an aphasia, the associated neurological disorders complicate the clinical features of the aphasia and therefore have important implications for the evaluation and treatment of aphasic patients.

Apraxia

Apraxia is a disorder of learnt movement in which the patient is unable to carry out, at will, a complex or skilled movement that they were previously able to perform, where that inability is not due to paralysis of the muscles, ataxia, sensory loss, comprehension deficits or inattention to commands (Geschwind, 1975). Although both developmental and acquired varieties of apraxia

have been identified, this chapter will describe only the acquired forms of the disorder.

Three major types of apraxia have been identified in the literature. These include ideomotor apraxia, ideational apraxia and limb-kinetic apraxia. In addition, a number of special types of apraxia are also recognized by some authors, including constructional apraxia, dressing apraxia, verbal apraxia and so on. It has been suggested by some authors (e.g. Benson, 1979), however, that many of these special types of apraxia represent either fixed motor or visuospatial disturbances and, therefore, cannot strictly be defined as apraxias.

Ideomotor apraxia

Ideomotor apraxia is the most common type of apraxia. It is essentially a disorder in which language alone is unable to initiate and direct correctly the performance of certain learnt motor tasks that the patient is otherwise able to perform under different circumstances and different sensory inputs. In other words, the patient is unable to carry out motor acts to verbal command but can carry out the same motor tasks at a reflex or automatic level. For example, the individual involved may be unable to carry out various facial expressions, such as a smile or a frown, in response to a verbal command and yet show normal facial expressions in spontaneous situations.

The disorder in movement in ideomotor apraxia cannot be accounted for by muscular weakness, disturbances in tone or posture, incoordination, sensory loss or incomprehension of the verbal command. Further, the disorder may be isolated to particular muscle groups such as the muscles in the buccofacial region (oral apraxia) or respiratory muscles, or it can involve the limbs (limb apraxia) either bilaterally or the non-dominant (left) limb unilaterally, depending on the location of the lesion.

Oral apraxia (buccofacial apraxia) was first described by Jackson (1932) in a patient with aphasia who could not protrude his tongue when asked to, but managed quite well to recover with his tongue a breadcrumb which remained stuck to his lip. Depending on the degree of severity, oral apraxia can interfere with a variety of voluntary non-speech movements of the tongue, pharynx and cheeks. For example, patients may be unable to move their tongues towards the corners of the mouth, the nose, the chin and so on when requested. They may also have trouble moving the tongue to make clicking sounds or the apicoden-

tal 'tsk-tsk'. Some patients with oral apraxia have problems whistling when requested or mimicking laughter and so on. Oral apraxia is commonly associated with Broca's aphasia.

According to Benson (1979), ideomotor apraxia can be demonstrated in as many as 40% of aphasic patients if correctly tested. Apraxia of both buccofacial and limb activities is seen frequently in Broca's aphasia, transcortical motor aphasia and conduction aphasia. Although clinically the presence of ideomotor apraxia in patients with aphasia is often overlooked, it is important that speech-language pathologists recognize that this finding has important implications for the evaluation and treatment of their aphasic patients. Of very real importance is the interference that apraxia produces in the testing of comprehension, particularly if comprehension is tested only through motor activities. For instance, ideomotor apraxia is recognized as another factor which may contribute to a patient's failure of the Token Test. On the other hand, a comprehension defect must be ruled out before an apraxia can be diagnosed.

Ideomotor apraxia is caused by an interruption of pathways between the centre for formulation of a motor act and the motor areas necessary for its execution. These pathways are depicted schematically in Figure 8.1. Briefly, the verbal

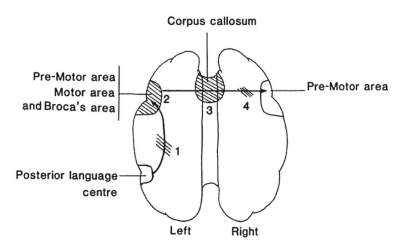

Figure 8.1 Horizontal section of the brain showing the major pathways thought to be involved in the performance of motor acts to strictly verbal commands. 1. Lesion involving the arcuate fasciculus → oral and bilateral limb apraxia. 2. Lesion involving the pre-motor area, motor area and Broca's area → oral and left limb apraxia. 3. Lesion involving the anterior portion of the corpus callosum → left limb apraxia. 4. Lesion in the subcortical white matter of the right hemisphere → left limb apraxia.

command is initially comprehended and interpreted in the posterior language centre and a response formulated. Information is then passed to the pre-motor cortex of the left hemisphere via the association fibres, including the arcuate fasciculus. In the pre-motor cortex, a programme is developed which determines the sequence of muscle contractions required to execute the command. Once developed, information regarding the programme is conveyed to the primary motor cortex of the left hemisphere, which in turn initiates the necessary nerve impulses that pass via the descending motor pathways to the muscles that execute the command. At the same time that information is passed to the primary motor cortex of the dominant hemisphere, the same information must also be directed to the motor areas of the non-dominant hemisphere so that the muscles on the left side of the body (e.g. the muscles of the left hand) can perform the skilled movement commanded if required. This transfer of information from the pre-motor cortex of the dominant hemisphere to the motor areas of the non-dominant hemisphere occurs through the anterior part of the corpus callosum.

Ideomotor apraxia can result from damage at any point along the pathways depicted in Figure 8.1. Depending on the point of disruption, however, the nature of the apraxic disturbance will vary. In the case of a lesion that involves the left inferior parietal lobe, particularly in the area of the supramarginal gyrus, it is likely that the arcuate fasciculus will be involved and a conduction aphasia will result (see Chapter 2). In addition, however, in most cases the patient will also have an ideomotor apraxia that involves all four limbs and the buccofacial muscles, since neither the right nor the left pyramidal motor system is able to receive information from the posterior language area. Depending on the extent of the lesion, in some cases the limbs are not affected or are only minimally involved.

A lesion involving the anterior language centre and primary motor strip of the left hemisphere, as may occur in cases of Broca's aphasia, precludes apraxia testing in the right limbs because of the presence of a concomitant right hemiplegia. In this instance, the patient exhibits a buccofacial and left-limb apraxia, since the right motor system is unable to receive information from the posterior language centre. On the other hand, a lesion in the anterior corpus callosum disconnects the right pre-motor and pyramidal motor cortices from the left hemisphere, thereby rendering the patient apraxic in the left limbs (callosal apraxia). Since the nuclei of the cranial nerves (with the exception of the nucleus supplying the lower part of the face) receive bilateral upper motor neurone innervation (see Chapter 9), the patient in this case should not exhibit buccofacial apraxia. Lesions located in the subcortical white matter of the right hemisphere which disconnect the fibres which have passed through the corpus callosum may also cause left-limb apraxia.

The motor performance of patients with ideomotor apraxia usually improves when they are asked to imitate the clinician's movements. Even so, the improvement in motor performance is usually only partial. In cases where the movement involves the use of an object (e.g. hammering), motor performance also usually improves if the patient is given the actual object to use. In these circumstances, the apraxic patient is able to bypass their language-motor disconnections through intact visual and somesthetic connections to the pyramidal motor cortices.

Patients with ideomotor apraxia do not present with any particular difficulties in performing spontaneous movements in everyday life. Consequently, the disorder does not produce any symptoms as such. Generally, the defective buccofacial and limb movements are only disclosed by specific testing.

Ideational apraxia

Ideational apraxia is a disorder of gestural behaviour which involves the loss of the ability to formulate the ideational plan for the execution of the components of a complex act (Liepmann, 1908). In this disorder, the individual component movements of a complex act cannot be synthesized into a purposeful plan, even though the simple isolated component movements may be performed normally. In some cases, the individual component movements may be performed in a faulty sequence, or portions only of the complex act may be performed. Occasionally, the patient with ideational apraxia may perform an action similar to, but not the same as, the one required. For example, patients affected with such an apraxia are incapable of carrying out a task such as making a cup of coffee, lighting a candle with a match and so on. One example described by Miller (1986) was that of a woman who, when attempting to light her gas stove, first lit the match, then blew it out and then turned on the gas, which she left going. According to Miller, she was only prevented from either gassing herself or causing an explosion by the intervention of a neighbour. On another occasion the same woman, again while lighting the gas stove, turned on the gas, then filled the kettle and finally struck a match causing a minor explosion. Clearly, in this case, although the woman was capable of performing each of the partial acts comprising the overall action, their sequencing and planification were deranged.

Unlike patients with ideomotor dyspraxia, where the disorder is not evident in everyday life, ideational apraxics stand out as being abnormal even in everyday activities. Clearly, owing to the poor sequencing of movements in a complex act, there is often a great potential for serious injury to be inflicted (e.g. the gas may be turned on prior to filling the kettle when making a cup of coffee; machinery may be started before safety procedures are performed). Patients with ideational apraxia are able to imitate an action in that, in such situations, the plan of the action is provided to them from outside.

Ideational apraxia is always manifested bilaterally and rarely occurs as an isolated phenomenon. Clinically, it is most often observed as a manifestation of diffuse brain disorders (e.g. cerebral arteriosclerosis), although in some cases it has been reported secondary to focal brain lesions (Poeck and Lehmkuhl, 1980). Ideational apraxia may co-occur with other apraxias (especially ideomotor apraxia), making it difficult to distinguish clinically and is most often seen by speech-language pathologists as part of either a severe aphasia or a dementia syndrome.

Limb-kinetic apraxia

Limb-kinetic apraxia (also called 'kinetic apraxia') was first described by Liepmann (1908) and is characterized by an inability to execute acquired fine-motor movements. The disturbance is often confined to one limb and in most cases affects the finer movements of the distal portions of one upper extremity. Furthermore, the impairment is present in automatic as well as volitional acts. Movements affected include those required for tasks such as writing, doing up buttons, sewing, playing musical instruments, opening a safety pin and so on.

Commonly seen as part of a Broca's aphasia, limb-kinetic apraxia is associated with lesions in the pre-motor area of the cerebral cortex. Consequently, it manifests unilaterally on the side contralateral to the corresponding lesion. It may co-occur with an ideomotor apraxia.

Liepmann (1908) suggested that limb-kinetic apraxia results from the loss of the so-called kinetic memories for a single limb. Subsequently, however, several authors have excluded it from the true apraxias (Kerschensteiner, Poeck and Lehmkuhl, 1975). Most contemporary authors regard it as a pyramidal movement disorder rather than an apraxia.

Constructional apraxia

In this type of apraxia, the patient is unable to form a construction in space. Miller (1986, p. 56), defined constructional apraxia as 'a disorder of planned movements for any kind of task involving the structuring or arranging of objects, parts of objects or lines in two and three dimensional space'. Patients with this disorder, therefore, are unable to copy simple geometric figures by drawing or by the arrangement of blocks, matches and so on. In the more severe cases, patients are not even able to draw such simple geometric figures as squares, circles and crosses. In general, patients are not aware of their inability to perceive spatial relationships.

In the majority of cases, constructional apraxia is associated with lesions in either of the parietal lobes, although constructional deficits have occasionally been described secondary to frontal lobe lesions. As an isolated disorder, it is more common following lesions of the non-dominant (right) hemisphere, in which case the disturbances associated with this condition also tend to be more severe. For instance, individuals with lesions in the right parietal lobe tend to produce drawings which, although elaborate, tend to be done hastily and without care. In addition, the presence of a model is of no help and disorientation on the page is marked and neglect of the left-hand side of the page is regularly observed. Further, the axes of the figures tend to be grossly disturbed.

In contrast, in those cases where the lesion involves the dominant (left) hemisphere, the individual involved tends to produce drawings which are carefully done but poor in content. With the aid of a model, however, the diagram may be more elaborate. In addition, the axes of the figures are more truly represented than in the drawings of patients with right parietal lesions. Neglect of the right-hand side of the page occurs without exception. Frequently there may be (associated with a constructional apraxia due to a lesion of the dominant hemisphere, in addition to an apraxia), all or some of the elements of a Gerstmann syndrome (see below).

Constructional apraxia is of importance to the speech-language pathologist in that, when it co-occurs with an aphasia, it has important implications for the assessment and clinical management of the aphasic patient. For instance, the presence of a constructional apraxia affects the performance of the aphasic individual on tests used by speech-language pathologists and related professionals and which require use of the patient's constructional abilities. For example, performance of the patient on the supplementary non-language tests of the Boston Diagnostic Aphasia Examination (Goodglass and Kaplan, 1983), which include construction of three-dimensional block designs, tests of drawing to command and stick constructions, could reasonably be expected to be influenced by the presence of a constructional apraxia.

Dressing apraxia

Dressing apraxia is a disturbance in which patients cannot dress because they are unable to relate the parts of the garment to the parts of their bodies. This disturbance is seen most frequently in association with lesions in the parietal lobe of the non-dominant (right) hemisphere, although it has also been reported to follow left parietal lesions. Dressing apraxia is often accompanied by a constructional apraxia and may co-occur with aphasia. In some cases the dressing apraxia is further complicated by the presence of a hemiplegia, hemianaesthesia, hemineglect and visual-field defects.

Apraxia of speech

Apraxia of speech is an acquired neurological speech disorder that is primarily characterized by articulatory disturbances (e.g. sound distortions and distorted sound substitutions), prolonged segment (i.e. vowel or consonant) and intersegment (i.e. time between sound, syllables, etc.) durations as well as a slow rate of speech, in the absence of neuromuscular deficits (e.g. reduced muscle tone, abnormal or absent reflexes, etc.) and language difficulties (McNeil, Robin and Schmidt, 1997; McNeil, Pratt and Fossett, 2004). Darley (1968) is often credited as being the first to introduce the term 'apraxia of speech' to describe a motor speech disorder that did not fit the accepted characteristics of the then recognized neurologically based speech production disorders, namely dysarthria and aphasia. Darley (1982) attributed apraxia of speech to a disorder of motor speech programming, describing it as 'a disorder in which the patient has trouble speaking because of a cerebral lesion that prevents his executing voluntarily and on command the complex motor activities in speaking, despite the fact that muscle strength is undiminished' (p. 10). Later, McNeil, Robin and Schmidt (1997) defined apraxia of speech as 'a phonetic-motoric disorder of speech production caused by inefficiencies in the translation of well-formed and filled phonologic frame to previously learned kinematic parameters assembled for carrying out the intended movement, resulting in intra- and interarticulator temporal and spatial segmental and prosodic distortions' (p. 329). Although there is now reasonable agreement on the features that differentiate apraxia of speech from dysarthria and aphasia (see sections below), researchers continue to disagree upon the underlying nature of apraxia of speech. While some researchers assert that apraxia of speech can be attributed to a phonological encoding deficit, others argue that its locus is motoric.

Clinical characteristics of apraxia of speech

Apraxia of speech is manifested primarily by errors in articulation and secondarily by what are thought by many researchers to be compensatory alterations of prosody (e.g. pauses, slow speech rate, equalization of stress, etc.). Articulation errors, therefore, are the primary features of this motor speech disorder. As they speak, patients with apraxia of speech struggle to correctly position their articulators. As they struggle, affected individuals appear to visibly and audibly grope to achieve the correct individual articulatory postures and sequence of articulatory postures to produce sounds and words, a problem thought to reflect difficulties in the spatial and temporal targeting of articulatory postures. The resulting articulation, however, is frequently off-target. As patients with apraxia of speech are aware of their articulatory mistakes, however, they usually attempt to correct them. Often, these attempted corrections are also erroneous, but importantly are not always the same as the original error in articulation. In fact, on a series of trials, the articulatory errors exhibited by individuals with apraxia of speech are highly variable. For example, the initial consonant v may, at different times, be produced by the same individual as v, z, p, f, r, b, h and w. Although on occasions patients with apraxia of speech are able to produce all phonemes correctly, at times the substitution of incorrect phonemes (literal paraphasias) as in-

dicated occurs frequently and inconsistently. It should be noted that, by using broad phonetic transcriptions to record what was heard with the naked ear, the majority of the original researchers who reported the perceptual features of apraxia of speech suggested that articulatory errors seen in these cases involve substitutions rather than the distortion of individual phonemes, as occurs in dysarthria (see Chapters 9, 10 and 11) (Johns and Darley, 1970; Trost and Canter, 1974; LaPointe and Johns, 1975). More recent studies, however, have disputed this finding, suggesting that vowel and consonant distortions, often caused by prolonged segment and intersegment durations, comprise the majority of apraxic speech errors (Odell *et al.*, 1990, 1991; McNeil, Robin and Schmidt, 1997; McNeil, Pratt and Fossett, 2004). The discrepancy between sound substitution errors and sound distortion errors may have been the result of 'phonemic false evaluation', whereby listeners classify phones in terms of categorical perception (i.e. listeners designate speech errors to an appropriate category and ignore those features not required for categorization). In addition, phonemic transcription was used as the basis of notation for phonemic errors in early investigations of apraxia of speech (LaPointe and Johns, 1975). Only phonetic transcription, however, is capable of detecting the sound distortions produced by participants with apraxia of speech (McNeil, Pratt and Fossett, 2004; Duffy, 2005). Thus, in the past, many of the sound-level distortions could have been incorrectly classified as sound substitution errors (McNeil, Pratt and Fossett, 2004). The differentiation between phonemic substitution errors and phonetic distortion errors is crucial to our understanding of the underlying nature of articulatory deficits in apraxia of speech. In contrast to phonemic substitution errors, which are generally assigned to the phonological encoding level of speech production models, phonetic distortion errors are considered to be of motoric nature (Odell *et al.*, 1990; McNeil, Pratt and Fossett, 2004). Indeed, McNeil, Pratt and Fossett (2004) postulated that 'sound distortions are at least partially a result of deficits in anticipatory coarticulation and extended segment and intersegment durations' (p. 396).

The number of articulatory errors exhibited by patients with apraxia of speech is greater during repetition than during conversational speech (Rosenbek, Kent and LaPointe, 1984). Consequently, apraxia of speech is most clearly illustrated when the patient is asked to repeat spoken language. Further, a number of studies have indicated that articulation in apraxia of speech is influenced by phonetic complexity, word position and word length with the number of articulatory errors produced by individuals with apraxia of speech increasing as the complexity of the articulatory exercise increases. Fewer errors, for instance, occur in the production of vowels than during the production of single consonants, with the greatest number of articulatory errors occurring during the production of consonant clusters (Trost and Canter, 1974; LaPointe and Johns, 1975; Burns and Canter, 1977; Dunlop and Marquardt, 1977; Wertz, LaPointe and Rosenbek, 1984). Repetition of a single consonant such as 'puh', 'tuh' or 'kuh' is ordinarily more easily accomplished by these patients than the repetition of the sequence puh–tuh–kuh (Rosenbek, Wertz and Darley, 1973). Further, some researchers have reported initial consonant phonemes to be misarticulated more often than final consonant phonemes (Johns and Darley, 1970; Trost and Canter, 1974; Odell *et al.*, 1991), while others have noted the word medial position to be most susceptible to error (Odell *et al.*, 1990).

Some authors have reported that palatal and dental consonants and low back vowels are significantly more susceptible to misarticulation than other phonemes are (e.g. alveolar, labiodental, bilabial and velar phonemes) in patients with apraxia of speech (LaPointe and Johns, 1975; Odell *et al.*, 1990, 1991). Also, phonemes occurring with a relatively high frequency in the English language tend to be more accurately articulated than phonemes which occur less often (Trost and Canter, 1974; Wertz, LaPointe and Rosenbek, 1984). The number of articulatory errors produced by these patients has also been found to increase as the length of the word increases with a higher incidence of articulatory errors being reported in the production of polysyllabic words than monosyllabic words (Johns and Darley, 1970; Deal and Darley, 1972). For example, as these patients produce a series of words with an increasing number of syllables (e.g. door, doorknob, doorkeeper, dormitory), more errors occur during the production of the longer words (Johns and Darley, 1970). Although speakers with apraxia of speech exhibit a high degree of inconsistency in their error productions, the majority of articulatory errors are reported to be close approximations to the target sound (Odell *et al.*, 1990).

In addition to the impairment in articulation, the prosodic features of the speech of patients with apraxia of speech are also disturbed. The prosodic deficits occur as a result of the fact that as these patients speak they slow down their rate of speech, space their words and syllables more evenly and stress each of them more equally in an attempt to avoid articulatory errors (Darley, Aronson and Brown, 1975). The non-fluent speech output observed in these patients is primarily caused by the pausing and hesitating that occurs as the person gropes for articulatory placement and makes repeated efforts to produce words correctly.

Patients with apraxia of speech display a marked discrepancy between their relatively good performance at automatic and reactive speech productions and their relatively poor volitional-purposive speech performance. These patients have been reported to sound normal when producing words and phrases that are well known to them through either practice or usage (Schuell, Jenkins and Jiminez-Pabon, 1964). For instance, on those occasions where these patients are either speaking off-hand or reciting an over-learnt expression or reacting to sudden stimulus, they may produce words without articulatory inaccuracy or groping (e.g. when counting, swearing, repeating rhymes and jingles, etc. and uttering greetings and farewells). In contrast, these same patients exhibit effortful and off-target groping in spontaneous speech when they are required to select a particular target word. Deal (1974) reported that patients with apraxia of speech exhibit both a consistency effect and an adaptation effect when required to read the same material repeatedly. Although during the performance of such a task these patients tend to produce their articulation errors in the same place from trial to trial, they also tend to make fewer errors on successive readings.

Neuropathology of apraxia of speech

Single left-hemisphere stroke has been identified as the most common cause of apraxia of speech (Duffy, 2005). Specifically, 41% of the 155 persons who had a primary speech pathology diagnosis of apraxia of speech had suffered a single stroke; lesions in the area of the left middle cerebral artery distribution were commonly associated with apraxia of speech (Duffy, 2005). An additional 8% of persons had endured multiple strokes that involved the left hemisphere, and the remaining 51% had disorders of degenerative or traumatic nature (20 and 15%, respectively), a tumour (15%) or a different cause (e.g. seizure disorder; 6%) (Duffy, 2005).

Recent evidence suggests that apraxia of speech is related to lesions in the left frontal, parietal and/or temporal cortex, and the left subcortex (i.e. striatal, capsular, caudate regions) (Square-Storer, Roy and Martin, 1997; Duffy, 2005). More specifically, Square-Storer, Roy and Martin (1997) outlined six areas that when lesioned could result in apraxia of speech. These included the pre-motor area and supplementary motor cortex, pars opercularis, insula, parietal lobe and lenticular nucleus (Square-Storer, Roy and Martin, 1997). There has been some suggestion that the insula must be implicated in order for apraxia of speech to occur (Dronkers, 1996; Ogar *et al.*, 2006); however, other studies have reported cases of apraxia of speech that have not involved insular damage (Hillis *et al.*, 2004).

Some researchers have reported lesion data for participants with apraxia of speech (Ziegler and von Cramon, 1986; McNeil *et al.*, 1990). Ziegler and von Cramon (1986) reported the site of lesion for eight patients with apraxia of speech. They noted that the anterior limb of the internal capsule ($n = 3$), the caudate nucleus ($n = 2$), putamen ($n = 3$), superior thalamic peduncle ($n = 3$), external capsules ($n = 6$) and the arcuate fascicle ($n = 8$) were the primary areas lesioned in their participant group. Similarly, McNeil *et al.* (1990) reported a combination of the following lesion sites for four participants with apraxia of

speech: the pre-motor cortex ($n = 1$), Broca's area ($n = 2$), pre-central gyrus ($n = 2$), post-central gyrus ($n = 3$), superior parietal ($n = 2$), supramarginal gyrus ($n = 2$), angular gyrus ($n = 1$), Wernicke's area ($n = 1$), middle temporal gyrus ($n = 1$), insula ($n = 2$), lenticular nuclei ($n = 1$) and posterior internal capsule ($n = 1$). As evident from these studies, apraxia of speech cannot be attributed to a single lesion site. Lesions of a subcortical and/or cortical nature could potentially result in apraxia of speech.

Differential diagnosis of apraxia of speech

Although apraxia of speech can be considered a unique disorder, it is important to recognize that pure apraxia of speech (i.e. apraxia of speech occurring in isolation) is extremely rare, the condition in most cases occurring in combination with other communication disorders (Duffy, 2005). Of 155 quasirandomly selected patients with a primary diagnosis of apraxia of speech, Duffy (2005) identified a concomitant aphasia in 72% of patients, and a concomitant dysarthria, most typically spastic dysarthria, in 29% of patients. Non-verbal oral apraxia was identified in 63% of 107 patients with a primary diagnosis of apraxia of speech (Duffy, 2005). Dronkers (1996) reported a higher incidence of concomitant aphasia and dysarthria. Specifically, aphasia was present in 92% of the 25 patients diagnosed with apraxia of speech, and dysarthria was present in 40% of cases (Dronkers, 1996). Non-verbal oral apraxia was detected in 48% of patients with apraxia of speech (Dronkers, 1996). Of 48 participants with a primary diagnosis of apraxia of speech between 1999 and 2001, Duffy (2005) reported that only four did not present with a concomitant communication deficit.

Apraxia of speech occurring in isolation, therefore, is unquestionably rare and the differential diagnosis of the condition complicated by the high incidence of comorbidity. This difficulty in differential diagnosis has to a large extent been responsible for the numerous and varied terminologies that have been used to describe apraxia of speech (Table 8.1) since the first reports of Paul Broca in 1861. Broca (1861) applied the term

Table 8.1 History of terminology used to describe apraxia of speech organized according to language or speech terminology.

Language	↔	Speech
Aphemia (Broca)	1861	
Aphasia (Trousseau)	1864	Speechlessness (Jackson)
Motor aphasia (Wernicke)	1874	
Subcortical motor aphasia (Lichtheim)	1885	
	1900	Motor apraxia of the glosso-labio-pharyngeal apparatus (Liepman)
	1906	Anarthria (Marie)
	1908	Apraxia of articulation (Wilson)
Pure motor aphasia (Dejerine)	1914	
Motor aphasia (von Monakow)		
Aphemia (Henschen)	1920	
Verbal aphasia (Head)	1923	
	1934	Pure word muteness (Kleist)
Predominantly expressive aphasia (Weisenberg and McBride)	1935	
	1939	Phonetic disintegration of speech (Alajouanine, Ombredane and Durand)
	1947	Apraxic dysarthria (Nathan)
Peripheral motor aphasia (Goldstein)	1948	
	1952	Articulatory dyspraxia (Critchley)
	1962	Cortical dysarthria (Bay)
	1963	Apraxia of speech sounds (Mayo Clinic)
	1964	Cortical dysarthria (Whitty)
	1965	Apraxia of vocal expression (Denny-Brown)
	1966	Phonetic disintegration (Shankweiler and Harris)
	1968	Apraxia of speech (Darley)
Afferent motor aphasia (Luria)	1970	
Phonematic aphasia (Hecaen)	1972	

'aphemia' to the speech disorder exhibited by two of his patients, Leborgne and Lelong, who were unable to produce any spontaneous speech, other than the perseverative utterance 'tan' in the former and a small set of monosyllables in the latter, in the absence of muscular paralysis, poor comprehension and reduced intelligence. Since that time, controversy has centred on the differentiation of apraxia of speech from aphasia, which has been reflected in the terminology used to describe apraxia of speech with a language bias by some authors and a speech bias by others (Table 8.1).

Differentiation of apraxia of speech from aphasia

Clinically, apraxia of speech is most frequently observed as part of an aphasia syndrome, particularly either a Broca's or conduction apha-
sia. When it occurs without aphasia, apraxia of speech is a 'uni-modality disorder', affecting speech out of proportion to other language modalities (Halpern, Darley and Brown, 1973). Tests of performance in various language modalities (i.e. reading, writing and speaking) reveal that, in these patients, speaking performance is significantly worse than performance in listening, reading and writing. On the other hand, in aphasic patients a more widespread disturbance of language function is seen, disturbances being evident in reading and writing as well as speaking. It was his observation of the disproportionate impairment of speaking in his two patients that led Broca (1861) to call this disorder 'aphemia' in an attempt to distinguish it from what he called 'verbal amnesia' in which there was considered to be a general impairment of language function.

According to Mohr (1976), although apraxia of speech has a number of features in common with Broca's aphasia, it is associated with a lesser degree of comprehension loss (there may be none demonstrable) and agrammatism. In addition, as indicated in Chapter 2, Mohr *et al.* (1975) have shown that apraxia of speech is associated with lesions restricted to Broca's area, whereas Broca's aphasia is produced by more extensive lesions, which usually involve the territory of the upper division of the middle cerebral artery.

Patients with apraxia of speech retain the ability to process meaningful linguistic units, and, although they may have difficulty in articulating a particular word, it can be easily demonstrated that the articulation problem is not related to a word-finding difficulty. For instance, the patient may be able to write the word that they have difficulty articulating. In addition, they are able to choose the word in question from among a group of words when given a choice. Halpern, Darley and Brown (1973) found that patients with apraxia of speech performed significantly better than aphasics did on auditory retention and naming tasks. These same authors also reported that apraxic patients were better than aphasics on writing to dictation and syntax and fluency tasks. Apraxia of speech, therefore, is an independent and separate disorder from aphasia (Darley, 1975), being a motor speech disorder rather than a language disorder.

In addition to occurring concurrently with an aphasic syndrome, apraxia of speech may also occur in association with an oral apraxia (i.e. an apraxia involving the muscles of the buccofacial area in non-speech movements). Although apraxia of speech may occur independently of oral apraxia, when an oral apraxia is demonstrated in patients, an apraxia of speech is also usually present.

Differentiation of apraxia of speech from dysarthria

Apraxia of speech and dysarthria are both motor speech disorders but each represents a breakdown at a different level of speech production. Apraxics, on neurological examination, show no significant evidence of slowness, weakness in coordination, paralysis or alteration of tone of the muscles of the speech mechanism that can account for the associated speech disturbance. Dysarthric patients, on the other hand, dependent on the type of dysarthria present, may exhibit either hyper- or hypotonus of the speech muscles, ataxia, a restricted range of movement and so on (see Chapters 9, 10 and 11). Whereas dysarthric patients show variable disturbances in all of the basic motor processes which underlie speech production, including respiration, phonation, resonation, articulation and prosody, in apraxia of speech the continuing impairment is specifically articulatory, with prosodic alterations at times occurring as compensatory phenomena.

One further difference between apraxia of speech and dysarthria lies in the nature of the articulatory errors seen in each disorder. In dysarthria, the articulatory errors are, characteristically, errors of simplification (e.g. distortions or omissions), whereas in apraxia of speech the articulatory errors largely take the form of complications of speech (e.g. substitution of one phoneme for another, additions of phonemes, repetition of phonemes and prolongations of phonemes).

Alexia and agraphia

Alexia and agraphia represent two separate disorders of written language. In general, disorders encountered in written language parallel those of the oral modalities in brain-damaged patients (Assal, Buttet and Jolivet, 1981). Dissociations between oral and written language disorder, however, have been reported, and reading and writing disturbances, although usually encountered as part of an aphasia syndrome, can occur as isolated language deficits (Hier and Mohr, 1977). When it occurs in isolation, a reading disturbance caused by brain damage is referred to as an 'alexia'. On the other hand, an isolated inability to write, as a result of brain damage, is called an 'agraphia'.

Four kinds of alexia are commonly described in the literature: alexia without agraphia, alexia with agraphia, frontal alexia and deep alexia.

Alexia without agraphia

Alexia without agraphia is a rare type of alexia which also goes by the names of occipital alexia, pure alexia, agnosic alexia and pure word blindness. The disorder is characterized in most cases by a severe reading disorder contrasted with preserved writing abilities. Patients with this disorder are unable to read aloud or cannot comprehend what they read but retain the ability to name seen objects, write spontaneously and copy written material slowly and slavishly despite being unable to read what they have written. These patients are better able to read letters than words, and letters in isolation better than letter strings. In some cases, the affected individual is able to understand commonly written words such as the name of the city where they live, their own name and commonly used language symbols. A colour-naming difficulty involving both an inability to name seen colours or match colours to a given name in the presence of an ability to sort and match colours normally and to use colour names in conversation is a variable finding in patients with alexia without agraphia.

Dejerine (1892) proposed that alexia without agraphia is caused by an inability to transfer visually perceived language stimuli from the primary visual areas to an area in the left hemisphere involved in the interpretation of visual language. This latter area is thought to be located in the angular gyrus of the left cerebral hemisphere. The underlying brain lesion in cases of alexia without agraphia usually involves the left medial occipital lobe (including the left primary visual cortex – Brodmann area 17) and either the splenium of the corpus callosum or the subcortical white matter adjacent and inferior to the splenium (Dejerine, 1891; Vignolo, 1983) (Figure 8.2). The usual pathology associated with the condition is a cerebrovascular accident involving occlusion of the posterior cerebral artery; however, the syndrome has also been described in association with tumours and arteriovenous malformations (Benson, 1979).

The lesion, as shown in Figure 8.2, disconnects the right posterior occipital lobe from communication with the left hemisphere via the splenium. In addition, the damage to the left primary vi-

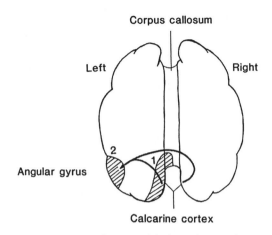

Figure 8.2 Horizontal section of the brain showing the major pathways connecting the primary visual cortex to the angular gyrus. 1. Lesion involving the left primary visual cortex and splenium of the corpus callosum → alexia without agraphia. 2. Lesion involving the angular gyrus of the dominant hemisphere → alexia with agraphia.

sual cortex produces a right hemianopia (defective vision or blindness in half of the visual field). The left visual cortex monitors events in the right visual field and hence, when damaged, as in patients with alexia without agraphia, is associated with the loss of the right visual field in each eye. As the right primary visual cortex is not involved in the lesion, however, patients are able to see in their left visual field. Owing to the involvement of the splenium, however, visual information perceived in the right primary visual cortex cannot be passed to the area in the left cerebral hemisphere involved in the interpretation of visual language (i.e. the angular gyrus). Consequently, even though patients are able to see written words with their left visual field, they are unable to comprehend the meaning of the words because of the disconnection between the right visual cortex and the left angular gyrus. Since the lesion does not involve the central or pericentral speech areas, no aphasic defects in spoken language occur and hence the patient with alexia without agraphia is able to spell words and recognize verbally spelt words. These patients can also recognize individual letters when they are drawn in the palm or when they are palpated from embossed blocks. Object-naming abilities are also preserved and, oddly enough, most of these patients are able to read Arabic numbers (Brown, 1974). However, these patients are unable to read sentences and passages they are able to write spontaneously unless they have been memorized.

Although the course of alexia without agraphia is variable, many patients show a slow and persistent improvement. Reading ability, however, rarely returns to normal.

Alexia with agraphia

Alexia with agraphia, also called 'parietal alexia' or 'parietal temporal alexia', was first described by Dejerine (1891). His case manifested an almost total inability to read, a limited writing ability, a mild aphasia and a calculation disturbance (acalculia). The loss of the ability to read is almost invariably severe in cases of alexia with agraphia, both the ability to read out loud and the ability to comprehend written language being disturbed. In addition, the reading disturbance often includes words, letters, numbers and musical notes, although the degree of impairment in the latter two categories varies from case to case (Benson, 1979). Unlike the majority of patients with alexia without agraphia, individuals with alexia with agraphia are unable to comprehend words spelt aloud (Brown, 1974). Likewise, they are unable to understand symbols such as letters and numbers presented via tactile means.

As suggested by the name of the condition, a writing disturbance is an important component of alexia with agraphia. In some cases it appears that writing is less disturbed than reading, while in others the reading and writing disorders are roughly equivalent in terms of severity. Usually, however, the writing disturbance is not so severe that the patient is unable to produce written letters. The writing is, however, invariably paragraphic, consisting of recognizable letters combined into unrecognizable words. Although patients with alexia with agraphia can produce written letters spontaneously, unlike persons with alexia without agraphia they are unable to write to dictation or at least produce a paragraphic output in this situation. Also in contrast to patients with alexia without agraphia, these patients show a significant disturbance in their ability to copy written material. While patients

with alexia without agraphia copy slowly and slavishly but correctly, persons with alexia with agraphia usually make mistakes in reproducing the actual form of the letters.

Dejerine (1891) localized the neuropathology in alexia with agraphia to the angular gyrus of the dominant (left) cerebral hemisphere. Although a variety of aetiologies, including cerebrovascular accidents, neoplastic disease and head trauma, may produce this syndrome, reports in the literature suggest that involvement of the dominant angular gyrus is a constant finding (Benson and Geschwind, 1969). The most common aetiology is a cerebrovascular accident which, in the majority of cases, involves occlusion of the angular branch of the left middle cerebral artery (Benson, 1979).

As the lesion associated with alexia with agraphia involves the posterior language centre, this syndrome is usually but not always accompanied by some form of aphasia. Often, the associated aphasic disturbance takes the form of an anomic aphasia; however, on occasions a Wernicke's aphasia is present in these cases. In addition to aphasia, a number of patients with alexia with agraphia exhibit either a full or a partial Gerstmann syndrome (see below). A visual-field defect in the form of either a hemianopia or quadrantanopsia, although not an invariable finding, is present in some cases.

The prognosis for recovery from alexia with agraphia varies depending on the underlying aetiology and size of the brain lesion. In some cases, a relatively rapid recovery of some or all reading skills occurs. The majority of these patients, however, show only a partial recovery.

Frontal alexia

Benson (1977) described a third kind of alexia which is present in individuals with frontal lobe pathology. Called 'frontal alexia', this syndrome differs in a number of ways from the two classical alexias first documented by Dejerine, which were described above. According to Benson (1979), the majority of patients with frontal alexia are able to comprehend some written material. In particular, these patients can usually read aloud and comprehend some individual words, especially nouns or action verbs, within a written sentence. As an example, Benson (1979) indicated that patients with frontal alexia in some cases are able to decipher newspaper headlines but are unable to understand the sentences that make up the article.

Although patients with frontal alexia are able to read some words, they have difficulty in reading (naming) individual letters within the words they can read. In other words, in contrast to patients with alexia without agraphia, these patients exhibit a literal alexia rather than a verbal alexia. Further, individuals with frontal alexia are unable to recognize most words spelt aloud, the few words they can recognize being primarily substantive words.

Frontal alexia is usually accompanied by a non-fluent aphasia usually in the form of a Broca's aphasia. A concomitant right hemiplegia or hemiparesis is also usually present and sensory changes and visual-field deficits are evidenced by some individuals with this disorder. Frontal alexics almost always demonstrate a severe writing disturbance. Their writing in most cases consists of poorly formed letters, and spelling errors are common. Their ability to copy written material is also impaired.

The lesion underlying frontal alexia involves the frontal lobe of the dominant (left) hemisphere. Benson (1979) describes the lesion as involving 'the posterior portion of the inferior frontal gyrus with extension into the subcortical tissues in the anterior insula' (p. 116). A cerebrovascular accident usually forms the underlying aetiology in most cases of frontal alexia.

Deep alexia

The concept of deep alexia (also called 'phonemic alexia') has arisen from research carried out since the late 1960s that has investigated alexia from either a linguistic or psycholinguistic point of view (Marshall and Newcombe, 1966, 1973). Deep alexia is characterized by the presence of semantic errors when the patient is reading aloud. The three major symptoms include: the presence of semantic substitution errors (e.g. 'child' being read as 'girl'; 'wed' as 'marry'; 'listen' as 'quiet',

etc.), the presence of derivational errors (e.g. 'direction' being read as 'directing') and the omission or misreading of grammatical morphemes during reading aloud (e.g. 'an' being read instead of 'you').

It appears that patients with deep alexia, when reading aloud, pass directly to the semantic value of a word, deriving a semantic impression from its printed form without appreciating the sound of the word in question (Kaplan and Goodglass, 1981). Consequently, the patients may produce a spoken word that is not exactly the equivalent of the written word, leading to semantic substitution errors. Likewise, as there is no semantic referent for grammatical morphemes, these cannot be dealt with by this information-processing route, thereby leading to their omission, or at least misreading. According to Kaplan and Goodglass (1981), the two problems central to deep dyslexia are that patients with this disorder are first unable to use graphophonemic recoding and, second, are unable to access the phonology of a word directly. In other words, these patients are no longer able to use a phonological reading system.

Components of a deep dyslexia may be observed in most types of aphasias. Most frequently, however, it is seen in association with a Broca's aphasia with agrammatism (Kaplan and Goodglass, 1981).

Agraphia

The various types of agraphia are largely delineated by their associations with other neuropsychological disorders. Consequently, the types of agraphia described in the literature include aphasic agraphia (agraphia with Broca's, Wernicke's and conduction aphasia, etc.), agraphia with alexia, constructional agraphia (agraphia with visuospatial disability), apraxic agraphia (agraphia associated with limb apraxia) and pure agraphia (agraphia in the absence of other neuropsychological deficits).

Pure agraphia, involving the selective impairment of written communication in isolation of other language disorders, is a condition that is only rarely described in the literature. In fact, the rarity of pure agraphia has led some authors to express doubts regarding the existence of this disorder as an autonomous entity (Kreindler and Fradis, 1968). Basso, Taborelli and Vignolo (1978) reported that, out of 500 brain damaged patients that they examined, only two cases exhibited a pure agraphia. One other case of pure agraphia was reported by Rosati and de Bastiani (1979) and a further case by Miceli, Silveri and Caramazza (1985). Chedru and Geschwind (1972) described the occurrence of pure agraphia in association with confusional states (e.g. dementia) and suggested that this mechanism may underlie the majority of cases of isolated agraphia reported in the literature to that time. Some reports of pure agraphia occurring secondary to focal brain lesions have also been reported in the literature (Basso, Taborelli and Vignolo, 1978; Rosati and de Bastiani, 1979; Miceli, Silveri and Caramazza, 1985).

Pure agraphia has been described in patients with lesions in multiple cerebral sites, including the second frontal convolution (Sinico, 1926; Hecaen and Albert, 1978; Kaplan and Goodglass, 1981), the superior parietal lobule (Basso, Taborelli and Vignolo, 1978), the posterior perisylvian region (Rosati and de Bastiani, 1979) and the region of the left caudate and internal capsule (Laine and Matilla, 1981).

Rather than as an isolated disorder, agraphia most commonly occurs as part of an aphasia syndrome (aphasic agraphia). A writing disturbance in one form or another occurs in each of the major clinically recognizable types of aphasia. (The nature of the writing disorder seen in each aphasia is described in Chapter 2.) Consequently, the aetiology of agraphia is similar to that of aphasia. In general, any brain disorder that affects the dominant hemisphere has the potential to cause agraphia, the only prerequisite being that the patient is able to write prior to becoming brain damaged. Therefore, cerebrovascular disorders of the brain, head trauma, tumours, encephalitis and atrophic brain disorders can all cause agraphia.

Agnosia

'Agnosia' refers to an inability to recognize familiar objects perceived by the senses owing to brain damage. It is important to note that the disorder of recognition in this condition does not result from sensory loss (e.g. visual-field defects; hemianaesthesia, etc.), mental deterioration, disorders of consciousness or attention or a non-familiarity with the object. Prior to a diagnosis of agnosia being made, therefore, it is necessary that the presence of these factors be ruled out. Agnosia usually affects recognition through only one sensory modality so that an object that cannot be recognized by one sensory route (e.g. vision) can be recognized by a different sensory system (e.g. touch).

The occurrence of agnosia is thought to be associated with lesions that involve the sensory association areas of the cerebral cortex. The sensory pathways connecting the sensory receptors to the cerebral cortex themselves remain intact, as does the primary receptive area for the particular sensory modality involved. According to Geschwind (1956a,b), the various agnosias represent isolated naming disturbances resulting from lesions that disconnect the perceptual recognition areas of the right or both hemispheres from the speech-language areas of the left hemisphere.

The three major types of agnosia are delineated according to the sensory modality involved. These include visual agnosia, auditory agnosia and tactile agnosia.

Visual agnosia

Visual agnosia is a rare condition characterized by an inability to visually recognize, describe or name objects. In addition, patients are unable to locate visually an object in their immediate environment when that object is named. Patients with visual agnosia are also unable to choose the correct name of a seen object if provided with a list of alternative names. Visual agnosics, however, are able to identify objects through other sensory modalities, a feature which distinguishes the naming deficit in this condition from that observed in anomic aphasia. In anomic aphasia, the naming of objects is affected in all sensory modalities. Also, in contrast with anomic aphasics, patients with visual agnosia not only fail to recognize seen objects but are also unable to describe what the object is used for. Anomic aphasics, on the other hand, although unable to name objects, can often describe the use of the object.

Visual agnosias may be specific for objects (visual object agnosia), colours (colour agnosia), faces (prosopagnosia), geometric figures and pictures (agnosia for images) plus a number of other factors. In general, the lesions associated with visual agnosia tend to be extensive and in most reported cases involve the occipital lobes bilaterally with the temporal and/or parietal lobe also being involved in some patients. Reports of visual agnosia occurring subsequent to unilateral lesions in either the right or the left hemisphere have also appeared in the literature.

Auditory agnosia

In this condition, although hearing is not impaired, the patient is unable to recognize or distinguish various sounds. For instance, provided no visual or tactile stimuli are provided, the patient cannot recognize familiar noises, such as the jingling of coins or keys. In some cases, this inability may also extend to speech.

Two different types of auditory agnosia which may occur independent of one another are currently recognized. First, an auditory agnosia for non-linguistic sounds (also called 'psychic deafness') has been described which involves an inability to recognize non-linguistic auditory stimuli such as animal noises, bells ringing and so on. Second, in some cases the auditory agnosia may selectively involve a failure to recognize linguistic stimuli. This latter condition has been referred to as 'auditory verbal agnosia' or 'pure word deafness' (subcortical word deafness). Pure word deafness is a rare disorder in which, although patients cannot comprehend verbal language and therefore cannot repeat words or write to dictation, their spontaneous speech, writing and reading abilities are not disrupted.

Although it is somewhat controversial, auditory agnosia for non-linguistic stimuli is thought to be caused by lesions which involve the auditory association cortex of both hemispheres but which spare Heschl's gyrus. Both bilateral and unilateral lesions have been described in association with the occurrence of pure word deafness. Where the disorder is the result of bilateral lesions, the damage has in most cases been described as being located in the mid-portion of the superior temporal gyri of both hemispheres. According to Geschwind (1965a,b), where the disorder results from a unilateral lesion, it is necessary that the lesion involve the subcortical area of the temporal lobe so as to prevent the posterior language area from receiving input from the primary auditory receptive areas of either hemisphere.

Tactile agnosia

A syndrome analogous to auditory and visual agnosia, which involved a failure to recognize objects by touch in the presence of a preserved ability to name objects on the basis of either auditory or visual stimuli, was reported by Beauvois *et al.* (1978). They referred to this syndrome as 'bilateral tactile aphasia'. Although sensation in the hands was otherwise normal in the case reported by them, the patient was unable to recognize objects placed in his hands unless he was allowed to see or hear them. The lesion was presumed to involve both parietal lobes.

Special forms of agnosia

Two special forms of agnosia that may co-occur with language disorders include autotopagnosia and anosognosia. 'Autotopagnosia' refers to the impaired recognition of body parts. Patients with this condition may deny that some body part such as the arm belongs to them. Autotopagnosia is thought to be caused by lesions in the posterior inferior portion of the parietal lobe.

Anosognosia involves a lack of awareness of disease or denial of disease. A patient with this disorder may for instance deny that they have a hemiplegia or may deny that they are blind (Anton's disease). The condition is associated with lesions of the parietal lobe in the region of the supramarginal gyrus.

Gerstmann syndrome

First described by Gerstmann (1931), this syndrome is characterized by four primary symptoms: a disability in calculation (acalculia), finger agnosia (an inability to recognize one's own fingers or the fingers of others), a right–left disorientation and agraphia. Gerstmann syndrome is usually associated with focal lesion of the dominant (left) cerebral hemisphere in the region of the angular gyrus and may occur independently or co-occur with aphasia. A partial Gerstmann syndrome is often seen in association with alexia and agraphia.

In that a full Gerstmann syndrome occurs only rarely in brain damaged individuals, a number of authors including Benton (1977) and Critchley (1966) have questioned the existence of this syndrome. Benson (1979) suggested that Gerstmann syndrome is only part of a larger disorder called 'angular gyrus syndrome', which includes, in addition to the symptoms of Gerstmann syndrome, anomic aphasia and alexia with agraphia.

Summary

Aphasia is often accompanied by a number of neurological disturbances that can complicate the assessment and treatment of affected patients. These include apraxia, agnosia, alexia, agraphia and Gerstmann syndrome. Individuals with apraxia are unable to carry out, at will, a complex or skilled movement that they were previously able to perform, where the inability is not caused by paralysis of the muscles, ataxia, sensory loss, comprehension deficits or inattention to commands. The major types of apraxia include ideomotor apraxia, ideational apraxia and limb-kinetic apraxia. Some special forms of apraxia have also been identified, including verbal apraxia (apraxia of speech), constructional apraxia and dressing apraxia among others. Apraxia of speech is of particular interest to speech-language pathologists and is thought to represent a disorder of motor speech programming manifested primarily by errors in articulation and secondarily by compensatory alterations of prosody (e.g. pauses, slow speech rate, equalization of stress, etc.).

Alexia represents a reading disorder caused by brain damage. The four most common types of alexia include alexia without agraphia, alexia with agraphia, frontal alexia and deep alexia. Agraphia, which represents a writing disorder resulting from brain damage, rarely occurs in isolation of other language disorders and most commonly occurs as part of an aphasia syndrome.

An inability to recognize familiar objects perceived by the senses as a consequence of brain damage is referred to as 'agnosia'. The three major types of agnosia are delineated according to the sensory modality involved and include visual agnosia, auditory agnosia and tactile agnosia. Visual agnosia is characterized by an inability to visually recognize, describe or name objects (visual object agnosia), colours (colour agnosia) or faces (prosopagnosia) among other factors. Likewise, in auditory agnosia, the affected individual is unable to recognize or distinguish various sounds even though their hearing is not impaired. Patients with tactile agnosia are unable to recognize familiar objects by touch alone, even though the same objects can be recognized via either visual or auditory stimuli.

Gerstmann syndrome may occur in isolation or may accompany aphasia. The four primary symptoms of this condition include acalculia, finger agnosia, right–left disorientation and agraphia.

References

Assal, G., Buttet, J. and Jolivet, R. (1981) Disassociations in aphasia: a case report. *Brain and Language*, **13**, 223–240.

Basso, A., Taborelli, A. and Vignolo, L.A. (1978) Dissociated disorders of speaking and writing in aphasia. *Journal of Neurology, Neurosurgery and Psychiatry*, **41**, 556–563.

Beauvois, M.F., Saillant, B., Meininger V. and Lhermitte, F. (1978) Bilateral tactile aphasia: a tacto-verbal dysfunction. *Brain*, **101**, 381–402.

Benson, D.F. (1977) The third alexia. *Archives of Neurology*, **34**, 327–331.

Benson, D.F. (1979) *Aphasia, Alexia and Agraphia*, Churchill Livingstone, New York.

Benson, D.F. and Geschwind, N. (1969) The alexias, in *Handbook of Clinical Neurology*, vol. **4** (eds P.J. Vinken and G.W. Bruyn), North-Holland Publishing Company, Amsterdam, pp. 284–298.

Benton, A.L. (1977) Reflections on the Gerstmann syndrome. *Brain and Language*, **4**, 45–62.

Broca, P. (1861) Portée de la parole. Ramollissement chronique et destruction partielle du lobe antérieur gauche du cerveau. *Bulletins de la Société d'anthropologie de Paris*, **2**, 219.

Brown, J.W. (1974) *Aphasia, Apraxia and Agnosia: Clinical and Theoretical Aspects*, Charles C. Thomas, Springfield, IL.

Burns, M.S. and Canter, G.J. (1977) Phonemic behaviour of aphasia patients with posterior cerebral lesions. *Brain and Language*, **4**, 492–507.

Chedru, F. and Geschwind, N. (1972) Writing disturbances in acute confusional states. *Neuropsychologia*, **10**, 343–353.

Critchley, M. (1966) The enigma of Gerstmann's syndrome. *Brain*, **89**, 183–198.

Darley, F.L. (1968) Apraxia of speech: 107 years of terminological confusion. Paper presented at the American Speech and Hearing Association, Denver.

Darley, F.L. (1975) Treatment of acquired aphasia, in *Advances in Neurology*, vol. 7 (ed. W.J. Friedlander), Raven Press, New York, pp. 311–329.

Darley, F.L. (1982) *Aphasia*, W.B. Saunders, Philadelphia.

Darley, F.L., Aronson, A.E. and Brown, J.R. (1975) *Motor Speech Disorders*, W.B. Saunders, Philadelphia.

Deal, J.L. (1974) Consistency and adaptation in apraxia of speech. *Journal of Communication Disorders*, 7, 135–140.

Deal, J.L. and Darley, F.L. (1972) The influence of linguistic and situational variables on phonemic accuracy in apraxia of speech. *Journal of Speech and Hearing Research*, **15**, 639–653.

Dejerine, J. (1891) Sur un cas de cécité verbale avec agraphie, suivi d'autopsie. *Comptes-Rendus Hebdomadaires des Séances et Mémoires de la Société de Biologie*, **3**, 197–201.

Dejerine, J. (1892) Contribution à l'étude anatomo-pathologique et clinique des différentes variétés de cécité verbale. *Comptes-Rendus Hebdomadaires des Séances et Mémoires de la Société de Biologie*, **4**, 61–90.

De Renzi, E. and Vignolo, L. (1962) The token test: a sensitive test to detect receptive disturbances in aphasia. *Brain*, **85**, 556–678.

Dronkers, N.F. (1996) A new brain region for coordinating speech articulation. *Nature*, **384**, 159–161.

Duffy, J.R. (2005) *Motor Speech Disorders: Substrates, Differential Diagnosis and Management*, 2nd edn, Mosby, St Louis.

Dunlop, J. and Marquardt, T. (1977) Linguistic and articulatory aspects of single word production in apraxia of speech. *Cortex*, **13**, 17–29.

Gerstmann, J. (1931) Zur symptomatologie der hirnläsionen im übergangsgebiet der unteren parietal-hund mittleren occipital windung. *Nervenarzt*, **3**, 691–695.

Geschwind, N. (1965a) Disconnection syndromes in animals and man. Part 1. *Brain*, **88**, 237–294.

Geschwind, N. (1965b) Disconnection syndromes in animals and man. Part 2. *Brain*, **88**, 585–644.

Geschwind, N. (1975) The apraxias: neural mechanisms of disorders of learned movements. *American Scientist*, **63**, 188–195.

Goodglass, H. and Kaplan, E. (1983) *The Assessment of Aphasia and Related Disorders*, Lea & Febiger, Philadelphia.

Halpern, H., Darley, F.L. and Brown, J.R. (1973) Differential language and neurologic characteristics in cerebral involvement. *Journal of Speech and Hearing Disorders*, **38**, 162–173.

Hecaen, H. and Albert, M.L. (1978) *Human Neuropsychology*, John Wiley & Sons, Inc., New York.

Hier, D.B. and Mohr, J.P. (1977) Incongruous oral and written naming. *Brain and Language*, **4**, 115–126.

Hillis, A.E., Work, M., Barker, P.B. *et al.* (2004) Re-examining the brain regions crucial for orchestrating speech articulation. *Brain*, **127**, 1479–1487.

Jackson, J.H. (1932) *Selected Writing*, Hodder and Stoughton, London.

Johns, D.F. and Darley, F.L. (1970) Phonemic variability in apraxia of speech. *Journal of Speech and Hearing Research*, **13**, 556–583.

Kaplan, E. and Goodglass, H. (1981) Aphasia-related disorders, in *Acquired Aphasia* (ed. M.T. Sarno), Academic Press, New York, pp. 151–172.

Kerschensteiner, M., Poeck, K. and Lehmkuhl, G. (1975) Die apraxien. *Aktuelle Neurologie*, **2**, 171–178.

Kreindler, A. and Fradis, A. (1968) *Performances in Aphasia: A Neurodynamical, Diagnostic and Psychological Study*, Gauthier-Villars, Paris.

Laine, T. and Matilla, R.J. (1981) Pure agraphia: a case study. *Neuropsychologia*, **19**, 311–316.

LaPointe, L.L. and Johns, D.F. (1975) Some phonemic characteristics in apraxia of speech. *Journal of Communication Disorders*, **8**, 259–269.

Liepmann, H. (1908) *Drei Aufsätze aus Dem Apraxiegebiet*, Karger, Berlin.

Marshall, J.C. and Newcombe, F. (1966) Syntactic and semantic errors in paralexia. *Neuropsychologia*, **4**, 169–176.

Marshall, J.C. and Newcombe, F. (1973) Patterns of paralexia: a psycholinguistic approach. *Journal of Psycholinguistic Research*, **2**, 175–199.

McNeil, M.R., Pratt, S.R. and Fossett, T.R.D. (2004) The differential diagnosis of apraxia of speech, in *Speech Motor Control in Normal and Disordered Speech* (eds B. Maassen, R.D. Kent, H.F.M. Peters *et al.*), Oxford Medical Publications, Oxford, pp. 383–413.

McNeil, M.R., Robin, D.A. and Schmidt, R.A. (1997) Apraxia of speech: definition, differentiation and treatment, in *Clinical Management of Sensorimotor Speech Disorders* (ed. M.R. McNeil), Thieme, New York, pp. 311–344.

McNeil, M.R., Weismer, G., Adams, S. and Mulligan, M. (1990) Oral structure nonspeech motor control in normal, dysarthric, aphasic and apraxic speakers: isometric force and static position control. *Journal of Speech and Hearing Research*, **33**, 255–268.

Miceli, G., Silveri, C. and Caramazza, A. (1985) Cognitive analysis of a case of pure dysarthria. *Brain and Language*. **25**, 187–212.

Miller, N. (1986) *Dyspraxia and its Management*, Croom Helm, London.

Mohr, J.P. (1976) Broca's area and Broca's aphasia, in *Studies in Neurolinguistics*, vol. **1** (eds H. Whitaker and H.A. Whitaker), Academic Press, New York, pp. 69–81.

Mohr, J.P., Funkenstein, H.H., Finkelstein, S. *et al.* (1975) Broca's area infarction versus Broca's aphasia. *Neurology*, **25**, 349.

Odell, K., McNeil, M.R., Rosenbek, J.C. and Hunter, L. (1990) Perceptual characteristics of consonant productions by apraxic speakers. *Journal of Speech and Hearing Disorders*, **55**, 345–359.

Odell, K., McNeil, M.R., Rosenbek, J.C. and Hunter, L. (1991) Perceptual characteristics of vowel and prosody production in apraxic, aphasic and dysarthric speakers. *Journal of Speech and Hearing Research*, **34**, 67–80.

Ogar, J., Willock, S., Baldo, J. *et al.* (2006) Clinical and anatomical correlates of apraxia of speech. *Brain and Language*, **97**, 343–350.

Poeck, K. and Lehmkuhl, G. (1980) Ideatory apraxia in a left-handed patient with right sided brain lesion. *Cortex*, **16**, 273–284.

Rosati, G. and de Bastiani, P. (1979) Pure agraphia: a discrete form of aphasia. *Journal of Neurology, Neurosurgery and Psychiatry*, **42**, 266–269.

Rosenbek, J.C., Kent, R.D. and LaPointe, L.L. (1984) Apraxia of speech and some perspectives, in *Apraxia of Speech: Physiology, Acoustics, Linguistics, Management* (eds J.C. Rosenbek, M.R. McNeil and A.R. Aronson), College Hill Press, San Diego, pp. 73–92.

Rosenbek, J.C., Wertz, R.T. and Darley, F.L. (1973) Oral sensation and perception in apraxia of speech and aphasia. *Journal of Speech and Hearing Research*, **16**, 22–36.

Schuell, H., Jenkins, J. and Jiminez-Pabon, E. (1964) *Aphasia in Adults*, Harper & Row, New York.

Sinico, S. (1926) Neoplasia della seconda circonvoluzione frontale sinistra: agrafia pura. *Gazzetta degli Ospedali e delle Cliniche (Milano)*, **47**, 627–631.

Square-Storer, P., Roy, E.A. and Martin, R.E. (1997) Apraxia of speech: another form of praxis disruption, in *Apraxia: the Neuropsychology of Action* (eds L.J.G. Rothi and K.M. Heilman), Psychology Press, Hove, pp. 173–206.

Trost, J.E. and Canter, G.J. (1974) Apraxia of speech in patients with Broca's aphasia: a study of phoneme production accuracy and error patterns. *Brain and Language*, **1**, 63–79.

Vignolo, L.A. (1983) Modality – specific disorders of written language, in *Localization in Neuropsychology* (ed. A. Kertesz), Academic Press, New York, pp. 119–135.

Wertz, R.T., LaPointe, L.L. and Rosenbek, J.C. (1984) *Apraxia of Speech in Adults: the Disorder and its Management*, Grune & Stratton, Orlando.

Ziegler, W. and von Cramon, D. (1986) Disturbed coarticulation in apraxia of speech: acoustic evidence. *Brain and Language*, **29**, 34–47.

Dysarthrias associated with upper and lower motor neurone lesions

9

Introduction

Darley, Aronson and Brown (1975) have defined dysarthria as 'a collective name for a group of related speech disorders that are due to disturbances in muscular control of the speech mechanism resulting from impairment of any of the basic motor processes involved in the execution of speech' (p. 2). According to this definition, the term 'dysarthria' is restricted to those speech disorders which have a neurogenic origin (i.e. those speech disorders that result from damage to the central or peripheral nervous system, and does not include those speech disorders associated with either somatic structural defects (e.g. cleft palate, congenitally enlarged pharynx, congenitally short palate and malocclusion) or psychological disorders (e.g. psychogenic aphonia).

Speech is a complex behaviour that requires the coordinated contraction of a large number of muscles for its production. This contraction is controlled by nerve impulses which originate in the motor areas of the cerebral cortex and then pass to the muscles by way of the motor pathways. Overall, the control of muscular ac-

tivity can be considered as if the nervous system involved a series of levels of functional activity in which the higher levels dominate the lower levels.

The lowest level of motor control is provided by the neurones which connect the central nervous system to the skeletal muscle fibres. These neurones, referred to as lower motor neurones, have their cell bodies located in either nuclei in the brainstem (in which case their axons run in the cranial nerves having a motor function) or the anterior horns of grey matter of the spinal cord (in which case their axons run in the various spinal nerves). The lower motor neurones form the only route by which nerve impulses can travel from the central nervous system to cause contraction of the skeletal muscle fibres and, for this reason, are also known as the final common pathway.

The motor areas of the cerebral cortex responsible for the initiation of voluntary muscle activity constitute the highest level of motor control. These areas are responsible for the initiation of voluntary muscle activity and can dominate the lower motor neurones arising from the brainstem and spinal cord, either via the direct descending motor pathways (also called the pyramidal system) or the indirect descending motor pathways

Table 9.1 Clinically recognized types of dysarthria together with their lesion sites.

Dysarthria type	Lesion site
Flaccid dysarthria	Lower motor neurones
Spastic dysarthria	Upper motor neurones
Hypokinetic dysarthria	Basal ganglia and associated brainstem nuclei
Hyperkinetic dysarthria	Basal ganglia and associated brainstem nuclei
Ataxic dysarthria	Cerebellum and/or its connections
Mixed dysarthria, for example	
Mixed flaccid/spastic dysarthria	Both lower and upper motor neurones (e.g. amyotrophic lateral sclerosis)
Mixed ataxic/spastic/flaccid dysarthria	Cerebellum/cerebellar connections, upper motor neurones and lower motor neurones (e.g. Wilson's disease)

(formerly called the extrapyramidal system).[1] The indirect pathways are so called because they are multisynaptic pathways and involve a multiplicity of connections with various subcortical structures, but particularly with the basal ganglia. The neurones that comprise the direct (pyramidal) and indirect (extrapyramidal) descending motor pathways are collectively referred to as upper motor neurones.

The type of dysarthria that results from damage to the neuromuscular system depends very much upon where in the neuromuscular system that damage is located. Parts of the neuromuscular system that can be affected include the lower motor neurones, upper motor neurones, extrapyramidal system, cerebellum, neuromuscular junction as well as the muscles of the speech mechanism themselves. Damage to each of these sites is associated with a particular type of dysarthria (Table 9.1).

Prior to looking in detail at the individual characteristics of the different types of dysarthria and attempting to explain the occurrence of the various deviant speech dimensions seen in association

with each, it is necessary that the reader have not only an understanding of neuropathology underlying each condition but also a knowledge of the neuroanatomy of the motor pathways.

Flaccid dysarthria (lower motor neurone dysarthria)

Lower motor neurones form the ultimate pathway through which nerve impulses are conveyed from the central nervous system to the skeletal muscles, including the muscles of the speech mechanism. The cell bodies of the lower motor neurones are located in either the anterior horns of the spinal cord or the motor nuclei of the cranial nerves in the brainstem. From this location, the axons of the lower motor neurones pass via the various spinal and motor cranial nerves of the peripheral nervous system to the voluntary muscles. Lesions of the motor cranial nerves and spinal nerves represent lower motor neurone lesions and interrupt the conduction of nerve impulses from the central nervous system to the muscles. As a consequence, voluntary control of the affected muscles is lost. At the same time, because the nerve impulses necessary for the maintenance of muscle tone are also lost, the muscles involved become flaccid (hypotonic).

In addition to loss of muscle tone, lower motor neurone lesions are characterized by muscle weakness, a loss or reduction of muscle reflexes, atrophy of the muscle involved and fasciculations (spontaneous twitches of individual

---

[1] The pyramidal system takes its name from the fact that the majority of the direct connections between the motor areas of the cerebral cortex and the lower motor neurones pass through the pyramids of the medulla oblongata. However, in that some of the direct pathways, namely the corticobulbar and corticomesencephalic tracts (see below) do not pass through the pyramids, the use of the term 'extrapyramidal system' to describe the indirect motor pathways has recently been discouraged

Table 9.2   Lower motor neurones associated with flaccid dysarthria.

Speech process	Muscle	Site of cell body	Nerves through which axons pass
Respiration	Diaphragm	Third–fifth cervical segments of spinal cord	Phrenic nerves
	Intercostal and abdominal	1st–12th thoracic and first lumbar segments of the spinal cord	Intercostal nerves. sixth thoracic to 1st lumber spinal nerves
Phonation	Laryngeal muscles	Nucleus ambiguus in medulla oblongata	Vagus nerves (X)
Articulation	Pterygoid, masseter, temporalis, and so on	Motor nucleus of trigeminal in pons	Trigeminal nerves (V)
	Facial expression, for example orbicularis oris	Facial nucleus in pons	Facial nerves (VII)
	Tongue muscles	Hypoglossal nucleus in medulla oblongata	Hypoglossal nerves (XII)
Resonation	Levator veli palatini	Nucleus ambiguus in medulla oblongata	Vagus nerves (X)
	Tensor veli palatini	Motor nucleus of trigeminal in pons	Trigeminal nerves (V)

muscle bundles – fascicles). All or some of these characteristics may be evidenced in the muscles of the speech mechanism in a patient with flaccid dysarthria. In particular, however, the degree of muscle atrophy may show some variability depending upon the nature of the underlying neurological disorder, and fasciculations are not manifest in all of the diseases that can cause damage to lower motor neurones.

Damage to either the lower motor neurones (including those that innervate the respiratory musculature and/or those that run in the cranial nerves to innervate the speech musculature) and/or the muscles of the speech mechanism results in speech changes collectively referred to as 'flaccid dysarthria', although the term 'peripheral dysarthria' has been used by some authors (Edwards, 1984). The actual name, flaccid dysarthria, is of course derived from the major symptom of lower motor neurone damage, flaccid paralysis. The speech characteristics of each patient with flaccid dysarthria, however, vary depending upon which particular nerves are affected and the relative degree of weakness resulting from the damage. The actual lower motor neurones which, if damaged, may be associated with flaccid dysarthria are listed in Table 9.2.

Innervation of the speech mechanism

With the exception of the muscles of respiration, the muscles of the speech mechanism are innervated by the motor cranial nerves which arise from the bulbar region (pons and medulla oblongata) of the brainstem. These nerves include cranial nerves V, VII, IX, X, XI and XII.

Trigeminal nerve (V)

The trigeminal nerves emerge from the lateral sides of the pons and are the largest of the cranial nerves (Figure 9.1). Each trigeminal nerve is composed of three branches, the ophthalmic branch, the maxillary branch and the mandibular branch. Of the three branches, the ophthalmic and maxillary are both purely sensory, while the mandibular is mixed sensory and motor. A large ganglion, the Gasserian ganglion, which is homologous to the dorsal root ganglion of the spinal nerve, is located at the point where the trigeminal divides into three branches.

The ophthalmic branch exits the skull through the superior orbital fissure and provides sensation from the cornea, ciliary body, iris, lacrimal gland, conjunctiva, nasal mucous membrane and the

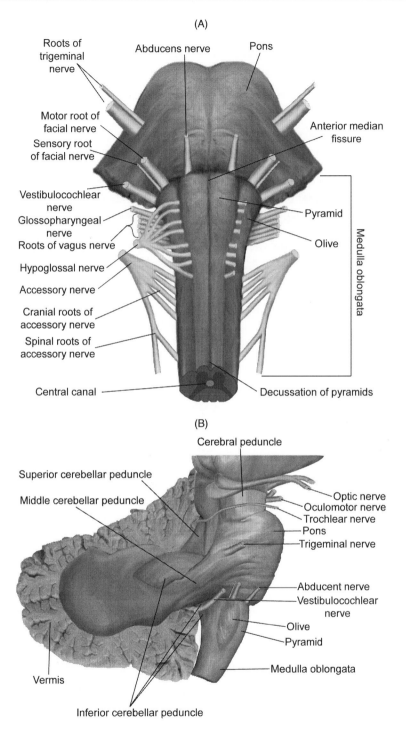

Figure 9.1   (A) Anterior view of the pons and medulla oblongata showing the origins of cranial nerves V to XII. (B) Lateral view of the brainstem (cerebellum partially removed) showing the origins of cranial nerves II to VIII.

skin of the eyelid, eyebrow, forehead and nose. The maxillary branch leaves the skull through the foramen rotundum and supplies sensory fibres to the skin of the cheek, lower eyelid, side of the nose and upper jaw, teeth of the upper jaw and mucous membrane of the mouth and maxillary sinus.

The mandibular branch unites with the motor root immediately after it has exited from the cranial cavity via the foramen ovale. The motor root arises from the motor nucleus of the trigeminal in the pons. Because the trigeminal nerve is mainly sensory, the motor root is much smaller than the sensory portion. Sensory fibres in the mandibular branch provide sensation from the skin of the lower jaw and the temporal region. In the mouth, they supply the lower teeth and gums and the mucous membrane covering the anterior two-thirds of the tongue. The motor fibres of the mandibular branch innervate the muscles of mastication, which include the temporalis, masseter and medial and lateral pterygoid muscles. In addition, the motor fibres also supply the mylohyoid, anterior belly of the digastric, the tensor veli palatini and the tensor tympani of the middle ear.

The functioning of the motor portion of the trigeminal nerve can be tested clinically by observing the movements of the mandible. Normally, when the mouth is opened widely, the mandible is depressed in the midline. In unilateral trigeminal lesions, however, the mandible deviates towards the paralysed side owing to the unopposed contraction of the pterygoid muscles on the active side (i.e. the side opposite to the lesion) when the mouth is opened. As a further test of trigeminal function, the masseter and temporalis muscles should be palpated while patients clench their teeth. In patients with unilateral lesions, it will be noted that the muscles of mastication on the same side as the lesion will either fail to contract or contract only weakly. Where bilateral trigeminal lesions are present, the muscles of mastication on both sides will undergo flaccid paralysis.

Facial nerve (VII)

Each facial nerve emerges from the lateral aspect of the brainstem at the lower border of the pons,

in the ponto-medullary sulcus, in the form of two distinct bundles of fibres of unequal size (Figure 9.1). The larger, more medial, bundle arises from the facial nucleus of the pons and carries motor fibres to the muscles of facial expression. The smaller, more lateral, bundle carries autonomic fibres and is known as the nervus intermedius. The two roots run together for a short distance in the posterior cranial fossa to enter the internal auditory meatus in the petrous temporal bone along with the VIIIth nerve (auditory nerve). Within the temporal bone, the facial nerve passes through the facial canal and eventually emerges from the skull at the stylomastoid foramen. From here, the motor fibres are distributed to the muscles of facial expression, including the occipito-frontalis, orbicularis oris and buccinators. Other muscles supplied by the facial nerve include the stylohyoid and the posterior belly of the digastric. Within the facial canal, a small number of motor fibres are given off to supply the stapedius muscle in the middle ear.

The autonomic fibres pass into two fine branches of the facial nerve which emerge independently from the temporal bone. One of these is the chorda tympani, which exits the skull via the petrotympanic fissure to join the lingual nerve, a branch of the mandibular division of the trigeminal nerve. The lingual nerve delivers the fibres of the chorda tympani to the submandibular ganglion. Here they synapse with post-ganglionic neurones which pass to the submandibular and sublingual salivary glands. The chorda tympani also convey taste sensation from the anterior two-thirds of the tongue. The second small branch which carries autonomic fibres supplies the lacrimal gland in the orbit and is known as the greater petrosal nerve.

The motor portion of the facial nerve is tested by observing the patient's face, both at rest and during the performance of a variety of facial expressions such as pursing the lips, smiling, corrugating the forehead, blowing out the cheeks, showing the teeth and closing the eyes against resistance. Normally, all facial movements should be equal bilaterally. Unilateral facial nerve lesions cause weakness or paralysis of the half of the face on the same side as the lesion. At rest, the face of patients with unilateral flaccid paralysis of the muscles of facial expression appears to be asymmetrical. The mouth on the affected side droops below that on the unaffected side and saliva may constantly drool from the corner. In addition, owing to loss of muscle tone in the orbicularis oris muscle, the lower eyelid may droop, causing the palpebral fissure on the affected side to be somewhat wider than on the normal side. When the patient smiles, the mouth is retracted on the active side but not on the affected side. Likewise, when asked to frown, the frontalis muscle on the contralateral side will corrugate the forehead; however, on the side ipsilateral to the lesion, no corrugation will occur.

In bilateral facial nerve paralysis, as might occur in Möbius syndrome, saliva may drool from both corners of the mouth. The seal produced by compression of the lips may be so weak that the patient cannot puff out their cheeks and the lips may be slightly parted at rest.

Glossopharyngeal nerve (IX)

Each glossopharyngeal nerve arises from the medulla oblongata as a series of rootlets at the upper end of the post-olivary sulcus. The IXth nerve leaves the cranial cavity via the jugular foramen along with the vagus and accessory nerves.

The glossopharyngeal nerve contains both sensory and motor as well as autonomic fibres. The motor fibres arise from the nucleus ambiguus and innervate the stylopharyngeus muscle. The sensory fibres provide sensation from the pharynx, the posterior one-third of the tongue, the fauces, tonsils and soft palate. They also carry the sense of taste from the posterior one-third of the tongue.

The autonomic fibres within the IXth nerve pass to the otic ganglion, where they synapse with post-ganglionic neurones, which in turn regulate secretion from the parotid salivary gland.

Vagus nerve (X)

Each vagus nerve arises from the lateral surface of the medulla oblongata by numerous rootlets which lie immediately inferior to those which give rise to the glossopharyngeal nerve. It then leaves the cranial cavity via the jugular foramen.

The vagus nerve contains sensory, motor and autonomic fibres and is the only cranial nerve to venture beyond the confines of the head and neck, supplying structures within the thorax and the upper parts of the abdominal cavity.

After emerging from the jugular foramen, the vagus receives additional motor fibres from the cranial portion of the accessory nerve. The motor fibres of the vagus arise from the nucleus ambiguus and in combination with those from the accessory nerve, supply the muscles of the pharynx, larynx and the levator veli palatini and musculus uvulae of the soft palate. The first branch of the vagus nerve important for speech is the pharyngeal nerve, which supplies the levator muscles of the soft palate. As the vagus descends in the neck, it gives off a second branch, the superior laryngeal nerve, which supplies the crico-thyroid muscle (the chief tensor muscle of the vocal cords). At a lower level in the neck, a third branch is given off, the recurrent laryngeal nerve, which supplies all of the intrinsic muscles of the larynx except for the crico-thyroid and is, therefore, responsible for regulating adduction of the vocal cords for phonation and abduction of the vocal cords for unvoiced phonemes and inspiration.

Prior to entering the larynx, the left recurrent laryngeal nerve descends into the thorax, loops under the aortic arch and then ascends along the lateral aspects of the trachea to enter the larynx from below and behind the left crico-thyroid joint. The right recurrent laryngeal nerve enters the larynx at the equivalent point on the right side but descends in the neck only as far as the right subclavian artery before commencing its ascent to the larynx. Looping of the left recurrent laryngeal nerve under the aortic arch makes it vulnerable to compression by intrathoracic masses (e.g. lung tumours) and aortic arch aneurysms.

The autonomic component of the vagus supplies organs in the thorax and abdomen, including the heart, lungs, major airways and blood vessels and the upper part of the gastrointestinal system.

Functioning of the vagus nerve can be easily checked clinically by noting (1) the quality of the patient's voice, (2) their ability to swallow and (3) the position and movements of the soft palate at rest and during phonation. Unilateral vagus nerve lesions cause paralysis of the ipsilateral vocal cord, leading to dysphonia. The paralysed cord can be neither abducted nor adducted. By asking patients to open their mouth and say /ah/, movements of the soft palate can be observed. Normally, the uvula and soft palate rise in the midline during phonation. However, unilateral lesions of the vagus nerve cause the palate to deviate to the contralateral side (the side opposite to the lesion) during phonation. In addition, the distance between the soft palate and the posterior pharyngeal wall is less on the paralysed side and the arch of the palate at rest will droop on the side of the lesion.

In bilateral lesions of the vagus nerves, both sides of the soft palate and vocal cords may be paralysed. Both sides of the soft palate rest at a lower level than normal, although their symmetry at rest may appear normal to inexperienced clinicians. However, despite the apparent symmetry, there is less space under the arches of the soft palate and the curvature is flatter. The extent of movement on phonation is reduced and in severe cases the palate may not rise at all. When observed by either direct or indirect laryngoscopy, abduction and adduction of both vocal cords is severely impaired.

Accessory nerve (XI)

There are two parts to each accessory nerve, a cranial portion which arises from the nucleus ambiguus in the medulla oblongata and a spinal portion which arises from the first five segments of the cervical region of the spinal cord (Figure 9.1). The cranial accessory emerges from the lateral part of the medulla oblongata in the form of four to five rootlets immediately below those that form the vagus nerve. Prior to leaving the cranial cavity via the jugular foramen, the cranial accessory is joined by the spinal accessory to form the accessory nerve. The spinal accessory fibres arise from the anterior horns of the first five cervical segments of the spinal cord. These fibres emerge from the lateral parts of the spinal cord and unite to form a single nerve trunk, which ascends alongside the spinal cord and enters the skull through the foramen magnum to join the cranial accessory.

After exiting through the skull, the cranial accessory leaves the spinal accessory and joins the vagus nerve and is distributed by that nerve to provide motor supply to the muscles of the pharynx, larynx, musculus uvulae and levator veli palatini muscles. The spinal accessory, on the other hand, provides the motor supply to the trapezius muscle and the upper portion of the sternocleidomastoid muscle.

Disorders of the cranial accessory are recognized clinically as disorders of the vagus nerve while disorders of the spinal accessory are evident in atrophy and paralysis of the trapezius and sternocleidomastoid muscles.

Hypoglossal nerve (XII)

Each hypoglossal nerve arises from motor cells in the hypoglossal nucleus and emerges from the medulla oblongata as a series of rootlets in the groove that separates the pyramid and olive. The nerves leave the cranial cavity via the hypoglossal canal, which lies in the margin of the foramen magnum.

The hypoglossal nerves provide the motor supply to the muscles of the tongue. Tongue muscles can be divided into two groups: the intrinsic muscles, which lie entirely within the substance of the tongue and are responsible for changes in its shape, and the extrinsic muscles. The latter muscles are attached at one end to structures outside the tongue and are responsible for moving the tongue within the mouth. The hypoglossal nerves innervate all of the tongue muscles, with the exception of the palatoglossus. Other muscles in the region of the neck also supplied by the hypoglossal nerves include the sternohyoid, sternothyroid, inferior belly of the omohyoid and the geniohyoid muscles.

Functioning of the hypoglossal nerves can be tested by observing the tongue at rest and during movement. Unilateral hypoglossal nerve damage is associated with atrophy and fasciculations in the ipsilateral side of the tongue. When observed in the mouth, the tongue on the side of the lesion may appear smaller and the surface corrugated, indicative of atrophy. Fasciculation of the tongue may in some cases be the earliest sign of lower motor neurone disease. When the patients are asked to protrude their tongue, it will deviate to the paralysed side. Another test for weakness of the tongue is to have patients press their tongue against their cheek while the examiner presses against the bulging cheek with the hand.

In bilateral hypoglossal involvement, both sides of the tongue may be atrophied and show fasciculations. Although protrusion occurs in the midline, the degree of protrusion may be severely limited by weakness and in the more severe cases the patient may not be able to extend the tongue far beyond the lower teeth. Elevation of the tip and body to contact the alveolar ridge or hard palate may be difficult or impossible.

Neurological disorders associated with lower motor neurone lesions

Flaccid paralysis of the muscles supplied by nerves arising from the bulbar region of the brainstem is commonly called 'bulbar palsy'. Diseases which cause bulbar palsy may affect either the cell body of the lower motor neurone or the axon of the lower motor neurone as it courses through the peripheral nerve. A variety of neurological diseases can cause damage to the lower motor neurones that innervate the muscles involved in speech production. Viral infections, tumours, cerebrovascular accidents, progressive degeneration and congenital conditions may impair the cranial nerve nuclei or anterior horn cells of the spinal cord. Traumatic head injuries, tumours, cardiovascular defects (aneurysms), bony prominences and toxins or infections that produce neuritis may affect the spinal and cranial nerves once they exit from the central nervous system.

Depending whether they affect the nerve in its peripheral course or involve the nerve cell bodies in either the cranial nerve nuclei or the anterior horns of the spinal cord, disorders of lower motor neurones which cause flaccid dysarthria can be divided into two groups. The major disorders of lower motor neurones which can cause flaccid dysarthria are listed in Table 9.3.

In addition to lesions in the lower motor neurones themselves, flaccid dysarthria can also be associated with either impaired nerve impulse transmission across the neuromuscular junction (e.g. myasthenia gravis) or disorders which involve the muscles of the speech mechanism themselves (e.g. muscular dystrophy and polymyositis).

Clinical characteristics of flaccid dysarthria

Flaccid dysarthria may be manifest in any or all of the major subsystems of the speech production apparatus, including the respiratory system, laryngeal valve, velopharyngeal valve and articulatory valve. Although the principal deviant speech characteristics vary according to the particular nerves and muscles affected, their occurrence has been attributed primarily to muscular weakness and reduced muscle tone and the effects of these on the speed, range and accuracy of the movements of the speech musculature. Darley, Aronson and Brown (1969a,b) found that the combination of speech characteristics that best distinguished flaccid dysarthria from other types of dysarthria were marked hypernasality often coupled with nasal emission of air, continuous breathiness in the voice and audible inspiration. Other prominent speech characteristics reported by these workers included imprecise consonants, monopitch, harsh voice quality, short phrases and monoloudness. The 10 main aspects of flaccid dysarthria listed by Enderby (1986) in rank order of frequency of occurrence are poor lip seal, abnormality of lips at rest, abnormality of spread of lips, dribbling, reduced elevation of tongue, abnormality of tongue at rest, poor alternating movements of tongue, reduced phonation time, poor intelligibility of repetition and poor intelligibility of description.

As indicated earlier, the particular speech characteristics exhibited by a patient with flaccid dysarthria depends upon which nerves and muscles are affected.

Phrenic and intercostal nerve lesions

The muscles of respiration are important for the motor production of speech in that the exhaled breath provides the power source for speech. It

Table 9.3 Neurological disorders of lower motor neurones causing flaccid dysarthria.

Site of lesion	Disorder	Aetiology	Signs and symptoms
Peripheral nerves (especially cranial nerves V, VII, IX, X, XI and XII	Polyneuritis	Inflammation of a number of nerves. Acute type – may follow viral infections, for example glandular fever. Chronic type – may be associated with diabetes mellitus and alcohol abuse	Sensory and lower motor neurone changes usually begin in the distal portion of the limbs and spread to involve other regions including the face, tongue, soft palate, pharynx and larynx. The muscles of respiration may also be involved. Bilateral facial paralysis may occur in idiopathic polyneuritis (Guillain–Barré syndrome)
	Compression of and damage to cranial nerves	Neoplasm, for example acoustic neuroma causing compression of the VIIth nerve. Aneurysm, for example compression of the left recurrent laryngeal nerve by an aortic arch aneurysm. Trauma, for example damage to the recurrent laryngeal nerve during thyroidectomy	Localized lower motor neurone signs dependent on the particular nerves involved
	Idiopathic facial paralysis (Bell's palsy)	Pathogenesis unknown in most cases but may be related to inflammatory lesions in the stylomastoid foramen. Approximately 80% of cases recover	Abrupt onset of unilateral facial paralysis
Cranial nerve nuclei and/or anterior horns of spinal cord	Brainstem cerebrovascular accidents	Lateral medullary syndrome (Wallenberg's syndrome) – caused by occlusion of the posterior inferior cerebellar artery, vertebral artery or lateral medullary artery	Damage of the nucleus ambiguus (origin of the IXth, Xth and cranial portion of the XIth nerve) leads to dysphagia, hoarseness and paralysis of the soft palate on the side of the lesion. Impaired sensation over the face, vertigo and nausea are also present
		Medial medullary syndrome – caused by occlusion of the anterior spinal or vertebral arteries	Damage to the hypoglossal nucleus leads to unilateral paralysis and atrophy of the tongue. A crossed hemiparesis (sparing the face) and sensory changes are also present
		Lateral pontine syndrome (Foville's syndrome) – caused by occlusion of the anterior inferior cerebellar artery or circumferential artery	Damage to the facial nucleus causes flaccid paralysis of the facial muscles on the side of the lesion. Other symptoms may include deafness, ataxic gait, vertigo, nausea and sensory changes

(Continued)

Table 9.3 *(Continued)*

Site of lesion	Disorder	Aetiology	Signs and symptoms
		Medial pontine syndrome (Millard–Gubler syndrome – caused by occlusion of the paramedian branch of the basilar artery	Symptoms include facial paralysis on the side of lesion, diplopia, crossed hemiparesis and impaired touch and position sense
	Progressive bulbar palsy	A type of motor neurone disease in which there is progressive degeneration of the motor cells in some cranial nerve nuclei	Progressive weakness and atrophy of the muscles of the speech mechanism
	Poliomyelitis	Viral infection which affects the motor nuclei of the cranial nerves and the anterior horn cells of the spinal cord	Paralysis and wasting of affected muscles will lower motor neurone signs. Paralysis may be widespread or localized and can affect the speech muscles, limb muscles and muscles of respiration
	Neoplasm	Brainstem tumours – these are more common in children than adults	Tumour may progressively involve the cranial nerve nuclei, causing gradual weakness and flaccid paralysis of the muscles of the speech mechanism
	Syringobulbia	Slowly progressive cystic degeneration in the lower brainstem in the region of the fourth ventricle. Congenital disorder with onset of symptoms usually in early adult life	As the cystic cavity develops there may be progressive involvement of the cranial nerve nuclei leading to the lower motor neurone signs in the muscles of the speech mechanism
	Möbius syndrome (congenital facial diplegia)	Congenital hyperplasia of the VIth and VIIth cranial nerve nuclei	Bilateral facial palsy (VII) and bilateral abducens palsy (VI)

follows, therefore, that interruption of the nerve supply to the respiratory muscles would interfere with normal speech production.

Lesions involving either the phrenic or the intercostal nerves may lead to respiratory hypofunction in the form of a reduced tidal volume and vital capacity and impaired control of expiration. Respiratory hypofunction may in turn affect the patient's speech resulting in speech abnormalities such as short phrases due to more rapid exhaustion of breath during speech and possibly to a reduction in pitch and loudness due to limited expiratory flow volume (Darley, Aronson and Brown, 1975; Darby, 1981).

Vagus nerve lesions

The vagus nerves supply the muscles of the larynx and the levator muscles of the soft palate. Consequently, lesions of the vagus can affect either the phonatory or resonatory aspects of speech production, or both, the speech abnormality exhibited by the patient varying according to the location of the lesion along the nerve pathway. Lesions which involve the nucleus ambiguus in the brainstem (as occurs in lateral medullary syndrome) or the vagus nerve near to the brainstem (e.g. in the region of the jugular foramen) cause paralysis of all muscles that are supplied by the vagus. In such cases, the vocal cord on the affected side is paralysed in a slightly abducted position, leading to flaccid dysphonia characterized by moderate breathiness, harshness and reduced volume. Additional voice characteristics that may also be present include diplophonia, short phrases and inhalatory stridor. Further, the soft palate on the same side is also paralysed, causing the presence of hypernasality in the patient's speech. If the lesion is bilateral, the vocal cords on both sides are paralysed and can be neither abducted nor adducted and elevation of the soft palate is also impaired bilaterally, causing more severe breathiness and hypernasality. The major clinical signs of bilateral flaccid vocal cord paralysis include: breathy voice (reflecting incomplete adduction of the vocal cords that results in excessive air escape), audible inhalation (inspiratory stridor – reflecting inadequate abduction of the vocal cords during inspiration) and abnormally short phrases during contextual speech (possibly as a consequence of excessive air loss during speech as a result of inefficient laryngeal valving). Other signs seen in some patients include monopitch and monoloudness.

Physiological and acoustic studies have tended to confirm the presence of the above perceptual features in patients with paralysis of one or both vocal cords. Consistent with the perception of breathiness, a number of studies based on aerodynamic assessments have identified increased phonatory airflow rates during speech in patients with either unilateral or bilateral vocal cord weakness (Iwata, von Leden and Williams, 1972; Till and Alp, 1991). A lack of firm glottal closure has been identified in patients with unilateral vocal cord paralysis by way of high-speed laryngeal photography and videostroboscopy. In addition, consistent with the expected effect of hypotonicity of the vocal cords, these latter techniques have also identified features such as greater vibratory amplitude and exaggerated mucosal waves in the affected cord. Acoustic studies of patients with unilateral vocal cord paralysis have identified a restriction in their fundamental frequency range and variability (Murry, 1978) consistent with the often reported perception of monopitch in flaccid dysarthria (Darley, Aronson and Brown, 1975).

Bilateral weakness of the soft palate is associated with hypernasality, audible nasal emission,

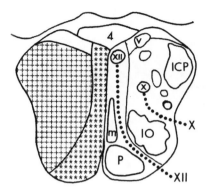

Figure 9.2 Transverse section through the medulla oblongata showing the structures affected in lateral medullary syndrome and medial medullary syndrome. ICP = inferior cerebellar peduncle; IO = inferior olive; m = medial lemniscus; P = pyramid; X = nucleus ambiguus and vagus nerve; XII = hypoglossal nucleus and hypoglossal nerve; ++ = lateral medullary syndrome; ** = medial medullary syndrome; 4 = fourth ventricle.

reduced sharpness of consonant production (as a consequence of reduced intraoral pressure due to nasal escape) and short phrases (reflecting premature exhaustion of expiratory air supply as a result of nasal escape).

Lateral medullary syndrome is one neurological disorder in which the origin of the vagus nerve in the brainstem can be affected, thereby leading to impaired phonation and resonation. Lateral medullary syndrome is caused by a cerebrovascular accident involving occlusion of the posterior inferior cerebellar artery, vertebral artery or lateral medullary artery and results in dysphagia, dysphonia, paralysis of the soft palate, nausea, vomiting and oscillopia (objects visually jump). The brainstem structures affected by lateral medullary syndrome are shown in Figure 9.2.

Lesions to the vagus nerve distal to the branch which supplies the soft palate (the pharyngeal branch) but proximal to the exit of the superior laryngeal nerve have the same affect on phonation as brainstem lesions. However, such lesions do not produce hypernasality, since functioning of the levator veli palatini is not compromised. Lesions limited to the recurrent laryngeal nerves (as may occur as a consequence of damage during thyroidectomy or as a result of compression of the vagus by intrathoracic masses or aortic arch aneurysms) are also associated with dysphonia. In this latter case, however, the crico-thyroid muscles (the principal tensor muscles of the vocal cords) are not affected and the vocal cords are paralysed closer to the midline (the paramedian position). Consequently, the voice is likely to be harsh and reduced in loudness, but with a lesser degree of breathiness, however, than seen in cases with brainstem lesions involving the nucleus ambiguus. Bilateral damage to the recurrent laryngeal nerves is rare. If present, bilateral paralysis of the vocal cords is more likely to have resulted from a brainstem lesion.

The presence or absence of hypernasality in combination with dysphonia, therefore, can provide valuable information about the location of the lesion along the course of the vagus nerve. The major lesion sites which may be associated with disruption of the vagus nerve together with their clinically recognizable effects on speech production are summarized in Figure 9.3.

Trigeminal, facial and hypoglossal nerve lesions

Together, the trigeminal, facial and hypoglossal nerves regulate the functioning of the articulators of speech. The trigeminal nerve controls the movements of the mandible. Unilateral trigeminal lesions have only a minor effect on speech, movements, such as elevation of the mandible, being impaired to only a minor extent. Bilateral trigeminal lesions, however, have a devastating effect on speech production in that the elevators of the mandible (e.g. masseter and temporalis muscles) may be too weak to approximate the mandible and maxilla, which may prevent the tongue and lips from making the necessary contacts with oral structures for the production of labial and lingual consonants and vowels. Lesions to the trigeminal nerves, however, rarely occur in isolation, with other cranial nerves also usually being involved. Almost any pathology involving the middle cranial fossa (e.g. arteriovenous malformations, stroke, infections, cerebellopontine angle tumours, etc.) can disrupt the trigeminal nerve, leading to sensory and/or motor disturbances in its distribution.

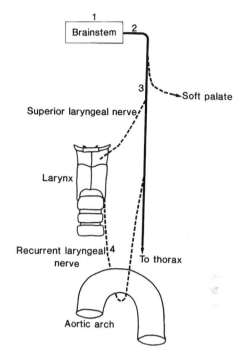

Figure 9.3 Distribution of the vagus nerve to the speech musculature showing the major lesion sites associated with disruption of speech. 1. Lesion in the nucleus ambiguus leading to impaired phonation and resonation. 2. Lesion in the region of the jugular foramen leading to impaired phonation and resonation. 3. Lesion distal to the origin of the pharyngeal nerve associated with impaired phonation and normal soft palate function. 4. Lesion of the left recurrent laryngeal nerve associated with flaccid paralysis of all left intrinsic laryngeal muscles except cricothyroid; as a consequence, abduction and adduction of the left vocal cord is impaired.

Unilateral flaccid paralysis of the muscles of facial expression, as occurs following lesions in one or other of the facial nerves, causes distortion of bilabial and labiodental consonants. As a result of weakness of the lips on the affected side, these patients are unable to seal their lips tightly and air escapes between the lips during the build-up of intraoral pressure. Consequently, the production of plosives, in particular, is defective. In patients with bilateral facial paralysis or paresis (e.g. in Möbius syndrome), the above situation is exaggerated. Bilateral weakness leads to speech impairments that range from distortion to complete obliteration of bilabial and labiodental consonants. In severe cases, some vowel distortion may also be evident owing to problems with either lip rounding or lip spreading. Lesions involving the VIIth nerve can occur in isolation or in combination with other cranial nerves, particularly the VIth (abducent) (e.g. lesions in the floor of the fourth ventricle) or VIIIth (vestibulocochlear) (e.g. acoustic neuromas) nerves. Common causes of facial nerve paralysis include vascular lesions, trauma, infections (e.g. mononucleosis, herpes zoster, otitic media, meningitis, Lyme disease, syphilis, sarcoidosis and inflammatory polyradiculoneuropathy) and tumours (e.g. cerebellopontine angle meningioma, acoustic neuroma). Bell's palsy is a condition involving facial weakness of the lower motor neurone type caused by idiopathic facial nerve involvement outside the central nervous system. Clinical examination reveals no abnormalities beyond the territory of the facial nerve. Weakness generally comes on abruptly but may progress over several hours or even several days. The cause is not known but may be related to reactivation of herpes simplex type 1 infection in the geniculate ganglion, injuring the facial nerve in some cases. The majority of patients recover without treatment over a period of days or months in some cases. Approximately, 10% of cases experience permanent facial weakness and disfigurement.

Lesions of the hypoglossal nerves cause disturbances in articulation by interfering with normal tongue movements. Both phonation and resonation, however, remain normal. Unilateral hypoglossal lesions as may occur in either brainstem conditions such as medial medullary syndrome (Figure 9.2) or peripheral nerve lesions such as submaxillary tumours compressing either the left or right hypoglossal nerve cause flaccid paralysis of the tongue on the same side as the lesion. Although this may be associated with mild temporary articulatory imprecision, especially during production of linguodental and linguopalatal consonants, in most cases the patient learns to compensate rapidly for the unilateral tongue weakness or paralysis (usually within a few days post-onset in acute conditions). More serious articulatory impairments, however, are associated with bilateral hypoglossal nerve lesions. Tongue movement in such cases may be severely restricted and speech sounds such as high front vowels and consonants that require elevation of

the tongue tip to the upper alveolar ridge or hard palate (e.g. /t/, /d/, /n/, /l/, etc.) may be grossly distorted. Lesions involving the XIIth nerve can be intramedullary, extramedullary or extracranial. The XIIth nerve is not usually involved in isolation but rather is affected in combination with other cranial nerves, particularly IX, X and XI. Aetiologies of XIIth nerve lesions include surgical trauma (e.g. during carotid endarterectomy), accidental trauma, carotid and vertebral artery aneurysms, tumours (e.g. in neck, salivary glands, base of tongue) and infections (including local and infectious mononucleosis).

Multiple cranial nerve lesions

The most severe form of flaccid dysarthria results from disruption of several cranial nerves simultaneously. In bulbar palsy the muscles supplied by cranial nerves V, VII, IX, X, XI and XII may simultaneously dysfunction. Consequently, in this condition the lips, tongue, jaw, palate and larynx are affected in varying combinations and with varying degrees of weakness. Disorders evident in the affected person's speech may include: hypernasality with nasal emission due to disruption of the palatopharyngeal valve; breathiness, harsh voice, audible inspiration, monopitch and monoloudness associated with laryngeal dysfunction; and distortion of consonant production due to impairment of the articulators.

Speech disorders in myasthenia gravis

Myasthenia gravis has been defined by Penn (1980) as 'a disorder of neuromuscular transmission, resulting from an auto-immune attack upon the nicotinic post-synaptic receptor for acetylcholine' (p. 382). The condition is characterized by muscle weakness that worsens as the muscle is used (fatigability) and rapidly recovers when the muscle is at rest. Females are more frequently affected than males and onset is usually in adult life between the ages of 20 and 50 years.

The abnormal muscular fatigability may, for a long time, be confined to, or predominate in, an isolated group of muscles. Ptosis (drooping) of one or both upper eyelids caused by weakness of

Table 9.4 Clinical signs of upper and lower motor neurone lesions.

Upper motor neurone lesions	Lower motor neurone lesions
• Hypertonus (spasticity)	• Hypotonus (flaccidity)
• Mild atrophy of disuse	• Atrophy of individual muscles
• Hyperactive muscle stretch reflexes (e.g. jaw-jerk)	• Muscle stretch reflexes decreased or absent
• Positive sucking reflex	• Negative sucking reflex
• Positive Babinski sign	• Negative Babinski sign

the levator palpebrae is often the first symptom of the condition. Facial, jaw, bulbar and neck muscle weakness ultimately develops in about 50% of cases. Symptoms include diplopia, dysarthria, a tendency for the jaw to hang open and difficulty chewing. There is also dysphagia, drooling and neck muscle weakness. Weakness of all facial muscles is common.

Darley, Aronson and Brown (1975) regarded myasthenia gravis as a special case of flaccid dysarthria because of the progression and increase in severity of speech difficulties with prolongation of speaking activity. As these patients speak, fatigue of the bulbar musculature becomes more and more evident in increased hypernasality, deterioration of articulation, onset and increase of dysphonia and reduction of loudness level (Darley, Aronson and Brown, 1975). Finally, the speech becomes unintelligible. Bannister (1985) suggested that the characteristic fatigability may be readily demonstrated by asking the patient to count up to 50, during which speech becomes progressively less distinct.

Spastic dysarthria (upper motor neurone dysarthria)

The term 'spastic dysarthria' was first used by Darley, Aronson and Brown (1969a,b) to describe the speech disturbance seen in association with damage to the upper motor neurones that convey nerve impulses from the motor areas of the cerebral cortex to the lower motor neurones originating from the bulbar cranial nerve nuclei. The lesions associated with spastic

dysarthria can involve either the cortical motor areas from which the descending motor pathways originate (primarily the pre-central gyrus and pre-motor cortex) or the descending tracts themselves as they pass through the internal capsule, cerebral peduncles or the brainstem. The speech characteristics of spastic dysarthria are presumed to reflect the effects of hypertonicity (spasticity) and weakness of the bulbar musculature in a way that slows movement and reduces its range and force (Murdoch, Thompson and Theodoros, 1997). The reference to 'spastic' in the term 'spastic dysarthria' is therefore a reflection of the clinical signs of upper motor neurone damage, which include spastic paralysis or paresis of the involved muscles, hyper-reflexia (e.g. hyperactive jaw-jerk), little or no muscle atrophy (except for the possibility of some atrophy associated with disuse) and the presence of pathological reflexes (e.g. sucking reflex). One of the basic features of upper motor neurone lesions is that reflex arcs remain anatomically intact, whereas in lower motor neurone lesions the reflex arc is disrupted and reflexes become absent or diminished. Table 9.4 compares the major signs associated with upper versus lower motor neurone lesions.

Neuroanatomy of the upper motor neurone system

The two major components comprise the upper motor neurone system, including a direct and an indirect component. The direct component, also known as the pyramidal system, comprises neurones that project their axons from their cell bodies located in the cortical motor areas directly to the level of the lower motor neurones without synapsing along the way. In contrast, the indirect component (previously referred to as the extrapyramidal system) involves multisynaptic pathways that originate from the motor cortex but then pass to the level of the lower motor neurones via multisynaptic connections that involve structures such as the basal ganglia, various brainstem nuclei, the reticular formation, cerebellum and thalamus. For instance, many of the extrapyramidal fibres descend from the motor cortex in the internal capsule and cerebral peduncles to the pons and are then relayed to the cerebellum, from which projections then pass to either the brainstem or the back of the cerebral cortex via the thalamus. Many other extrapyramidal fibres descend from the motor cortex via the internal capsule to the basal ganglia, where they are relayed by a variety of pathways to the excitatory and inhibitory centres of the brainstem. Overall, the extrapyramidal system is said to comprise all of those tracts, besides the pyramidal system, that transmit motor signals from the cortical motor areas to the lower motor neurones. The final pathways for transmission of extrapyramidal signals to the lower motor neurones include the vestibulospinal tracts, the tectospinal tracts, the rubospinal tracts and the reticulospinal tracts (Figure 9.4).

The extrapyramidal system appears to be primarily responsible for postural arrangements and the orientation of movement in space, whereas the pyramidal system is chiefly responsible for controlling the far more discrete and skilled voluntary aspects of a movement. Because in most locations (e.g. internal capsule) the two systems lie in close anatomical proximity, lesions that affect one component will usually also involve the other component. The term 'upper motor neurone lesion' is usually not applied to disorders affecting only the extrapyramidal system (e.g. in basal ganglia lesions). Such disorders are termed 'extrapyramidal syndromes' and are discussed further in Chapter 10.

The pyramidal system

Based on their projections to the spinal cord, midbrain or bulbar region of the brainstem, three

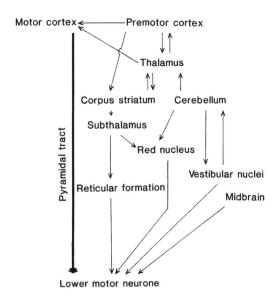

Figure 9.4 Schematic diagram of the direct (pyramidal) and indirect (extrapyramidal) motor pathways.

major fibre groups are recognized as comprising the pyramidal system. These groups include: the corticospinal tracts (pyramidal tracts proper), the cortico-mesencephalic tracts and the corticobulbar tracts.

Corticospinal tracts. The corticospinal tracts descend from the cerebral cortex to various levels of the spinal cord, where they synapse with lower motor neurones. Although the greatest proportion of fibres arise from the motor cortex (primarily the pre-central gyrus), the corticospinal tracts originate from both the motor and sensory areas of the cerebral cortex. The corticospinal tract in each cerebral hemisphere enters the subcortical white matter from the cortex in a fan-shaped distribution of fibres called corona radiata (radiating crown). The common central mass of white matter in each cerebral hemisphere, which contains commissural, association and projection fibres and into which the pyramidal fibres pass, has an oval appearance in horizontal sections of the brain and is, therefore, called the centrum semiovale. From the corona radiata the fibres of the corticospinal tracts converge into the posterior limb of the internal capsule (see Chapter 3) and then pass via the cerebral peduncles of the midbrain to the pons. As the fibres of the corticospinal tracts are closely grouped together as they pass through the internal capsule, even small lesions in this area can have a devastating effect on the motor control of the limbs on one half of the body. After traversing the pons, the fibres group together to form the pyramids of the medulla oblongata. It is from the pyramids that the term 'pyramidal tracts' is derived. Near to the junction of the medulla oblongata and the spinal cord, the majority (85–90%) of the fibres in each pyramid cross to the opposite side, interlacing as they do so and forming the decussation of the pyramids. It is this crossing that provides the contralateral motor control of the limbs, the motor cortex controlling movement of the right limbs and vice versa. The fibres that cross then descend in the lateral funiculus of the spinal cord as the lateral corticospinal tracts. Of those fibres that remain uncrossed, most descend in the ventral funiculus as the anterior corticospinal tracts. Most of these latter fibres descussate to the opposite side further down the spinal cord.

Corticomesencephalic tracts. The corticomesencephalic tracts comprise fibres which descend from the cerebral cortex to the nuclei of cranial nerves III, IV and VI which provided the motor supply to the extrinsic muscles of the eye. These fibres arise from the frontal eye field which is that part of the cerebral cortex of the frontal lobe that lies immediately anterior to the pre-motor cortex.

Corticobulbar Tracts. The fibres of the corticobulbar tracts start out in company with those of the corticospinal tracts but take a divergent route at the level of the midbrain. They terminate by synapsing with lower motor neurones in the nuclei of cranial nerves V, VII, IX, X and XII. For this reason, they form the most important component of the pyramidal system in relation to the occurrence of spastic dysarthria. Although the majority of corticobulbar fibres cross to the contralateral side, uncrossed (ipsilateral) connections also exist. In fact, most of the motor nuclei of the cranial nerves in the brainstem receive bilateral upper motor neurone connections. Consequently, although to a varying degree the predominance of upper motor neurone innervation to the cranial nerve nuclei comes from the contralateral hemisphere, in most instances there is also considerable ipsilateral upper motor neurone innervation.

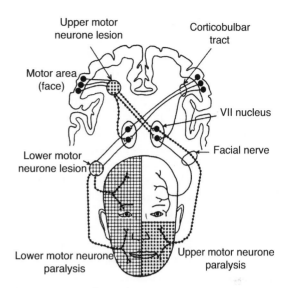

Figure 9.5 The effects of unilateral disruption to the upper and lower motor neurone supply to the muscles of facial expression.

One important exception to the above upper motor neurone innervation of the cranial nerve nuclei is that part of the facial nucleus that gives rise to the lower motor neurones that supply the lower half of the face. It appears to receive only a contralateral upper motor neurone connection (Sears and Franklin, 1980; Snell, 1980). (See Figure 9.5.)

Clinically, the presence of a bilateral innervation to most cranial nerve nuclei has important implications for the type of speech disorder that follows unilateral upper motor neurone lesions. Although a mild and usually transient impairment in articulation may occur subsequent to unilateral corticobulbar lesions, in general bilateral corticobulbar lesions are required to produce a permanent dysarthria.

Unilateral upper motor neurone lesions located in either the motor cortex or the internal capsule and so on cause a spastic paralysis or weakness in the contralateral lower half of the face but not the upper part of the face, which may be associated with a mild, transient dysarthria owing to weakness of orbicularis oris. There is no weakness of the forehead, muscles of mastication, soft palate (i.e. no hypernasality), pharynx (i.e. no swallowing problems) or larynx (i.e.

no dysphonia). A unilateral upper motor neurone lesion may, however, produce a mild unilateral weakness of the tongue on the side opposite the lesion. In the case of such a unilateral lesion, it appears, therefore, that the ipsilateral upper neurone is adequate to maintain near normal function of most bulbar muscles, except those in the tongue. Although most authors agree that the hypoglossal nucleus receives bilateral upper motor neurone innervation, for some reason the ipsilateral connection appears to be less effective than in the case of other cranial nerve nuclei. Snell (1980) suggested that the part of the hypoglossal nucleus that supplies the genioglossus muscle (the only muscle that can protrude the tongue) receives upper motor neurone innervation from only the contralateral cerebral hemisphere.

Neurological disorders associated with upper motor neurone lesions

Two major syndromes can be attributed to upper motor neurone damage: pseudobulbar palsy (also known as 'supranuclear bulbar palsy') and spastic hemiplegia. Both are characterized by spasticity and impairment or loss of voluntary movements.

Pseudobulbar palsy

Pseudobulbar palsy takes its name from its clinical resemblance to bulbar palsy ('pseudo' means 'false') and is associated with a variety of neurological disorders which bilaterally disrupt the upper motor neurone connections to the bulbar cranial nerves. In this condition, the bulbar muscles, including the muscles of articulation, the velopharynx and larynx are hypertonic and exhibit hyper-reflexia. In addition, there is a reduction in the range and force of movement of the bulbar muscles as well as slowness of individual and repetitive movements. The rhythm of repetitive movements, however, is regular and the direction of movement normal. Symptoms of pseudobulbar palsy include bilateral facial paralysis, dysarthria, dysphonia, bilateral hemiparesis, incontinence and bradykinesia. Drooling from the corners of the mouth is common and many of these patients exhibit lability. A hyperactive jaw

reflex and positive sucking reflex are also evident, and swallowing problems are a common feature. This syndrome is the neurological disorder with which spastic dysarthria is most commonly associated in that persistent spastic dysarthria is caused by bilateral disruption of the upper motor neurone supply to the bulbar cranial nerve nuclei.

The aetiology of pseudobulbar palsy varies, but may include bilateral cerebrovascular accidents, brain damage sustained as the result of head injuries acquired in accidents, extensive brain tumours, cerebral palsy of infancy or degenerative neurological conditions such as multiple sclerosis or motor neurone disease. Lesions that cause spastic dysarthria can be located in a number of different regions of the brain, including the cortical motor areas from which the descending motor pathways originate (primarily the pre-central gyrus and pre-motor cortex) and the descending tracts themselves as they pass through the internal capsule, the cerebral peduncles or the brainstem.

All aspects of speech production, including phonation, resonation, articulation and respiration, are affected in pseudobulbar palsy but to varying degrees. Bilateral spastic paralysis of the laryngeal muscles causes narrowing of the glottis thereby increasing the resistance to airflow at this point. It should be noted that hypertonic changes in the vocal cords cannot easily be visualized, and so laryngoscopy of patients with bilateral upper motor neurone lesions often does not reveal any obvious abnormality in their structure or function. Evidence of vocal cord dysfunction, however, will be present in the patient's voice as a harsh voice quality and strained/strangled sound, associated with the exhaled breath during speech being squeezed with difficulty through the narrow glottis. This is the reverse of what is found in flaccid dysarthria. The range of movement of the vocal cords may also be reduced by hypertonus, thereby causing changes in prosody. The vocal pitch of patients with pseudobulbar palsy is lower than that of normals'.

The major articulatory disorder evidenced by patients with pseudobulbar palsy is the production of imprecise consonants, although in severe cases vowel distortions may also be present. A slow rate of articulation is frequently observed in these cases. An oromotor examination usually reveals weakness of the tongue and lips. Although the tongue is of normal size and not atrophied, movement of the tongue in and out of the mouth is performed slowly and the extent of tongue protrusion limited. In some cases, the patient may be unable to protrude the tongue beyond the lower teeth, and lateral movements are restricted. Voluntary lip movements are also slow and restricted in range. According to Darley, Aronson and Brown (1969a,b), the production of syllable repetitions is usually slow but rhythmic.

Hypernasality is a usual finding in pseudobulbar palsy. During phonation, the soft palate can be seen to elevate symmetrically, however, the elevation is slow and may be incomplete. Swallowing problems are also a common feature of the disorder and there is a definite danger of choking in the more severe cases.

Spastic hemiplegia

Unilateral upper motor neurone lesions produce spastic hemiplegia, a condition in which the muscles of the lower face and extremities on the opposite side of the body are primarily affected. The bulbar muscles are not greatly affected, with weakness being confined to the contralateral lips, lower half of the face and tongue. In addition, the forehead, palate, pharynx and larynx are largely unaffected. Consequently, unlike pseudobulbar palsy, spastic hemiplegia is not associated with problems in mastication, swallowing, velopharyngeal function or laryngeal activity. The tongue appears normal in the mouth but deviates to the weaker side on protrusion. Only a transitory dysarthria comprising a mild articulatory imprecision rather than a persistent spastic dysarthria is present.

Clinical characteristics of spastic dysarthria

Darley, Aronson and Brown (1975) identified four major symptoms of muscular dysfunction subsequent to disruption of the upper motor neurone supply to the speech musculature that reflect in the speech output: spasticity, weakness, lim-

ited range of movement and slowness of movement. Consequently, these physiological features are characteristically identified as the underlying basis of the majority of the deviant speech behaviours observed in individuals with spastic dysarthria, a condition characterized by slow, dragging, laboured speech which is produced with some effort.

Perceptual features of spastic dysarthria

The most prominent perceptible speech deviations reported by Darley, Aronson and Brown (1969a,b) to be associated with spastic dysarthria include: imprecise consonants, monopitch, reduced stress, harsh voice quality, monoloudness, low pitch, slow rate, hypernasality, strained/strangled voice quality, short phrases, distorted vowels, pitch breaks, continuous breathy voice and excess and equal stress. The deviant speech characteristics clustered primarily in the areas of articulatory/resonatory incompetence, phonatory stenosis and prosodic insufficiency. Chenery, Murdoch and Ingram (1992) identified a similar set of deviant perceptual features in their group of subjects with pseudobulbar palsy, thereby confirming that subjects with spastic dysarthria present with deficits in all aspects of speech production (i.e. respiration, phonation, resonation, articulation and prosody), albeit to varying degrees.

In addition to the perceptual speech characteristics, oromotor examinations of subjects with spastic dysarthria also reveal a characteristic pattern of deficits. Oromotor assessment usually reveals the presence of weakness in the muscles of the lip and tongue with movement of the tongue in and out of the mouth usually performed slowly. The extent of tongue movement is often very limited, such that the patient may be unable to protrude their tongue beyond the lower teeth. Lateral movements of the tongue are also restricted, although the tongue is of normal size. Voluntary lip movements are also usually slow and restricted in range. Based on an assessment using the Frenchay Dysarthria Assessment, Enderby (1986) identified the major characteristics of spastic dysarthria to be (in decreasing order of frequency of occurrence): poor movement of the tongue in speech, slow rate of speech, poor phonation and intonation, poor intelligibility in conversation, reduced alternating movements of the tongue, poor lip movements in speech, reduced maintenance of palatal elevation, poor intelligibility of description, hypernasality and lack of control of volume.

In support of the findings of Darley, Aronson and Brown (1969a,b), other groups of researchers have also identified a slow rate of speech in spastic dysarthric speakers based on their performance when reading a standard passage (Linebaugh and Wolfe, 1984; Ziegler and von Cramon, 1986). As a measure of articulation rate, Linebaugh and Wolfe (1984) used the mean syllable duration, which was obtained by dividing the audible speech emission time by the number of syllables produced during a standard reading passage. Using this method, they found that spastic dysarthric speakers had significantly longer mean syllable durations than normal speakers and that the mean syllable duration significantly correlated with both intelligibility and naturalness for spastic dysarthric speakers. In an attempt to make Darley, Aronson and Brown's (1969a,b) concepts of 'slow rate', 'imprecise consonants' and 'distorted vowels' more precise and quantifiable, Ziegler and von Cramon (1986), using a computerized signal processing technique, reported spastic dysarthric speakers to have increased word and syllable durations (indicative of a slow rate), a reduction of sound pressure level contrast in consonant articulation (indicative of imprecise consonants) and centralization of vowel formants (indicative of distorted vowels). In addition to a slower rate of speech, spastic dysarthric speakers have also been reported to have significantly slower syllable repetition rates than normal subjects (Portnoy and Aronson, 1982; Dworkin and Aronson, 1986).

Portnoy and Aronson (1982) investigated the feature of slow diadochokinetic rate in a group of patients with spastic dysarthria using computerized instrumentation. They found that patients with spastic dysarthria not only had significantly slower syllable repetition rates than normal subjects but also had significantly more variable than normal syllable repetition rates. This latter quantitative result is inconsistent with the perceptual analysis of Darley, Aronson and Brown (1969a,b), who described spastic dysarthric subjects as having a regular rhythm of syllable repetition.

Physiological and acoustic features of spastic dysarthria

Although perceptual analysis remains the foundation of day-to-day dysarthria assessment, the inherent inadequacies of this approach casts serious doubts over the suitability of perceptual analysis as the primary tool in the differential diagnosis and treatment of dysarthria. Orlikoff (1992) proposed that the identification of abnormal perceptual features through perceptual analysis merely defines the presence of the disorder and documents the overall speech disability. It does not, however, define the nature of the underlying pathophysiological dysfunction. Murdoch, Thompson and Theodoros (1997) proposed that dysarthria treatment should be based on a thorough pathophysiological assessment to determine the status of muscular impairment in each of the speech production subsystems. Physiological assessment should be used not only to explain and quantify speech impairments but also to help parse the subsystems of the speech mechanism that are disordered. Understanding the underlying pathophysiological deficits contributing to the speech disorder, through a combined perceptual, acoustic and physiological approach, can lead to more efficient and effective treatment strategies by enabling clinicians, first, to better define the loci of the speech deficits (i.e. articulatory, velopharyngeal, laryngeal or respiratory) and, second, to identify those features of the speech disorder whose improvement would lead to the greatest gains with treatment. Roy *et al.* (2001) used a combined perceptual, acoustic and physiological approach to plot the recovery of an individual with severe spastic dysarthria and confirmed the benefits of this approach to diagnosis and treatment and for tracking the effects of interventions.

Unfortunately, to date, very few instrumental investigations have been conducted to examine physiological impairments underlying the deviant perceptual speech dimensions observed in persons with spastic dysarthria. Further, in that the majority of reported studies have used very small subject groups (in most cases $n < 5$), included subjects with a variety of dysarthria severity levels or used subjects with congenital spastic dysarthria (which may or may not be comparable to the performance of subjects with acquired neurological damage), in most instances it is difficult to make conclusive statements regarding the nature of the physiological deficits associated with spastic dysarthria. The following sections provide a summary of the major findings from the relatively few physiological and acoustic investigations of subjects with spastic dysarthria reported to date.

Articulatory function in spastic dysarthria. Deficits in articulatory function, particularly reduced movement of the lips and tongue (Enderby, 1986), have been identified as a characteristic feature of subjects with spastic dysarthria. Instrumental studies have also confirmed a reduced range of articulatory movement and a slowing down in the rate of speech in patients with spastic dysarthria. Hirose, Kiritani and Sawashima (1980, 1982) used cineradiography and an X-ray microbeam system, fibreoptic and photoglottographic recording, ultrasonic techniques, and a position sensor detector as well as electromyographic assessment to analyse the articulatory dynamics of two patients with pseudobulbar palsy. It was found that the single and repetitive articulatory movements of these subjects were very slow with a limited range of movement; however, the consistency of the dynamic pattern of articulatory movements as observed in syllable repetition tasks tended to be preserved. This latter finding is consistent with the perceptual findings of Darley, Aronson and Brown (1975) that spastic dysarthric patients repeat syllables at a slower than normal rate but with normal rhythm. Hirose, Kiritani and Sawashima's (1980, 1982) investigations also revealed that lip and tongue articulation was often accompanied by jaw displacement, which was taken to indicate voluntary compensatory articulation strategies. Post-recording analysis of the data demonstrated that after removal of the influence of jaw movement from the articulatory traces the range of independent tongue tip movement was very limited (Hirose, Kiritani and Sawashima, 1980, 1982).

As indicated previously, Ziegler and von Cramon (1986), using acoustic evaluation, confirmed the perception of a reduced speech rate in persons with spastic dysarthria. They attributed the presence of increased word and syllable durations to reduced movement velocity of the tongue, lips, jaw and velum. In addition to an altered rate of speech production, a marked reduction in sound pressure level contrast in consonant articulation and a centralization of vowel formants have been noted in the speech of subjects with spastic dysarthria (Ziegler and von Cramon, 1986). These findings represent acoustic evidence to support the perception of imprecise consonants and imprecise vowels in the speech of these subjects. Acoustic investigations of a short segment of speech from a subject with spastic dysarthria have also revealed a number of other acoustic correlates of the perceptual features of 'imprecise articulation', including relative weak frication intensity noise and a shift in aperiodic energy during the production of sounds 's' and 'sh' (Weismer, 1984).

Platt, Andrews and Howie (1980a) and Platt *et al.* (1980b) carried out a study of the phonological production of 50 cerebral palsy adults, 32 of whom had spastic dysarthria. Sounds which proved most difficult were post-alveolar fricatives /s/, /z/ affricates /ts/, /dz/ and labiodental consonants /v/. There were more word final consonant errors than word initial consonant errors and the three vowels which represent the extremes of the vowel quadrilateral /i/, /a/, /ʊ/ were difficult. Diadochokinetic rates were about half of that expected of a normal population. It is not known whether the speech patterns of cerebral palsy adults who have had spastic dysarthria from birth are similar to patients who have acquired a pseudobulbar palsy much later in life. Therefore, these phonological findings may not be directly applicable to the type of acquired disorders discussed so far.

The articulatory movements of dysarthric subjects has also been examined using electropalatography. Hardcastle, Morgan-Barry and Clark (1985) examined the lingual movements of three subjects, one dyspraxic and two dysarthric – one of whom had moderate spastic dysarthria. The results of this investigation revealed that the dysarthric subjects produced distortions in target configurations for consonant sounds manifest mainly by a reduction in spatial goals (e.g. incomplete closures for stops). The subject with spastic dysarthria also demonstrated an overshoot of target goals (Hardcastle, Morgan-Barry and Clark, 1985). On the basis of these findings, it was concluded that the dysarthric subjects demonstrated an inadequate control over muscle-tension requirements for consonant articulation (Hardcastle, Morgan-Barry and Clark, 1985).

From these investigations it can be determined that the presence of imprecise consonants in the speech of subjects with spastic dysarthria appears to be the result of physiological impairments in the function of the articulators. Indeed, investigations of articulatory function have revealed specific strength and motor control deficits in subjects with spastic dysarthria. Dworkin and Aronson (1986) used a semiconductor strain-gauge force transducer to assess tongue strength in a group of 18 dysarthric subjects that included three subjects with spastic dysarthria. They found that the dysarthric group had weaker tongue strength, as well as reduced and unsustained levels of maximum tongue strength effort compared to normal controls during sustained effort tasks.

The investigation of the lingual function of a group of 16 subjects with spastic dysarthria similarly revealed deficits in maximum tongue pressure following upper motor neurone damage (Thompson, Murdoch and Stokes, 1995a). In addition, these assessments revealed an impaired rate of repetitive tongue movement in the dysarthric group as well as evidence of fatigue during sustained effort tasks in comparison to the performance of a group of age-matched control subjects (Thompson, Murdoch and Stokes, 1995a). Similarly, impairments in maximum force, repetition rate and endurance capabilities were also observed in the labial function of subjects with upper motor neurone damage (Thompson, Murdoch and Stokes, 1995b).

In addition to reductions in the maximum force/pressures generated by the articulators of subjects with spastic dysarthria, a number of investigations have also identified deficits in force control (Abbs, Hunker and Barlow, 1983) and a reduction in the rate of force change (Barlow and

Abbs, 1986) of the articulators of these subjects. Abbs, Hunker and Barlow (1983) detailed the results of articulatory function in a subject with congenital spasticity. Assessment revealed force control deficits in the lip, tongue and jaw of this subject, with the lips and tongue having the most instability at maximum force levels, while jaw instability was greatest at very low force levels (Abbs, Hunker and Barlow, 1983). The reduced capacity to recruit muscle forces at normal rates is also recognized as a fundamental pathophysiological feature of orofacial control in patients with the upper motor neurone syndrome (Barlow and Abbs, 1986). Barlow and Abbs (1986) examined fine force and position control in six normal males and five adults with congenital cerebral palsy of a predominantly spastic form and the results of their investigation revealed reductions in the average rate of force change in the lips, tongue and jaw of these dysarthric subjects.

Determination of the exact nature of the physiological mechanisms underlying the impairments identified in the articulators of subjects with spastic dysarthria is an area in need of further investigation. In the light of the suggestions made by Barlow and Abbs (1984), the reduction in maximum tongue strength demonstrated by subjects with spastic dysarthria may be best explained simply by muscle weakness that is due to the disruption of the motor control signals descending from the motor cortex. Upper motor neurone lesions invariably reduce muscle strength because fewer lower motor neurones are activated and hence fewer motor units are firing (Sahrman and Norton, 1977). There is also evidence that upper motor neurone damage can cause weakness due to secondary lower motor neurone degeneration resulting from limitations in firing frequency (Sahrman and Norton, 1977).

Velopharyngeal function in spastic dysarthria. Velopharyngeal function is usually compromised in spastic dysarthria, and hypernasality is, therefore, a common feature of the speech disorder associated with pseudobulbar palsy, although to a lesser degree than in conditions such as bulbar palsy that involve damage to lower motor neurones. The movement pattern of the velopharyngeal musculature in the spastic dysarthric group has been described as symmetrical, with the rate of elevation of the soft palate during phonation being slow and sometimes incomplete. The palate usually responds reflexively when stimulated with a tongue depressor.

Thompson and Murdoch (1995) investigated the presence of nasality disturbances in a group of 18 dysarthric subjects with upper neurone motor damage following cerebrovascular accidents. They used an accelerometric assessment technique to indirectly evaluate the functioning of the velopharyngeal component of the speech mechanism in these subjects. The results of their investigation revealed that the cerebrovascular accident subjects as a group produced a significantly higher degree of nasality on the production of non-nasal speech tasks than the control subjects. No significant difference, however, was observed between the two groups on the production of nasal utterances. Consequently, the results of the instrumental investigation confirmed the presence of hypernasal resonance in the group of subjects with spastic dysarthria. The results of the individual evaluation of each subject, however, revealed that less than half of the subjects presented with disorders of nasal resonance, indicating a relatively low incidence of nasality disorders in subjects with predominantly mild and mild/moderate degrees of spastic dysarthria. No subject was found to have hyponasality on the basis of the instrumental assessment.

The presence of hypernasality in the speech of subjects with spastic dysarthria has been attributed to the presence of a slow and incomplete elevation of the soft palate (Chenery, Murdoch and Ingram, 1992). Based on personal observations made during cineradiography, Aten (1983) reported that, following initial elevation, there is a progressive failure of velar closure in spastic dysarthric patients when counting or during the production of serial speech. In subjects with more severe resonance disorders, Aten (1983) describes an 'inertia in initiating speech activities' (p. 70), which is not actually weakness but rather 'a rapid onset of increased resistance to stretch' (p. 70) which blocks the normal movement of the velum (Aten, 1983).

Hirose, Kiritani and Sawashima (1982) used an X-ray microbeam system to analyse the articulatory dynamics of two patients with pseudobulbar palsy and two with amyotrophic lateral sclerosis. In their observations of articulatory movements during repetition of the word 'ten', it was found that the degree of velum elevation during the /t/ section of the utterance became lowered with repetition of the utterance. The tendency towards the lowering of the velum during the repetition was determined to be indicative of the effects of fatigue, and the underlying basis for the presence of hypernasal voice quality in these patients. This observed pattern of behaviour is consistent with the personal observations of Aten (1983) noted previously.

At present, it is assumed that the noted reduction in speed and range of movements of the palate, such as those reported by Aten (1983), are the product of spasticity in the muscles responsible for palatal elevation. Unfortunately, however, there has been a lack of systematic, direct investigations of palatal movement in subjects with spastic dysarthria. Consequently, in order to more fully understand the mechanisms underlying the hypernasality identified in this subject group, there is a need for more detailed physiological investigations of velopharyngeal function to be conducted, incorporating endoscopic, X-ray microbeam and electromyographic investigations of the velar mechanism both at rest and during connected speech.

Laryngeal function in spastic dysarthria. Since the descriptions of the perceptual features of spastic dysarthria provided by Darley, Aronson and Brown (1969a,b), it has been presumed that bilateral upper motor neurone lesions are manifest at the laryngeal level primarily by the increased tone of the laryngeal muscles leading to a narrowing of the laryngeal aperture (phonatory stenosis). This narrowing is supposedly the result of a hyperadduction of the vocal cords. Hypertonic changes in the vocal cords, however, cannot be easily visualized so that laryngoscopy of pseudobulbar cases often does not reveal any obvious abnormality in their structure and function. The presence of hypertonicity in the laryngeal adductor muscles is suggested, however, by the observed harsh voice quality and strained/strangled sound of the voice in pseudobulbar palsy.

Given the speculated presence of laryngeal hyperadduction, it would be expected that physiological investigations of the laryngeal function of subjects with spastic dysarthria would reveal behaviours characteristic of laryngeal hyperfunction. In the case of aerodynamic measures of vocal function, the presence of laryngeal hyperfunction would be expected to manifest as increased resistance, increased pressure, decreased laryngeal airflow during phonation and a decrease in the ad/abduction rate of the vocal folds (Smitheran and Hixon, 1981; Hillman *et al.*, 1989). Investigations of the vocal fold vibratory cycle have also indicated that increased vocal fold tension associated with laryngeal hyperfunction results in an increased fundamental frequency (Hollien, 1960) and corresponding decreases in the duty cycle and closing times (Kitzing, Carlborg and Löfqvist, 1982: Hanson, Gerratt and Ward, 1983; Frokjaer-Jensen and Thyme-Frokjaer, 1989; Hillman *et al.*, 1989). Consequently, electroglottographic investigation of the laryngeal function of spastic dysarthria would expect to identify an increased fundamental frequency and a decreased duty cycle and closing time.

The results of an investigation (Murdoch, Thompson and Stokes, 1994) into the laryngeal function of subjects with predominantly mild to moderate spastic dysarthria following cerebrovascular accidents, however, was found to only partly confirm the presence of these laryngeal parameters in subjects with spastic dysarthria. Using both electroglottographic and aerodynamic techniques, Murdoch, Thompson and Stokes (1994) found that only 50% of their group of dysarthric subjects exhibited a predominance of features classically associated with hyperfunctional laryngeal activity, including increased resistance, elevated pressures and decreased laryngeal airflow. Even then, not all of these features were always evident in the same subject, with the results of a cluster analysis identifying three different subgroups with varying combinations of hyperfunctional features. The remaining 50% of the cerebrovascular accident subjects in the Murdoch, Thompson and Stokes (1994) investigation were collected into a single 'hypofunctional' subgroup, their performance on the instrumental measures demonstrating lower than normal resistance and higher than normal airflow during phonation, features more frequently associated with laryngeal hypofunction.

Although this was an unexpected finding, Murdoch, Thompson and Stokes (1994) suggested a number of theories or situations in which hyperfunctional laryngeal behaviour may in fact have resulted in the hypofunctional parameters identified in 50% of the subject group. One explanation was that, owing to hypertonus, the movements of the vocal cords of the midline during phonation is sufficiently slowed to allow some air wastage. The existence of vocal muscles stiffness due to hyperfunction could, therefore, possibly account for the increased flow and reduced resistance noted in the hypofunctional group of subjects. It was also suggested that the presence of hypofunctional laryngeal parameters such as increased laryngeal airflow could possibly be explained as the result of the subject adopting compensatory laryngeal behaviours to reduce the muscular effort needed to produce speech against hypertonic vocal cords (Murdoch, Thompson and Stokes, 1994). In the absence of direct laryngeal examination, however, the mechanisms underlying the laryngeal behaviours identified in this group remain purely speculative. Replication of this investigation including subjects with more severe degrees of spastic dysarthria, and incorporating a direct examination of laryngeal behaviour and electromyographic recordings of vocal muscle tone, would provide greater insight into the laryngeal behaviours of this subject group.

Respiratory function in spastic dysarthria. Impaired respiratory support for speech has been identified as one of the predominant perceptual features of speech disorders associated with upper motor neurone damage (Darley, Aronson and Brown, 1975; Enderby, 1983; Chenery, Murdoch and Ingram, 1992). As in the case of laryngeal function, few quantitative instrumental studies have been reported on speech respiration in pseudobulbar palsy.

Murdoch *et al.* (1989) investigated the respiratory function of five subjects with pseudobulbar palsy using both spirometric and kinematic assessments. Of their subject group, four subjects exhibited reduced vital capacities on standard spirometric assessments. The kinematic assessment of the dysarthric group revealed irregularities in the chest wall movements of the diaphragm and abdomen which occurred during vowel and syllable production tasks but not during reading tasks (Murdoch *et al.*, 1989). Volume excursions during reading and conversation tasks were also found to be reduced. On the basis of these findings, it was concluded that the identified respiratory impairments had the potential to interfere with speech production, particularly where speech is associated with respiratory effort above normal tidal volume (Murdoch *et al.*, 1989).

In a subsequent study (Thompson, 1995), the respiratory function and speech breathing abilities of a group of 18 subjects with mild to moderate spastic dysarthria following cerebrovascular accident were investigated. In contrast to the results of Murdoch *et al.* (1989), the results of the kinematic assessments conducted by Thompson (1995) revealed that the dysarthric subjects had normal respiratory parameters during reading and conversational speech tasks. Analysis of the kinematic patterns during the production of the maximum effort speech tasks, however, identified reduced lung volumes in the cerebrovascular accident group, consistent with the Murdoch *et al.* (1989) study. Particularly during the production of maximum effort tasks, there was evidence to suggest that the reduced lung volumes observed in the cerebrovascular accident group were contributed to by reduced rib cage and abdominal expansion during inspiration as well as reduced abdominal contraction during expiration, possibly as a result of the presence of spasticity or weakness of the chest wall muscles. Spirometric analysis also confirmed reduced lung volumes and capacities in the dysarthric subject group (Thompson, 1995).

Based on the above information, it would appear, therefore, that a decrease in the excursion of the chest wall muscles during both the inspiratory and expiratory phases of respiration contributes to a reduction in the volumes exchanged during maximum respiratory efforts in spastic dysarthric speakers. Dependent on the severity of the dysarthria, this reduction in lung volume excursion may or may not influence the volume exchanges during speech breathing. At this point, without the benefit of electromyographic inves-

tigations of the chest wall musculature of these subjects, it is presumed that the reduced chest wall movement is the result of spasticity and weakness.

Summary of perceptual, acoustic and physiological investigations of spastic dysarthria. In general, the acoustic and physiological studies that have been carried out tend to support the perceptual analysis of spastic dysarthria reported by Darley, Aronson and Brown (1969a,b). These studies have shown that spastic dysarthric speakers have a slow rate of speech most probably caused by longer durations of syllables and perhaps longer pauses within and between words. There is evidence that the articulators move through a reduced range and that tongue strength in spastic dysarthria is reduced compared to normal. Although observations made during cineradiography of spastic dysarthric speakers suggest that velopharyngeal function is impaired, objective instrumental validation is needed. Those instrumental studies reported to date have indicated that impairments in speech breathing may contribute to the overall speech problem in spastic dysarthria. Although it is thought that the disturbed functioning of the various components of the speech mechanism is the product of spasticity associated with bilateral upper motor neurone lesions, this interpretation remains speculative and further objective validation of this hypothesis is needed.

Summary

The term 'dysarthria' is the name applied to a group of related speech disorders caused by damage to the central and/or peripheral nervous systems. Clinically, six major types of dysarthria are recognized: flaccid dysarthria, spastic dysarthria, ataxic dysarthria, hypokinetic dysarthria, hyperkinetic dysarthria and mixed dysarthria. The type of dysarthria resulting from damage to the nervous system is dependent upon the site of damage to the neuromuscular system. Parts of the neuromuscular system that can be affected are the lower motor neurones, upper motor neurones, extrapyramidal (indirect) system, cerebellum and neuromuscular junction as well as the muscles of the speech production mechanism themselves.

Flaccid dysarthria is associated with lower motor neurone lesions and takes its name from the major symptom of lower motor neurone damage, flaccid paralysis. The symptoms of flaccid dysarthria, however, vary depending on the specific nerves affected. The peripheral nerves that carry lower motor neurones to the muscles of the speech mechanism and which, if damaged, can lead to flaccid dysarthria include cranial nerves V, VII, XI, X, XI and XII and the spinal nerves supplying the muscles of respiration (phrenic nerves and intercostal nerves). A variety of neurological conditions can cause flaccid dysarthria, including cerebrovascular accidents, infectious disorders, tumours, cardiovascular defects (aneurysms), traumatic head injuries and toxic conditions.

Spastic dysarthria is associated with damage to the upper motor neurones that convey nerve impulses from the motor areas of the cerebral cortex to the lower motor neurones. The condition takes its name from the principal symptom of upper motor neurone lesions, spastic paralysis. Lesions of upper motor neurones that lead to spastic dysarthria commonly involve the cerebral cortex, the internal capsule or the cerebral peduncles of the brainstem. In general, bilateral upper motor neurone lesions are required to produce a significant and persistent spastic dysarthria. Consequently, spastic dysarthria is most commonly associated with pseudobulbar palsy, a condition characterized by spastic paralysis of the bulbar musculature as a result of bilateral upper motor neurone lesions. Spastic dysarthria is characterized by slow, dragging, laboured speech which is produced only with considerable effort.

References

Abbs, J.H., Hunker, C.J. and Barlow, S.M. (1983) Differential speech motor subsystem impairments with suprabulbar lesions: neurophysiological framework and supporting data, in *Clinical Dysarthria* (ed. W.R. Berry), College Hill Press, San Diego, pp. 21–56.

Aten, J.A. (1983) Treatment of spastic dysarthria, in *Current Therapy of Communication Disorders: Dysarthria and Apraxia* (ed. W.H. Perkins), Thieme-Stratton, New York, pp. 69–77.

Bannister, R. (1985) *Brain's Clinical Neurology*, Oxford University Press, Edinburgh.

Barlow, S.M. and Abbs, J.H. (1984) Oro-facial fine motor control impairments in congenital spasticity: evidence against hypertonus-related performance deficits. *Neurology*, **34**, 145–150.

Barlow, S.M. and Abbs, J.H. (1986) Fine force and position control of select orofacial structures in the upper motor neurone system. *Experimental Neurology*, **94**, 699–713.

Chenery, H.J., Murdoch, B.E. and Ingram, J.C.L. (1992) The perceptual speech characteristics of persons with pseudobulbar palsy. *Australian Journal of Human Communication Disorders*, **20**, 21–31.

Darby, J.K. (1981) The interaction between speech and disease, in *Speech Evaluation in Medicine* (ed. J.K. Darby), Grune & Stratton, New York, pp. 35–46.

Darley, F.L., Aronson, A.E. and Brown, J.R. (1969a) Differential diagnostic patterns of dysarthria. *Journal of Speech and Hearing Research*, **12**, 246–269.

Darley, F.L., Aronson, A.E. and Brown, J.R. (1969b) Clusters of deviant speech dimensions in the dysarthrias. *Journal of Speech and Hearing Research*, **12**, 462–496.

Darley, F.L., Aronson, A.E. and Brown, J.R. (1975) *Motor Speech Disorders*, W.B. Saunders, Philadelphia.

Dworkin, J.P. and Aronson, A.E. (1986) Tongue strength and alternate motion rates in normal and dysarthric subjects. *Journal of Communication Disorders*, **19**, 115–132.

Edwards, M. (1984) *Disorders of Articulation: Aspects of Dysarthria and Verbal Dyspraxia*, Springer-Verlag, Vienna.

Enderby, P. (1983) *Frenchay Dysarthria Assessment*, College Hill Press, San Diego.

Enderby, P. (1986) Relationships between dysarthric groups. *British Journal of Disorders of Communication*, **21**, 189–197.

Frokjaer-Jensen, B. and Thyme-Frokjaer, K. (1989) Changes in respiratory and phonatory efficiency during an intensive voice training course. Paper presented at the *Congress of the International Association of Logopaedics and Phoniatrics*, Prague.

Hanson, D.G., Gerratt, B.R. and Ward, P.H. (1983) Glottographic measurement of vocal dysfunction: a preliminary report. *Annals of Otology, Rhinology and Laryngology*, **92**, 413–420.

Hardcastle, W.J., Morgan-Barry, R.A. and Clark, C.J. (1985) Articulatory and voicing characteristics of adult dysarthic and verbal dyspraxic speakers: an instrumental study. *British Journal of Disorders of Communication*, **20**, 249–270.

Hillman, R.E., Holmberg, E.B., Perkell, J.S. *et al.* (1989) Objective assessment of vocal hyperfunction: an experimental framework and initial results. *Journal of Speech and Hearing Research*, **32**, 373–392.

Hirose, H., Kiritani, S. and Sawashima, M. (1980) Patterns of dysarthric movements in patients with amyotrophic lateral sclerosis and pseudobulbar palsy. *Annual Bulletin of the Research Institute for Logopaedics and Phoniatrics*, **14**, 263–272.

Hirose, H., Kiritani, S. and Sawashima, M. (1982) Patterns of dysarthric movements in patients with amyotrophic lateral sclerosis and pseudobulbar palsy. *Folia Phoniatrica et Logopaedica*, **34**, 106–112.

Hollien, H. (1960) Vocal pitch variation related to changes in vocal fold length. *Journal of Speech and Hearing Research*, **3**, 150–156.

Iwata, S., von Leden, H. and Williams, D. (1972) Air flow measurements during phonation. *Journal of Communication Disorders*, **5**, 67.

Kitzing, P., Carlborg, B. and Löfqvist, A. (1982) Aerodynamic and glottographic studies of the laryngeal vibratory cycle. *Folia Phoniatrica et Logopaedica*, **34**, 216–224.

Linebaugh, C.W. and Wolfe, V.E. (1984) Relationships between articulation rate, intelligibility and naturalness in spastic and ataxic speakers, in *The Dysarthrias: Physiology, Acoustics, Perception, Management* (eds M.R. McNeil, J.C. Rosenbek and A.E. Aronson), College Hill Press, San Diego, pp. 197–205.

Murdoch, B.E., Noble, J., Chenery, H. and Ingram, J. (1989) A spirometric and kinematic analysis of respiratory function in pseudobulbar palsy. *Australian Journal of Human Communication Disorders*, **17**, 21–35.

Murdoch, B.E., Thompson, E.C. and Stokes, P.D. (1994) Phonatory and laryngeal dysfunction following upper motor neurone vascular lesions. *Journal of Medical Speech-Language Pathology*, **2**, 177–189.

Murdoch, B.E., Thompson, E.C. and Theodoros, D.G. (1997) Spastic dysarthria, in *Clinical Management of Sensorimotor Speech Disorders* (ed. M.R. McNeil), Thieme, New York, pp. 287–310.

Murry, T. (1978) Speaking fundamental frequency characteristics associated with voice pathologies. *Journal of Speech and Hearing Disorder*, **43**, 374–378.

Orlikoff, R.F. (1992) The use of instrumental measures in the assessment and treatment of motor speech disorders. *Seminars in Speech and Language*, **13**, 25–37.

Penn, A.S. (1980) Myasthenia gravis, in *Neurology*, vol. 5 (ed. R.W. Rosenberg), Grune & Stratton, New York, pp. 382–391.

Platt, L.J., Andrews, G. and Howie, P.M. (1980a) Dysarthria of adult cerebral palsy: II. Phonemic analysis of articulation errors. *Journal of Speech and Hearing Research*, **23**, 41–55.

Platt, L.J., Andrews, G., Young, M. and Quinn, P.T. (1980b) Dysarthria of adult cerebral palsy: I. Intelligibility and articulatory impairment. *Journal of Speech and Hearing Research*, **23**, 28–40.

Portnoy, R.A. and Aronson, A.E. (1982) Diadochokinetic syllable rate and regularity in normal and in spastic and ataxic dysarthric subjects. *Journal of Speech and Hearing Disorders*, **47**, 324–328.

Roy, N., Leeper, H.A., Blomgren, M. and Cameron, R.M. (2001) A description of phonetic, acoustic and physiological changes associated with improved intelligibility in a speaker with spastic dysarthria. *American Journal of Speech-Language Pathology*, **10**, 274–288.

Sahrman, S.A. and Norton, B.J. (1977) The relationship of voluntary movement to spasticity in the UMN syndrome. *Annals of Neurology*, **2**, 460–465.

Sears, E.S. and Franklin, G.M. (1980) Diseases of the cranial nerves, in *Neurology*, vol. 5 (ed. R.N. Rosenberg), Grune & Stratton, New York, pp. 471–493.

Smitheran, J.R. and Hixon, T.J. (1981) A clinical method for estimating laryngeal airway resistance during vowel production. *Journal of Speech and Hearing Disorders*, **46**, 138–146.

Snell, R.S. (1980) *Clinical Neuroanatomy for Medical Students*, Little, Brown and Company, Boston.

Thompson, E.C. (1995) The physiological approach to dysarthria assessment and treatment: an examination in upper motor neurone dysarthria. Unpublished doctoral thesis, University of Queensland, Australia.

Thompson, E.C. and Murdoch, B.E. (1995) Disorders of nasality in subjects with upper motor neurone type dysarthria following cerebrovascular accident. *Journal of Communication Disorders*, **28**, 261–276.

Thompson, E.C., Murdoch, B.E. and Stokes, P.D. (1995a) Tongue function in subjects with upper motor neuron type dysarthria following cerebrovascular accident. *Journal of Medical Speech-Language Pathology*, **3**, 27–40.

Thompson, E.C., Murdoch, B.E. and Stokes, P.D. (1995b) Lip function in subjects with upper motor neurone type dysarthria following cerebrovascular accident. *European Journal of Disorders of Communication*, **30**, 451–466.

Till, J.A. and Alp, L.A. (1991) Aerodynamic and temporal measures of continuous speech in dysarthric speakers, in *Dysarthria and Apraxia of Speech: Perspectives on Management* (eds C.A. Moore, K.M. Yorkston and D.R. Beukelman), Paul H. Brooks, Baltimore, MD.

Weismer, G. (1984) Acoustic descriptions of dysarthric speech: perceptual correlates and physiological inferences. *Seminars in Speech and Language*, **5**, 293–313.

Ziegler, W. and von Cramon, D. (1986) Spastic dysarthria after acquired brain injury: an acoustic study. *British Journal of Disorders of Communication*, **21**, 173–187.

Dysarthrias associated with extrapyramidal syndromes 10

Introduction

The term 'extrapyramidal system' was first used by Wilson (1912) to refer to those parts of the central nervous system concerned with motor function but which are not a part of the pyramidal system. The extrapyramidal system, as described in Chapter 9, consists of a complex series of multisynaptic pathways which indirectly connect the motor areas of the cerebral cortex to the level of the lower motor neurones. The major components of the extrapyramidal system include the basal ganglia (see Chapter 3) within the cerebral hemispheres plus the various brainstem nuclei that contribute to motor functioning. These latter nuclei include the paired substantia nigra, the red nuclei and the subthalamic nuclei.

Diseases which selectively affect the extrapyramidal system without involving the pyramidal pathways are referred to as 'extrapyramidal syndromes' and include a number of clinically defined disease states of diverse aetiology and often obscure pathogenesis. Extrapyramidal syndromes share a number of related symptoms and the major pathological changes noted in these disorders are located within the various extrapyramidal nuclei. Movement disorders are the pri-

mary features of the extrapyramidal syndromes and, where the muscles of the speech mechanism are involved, disorders of speech may occur. The clinical signs and symptoms that characterize extrapyramidal syndromes and help tie these various disorders together fall into the following four groups: (1) hypokinesia (akinesia) – slowness and poverty of spontaneous movement; (2) hyperkinesia – abnormal involuntary movements; (3) rigidity of the muscles; and (4) loss of normal postural reactions.

Overall, the extrapyramidal system appears to control muscle tone for the maintenance of posture and for supporting movements (i.e. those muscle actions which provide a firm base of support against which skilled voluntary acts can take place).

As in the case of movement disorders of basal ganglia origin affecting limb and trunk muscles, dysarthrias associated with lesions in the basal ganglia take the form of hypo- and hyperkinetic movement disorders. In general, hypokinetic disorders (e.g. Parkinson's disease) are associated with increased basal ganglia output, whereas hyperkinetic movement disorders (e.g. Huntington's disease) are associated with decreased output. Hypokinetic disorders are characterized by significant impairments in movement initiation (akinesia) and reduction in the velocity of voluntary movements (bradykinesia) and are usually accompanied by muscular rigidity and tremor at rest. By contrast, hyperkinetic disorders are characterized by excessive motor activity in the form of involuntary movements (dyskinesia) with varying degrees of hypotonia. With regard to their effect on the speech production mechanism, these disorders manifest as hypokinetic dysarthria (classically associated with Parkinson's disease) and hyperkinetic dysarthria (seen in association with a range of hyperkinetic conditions such as Huntington's disease, dystonia, etc.).

Models of hypokinetic and hyperkinetic movement disorders

Although the connections for the basal ganglia are not yet fully understood, with new findings continuing to be made, the basic anatomy of the circuitry connecting these structures was clearly described by Alexander, DeLong and Strick (1986). Essentially, according to their description, information originating in the cerebral cortex passes through the basal ganglia and returns via the thalamus to specific areas of the frontal lobe, this feedback circuit often being referred to as the cortico-striato-pallido-thalamo-cortical loop. (For a detailed description of the neuroanatomy of the basal ganglia, see Chapter 3.)

Alexander, DeLong and Strick (1986) identified at least five separate, parallel cortical–basal ganglia circuits according to the specific region of the frontal lobe that serves as a target for their thalamocortical projections. One of these cortical–basal ganglia circuits projected to the skeletomotor areas of the frontal cortex while another projected to the oculomotor areas. The three remaining circuits projected to non-motor areas of the frontal cortex: the dorsolateral prefrontal area (Brodmann area 46), the lateral orbitofrontal cortex (Brodmann area 12) and the anterior cingulated/medial orbitofrontal cortices (Brodmann areas 24 and 13). Importantly, these circuits appear to be, to a large extent, functionally segregated (Alexander, DeLong and Strick,

1986), suggesting that structural convergence and functional integration occur within, rather than between, each of the identified circuits.

The cortical–basal ganglia circuit that has received the greatest attention in the literature, and which is of greatest relevance to movement disorders associated with motor speech impairments is the skeletomotor circuit. At the cortical level, this circuit comprises the pre- and post-central sensorimotor areas and, at the subcortical level, the sensorimotor areas in the basal ganglia and the ventral anterior and ventral lateral thalamus. Cortical projections of the motor circuit terminate largely in the putamen. According to current models of the organization of the basal ganglia, putaminal output is directed over two separate projection systems, the so-called direct and indirect pathways. The direct pathway originates from striatal neurones that contain gamma aminobutyric acid (GABA) plus the peptide substance P and/or dynorphin and conveys activity from the neostriatum monosynaptically to the internal segment of the globus pallidus and substantia nigra pars reticulata (SNPR). In contrast, the indirect pathway arises from striatal neurones that contain GABA and enkephalin and conveys activity to the internal segment of the globus pallidus and SNPR polysynaptically via a sequence of connections involving the external segment of the globus pallidus and the subthalamic nucleus. In both cases the returning thalamocortical connections seem to reach precisely the regions of the frontal cortex that contribute as inputs to the neostriatum (Strick, Dunn and Picard, 1995). A diagrammatic representation of the basis circuitry of the basal ganglia is presented in Figure 10.1.

Imbalance between the activity in the direct and indirect pathways and the resulting alterations in the activity of the internal segment of the globus pallidus and SNPR are thought to account for the hypo- and hyperkinetic features of basal ganglia disorders, including hypo- and hyperkinetic dysarthria. The possible roles of the direct and indirect pathways to the development of hypo- and hyperkinetic movement disorders are discussed further below.

Hypo- and hyperkinetic movement disorders represent the extreme ends of the clinical spectrum of basal ganglia associated motor

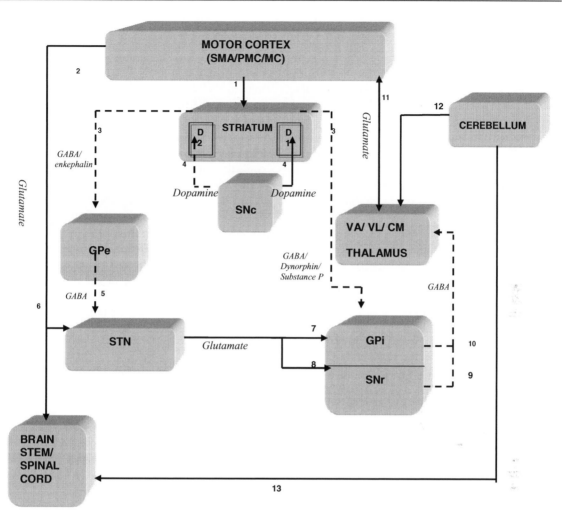

Figure 10.1 Modified schematic diagram of skeletomotor circuit under normal conditions based on DeLong (1990) and Mink (2007). SMA = supplementary motor area; PMC = pre-motor cortex; MC = motor cortex; D1 = striatal output neurone receptor type D1; D2 = striatal output neurone receptor type D2; SNc = substantia nigra compacta; GPe = globus pallidus externus; STN = subthalamic nucleus; GPi = globus pallidus internus; SNr = substantia nigra reticulata; VA = ventral anterior nucleus of thalamus; VL = ventral lateral nucleus of thalamus; CM = centrum medianum; ⟶ excitatory pathway; ----▶ = inhibitory pathway. 1 = corticostriatal pathway; 2 = corticobulbar and corticospinal pathways; 3 = striatopallidal pathways; 4 = nigrostriatal pathways; 5 = pallido-subthalamic pathway, 6 = cortico-subthalamic pathway; 7 = subthalamo-pallidal pathway; 8 = subthalamo-nigral pathway; 9 = nigrothalamic pathway; 10 = pallidothalamic pathway; 11 = thalamocortical and corticothalamic pathways; 12 = cerebellothalamic pathway; 13 = cerebellorubral pathway. Glutamate, GABA (gamma aminobutyric acid), enkephalin, dynorphin, and substance P = active neurotransmitters.

disturbances. Parkinsonism is characterized by a reduction in striatal dopaminergic transmission, leading to increased basal ganglia output to the thalamus. In contrast, the major hyperkinetic syndromes such as chorea, athetosis, dystonia and so on are all characterized by reduced basal ganglia output to the thalamus, leading to the disinhibition of the thalamocortical neurones, which in turn leads to the development of involuntary movements. DeLong (1990) suggested that hypo- and hyperkinetic movement disorders can be explained using a functional model of the basal ganglia–thalamocortical circuit derived from findings of experiments involving monitoring the neuronal activity of various basal ganglia sites in primates treated with MPTP (1-methyl-4-phenyl-1,2,3,6-tetrahydropyridine). In primates treated with MPTP, the dopaminergic cells in the substantia nigra pars compacta (SNPC) degenerate, and the animals subsequently develop a clinical syndrome that closely resembles human Parkinsonism (Miller and DeLong, 1987). What the findings of these studies suggest is that the hypokinetic movement disorders associated with Parkinson's disease may result from increased inhibition of the thalamocortical neurones that renders the cortical projection areas less responsive to other inputs normally involved in initiating movements.

Model of hypokinetic movement disorders

Briefly, according to the model of hypokinetic movement disorders proposed by DeLong (1990) (Figure 10.2), loss of striatal dopamine leads to excessive inhibition of the globus pallidus, leading to disinhibition of the subthalamic nucleus, which in turn provides excessive excitatory drive to the basal ganglia output nuclei (i.e. the internal segment of the globus pallidus and SNPR) via the indirect pathway, leading to thalamic inhibition. This effect is reinforced by reduced inhibitory input to the basal ganglia output nuclei through the direct pathway, also leading to inhibition of thalamocortical neurones. According to DeLong (1990), these effects are postulated to result in a reduction in the usual reinforcing influence of the subcortical motor circuit upon cortically initiated movements, leading to symptoms such as akinesia and bradykinesia. The model proposed by DeLong (1990) is supported by data based on microelectrode recordings of basal ganglia neurone activity in MPTP-treated primates (Filion, Tremblay and Bedard, 1988; Filion and Tremblay, 1991), which have shown that neurones in the subthalamic nucleus and internal segment of the globus pallidus of these primates have higher discharge rates and show prominent changes in their discharge patterns, including a greater tendency to discharge in bursts. Further support has been derived from metabolic studies based on positron

emission tomography (PET), which have demonstrated that the changes in basal ganglia discharge that results from dopamine depletion alter the neuronal activity in the thalamus and brainstem as well as cortical metabolic activity consistent with the hypokinetic model (Brooks, 1991; Eidelberg, 1992; Calne and Snow, 1993; Leenders, 1997). Given that, according to the above hypokinetic model, motor disturbances in Parkinson's disease are postulated to result in large part from increased thalamic inhibition due to excess excitatory drive from the subthalamic nucleus to the output nuclei of the basal ganglia, it has been speculated that induced lesions in the subthalamic nucleus would ameliorate symptoms such as bradykinesia and akinesia (DeLong, 1990). Experiments involving selective lesioning of the subthalamic nucleus with ibotenate (a fibre-sparing neurotoxin) in MPTP-treated monkeys have confirmed this hypothesis (DeLong, 1990).

Model of hyperkinetic movement disorders

In addition to the model of hypokinetic movement disorders, DeLong (1990) also proposed a functional model to explain hyperkinetic movement disorders. Evidence is available to suggest that a common mechanism underlies the various hyperkinetic movement disorders, such as the choreiform movement in Huntington's disease and dyskinetic movements seen in hemiballismus. In fact, it has been suggested that these dyskinesias differ only by the intensity and amplitude of the movements. It is known that, early in the course of Huntington's disease, there is a selective loss of striatal GABA/enkephalin neurones that give rise to the indirect pathway. Experiments involving neurotoxin (ibotenate) induced lesions in the subthalamic nucleus of monkeys suggest ballismus is associated with disinhibition of the thalamus as a result of subthalamic nucleus lesions. According to the model of hyperkinetic movement disorders proposed by DeLong (1990), reduced excitatory projections from the subthalamic nucleus to the internal segment of the globus pallidus owing to either subthalamic nucleus lesions (as in ballismus) or reduced striatopallidal

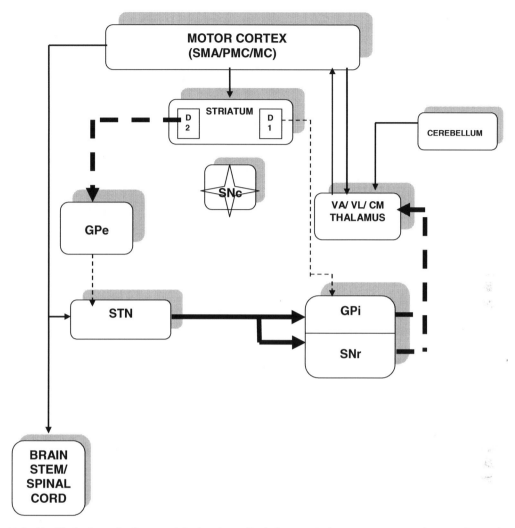

Figure 10.2 Modified schematic diagram of the basal ganglia thalamocortical motor circuit in Parkinson's disease based on DeLong (1990). SMA = supplementary motor area; PMC = pre-motor cortex; MC = motor cortex; D1 = striatal output neurone receptor type D1; D2 = striatal output neurone receptor type D2; SNc = substantia nigra compacta; GPe = globus pallidus externus; STN = subthalamic nucleus; GPi = globus pallidus internus; SNr = substantia nigra reticulata; VA = ventral anterior nucleus of thalamus; VL = ventral lateral nucleus of thalamus; CM = centrum medianum; ⟶ = excitatory pathway; ----▶ = inhibitory pathway; ✦ = lesion site.

inhibitory influences along the indirect pathway (as in Huntington's disease) (Figure 10.3) lead to reduced inhibitory outflow from the internal segment of the globus pallidus/SNPR and excessive disinhibition of the thalamus. Dystonia has been likened to Parkinson's disease with evidence of excessive indirect pathway activity, yet differs in that direct pathway activity is also excessive, producing an overall reduction in output from the

internal segment of the globus pallidus (Figure 10.4). In the case of levodopa-induced dyskinesias, disinhibition of the thalamus is thought to result from excessive dopaminergic stimulation of the striatal GABA/substance P neurones that send inhibitory projections to the output nuclei of the basal ganglia via the direct pathway (Figure 10.5). The proposed overall effect is that of excessive positive feedback to the pre-central motor fields

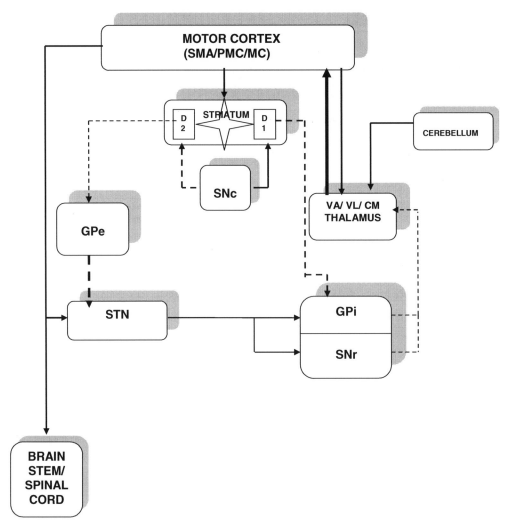

Figure 10.3 Modified schematic diagram of the basal ganglia thalamocortical motor circuit in Huntington's disease based on DeLong (1990). SMA = supplementary motor area; PMC = pre-motor cortex; MC = motor cortex; D1 = striatal output neurone receptor type D1; D2 = striatal output neurone receptor type D2; SNc = substantia nigra compacta; GPe = globus pallidus externus; STN = subthalamic nucleus; GPi = globus pallidus internus; SNr = substantia nigra reticulata; VA = ventral anterior nucleus of thalamus; VL = ventral lateral nucleus of thalamus; CM = centrum medianum; ⟶ = excitatory pathway; ----▶ = inhibitory pathway; ✦ = lesion site.

engaged by the skeletomotor circuit, resulting in hyperkinetic movements (DeLong, 1990).

Hypokinetic dysarthria

Hypokinetic dysarthria is most commonly associated with Parkinson's disease. In fact the term 'hypokinetic dysarthria' was first used by Darley, Aronson and Brown (1969a,b) to describe the resultant complex pattern of perceptual speech characteristics associated with Parkinsonism. More recently, an acoustically similar form of dysarthria has also been observed in persons with progressive supranuclear palsy (Steele–Richardson–Olszewski syndrome) (Hanson and Metter, 1980; Metter and Hanson, 1986).

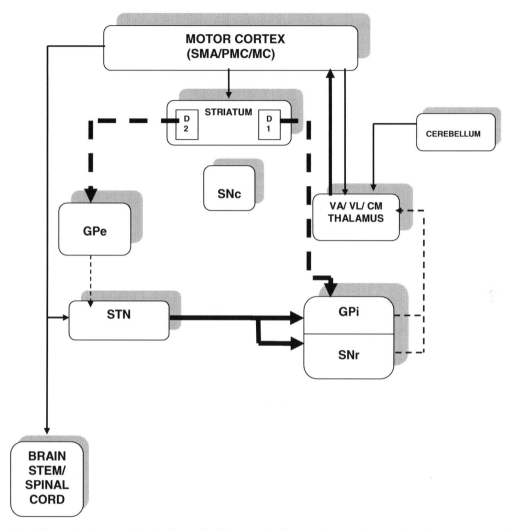

Figure 10.4 Schematic diagram of the basal ganglia thalamocortical motor circuit in dystonia based on Starr, Rau and Davis (2005). SMA = supplementary motor area; PMC = pre-motor cortex; MC = motor cortex; D1 = striatal output neurone receptor type D1; D2 = striatal output neurone receptor type D2; SNc = substantia nigra compacta; GPe = globus pallidus externus; STN = subthalamic nucleus; GPi = globus pallidus internus; SNr = substantia nigra reticulata; VA = ventral anterior nucleus of thalamus; VL = ventral lateral nucleus of thalamus; CM = centrum medianum; ⎯⎯➤ = excitatory pathway; ----➤ = inhibitory pathway.

Parkinson's disease

Parkinson's disease is a progressive, degenerative, neurological disease associated with selective loss of dopaminergic neurones in the pars compacta of the substantia nigra (Uitti and Calne, 1993). The condition arises from nigrostriatal dopaminergic cell degeneration (Obeso, Guridi and DeLong, 1997), which produces an activity imbalance within dopamine-regulated pathways of the basal

ganglia, namely an increase in indirect pathway activity and a decrease in direct pathway activity (Wichmann and Delong, 1998) (Figure 10.2). Aetiological influences remain undetermined; however, current consensus espouses environmental influences in tandem with a genetic susceptibility as the potential underlying cause of Parkinson's disease (Guttman, Kish and Furukawa, 2003). A clinical presentation of bradykinesia – plus one of the following: rigidity, tremor or postural

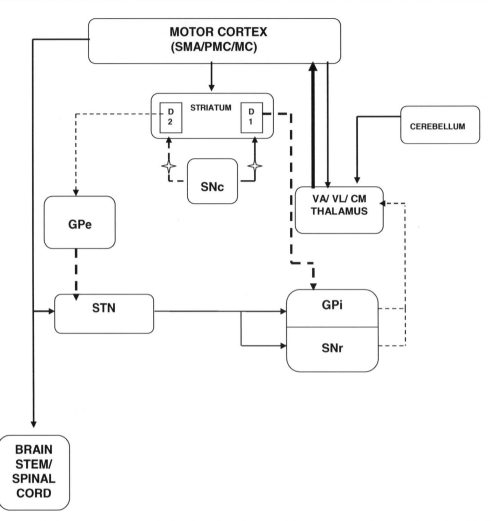

Figure 10.5   Modified schematic diagram of the basal ganglia thalamocortical motor circuit subserving drug-induced dyskinesias based on DeLong (1990). SMA = supplementary motor area; PMC = pre-motor cortex; MC = motor cortex; D1 = striatal output neurone receptor type D1; D2 = striatal output neurone receptor type D2; SNc = substantia nigra compacta; GPe = globus pallidus externus; STN = subthalamic nucleus; GPi = globus pallidus internus; SNr = substantia nigra reticulata; VA = ventral anterior nucleus of thalamus; VL = ventral lateral nucleus of thalamus; CM = centrum medianum; ⟶ = excitatory pathway; ----▶ = inhibitory pathway; ✧ = excessive dopaminergic stimulation of GABA/substance P neurones.

instability – confirms the diagnosis of Parkinson's disease (Valls-Sole, 2007). As previously defined, 'bradykinesia' refers to abnormal reductions in the amplitude and velocity of voluntary movement (DeLong, 1990); 'rigidity' refers to general increase in muscle tone, or resistance to passive movement (Adams and Jog, 2008); 'Parkinsonian tremor' is typically present at rest; and 'postural instability' is characterized by an unsteadiness in gait and poor balance (Adams and Jog, 2008).

The annual incidence of Parkinson's disease is estimated to be 20 per 100 000. The cumulative lifetime risk for Parkinsonism is > 1 in 40, making it one of the more common neurological diseases. Onset is insidious and the course is that of a slow progression of disability over many years. The degree and rate of progression, however, does vary from patient to patient. Parkinson's disease begins most commonly after age 40 with the mean age of onset between 58 and 62 years. The age-specific incidence of Parkinson's disease peaks in the age group 70–79 years (Martilla and Rinne, 1991). The cardinal signs of Parkinson's disease include akinesia/bradykinesia, rigidity, tremor at rest and postural reflex impairment. The degree to which each of these signs is present varies from patient to patient. Affected persons may complain of rigidity and tremor, immobility of facial expression, slowness of movements and diminished swinging of the arms and heaviness of the limbs when walking. Posture is often stooped forward, with the arms at the sides, elbows slightly flexed and fingers adducted. The patients often exhibit a characteristic gait, which involves short, slow, shuffling steps. In addition, as they walk, affected persons tend to stoop forward and develop an increasing speed (festinating gait). Dementia occurs in approximately 41% of Parkinsonian cases. A speech disorder may in some cases be the first symptom to emerge (Hoehn and Yahr, 1967). Gracco, Marek and Gracco (1993) and Hanson (1991) found laryngeal dysfunction to be readily observable in subjects with early Parkinson's disease, and indicated that it may precede the appearance of symptoms elsewhere. It has been estimated that 60–80% of patients with Parkinson's disease exhibit a hypokinetic dysarthria, with the prevalence increasing as the disease advances (Scott, Caird and Williams, 1985; Johnson and Pring, 1990).

The most common form of Parkinsonism is idiopathic Parkinson's disease, a form of the disorder in which no immediate cause is obvious. In these cases the disease has been ascribed by various authors to the degeneration of nerve cells and tracts in either the corpus striatum or substantia nigra (including the nigrostriatal pathways), although it is now agreed that the most important lesions are those located in the substantia nigra. The degenerative changes in these structures appear to be associated with a deficiency of a neurotransmitter substance called dopamine. Abnormally low concentrations of dopamine in the basal ganglia and substantia nigra have been reported upon post-mortem examination of brains of patients with idiopathic Parkinsonism. In addition to the idiopathic variety, Parkinson's disease may also be precipitated by an attack of epidemic encephalitis or may be the outcome of cerebral arteriosclerosis, carbon monoxide or manganese poisoning, traumatic head injury, neurosyphilis, cerebrovascular accidents or drug toxicity.

The medical management of Parkinson's disease has conventionally involved the administration of dopamine replacement (e.g. levodopa) and dopamine enhancement (e.g. dopamine receptor agonists) drug therapies (Schapira, 2005), with the modulation of depleted dopamine stores producing an improvement in motor function, at least for the short term. Recognized limitations in relation to dopaminergic pharmacotherapy such as the development of dyskinesias and on/off states, however, prompted a re-evaluation and more general application of neurosurgical techniques such as pallidotomy, thalamotomy and deep brain stimulation to treat the Parkinsonian symptom complex (Obeso, Guridi and DeLong, 1997).

Progressive supranuclear palsy

Progressive supranuclear palsy is conventionally taken to refer to the subcortical degenerative syndrome of unknown aetiology that produces an akinetic-rigid form of Parkinson's disease first described by Steele, Richardson and Olszewski (1964). Affected persons have an akinetic-rigid syndrome, pseudobulbar palsy and dementia of frontal-lobe type associated with lesions located in the basal ganglia (including the globus pallidus, caudate nucleus and subthalamic nucleus), brainstem and cerebellar nuclei. Hypokinetic dysarthria is the prominent dysarthria type in progressive supranuclear palsy; however, in the early stages of the disorder, the dysarthria is often mixed with hypokinetic, spastic and ataxic components (Kluin *et al.*, 1993). Onset of the disorder is usually in middle to later life and the condition is rapidly progressive, resulting in marked incapacity of the patient in 2–3 years.

Clinical characteristics of hypokinetic dysarthria

In contrast to other forms of dysarthria, the clinical characteristics of hypokinetic dysarthria were identified by a systematic analysis of patients with a specific disease, namely idiopathic Parkinson's disease. Overall, the speech characteristics associated with hypokinetic dysarthria follow largely from the generalized pattern of hypokinetic motor disorders, which includes marked reductions in the amplitude of voluntary movement (akinesia), initiation difficulties, slowness of movement (bradykinesia), muscular rigidity, tremor at rest and postural reflex impairments. According to Darley, Aronson and Brown (1975), marked limitation of the range of movement of the muscles of the speech mechanism is the outstanding characteristic of hypokinesia as it affects speech. These authors stated that the reduced mobility, restricted range of movement and supranormal rate of the repetitive movements of the muscles involved in speech production lead to the various manifestations of hypokinetic dysarthria.

Although impairments in all aspects of speech production (i.e. respiration, phonation, resonance, articulation and prosody) involving the various subsystems of the speech production mechanism have been identified in individuals with Parkinson's disease, these individuals are most likely to exhibit disturbances of prosody, phonation and articulation (Darley, Aronson and Brown, 1975; Chenery, Murdoch and Ingram, 1988; Zwirner and Barnes, 1992). The reported features of the speech disturbance in Parkinson's disease commonly include monopitch and monoloudness, decreased use of all vocal parameters for effecting stress and emphasis, breathy and harsh voice quality, reduced vocal intensity, variable rate including short rushes of speech or accelerated speech, consonant imprecision, impaired breath support for speech, reduction in phonation time, difficulty in the initiation of speech activities and inappropriate silences (Darley, Aronson and Brown, 1969a,b; Ludlow and Bassich, 1983, 1984; Scott, Caird and Williams, 1985; Chenery, Murdoch and Ingram, 1988). Reduced pitch and loudness variation were among the most prominent speech deficits observed in patients with Parkinson's disease in the perceptual-based studies of Darley, Aronson and Brown (1969a, b, 1975). Based on their average perceptual rating scores, the following hierarchy of deviant speech dimensions was observed in 32 patients

with Parkinson's disease: (1) monopitch, (2) reduced stress, (3) monoloudness and (4) imprecise consonants.

The reported findings, however, have not always been consistent with respect to the type of disturbances, the frequency of occurrence and the degree of severity of the abnormal perceptual, acoustic and physiological features present in the speech of persons with hypokinetic dysarthria. For example, Darley, Aronson and Brown (1975) reported that, in 15 of their 32 patients with Parkinson's disease, the average perceived speech loudness levels were lower than those of other dysarthric groups, suggesting that reduced speech loudness is a distinctive feature of speech in Parkinson's disease and as such may have a useful role in the differential diagnosis of hypokinetic dysarthria. Nevertheless, reduced speech loudness does not appear to be present in all dysarthric patients with Parkinson's disease. Ludlow and Bassich (1984) reported that only 42% (5/12) of their dysarthric patients with Parkinson's disease were perceived to have reduced speech loudness. Similarly, in a later study Gamboa *et al.* (1997) reported that only 49% of dysarthric patients with Parkinson's disease (20/41) self-reported they had developed hypophonia. It has been suggested that these values may underestimate the actual proportion of dysarthric patients with Parkinson's disease who are hypophonic, given that many of these people appear to be able to compensate for their hypophonia during formal speech testing. Further patients with Parkinson's disease may have perceptual deficits that make it difficult for them to accurately identify hypophonia in their own speech (Ho, Bradshaw and Iansek, 2000).

Respiratory function in hypokinetic dysarthria

A number of the perceptual features identified in hypokinetic dysarthria, such as reduction in overall loudness, decay of loudness, reduced phrase length, short rushes of speech and reduced phonation time, have been attributed to the impairment of respiration (Darley, Aronson and Brown, 1975). In support of these assumptions, Chenery, Murdoch and Ingram (1988) identified a mild impairment of respiratory support for speech in the majority (89%) of their subjects with Parkinson's disease. In addition, more than half of their subjects demonstrated reductions in phrase lengths, short rushes of speech, reduced loudness and decay of loudness during speech. Similarly, Ludlow and Bassich (1984) identified a reduction in overall loudness in 42% of their subjects, and the majority of the cases with Parkinson's disease demonstrated a variable rate of speech which could be partially attributed to respiratory insufficiency.

Patients with Parkinson's disease have been identified by several investigators to exhibit significant reductions in their vital capacity (Cramer, 1940; De La Torre, Mier and Boshes, 1960). In particular, De La Torre, Mier and Boshes (1960) found that two-thirds of their subjects with Parkinson's disease recorded vital capacities 40% below the expected values. Laszewski (1956) reported that the majority of his subjects exhibited a marked reduction in vital capacity, with little measurable thoracic excursion during inhalation or exhalation. During a sustained phonation task, Mueller (1971) found that subjects with Parkinson's disease expended significantly smaller volumes of air than control subjects. Using spirographic analysis, Hovestadt *et al.* (1989) revealed that, on non-speech tasks, peak inspiratory and expiratory flow and maximum expiratory flow at a 50% level were significantly below normal for patients with relatively severe Parkinson's disease. In contrast, neither Murdoch *et al.* (1989) nor Solomon and Hixon (1993) identified significant overall reductions in vital capacity and lung volumes in their groups of subjects with Parkinson's disease.

Recent studies involving kinematic investigations of respiratory function in Parkinson's disease have also identified incoordinaton of the components of the chest wall during speech breathing. Murdoch *et al.* (1989) identified irregularities in chest wall movement during the production of sustained vowels and syllable repetitions. These abnormal chest wall movements took the form of abrupt changes in the relative contribution of the chest wall components and featured both ribcage and abdominal paradoxical movements. In addition, Murdoch *et al.* found that the subjects with Parkinson's disease

demonstrated a wide range of relative volume contributions of the ribcage and abdomen during speech breathing, with a predominance of ribcage involvement. Solomon and Hixon (1993), using different instrumentation, however, recorded smaller ribcage than abdominal contribution to lung volume change in speech breathing of patients with Parkinson's disease and found that ribcage and abdominal paradoxical movements were not specific to subjects with Parkinson's disease alone. Both studies, however, identified a significantly greater breathing rate and minute ventilation in subjects with Parkinson's disease compared with control subjects.

Laryngeal function in hypokinetic dysarthria

Phonatory disturbance is often the initial symptom of the ensuing speech disorder associated with Parkinson's disease. In fact, Logemann *et al.* (1978) identified laryngeal problems as being the most prominent deviant features in their group of 200 subjects with Parkinson's disease, occurring in 89% of cases. Similarly, about half of the deviant speech dimensions identified by Darley, Aronson and Brown (1975) and Ludlow and Bassich (1983) as being the most distinguishing features of hypokinetic dysarthria related to phonatory disturbance. The deviant perceptual features associated with laryngeal dysfunction in Parkinson's disease include disorders of vocal quality and impairment of the overall levels and variability of pitch and loudness.

Descriptions of the vocal quality of the hypokinetic speaker have included a number of deviant vocal parameters, including hoarseness, harshness, breathiness, vocal tremor and glottal fry. Inconsistencies in the frequency of occurrence of these deviant phonatory features are apparent across many of the reported perceptual studies. In relation to hoarseness and harshness, the perceptual findings would appear to be equivocal with respect to the prominence of either feature in the vocal output of persons with hypokinetic dysarthria. Hoarseness was perceived to be present in 45% of patients in Logemann *et al.*'s (1978) study, one-third of subjects examined by Ludlow and Bassich (1984), in each subject in the Chenery, Murdoch and Ingram (1988) study and in 84% of the subjects with Parkinson's disease assessed by Murdoch *et al.* (1995). Hoarseness, however, was not found to be a prominent deviant dimension in the study reported by Darley, Aronson and Brown (1975). Instead, harshness was listed among the ten most deviant speech features identified by these latter authors. A harsh vocal quality has been perceived to be present in 77–84% of patients with hypokinetic dysarthria (Ludlow and Bassich, 1984; Chenery, Murdoch and Ingram, 1988; Zwirner and Barnes, 1992). Although there is some degree of inconsistency in the reported frequency of occurrence of breathiness in hypokinetic dysarthria, it would appear that a breathy vocal quality is also a relatively common characteristic of this type of dysarthria (Darley, Aronson and Brown, 1975). Breathiness has been reported to occur in approximately 50–95% of patients with hypokinetic dysarthria (Chenery, Murdoch and Ingram, 1988; Zwirner and Barnes, 1992; Murdoch *et al.*, 1995). Glottal fry has been identified in 60–85% of cases with hypokinetic dysarthria, while pitch unsteadiness or vocal tremor has been reported to be present in approximately 65% of subjects with Parkinson's disease (Chenery, Murdoch and Ingram, 1988; Murdoch *et al.*, 1995). The findings of acoustic studies suggest that the disorders of vocal quality perceived to be present in patients with Parkinson's disease result from phonatory inefficiency due to abnormal positioning of the vocal folds, irregular vocal fold activity and problems with the synchronization of phonation and articulation.

In addition to deviations in vocal quality, the hypokinetic dysarthria associated with Parkinson's disease is characterized perceptually by the presence of monopitch and monoloudness and a reduction in overall pitch and loudness levels. Darley, Aronson and Brown (1975) identified monopitch and monoloudness as prominent features of the verbal output of subjects with Parkinson's disease, being, respectively, the first and third most deviant perceptual speech features of hypokinetic dysarthria. Later perceptual studies have confirmed the presence of monopitch and monoloudness in the majority of subjects with Parkinson's disease (Ludlow and Bassich, 1984; Chenery, Murdoch and Ingram, 1988; Zwirner and Barnes, 1992). Similarly, acoustic findings

have provided consistent evidence of a reduction in the variability of pitch and loudness in the speech output of these subjects (Metter and Hanson, 1986; Flint, Black and Campbell-Taylor, 1992; King *et al.*, 1994).

Unfortunately, few studies reported in the literature have been based on physiological investigation of laryngeal function in persons with Parkinson's disease. Collectively, those studies that have been reported have shown that individuals with Parkinson's disease demonstrate abnormal vocal fold posturing and vibratory patterns and laryngeal aerodynamics (Hanson, Gerratt and Ward, 1983; Hirose, Sawashima and Niimi, 1985; Gerratt, Hanson and Berke, 1987; Murdoch *et al.*, 1995). Physiological studies utilizing photoglottography (PGG) and electroglottography (EGG) have identified abnormal vocal fold vibratory patterns in patients with Parkinson's disease (Hanson, Gerratt and Ward, 1983; Gerratt, Hanson and Berke, 1987). Essentially, these studies have demonstrated a proportionately greater amount of time spent in opening relative to closing duration with no well-defined closed period (Hanson, Gerratt and Ward, 1983; Gerratt, Hanson and Berke, 1987). Hanson, Gerratt and Ward (1983) noted that only 15% of the glottal cycle was spent in the 'closed period'. In addition these latter authors found that the waveform shape varied widely from cycle to cycle, suggesting variability in the control of vocal fold posture. Abnormalities in the laryngeal aerodynamics of persons with Parkinson's disease as identified by instrumental studies are also generally consistent with impaired laryngeal function in this group. Murdoch *et al.* (1995) identified a hyperfunctional pattern of laryngeal activity in subjects with Parkinson's disease characterized by increased glottal resistance and reduced subglottal pressure, average phonatory sound pressure level and phonatory flow rate compared to matched control subjects. Murdoch *et al.* suggested that the aerodynamic findings in their study reflected the presence of rigidity in the laryngeal musculature. In addition, their study indicated that dysarthric speakers with Parkinson's disease were not homogeneous, but rather exhibited differential impairment within the laryngeal subsystem. Overall, the laryngeal subsystem of the speech production mechanism in subjects with Parkinson's disease would appear to demonstrate a greater degree of variability in perceptual, acoustic and physiological features than other subsystems of the speech production apparatus.

Velopharyngeal function in hypokinetic dysarthria

Controversy surrounds the existence of a resonatory disturbance in persons with Parkinson's disease. Several authors have reported low incidences of perceived hypernasality in groups of subjects with Parkinson's disease (Darley, Aronson and Brown, 1975; Logemann *et al.*, 1978; Theodoros, Murdoch and Thompson, 1995). At the same time, hypernasality has been identified as one of the most useful perceptual features for differentiating between hypokinetic dysarthria and normal speech (Ludlow and Bassich, 1983). For some individuals with Parkinson's disease, hypernasality has been found to be the most prominent deviant speech feature (Hoodin and Gilbert, 1989a,b).

The physiological evaluation of velopharyngeal functioning using a variety of direct and indirect instrumental techniques has provided objective evidence of dysfunction of the velopharyngeal valve in subjects with Parkinson's disease. Hirose *et al.* (1981) conducted a study in which velar movements were directly observed by means of an X-ray microbeam system that tracked a lead pellet attached to the nasal side of the velum. During the rapid repetition of the monosyllable /ten/, Hirose *et al.* identified a gradual decrease in the degree of displacement of the velum. In effect, the lowering and elevation of the velum for the nasal and non-nasal consonants, respectively, were found to be incomplete towards the end of the speech task. At a rapid rate of repetition, the interval between each utterance was noted to be inconsistent and the displacement and rate of velar movements were found to be markedly reduced (Hirose *et al.*, 1981).

In a study involving the use of videofluoroscopy to examine velar movements during speech in patients with Parkinson's disease, Robbins, Logemann and Kirshner (1986) identified a significant reduction in velar elevation, which was

considered to reflect a reduced range of velar movement. Nasal accelerometry has also revealed a significantly greater degree and increased frequency of hypernasality in the speech output of a group of hypokinetic speakers with Parkinson's disease (Theodoros, Murdoch and Thompson, 1995). Specifically, the individuals with Parkinson's disease, as a group, recorded significantly higher Horii Oral Nasal Coupling (HONC) indices compared with the controls. Of the 23 individuals with Parkinson's disease, 17 (74%) were identified by Theodoros, Murdoch and Thompson (1995) as exhibiting increased nasality.

Clinicians, therefore, should be alert to the existence of resonatory disturbance in Parkinson's disease and be aware that this abnormality may manifest itself, to varying degrees, in some individuals and not others. Further research, involving the simultaneous use of both direct and indirect instrumental measures together with perceptual evaluation, is required to determine the exact nature of velopharyngeal function in hypokinetic dysarthria.

Articulatory function in hypokinetic dysarthria

By far the majority of speakers with hypokinetic dysarthria exhibit disorders of articulation. Articulatory impairments such as consonant and vowel imprecision and prolongation of phonemes have been observed, with consonant imprecision identified as the most common articulatory disturbance (Darley, Aronson and Brown, 1975; Logemann *et al.*, 1978; Chenery, Murdoch and Ingram, 1988; Zwirner and Barnes, 1992). Consonant articulation has been found to be characterized by errors in the manner of production involving incomplete closure for stops and partial construction of the vocal tract for fricatives, resulting in the abnormal production of stop-plosives, affricates and fricatives (Canter, 1965; Logemann and Fisher, 1981).

In addition to abnormalities of articulation, disordered speech rate is also frequently observed in patients with Parkinson's disease. Perceptually, individuals with Parkinson's disease have been noted to demonstrate both a faster (Darley, Aronson and Brown, 1975; Enderby, 1986; Chenery, Murdoch and Ingram, 1988; Zwirner and Barnes, 1992) and a slower (Chenery, Murdoch and Ingram, 1988; Zwirner and Barnes, 1992) overall rate of speech than normal, with most studies suggesting that the speech rate of these patients is generally variable (Ludlow and Bassich, 1983; Scott, Caird and Williams, 1985; Hoodin and Gilbert, 1989a). In addition, subjects with Parkinson's disease have been noted to demonstrate short rushes of speech, or what is perceived as an 'accelerated' speech pattern (Darley, Aronson and Brown, 1975; Chenery, Murdoch and Ingram, 1988; Zwirner and Barnes, 1992). The production of short rushes of speech in the verbal output of speakers with Parkinson's disease was found by Darley, Aronson and Brown (1975) to be one of the most prominent features of hypokinetic dysarthria. Furthermore, this deviant speech dimension was identified in 84% of the subjects with Parkinson's disease assessed by Chenery, Murdoch and Ingram (1988). In some cases, a progressive acceleration of speech within a speech segment has also been perceived to be present (Scott, Caird and Williams, 1985; Chenery, Murdoch and Ingram, 1988).

Acoustic analysis of the speech rate disturbance in Parkinson's disease has generally confirmed the perceptual impression of a variety of rate disturbances being evident in these subjects. Studies have demonstrated a normal rate of speech production (Ackermann and Ziegler, 1991; Flint, Black and Campbell-Taylor, 1992), a normal to increased rate (Kent and Rosenbek, 1982; Weismer, 1984) and an increased rate (Hammen, Yorkston and Beukelman, 1989; Lethlean, Chenery and Murdoch, 1990), while some groups of subjects with Parkinson's disease have been found to exhibit rate disturbance on a continuum from slower to faster than normal (Metter and Hanson, 1986). Interestingly, however, while many individuals with Parkinson's disease demonstrate a faster than normal rate of speech, Ludlow and Bassich (1984) found that, when specifically required to increase their speech rate, the subjects were often unable to do so.

Physiological investigations of the articulatory function of patients with Parkinson's disease have identified the presence of abnormal patterns of muscle activity, reductions in the range and velocity of articulatory movement, impaired strength, endurance and fine force control of the articulators and tremor in the orofacial structure. These investigations have included a wide variety of instrumental techniques, including direct recordings of muscle activity such as electromyography (Hunker, Abbs and Barlow, 1982; Hirose, 1986; Moore and Scudder, 1989), and a range of kinematic procedures, including strain-gauge transduction systems (Abbs, Hunker and Barlow, 1983; Connor, Ludlow and Schulz, 1989), lead-pellet tracking (Hirose, Kiritani and Sawashima, 1982), electromagnetic articulography (Ackermann *et al.*, 1993) and optoelectrics (Svensson, Henningson and Karlsson, 1993). Overall, the most common physiological findings relating to the articulatory subsystem of subjects with Parkinson's disease include a reduction in the amplitude of displacement of the articulators and a decrease in velocity of movement (Forrest and Weismer, 1995). The physiological findings of reduced amplitude and velocity of the articulatory movements provide support for the 'articulatory undershoot' hypothesis proposed to explain the articulatory imprecision evident in persons with Parkinson's disease (Hunker, Abbs and Barlow, 1982).

In summary, the findings of the perceptual, acoustic and physiological studies relating to articulatory function in Parkinson's disease have generally been consistent in identifying articulatory deficits in this group. Further research, however, is needed to determine the specific relationships among the deviant perceptual, acoustic and physiological speech features to define the precise nature of articulatory dysfunction. Such an approach requires a comprehensive perceptual, acoustic and physiological assessment of the articulatory subsystem of individual speakers with hypokinetic dysarthria.

Prosodic function in hypokinetic dysarthria

According to Darley, Aronson and Brown (1975), prosodic disturbances constitute the most prominent features of hypokinetic dysarthria. Descriptions of the speech of persons with Parkinson's disease frequently refer to the dysprosodic aspects of speech production in relation to stress and intonation, fluency and rate. Impairment of stress patterning, variable rate, short rushes of speech or 'accelerated' speech, difficulty in the initiation of speech, phoneme repetition, palilalia, inappropriate silences and monopitch and monoloudness have been identified in these individuals (Darley, Aronson and Brown, 1975; Ludlow and Bassich, 1983, 1984; Chenery, Murdoch and Ingram, 1988; Zwirner and Barnes, 1992).

Hyperkinetic dysarthria

Hyperkinetic dysarthria is the collective name for a diverse group of speech disorders in which the deviant speech characteristics are the product of abnormal involuntary movements that disturb the rhythm and rate of motor activities, including those involved in speech production. These involuntary movements, which may involve the limbs, trunk, neck, face and so on, may be rhythmic or irregular and unpredictable, rapid or slow. The abnormal involuntary movements involved vary considerably in their form and locus across the different diseases of the basal ganglia. Consequently, there is considerable heterogeneity in the deviant speech dimensions that manifest as the speech disorders termed 'hyperkinetic dysarthria'. Any or all of the major subcomponents of the speech production apparatus may be involved, including the respiratory system, phonatory valve, resonatory valve and articulatory valve. Disturbances in prosody are also present.

In that the various different types of hyperkinetic dysarthria are each associated with one of the hyperkinetic movement disorders (Freed, 2000), clinically the hyperkinetic dysarthrias are usually described in the context of the underlying movement disorders causing the speech disturbance. With this construct in mind, Darley, Aronson and Brown (1975) distinguished between two categories of hyperkinetic disorders: quick hyperkinesias and slow hyperkinesias. Quick hyperkinesias include myoclonic jerks (e.g. palatopharyngolaryngeal myoclonus), tics, chorea and ballism, and are characterized by rapid, abnormal, involuntary movements that are either unsustained or sustained only very briefly,

and are random in occurrence with respect to the particular body part affected. In contrast, the abnormal involuntary movements seen in slow hyperkinesias build up to a peak slowly and are sustained for at least one second or longer. In some instances, the abnormal muscle contractions seen in association with slow hyperkinesias are sustained for many seconds or even minutes, with muscle tone waxing and waning to produce a variety of distorted postures. The three major conditions included in the category of slow hyperkinesias are athetosis, dyskinesia (lingual-facial-buccal dyskinesia) and dystonia. The major types of hyperkinetic disorders are outlined in Table 10.1.

Quick hyperkinesias: myoclonic jerks

Myoclonic jerks are abrupt, sudden, unsustained muscle contractions that occur irregularly. These involuntary muscle contractions may occur as single jerks of a body part or may be repetitive, with the muscles of the limbs, face, oral cavity, soft palate, larynx and diaphragm being affected among others. In those instances where the involuntary movements are repetitive, they can be either rhythmic or non-rhythmic in nature. According to Simon, Arminoff and Greenberg (1999), myoclonic jerks are classified according to their distribution, relationship to precipitating stimuli or aetiology. Although myoclonic jerks are sometimes focal, involving only isolated muscles (focal myoclonus), they may also be multifocal, occurring simultaneously in larger groups of muscles (generalized myoclonus).

Myclonic jerks may occur as a normal phenomenon in healthy persons as an isolated abnormality, or in association with lesions located in a variety of different sites in the central nervous system, ranging from the cerebral cortex (cortical reflex myoclonus) to the spinal cord (spinal myoclonus). Myoclonus may also occur as part of a convulsive disorder (epilepsy) or in association with diffuse metabolic, infectious or toxic disturbances of the nervous system, such as diffuse encephalitis and toxic encephalopathies. Although often occurring spontaneously, myoclonic jerks may also be induced by various sensory stimuli

Table 10.1 Major types of hyperkinetic disorder.

Disorder	Symptoms	Effect on speech
Myoclonic jerks	Characterized by abrupt, sudden, unsustained muscle contractions which occur irregularly. Involuntary contractions may occur as single jerks of the body or may be repetitive. Two forms may affect speech: palatal myoclonus and action myoclonus.	Speech disorder in palatal myoclonus usually characterized by phonatory, resonatory and prosodic abnormalities, for example vocal tremor, rhythmic phonatory arrests, intermittent hypernasality, prolonged intervals and inappropriate silences.
Tics	Tourette's disorder characterized by development of motor and vocal tics plus behavioural disorders. Vocal tics include simple vocal tics (e.g. grunting, coughing, barking, hissing, etc.) and complex vocal tics (e.g. stuttering-like repetitions, palilalia, echolalia and coprolalia). Brief, unsustained, recurrent, compulsive movements. Usually involve a small part of the body, for example facial grimace.	Action myoclonus – speech disrupted as a result of fine, arrhythmic, erratic muscle jerks, triggered by activity of the speech musculature.
Chorea	A choreic movement consists of a single, involuntary, unsustained, isolated muscle action producing a short, rapid, uncoordinated jerk of the trunk, limb, face, tongue, diaphragm, and so on. Contractions are random in distribution and timing is irregular. Two major forms: Sydenham's chorea and Huntington's disease.	A perceptual study of 30 patients with chorea demonstrated deficits in all aspects of speech production (Darley, Aronson and Brown, 1969a).
Ballism	Rare hyperkinetic disorder characterized by involuntary, wide-amplitude, vigorous, flailing movements of the limbs. Facial muscles may also be affected.	Least important hyperkinetic disorders with regard to occurrence of hyperkinetic dysarthria.
Athetosis	Slow hyperkinetic disorder characterized by continuous, arrhythmic, purposeless, slow, writhing-type movements that tend to flow one into another. Muscles of the face, neck and tongue are involved, leading to facial grimacing, protrusion and writhing of the tongue and problems with speaking and swallowing.	Descriptions of the speech disturbance in athetosis largely related to athetoid cerebral palsy rather than hyperkinetic dysarthria in adults.
Dyskinesia	Two dyskinetic disorders are included under this heading: tardive dyskinesia and levodopa-induced dyskinesia. Basic pattern of abnormal involuntary movement in both of these conditions is one of slow, repetitive, writhing, twisting, flexing and extending movements often with a mixture of tremor. Muscles of the tongue, face and oral cavity most often affected.	Accurate placement of the articulators of speech may be severely hampered by the presence of choreoathetoid movements of the tongue, lip pursing and smacking, tongue protrusion, and sucking and chewing behaviours.
Dystonia	Characterized by abnormal involuntary movements that are slow and sustained for prolonged periods. Involuntary movements tend to have an undulant, sinuous character that may produce grotesque posturing and bizarre writhing, twisting movements.	Dystonias affecting the speech mechanisms may result in respiratory irregularities and/or abnormal movement and bizarre posturing of the jaw, lips, tongue, face and neck. In particular, focal cranial/orolingual-mandibular dystonia and spasmodic torticollis have the most direct effect on speech function.

(e.g. visual, auditory or tactile stimuli) or in some instances by voluntary muscle activity (action myoclonus).

The muscles of the speech mechanism may be affected by myoclonic jerks in the same way as the muscles of the limbs. Myoclonic jerks may involve the muscles of the soft palate, larynx and diaphragm either individually or in combination. In those rare cases where it occurs in isolation, palatal myoclonus usually involves the rhythmical contraction of the soft palate, which may result in temporary hypernasality and articulatory imprecision. Laryngeal myoclonus most frequently occurs in combination with palatal myoclonus (Drysdale, Ansell and Adeley, 1993) where it can have the additional effect of temporarily interrupting phonation. Diaphragmatic myoclonus can cause slight interruptions to airflow and is usually most easily detected in sustained phonation tasks.

In particular, two forms of myoclonus have a marked effect on speech: palatopharyngolaryngeal myoclonus (sometimes simply referred to as 'palatal myoclonus') and action myoclonus. Palatopharyngolaryngeal myoclonus is characterized by continuous synchronous jerks of the soft palate at the rate of 1–4 Hz with other brainstem-innervated muscles, particularly the larynx and pharynx usually involved. The condition can be either symptomatic or idiopathic (essential rhythmical palatal myoclonus), with the symptomatic condition most often the result of cerebrovascular lesions involving the brainstem or cerebellum (Deuschl, Mischke and Schenck, 1990). However, a variety of other conditions, including tumours, multiple sclerosis, encephalitis and degenerative diseases, can also lead to palatal myoclonus. Hyperkinetic dysarthria due to palatopharyngolaryngeal myoclonus rarely exists as an isolated speech disturbance, but more frequently occurs in conjunction with another type of dysarthria. Although palatopharyngolaryngeal myoclonus has direct effects on the speech musculature, speech deficits may not be readily perceived during conversational speech because of the low amplitude and brevity of the myoclonic movements (Duffy, 1995). Where a speech disturbance is apparent, it is usually characterized by phonatory, resonatory and prosodic abnormalities, such as vocal tremor, momentary rhythmic phonatory arrests, intermittent hypernasality, prolonged intervals and inappropriate silences (Darley, Aronson and Brown, 1975; Aronson, 1990).

Action myoclonus is differentiated from other myoclonic conditions, such as palatopharyngolaryngeal myoclonus, by the fact that it is triggered by muscle activity. In this condition speech function is disrupted as a result of fine, arrhythmic, erratic muscle jerks that are triggered by muscle activity associated with a conscious attempt at a task requiring precision of movement (e.g. speech production) (Lance and Adams, 1963). The muscle jerks may present one at a time or in a series and are usually less than 200 ms in duration (Lance and Adams, 1963). Documentation of the speech impairment associated with action myoclonus is restricted to one unpublished report. Aronson *et al.* (1984), cited in Duffy, 1995), identified articulatory and phonatory impairments in a study of four cases. Despite demonstrating normal orofacial features at rest, myoclonic spasms of the lips were evident when speech was attempted, resulting in a reduced speech rate. Phonatory disturbances observed in these four cases included repetitive fluctuations in phonation and adductor vocal arrests that were synchronized with the myoclonic jerks of the lip muscles.

Quick hyperkinesias: tics

Tics are brief, unsustained, recurrent, compulsive movements that involve a relatively small part of the body and occur out of a background of normal motor activity. They usually occur spontaneously without provocation by any particular stimulus and are generally considered as involuntary movements. Although tics may be briefly controlled voluntarily, such periods of suppression are often followed by a period of more intensive involuntary contraction.

Tics can be classified into four groups depending on whether they are simple or multiple and transient or chronic. Transient simple tics are very common in children, usually terminating spontaneously within one year and generally requiring no treatment. Chronic simple tics can develop at any age but often begin in childhood and treatment is not necessary in most cases. The syndrome of multiple motor and vocal tics is generally referred to as 'Tourette's disorder'. First described by Frenchman Gilles de la Tourette in 1885, the first signs of Tourette's disorder consist of motor tics in 80% of cases and vocal tics in 20% (Simon, Arminoff and Greenberg, 1999; Alsobrook and Pauls, 2002). The condition primarily affects boys (4 : 1 ratio) and the development of motor and vocal tics is accompanied by a variety of behavioural disorders, including obsessive–compulsive disorder, attention-deficit hyperactivity disorder and other forms of general behavioural disturbances, such as conduct disorder, panic disorder, multiple phobias, mania and so on. In those cases where the initial sign is a motor tic, it most commonly involves the face, taking the form of sniffing, barking, blinking or forced eye closure. The motor tics progressively involve the face, neck, upper limbs and eventually the entire body. Vocal tics include both simple and complex vocal tics. Simple vocal tics include grunting, coughing, barking, throat clearing, hissing and snorting (Serra-Mestres, Robertson and Shetty, 1998). This may occur as isolated events or be embedded with involuntary verbal utterances. In addition, complex vocal tics such as stuttering-like repetitions, unintelligible sounds, palilalia (repetition of self-generated words or phrases) and echolalia have also been reported. Copralalia (involuntary, compulsive swearing), although not universal, is another characteristic complex vocal tic observed in Tourette's disorder. Soft neurological signs, such as mild incoordination in motor skills and slight asymmetry of motor function, including deep tendon reflexes, are also occasionally evident on examination of the child. The incidence of Tourette's disorder is < 1 in 100 000 (Friedhoff, 1982) and drug therapy utilizing antidopaminergic agents has been shown to be effective in some cases.

Quick hyperkinesias: chorea

The term 'chorea' is derived from the Greek word for 'dance' and was originally applied to the dance-like gait and continual limb movements seen in acute infectious chorea. A choreic (or choreiform) movement consists of a single, unsustained, isolated muscle action producing a short, rapid, uncoordinated jerk of the trunk, limb, face, tongue, diaphragm and so on. They are random in their distribution and their timing is irregular and unpredictable. Choreiform movements range in severity from gross displacements of body parts to subtle abnormal involuntary movements. Choreiform contractions are slower than myoclonic jerks, each lasting from 0.1 to 1 second and can occur at rest, during sustained postures or may be superimposed on voluntary movements. When superimposed on normal movements, the abnormal involuntary movements can cause characteristic symptoms, such as dance-like gait. When superimposed on the normal movements of the speech mechanism during speech production, choreic movements can cause momentary disturbances in the course of contextual speech.

A variety of different conditions may be associated with the occurrence of chorea, including metabolic and toxic conditions (e.g. hepatic encephalopathy, Wilson's disease, hyperthyroidism, dopaminergic medications), inflammatory/infectious disorders (e.g. Sydenham's chorea, encephalitis), vascular lesions involving the basal ganglia or thalamus and degenerative conditions (e.g. Huntington's disease). Pregnant women can also on occasion manifest choreiform movements. Chorea can also occur as an idiopathic disorder. Two of the most common choreiform disorders are Sydenham's chorea and Huntington's disease. Sydenham's chorea occurs principally in children and adolescents, and Huntington's disease occurs principally in adults. Both disorders are characterized by hyperkinesia, as well as speech, language, cognitive and psychiatric disorders.

Sydenham's chorea

First described by Thomas Sydenham in 1686 as 'St Vitus' dance', Sydenham's chorea is a movement disorder occurring primarily in association with β-haemolytic streptococcal throat infections or with rheumatic heart disease (Goldenberg *et al.*, 1992; Simon, Arminoff and Greenberg, 1999). The symptom complex of the condition includes involuntary, purposeless, rapid movements which are often associated with incoordination, muscle weakness and/or behavioural abnormalities. These spontaneous movements may involve any portion of the body and occur at rest but disappear during sleep. The condition usually occurs in childhood or adolescence, with onset usually being noted between the ages of five and 10 years. Females are affected more than males and the onset of choreic involuntary movements may be either acute or insidious. The prognosis for Sydenham's chorea is good and recovery is the general rule, with symptoms usually subsiding within four to six months (Simon, Arminoff and Greenberg, 1999). The course of the condition, however, is extremely variable with some cases recovering within a few weeks while others have persistence of the abnormal involuntary movements over a period of years. Frequent relapses occur in some patients with Sydenham's chorea. Pathological changes in Sydenham's chorea have been variously reported in the cerebral cortex, cerebellum, thalamus, caudate nucleus, putamen and midbrain. These changes consist of widespread neuronal degeneration, vascular changes and, rarely, focal brain lesions from embolization resulting from endocarditis. Neuropathological and radiological findings in the acute stage are rare and no consistent neuropathological lesions have been identified in Sydenham's chorea.

Hyperkinetic dysarthria associated with Sydenham's chorea has received little attention in the research literature. Further, the few studies reported have largely only documented the presence of dysarthria in persons with Sydenham's chorea rather than providing specific details as to the clinical features of the condition. Nausieda *et al.* (1980) reported the findings of a retrospective study of 240 individuals with Sydenham's chorea noting that 39% had dysarthria. Swedo *et al.* (1993) examined 11 moderately affected children reporting that all exhibited a dysarthria which manifested as 'slurred or incoherent speech ... with two children rendered mute' (p. 707). In all but two of the children, the dysarthria subsided within months of the initiation of medical treatment and was noted to not be present at an 18-month follow-up assessment. Further studies reporting the presence of dysarthria in Sydenham's chorea were conducted by Goldenberg *et al.* (1992), who examined 187 children in Brazil, and Kulkarni and Anees (1996), who examined 60 children in India.

Huntington's disease

Huntington's disease is an autosomal dominant neurodegenerative genetic condition which causes pathologic changes in the striatum (in particular the head of the caudate nucleus) (Martin and Gusella, 1986), namely the loss of the gamma aminobutyric acid (GABA) neurones (Albin, Young and Penney, 1989). In relation to basal ganglia circuitry, the preferential loss of GABAergic striatal neurones within the indirect pathway (Hedreen and Folstein, 1995) results in the disinhibition of the inhibitory external segment of the globus pallidus projections to the subthalamic nucleus and, consequently, reduced inhibitory output from the SNPR/internal segment of the globus pallidus, leading to superfluous excitation of thalamocortical projection neurones (DeLong, 1990) (Figure 10.3). Clinical symptoms typically present after 30 years of age and characteristically include choreic body movements (i.e. involuntary writhing movements), which may produce the follow-on effects of abnormal gait, dysarthria and swallowing difficulties (Enderby, 2008). Ataxia, dystonia, bruxism, myoclonus, tics, Tourettism and Parkinsonism have also been observed in Huntington's disease, and cognitive, psychiatric and behavioural disturbances are common as well (Adam and Jankovic, 2008). Motor symptoms may be further divided into impaired accessory/involuntary (e.g. chorea, dystonia, rigidity) and voluntary movements (e.g. speech, gait, swallowing), with evidence of a disproportionate exacerbation in voluntary versus involuntary movement impairments over the course of the disease, associated with greater levels of functional disability (Folstein, 1989).

The medical management of Huntington's disease has conventionally involved the symptomatic treatment of chorea and dystonia, with neuroleptic (e.g. haloperidol, pimozide, fluphenazine, thioridazine, sulpiride, tiapride, olanzapine) and dopamine-depleting (e.g. tetrabenazine) medications (Jankovic, 2006a; Bonelli and Hoffman, 2007). Of particular note, it has been observed that effective antichoreic medications may exacerbate voluntary movement impairments such as speech and/or swallowing (Bonelli, Wenning and Kapfhammer, 2003), with evident implications for speech pathology management.

In the advanced stages of Huntington's disease the clinical picture includes facial grimacing (involving the lips, tongue and cheeks), jerks of the head, weaving movements of the arms and shoulders, twists and jerks of the body, as well as superimposed voluntary movements (e.g. an involuntary upward jerk of the arm may be fused into a scratching of the head). The patient's gait at this stage is often markedly involved, consisting of jerky lurching steps that represent a combination of voluntary and involuntary movements. Muscular strength, however, is unimpaired. Unlike Parkinson's disease, the ability to initiate voluntary movements is intact. However, the conduct of a continuous movement (e.g. walking or speech production) is frequently impeded by superimposed muscle jerks.

The pervasive choreiform movements evident in patients with Huntington's disease and other forms of chorea have a profound effect on the individual's attempts at speech production because of the sudden, rapid and unpredictable nature of the involuntary movements which interfere with respiratory, laryngeal, velopharyngeal and articulatory speech activity. The laboured and effortful speech is presumed to be a manifestation of inaccuracy in the direction of movement, irregularity in rhythm, range, force and muscle tone, and a reduced rate of individual and repetitive movements of the muscles of the speech mechanism (Darley, Aronson and Brown, 1969b). Hyperkinetic dysarthria associated with chorea is distinguished from other types of dysarthria by the sporadic and transient nature of the abnormal speech features. Individuals with chorea may, in fact, demonstrate normal speech intelligibility, punctuated by distorted speech production during the periods of hyperkinesias.

Clinical features of hyperkinetic dysarthria in Huntington's disease. To date, relatively few studies based on perceptual, acoustic and/or physiological assessments have documented the clinical features of hyperkinetic dysarthria associated with Huntington's disease. The most comprehensive perceptual study to have been reported was performed by Darley, Aronson and Brown (1969a). They reported that all basic motor-speech processes were disturbed. The 10 most deviant speech dimensions observed in patients with chorea by Darley, Aronson and Brown (1969a) were, in rank order: (1) imprecise consonants, (2) prolonged intervals, (3) variable speaking rate, (4) monopitch, (5) harsh voice quality, (6) inappropriate silences, (7) distorted vowels, (8) excess loudness variation, (9) prolonged phonemes and (10) monoloudness. In particular, they reported that choreic patients were most distinctive from other patients with dysarthria in the area of prosodic alterations, being more deviant than any other neurological group on the speech dimensions of excess loudness variation, variable rate and prolonged intervals. According to Darley, Aronson and Brown (1975), the prosodic changes appear to represent an attempt by the choreic speaker to avoid articulatory and phonatory interruptions by variably altering their rate of speech, prolonging their phonemes and prolonging the intervals between words, equalizing the stress on syllables and introducing inappropriate silences.

Hartelius *et al.* (2003) also examined the speech of speakers with mild and moderate Huntington's disease and, consistent with Darley, Aronson and Brown (1969a,b), observed significant speech deviations in all areas of speech production tested. The most severe speech deviations observed by this group were in phonation, oromotor performance including oral diadochokinesis and prosody. Although no correlation was found between age or gender and severity of dysarthria, a significant difference in the severity of dysarthria was found between the group with mild Huntington's disease and the group with moderate Huntington's disease. The most frequently occurring perceptual deviations found in continuous speech were mainly related to speech timing and phonation and were hypothesized to reflect the underlying excessive and involuntary movement pattern.

Imprecise consonant and distorted vowel production and irregular articulatory breakdowns have been reported to characterize the articulation of patients with chorea (Darley, Aronson and Brown, 1975) and are consistent with the expected adverse effects of choreiform movements on lip, tongue and jaw function. Support for this conclusion has been provided by several acoustic studies of the speech output of patients with Huntington's disease. Zwirner and Barnes (1992) identified greater than normal variability in the first and second formants of a sustained vowel, reflecting abnormal jaw movements (first formant) and aberrations of tongue position and shape (second formant). In addition, Ackermann, Hertrich and Hehr (1995) found that, on an oral diadochokinetic task, their patients with Huntington's disease exhibited increased syllable durational variability and, in some cases, incomplete articulatory gestures which could be attributed to the effects of choreic activity.

The excessive loudness variation exhibited by patients with Huntington's disease was considered a characteristic of this form of hyperkinetic dysarthria by Darley, Aronson and Brown (1969a,b). In some cases, voice stoppages or arrests were observed in these patients. Objective acoustic assessments of voice in patients with Huntington's disease have identified high phonatory instability (increased variability in fundamental frequency and sudden reductions in frequency of approximately one octave) consistent with involuntary laryngeal movements (Ramig, 1986; Ramig *et al.*, 1988; Zwirner, Murry and Woodson, 1991; Zwirner and Barnes, 1992).

Hypernasality when present in patients with Huntington's disease is usually only mild and intermittent, reflecting the variable nature of the choreiform movements affecting soft palate function. Darley, Aronson and Brown (1969a) reported that only approximately 40% of their patients with Huntington's disease exhibited hypernasality. Likewise, these researchers only observed abnormal respiratory patterns in six of their 30 patients with chorea, the abnormal respiratory pattern taking the form of sudden, forced and involuntary inspiration and/or expiration.

However, Darley, Aronson and Brown (1969a) found this abnormal respiratory pattern to be unique to this form of hyperkinetic dysarthria.

Quick hyperkinesias: ballism (hemiballismus)

Hemiballismus is a rare hyperkinetic movement disorder characterized by involuntary, wide-amplitude, vigorous, flailing movement of the limbs, particularly the arm, on one side of the body. Facial muscles may also be affected. The most consistent neuropathological finding associated with hemiballismus is vascular damage to the subthalamic nucleus or its immediate connections on the side contralateral to the involuntary movement disorder. Ballism can also be caused by other conditions, including infections, drugs, autoimmune disorders, primary brain tumours and acquired immunodeficiency syndrome (AIDS). Ballism is the least important of all the quick hyperkinesias in relation to the occurrence of hyperkinetic dysarthria.

Slow hyperkinesias: athetosis

Athetosis is a slow hyperkinesia characterized by continuous, arrhythmic, purposeless, slow, writhing-type movements that tend to flow one into the other. The abnormal movements cease only during sleep and the affected muscles are always hypertonic and may show transient stages of spasms. Athetoid movements particularly involve the distal musculature of the limbs. The muscles of the face, neck and tongue, however, may also be affected, leading to facial grimacing, protrusion and writhing of the tongue and problems with speaking and swallowing.

Athetosis occurs most often as part of a congenital complex of neurological signs that results from a disordered development of the brain, birth injury or other aetiological factors and represents a subcategory of cerebral palsy (Morris *et al.*, 2002). The term, therefore, is rarely used to describe movement disorders acquired in adulthood, with many neurologists regarding athetosis as synonymous with dystonia when referring to the acquired condition. Consequently, the majority of reports in the literature relating to the occurrence and nature of speech disorders associated with athetosis are largely based on studies of children or adults with cerebral palsy. Intelligibility of connected speech has been reported to be markedly decreased though phonemic competence is intact, suggesting that athetoid individuals lack the neuromuscular control for articulatory precision (Platt, Andrews and Howie, 1980). The articulatory abnormalities noted in individuals with athetosis include wide-ranging jaw movements, inappropriate tongue placement, intermittent velopharyngeal closure, retrusion of the lower lip and prolonged transition time for articulatory movements (Kent and Netsell, 1978).

Slow hyperkinesias: dyskinesia (lingual-facial-buccal dyskinesia

The term 'dyskinesia' is often used in a general way to refer to abnormal, involuntary, hyperkinetic movements without regard to aetiology (Miller and Jankovic, 1990). Although when used in this way all involuntary movements could be described as 'dyskinetic', only two dyskinetic disorders are usually considered under this heading: tardive dyskinesia and levodopa-induced dyskinesia. As both of these conditions may be limited to the bulbar musculature, they are sometimes referred to as 'focal dyskinesias'. Further, because the muscles of the tongue, face and oral cavity are most often affected, these two disorders are also termed 'lingual-facial-buccal dyskinesias'. The basic pattern of abnormal involuntary movement in both of these conditions is one of slow, repetitive, writhing, twisting, flexing and extending movements, often with a mixture of tremor.

Tardive dyskinesia

Tardive dyskinesia is a late-onset, acquired movement disorder resulting from long-term neuroleptic treatment (treatment with a pharmacological agent having antipsychotic action) (Jeste and Wyatt, 1982). Although neuroleptic drugs have been prescribed for psychiatric disorders since

the 1930s, the condition was first described by Schonecker (1957), when the term 'tardive dyskinesia' was coined. Also sometimes referred to as 'Meige syndrome', tardive dyskinesia is regarded by some neurologists as a form of focal dystonia involving the craniocervical region (Ferguson, 1992). The syndrome occurs relatively late in the course of neuroleptic therapy.

The abnormal involuntary movements seen in tardive dyskinesia are usually of the choreoathetoid type, are sometimes stereotyped and principally affect the tongue, lips and jaw and, to a lesser degree, the larynx and respiratory musculature (Feve, Angelard and Lacau St Guily, 1995). The limbs and trunk are also occasionally involved. A combination of tongue twisting and protrusion, lip smacking and puckering and chewing movement in a repetitive and stereotypic fashion is often observed (Jankovic, 1995). In addition, the soft palate may also elevate and lower involuntarily. When asked to do so, patients with tardive dyskinesia may be able to suppress involuntary mouth movements. These movements may also be suppressed by voluntary actions such as putting food in the mouth or talking.

In relation to medical management, the subcutaneous injections of botulinum toxin into effected facial muscles has been successful in relieving the associated dystonia (Drummond, 2008), yet the greatest improvements in speech symptoms have been identified upon the termination of antipsychotic treatment (Drummond and Fitzpatrick, 2004).

Speech production is often markedly affected in tardive dyskinesia owing to the abnormal involuntary, rhythmic movements of the orofacial, lingual and mandibular structures. The accurate placement of the articulators of speech may be severely hampered by the presence of choreoathetoid movements of the tongue, lip pursing and smacking, tongue protrusion, and sucking and chewing behaviours (Matthews and Glaser, 1984; Vernon, 1991). According to Darley, Aronson and Brown (1969a,b), articulatory deviations were the most prominent features of the hyperkinetic dysarthria exhibited by their patients with tardive dyskinesia. Other perceptually based studies have also identified prosodic, phonatory and respiratory impairments, in addition to articulatory disorders, in small groups of subjects with tardive dyskinesia (Gerratt, 1983; Gerratt, Goetz and Fisher, 1984). In a perceptual study of 12 patients with tardive dyskinesia, Gerratt, Goetz and Fisher (1984) reported that these patients exhibited marked disturbances in the temporal organization of speech (prosodic impairment) and phonation, while articulatory deficits (irregular articulatory breakdowns and imprecise consonants) were perceived to be less severely impaired. Respiratory dysfunction, involving respiratory dysrhythmia, involuntary grunts and gasping sounds, have also been reported in patients with tardive dyskinesia (Weiner *et al.*, 1978; Faheem *et al.*, 1982).

The most comprehensive perceptual study of the hyperkinetic dysarthria associated with tardive dyskinesia was conducted by Khan *et al.* (1994). They reported that the 17 male psychiatric patients with tardive dyskinesia examined in their study demonstrated significantly reduced phonation times, levels of speech intelligibility and speech rate compared to 10 neuroleptically treated patients without tardive dyskinesia. La Porta *et al.* (1990) phonetically analysed the speech of two subjects with tardive dyskinesia during reading, sentence repetition and spontaneous conversation tasks. Both cases were found to produce high frequencies of abnormal consonants, compared to a single control subject who had received long-term neuroleptic treatment but did not exhibit tardive dyskinesia. Specifically, the two patients with tardive dyskinesia made the most number of errors on alveolar, alveodental and palatal phonemes, consistent with abnormal movements of the tongue in tardive dyskinesia. Interestingly, La Porta *et al.* (1990) found that vowel production was unimpaired in these two subjects.

Support for the above perceptual findings in relation to articulation and phonation has come from acoustic investigations of the dysarthria associated with tardive dyskinesia. For example, Gerratt (1983) investigated motor steadiness of the vocal tract musculature superior to the glottis during vowel production in five subjects with tardive dyskinesia using a measure of formant frequency fluctuation as an indicator of changes in vocal tract configuration. Consistent with the articulatory and phonatory deficits identified perceptually by La Porta *et al.* (1990) and Khan *et al.* (1994), their results indicated that formant frequency fluctuations were markedly higher for four of the five subjects compared to normal controls, reflecting a reduction in motor steadiness supraglottally.

Physiological investigations of the speech mechanism in patients with tardive dyskinesia have involved objective analyses of buccolingual, tongue and respiratory function using a variety of instrumental techniques. Caligiuri, Harris and Jeste (1988), using a head-mounted transduction system and a pursuit tracking paradigm, evaluated the fine-motor control of lip, jaw and tongue movements in 11 patients with tardive dyskinesia. Greater tracking errors were demonstrated by the patients with tardive dyskinesia for the lip (31%), tongue (36%) and jaw (31%) compared with non-tardive-dyskinetic patients (lip 12%, tongue 12%, jaw 13%). Using position transducers, Caligiuri, Jeste and Harris identified greater motor instability in the tongue in 13 patients with tardive dyskinesia compared to control subjects and non-tardive-dyskinetic patients. Physiological assessment of respiratory function in patients with tardive dyskinesia, using respiratory inductance plethysmography, has confirmed perceptual observations of respiratory impairments in these patients. Wilcox *et al.* (1994) found that patients with tardive dyskinesia demonstrated rapid, shallow breathing characterized by irregular tidal breathing patterns, with greater variability in both tidal volume and time of the total respiratory cycle than that of control subjects.

As indicated above, tardive dyskinesia occurs later in the course of neuroleptic therapy, often after a decrease in the drug dosage or discontinuation of the drug therapy. The involuntary lingual-facial-buccal movements often persist for months or years after the neuroleptic therapy has been discontinued. If recognized early, however, the symptoms of tardive dyskinesia (including the associated hyperkinetic dysarthria) may recede with the discontinuation of neuroleptic treatment (Drummond and Fitzpatrick, 2004).

Levodopa-induced dyskinesia

Combined lingual-facial-buccal dyskinesia is not unique to tardive dyskinesia but may also be seen as part of the hyperkinesia of Huntington's disease and following high-dose levodopa therapy in Parkinson's disease. As in tardive dyskinesia, the abnormal involuntary movements seen in the latter condition are also typically choreic and characteristically involve the muscles of the tongue, face and mouth. The tongue may demonstrate 'fly-catcher' movements in which it involuntarily moves in and out of the mouth repeatedly. Simultaneously, the lips may pucker and retract while the jaw may open and close or move from side to side spontaneously. The induction of lingual-facial-buccal dyskinesia by levodopa therapy is consistent with the proposal of Ludlow and Bassich (1984) that patients with Parkinson's disease treated with levodopa have a speech disorder resembling a hyperkinetic rather than a hypokinetic dysarthria.

Slow hyperkinesias: dystonia

'Dystonia' is a collective term for a variety of neurogenic movement and posture disorders characterized by abnormal, involuntary muscle contractions which may be accompanied by irregular repetitive movements. Dystonic movements are abnormal, involuntary movements which are slow and sustained for prolonged periods. Affected muscles are hypertonic and the involuntary movements tend to have an undulant, sinuous character which may produce grotesque posturing and bizarre writhing movements. Dystonia tends to involve large parts of the body, particularly the muscles of the trunk, neck and proximal parts of the limbs. However, the muscles of the speech mechanism may also be involved, in which case the patient may exhibit spasms of the face, producing facial grimacing, forceful spasmodic eye closing (blepharospasm), pursing of the lips, jaw spasm, involuntary twisting and protrusion of the tongue and respiratory irregularities. The most distinguishing feature of dystonia involves the maintenance of an abnormal or altered posture, on some occasions involving only a single focal part of the body while on others involving a diffuse region of the body. The abnormal involuntary contractions usually build up slowly, produce a prolonged distorted posture such as twisting of the trunk about the long axis (torsion spasm) and then gradually recede. Occasionally, dystonic movements begin with a jerk and then build up to a peak before subsiding.

The medical management of dystonia typically involves the administration of dopaminergic, anticholinergic and GABA agonist medications (Jankovic, 2006b), which alter GABA-mediated inhibition, dopaminergic and muscarinic cholinergic neurotransmission within dystonic brains (Breakefield *et al.*, 2008). In addition, intramuscular injections of botulinum toxin within effected muscles may also provide relief in more focal cases by blocking the release of acetylcholine from motor neurones, thereby reducing excessive muscle activity (Breakefield *et al.*, 2008). Similarly, to Parkinson's disease, deep brain stimulation of the internal segment of the globus pallidus providing functional manipulation of dystonic motor circuits has also been successful in alleviating some cases of dystonia (Breakefield *et al.*, 2008).

A variety of conditions may lead to dystonia, including encephalitis, head trauma, vascular diseases and drug toxicity. In addition, various progressive degenerative diseases of the central nervous system such as Wilson's disease and Huntington's disease often manifest dystonic features at some time in their course. One type of dystonia, dystonia musculorum deformans, is an inherited disease. In many cases, however, the cause of dystonia is unknown. Although it is often reported that dystonia is a disorder of the basal ganglia, no consistent and specific pathophysiology or pathomorphologic alteration in the brain has been identified.

Depending on the distribution of the abnormal involuntary movements, dystonia can be classified into several subtypes:

- focal dystonia (involving only a single segment or part of the body);
- segmental dystonia (involving two or more contiguous body segments);

- multifocal dystonia (involving two non-contiguous body parts);
- generalized dystonia (involving one or both legs plus another area of the body).

Focal dystonias that may affect speech and voice include orolingual-mandibular dystonia, laryngeal dystonia and cervical dystonia (also known as 'spasmodic torticollis'). Patients with orolingual-mandibular dystonia have abnormal movements of the vocal tract, including sustained tongue movements, clenched jaw or forced jaw opening (Yoshida *et al.*, 2002; Yoshida and Iizuki, 2003). These signs often occur with blepharospasm, and this complex has been referred to as 'focal cranial dystonia' or 'Meige syndrome' (Jankovic, 1988). According to Darley, Aronson and Brown (1975), articulation, phonation and prosody may all be significantly disturbed in patients with dystonia. In a study of 30 dystonia cases, Darley, Aronson and Brown (1969a) found that the deviant speech dimensions of imprecise consonants, disturbed vowels, harsh voice quality, irregular articulatory breakdown, strained/strangled voice quality, monopitch, monoloudness, inappropriate silence, short phrases and prolonged intervals to be the 10 major features of the hyperkinetic dysarthria seen in dystonia. Notably, three of the four most prominent deviant characteristics were related to articulatory disturbance. Resonatory disturbances have not been found to be characteristic features of dysarthria associated with dystonia. Approximately 30% of cases have been found to demonstrate hypernasality, with the majority of subjects exhibiting this abnormality to a mild degree (Darley, Aronson and Brown, 1969a,b; Golper *et al.*, 1983). Likewise, except for two patients in Golper *et al.*'s (1983) study who were perceived to exhibit respiratory muscle spasms, studies of the speech output of patients with dystonia have generally failed to identify specific impairments of respiration. A number of perceptual features identified in this population, such as excessive loudness variations, short phrases and alternating loudness, could, however, reflect the contribution of respiratory impairment in this population.

As a reflection of the phenomenon of laryngospasm during phonation, laryngeal dystonia is referred to as 'spasmodic dysphonia'. Three subtypes of spasmodic dysphonia are recognized based on the specific aspect of vocal fold movement impaired. These subtypes include adductor, abductor and mixed spasmodic dysphonia of which adductor is by far the most common (Blitzer and Brin, 1992). Three syllable-level adductor spasmodic dysphonia signs have been identified by various researchers as being key to the classification of the adductor spasmodic dysphonia voice: pitch shift (Sapienza, Walton and Murry, 1999, 2000), phonatory break (Langeveld *et al.*, 2000) and aperiodicity (Sapienza, Walton and Murry, 1999, 2000).

Spasmodic torticollis – a condition in which tonic or clonic spasm in the neck muscles (especially the sternocleidomastoid and trapezius muscles) cause the head to be deviated to the right or left, or sometimes forwards (antecollis) and backwards (retrocollis) – has also been reported to disrupt speech production (Case, LaPointe and Duane, 1990; LaPointe, Case and Duane, 1993; Zraick *et al.*, 1993). Acoustic speech/voice characteristics of the hyperkinetic dysarthria associated with spasmodic torticollis include reduced maximum phonation duration, slower sequential articulatory movement rates, slower alternate articulatory movement rates, longer phonatory reaction time, slower reading rate (in words per minute), lower overall intelligibility rating, increased jitter, increased shimmer, increased harmonic-to-noise ratio (females), lower habitual fundamental frequency (females), lower ceiling fundamental frequency (females) and restricted frequency range (females).

Essential voice tremor

Tremors are involuntary movements resulting from the contraction of opposing muscle groups, which produces rhythmic or alternating movement of a joint or group of joints. A number of different types of tremor are recognized, which include:

- physiological tremor (e.g. tremor associated with cold or nervousness);

- essential tremor (e.g. familial, action and senile);
- toxic tremor (e.g. tremor in thyrotoxicosis and alcoholism);
- pathological tremor (e.g. intention tremor in cerebellar disorders and rest tremor in Parkinson's disease).

Essential tremor is a hyperkinetic movement disorder that most often affects the head, arms or hands. It is the most common of the movement disorders, with approximately 50% of cases being familial, with the bulk of the rest being idiopathic (Duffy, 1995). The condition is usually regarded as an exaggeration of normal physiological tremors. Although often referred to as a 'benign disorder', the symptoms of essential tremor are typically progressive and potentially disabling and may force affected persons to change jobs or seek early retirement. This type of tremor is absent at rest and appears when the patient acts to move or support a body part (hence the name 'action tremor'). Essential tremor is not associated with other evidence of neurological disease.

Pharmacotherapeutics provide the primary treatment regime for essential tremor. A range of anti-tremor agents have been shown to be effective (Evidente, 2000), including beta blockers (e.g. propranolol, metoprolol, nadolol); anticonvulsants (e.g. primidone); benzodiazepines (e.g. diazepam, clonazepam, alprazolam); carbonic anhydrase inhibitors particularly methazolamide in the case of head and voice tremor (Muenter, Daube and Caviness, 1991) and botulinum toxin injections, again, particularly in the case of hand, voice and head movements (Wasielewski, Burns and Koller, 1998). Similarly to Parkinson's disease, however, in the case of drug-resistant or severe essential tremor, thalamotomy and thalamic deep brain stimulation have been reported to successfully alleviate tremor (Schuurman, Bosch and Bossuyt, 2000).

Essential or organic voice tremor is a focal presentation of essential tremor (Murdoch, 1990). The typical form of essential voice tremor occurs when the alternating contractions of the adductors and abductors of the vocal folds are of equal strength, in contrast to other presentations such as adductor and abductor spasmodic dysphonia where either the adductor or abductor movements of the vocal folds are disproportionately stronger. During contextual speech, essential voice tremor may not be apparent, especially when the tremor is mild. Vowel prolongation is typically the best task for eliciting voice tremor (Aronson, 1990), which can be perceived as rhythmical frequency modulations of 4–7 Hz, sometimes accompanied by fluctuations in loudness. Although essential voice tremor may occur in isolation, it is usually accompanied by head or extremity tremor.

Summary

Extrapyramidal syndromes include a range of neurological diseases that can broadly be classified as either hypokinetic or hyperkinetic disorders. Hypokinetic disorders are characterized by significant impairments in movement initiation (akinesia) and reduction in the velocity of voluntary movements and are usually accompanied by muscular rigidity and tremor at rest. Hyperkinetic disorders, in contrast, are characterized by excessive motor activity in the form of involuntary movement (dyskinesia) with varying degrees of hypotonia.

Hypokinetic dysarthria is classically associated with Parkinson's disease but may also occur in progressive supranuclear palsy. Overall, the speech characteristics associated with hypokinetic dysarthria follow the generalized pattern of hypokinetic motor disorders, including marked reductions in the amplitude of voluntary movement, initiation difficulties, slowness of movement (bradykinesia), muscular rigidity and tremor at rest. Although all aspects of speech production may be impaired, individuals with hypokinetic dysarthria most commonly exhibit disturbances of prosody, phonation and articulation.

Hyperkinetic dysarthria can occur in association with a range of different hyperkinetic movement disorders, including myoclonic jerks, tics, chorea, ballism, athetosis, dyskinesia and dystonia. In each case the speech characteristics are the product of abnormal involuntary movements that disturb the rhythm and rate of motor activities, including those involved in speech production. In some instances, these involuntary movements are rapid and unsustained or sustained only briefly (e.g. myoclonic jerks, tics, chorea) and are referred to as 'quick hyperkinesias', while in others the involuntary movements are slow and sustained for many seconds or minutes (e.g. dystonia). This latter group of hyperkinetic disorders is referred to as 'slow hyperkinesias'. The clinical characteristics of hyperkinetic dysarthria vary according to the specific hyperkinetic disorder exhibited by the patient.

References

Abbs, J.H., Hunker, C.J. and Barlow, S.H. (1983) Differential speech motor subsystem impairment with supranuclear lesions: neurophysiological framework and supporting data, in *Clinical Dysarthria* (ed. W.R. Berry), College Hill Press, San Diego, pp. 21–56.

Ackermann, H., Hertrich, I. and Hehr, T. (1995) Oral diadochokinesis in neurological dysarthrias. *Folia Phoniatrica et Logopaedica*, **47**, 15–23.

Ackermann, H., Grone, B.F., Hoch, G. and Schonle, P.W. (1993) Speech freezing in Parkinson's disease: a kinematic analysis of orofacial movements by means of electromagnetic articulography. *Folia Phoniatrica et Logopaedica*, **45**, 84–89.

Ackermann, H. and Ziegler, W. (1991) Articulatory deficits in Parkinson's dysarthria: an acoustic analysis. *Journal of Neurology, Neurosurgery and Psychiatry*, **54**, 1093–1098.

Adam, O.R. and Jankovic, J. (2008) Symptomic treatment of Huntington disease. *Neurotherapeutics: the Journal of American Society for Experimental Neurotherapeutics*, **5**, 181–197.

Adams, S.G. and Jog, M. (2008) Parkinson's disease, in *Clinical Management of Sensorimotor Speech Disorders*, 2nd edn (ed. M.R. McNeil), Thieme, New York, pp. 365–368.

Albin, R.L., Young, A.B. and Penney, J.B. (1989) The functional anatomy of basal ganglia disorders. *Trends in Neuroscience*, **12**, 366–375.

Alexander, G.E., DeLong, M.R. and Strick, P.L. (1986) Parallel organization of functionally segregated circuits linking basal ganglia and cortex. *Annual Review of Neuroscience*, **9**, 357–381.

Alsobrook, J.P. and Pauls, D.L. (2002) A factor analysis of tic symptoms in Gilles de la Tourette's syndrome. *American Journal of Psychiatry*, **159**, 291–296.

Aronson, A.E. (1990) *Clinical Voice Disorders*, Georg Thieme, New York.

Blitzer, A. and Brin, M.F. (1992) The dystonic larynx. *Journal of Voice*, **6**, 294–297.

Bonelli, R. and Hoffman, P. (2007) A systematic review of the treatment studies in Huntington's disease since 1990. *Expert Opinion in Pharmacotherapy*, **8**, 141–153.

Bonelli, R., Wenning, G.K. and Kapfhammer, H.P. (2003) Huntington's disease: present treatments and future therapeutic modalities. *International Clinical Psychopharmacology*, **19**, 51–62.

Breakefield, X.O., Blood, A.J., Li, Y. *et al.* (2008) The pathophysiological basis of dystonias. *Nature Reviews: Neuroscience*, **9**, 222–234.

Brooks, D.J. (1991) Detection of preclinical Parkinson's disease with PET. *Neurology*, **41** (Suppl. 2), 24.

Caligiuri, M.P., Harris, M.J. and Jeste, D.V. (1988) Quantitative analyses of voluntary orofacial motor control in schizophrenia and tardive dyskinesia. *Biological Psychiatry*, **24**, 787–800.

Caligiuri, M.P., Jeste, D.V. and Harris, M.J. (1989) Instrumental assessment of lingual motor instability in tardive dyskinesia. *Neuropsychopharmacology*, **2**, 309–312.

Calne, D. and Snow, B.J. (1993) PET imaging in Parkinsonism. *Advances in Neurology*, **60**, 484.

Canter, G. (1965) Speech characteristics of patients with Parkinson's disease. II. Physiological support for speech. *Journal of Speech and Hearing Disorders*, **30**, 44–49.

Case, J., LaPointe, L. and Duane, D. (1990) Speech and voice characteristics in spasmodic torticollis. Paper presented at the *International Congress of Movement Disorders*, Washington, DC.

Chenery, H.J., Murdoch, B.E. and Ingram, J.C.L. (1988) Studies in Parkinson's disease. I. Perceptual speech analysis. *Australian Journal of Human Communication Disorders*, **16**, 17–29.

Connor, N.P., Ludlow, C.L. and Schulz, G.M. (1989) Stop consonant production in isolated and repeated syllables in Parkinson's disease. *Neuropsychologia*, **27**, 829–838.

Cramer, W. (1940) De spraak bij Patienten met Parkinsonisme. *Logopaedie en Phoniatrie*, **22**, 17–23.

Darley, F.L., Aronson, A.E. and Brown, J.R. (1969a). Differential diagnostic patterns of dysarthria. *Journal of Speech and Hearing Research*, **12**, 246–269.

Darley, F.L., Aronson, A.E. and Brown, J.R. (1969b). Clusters of deviant speech dimensions in the dysarthrias. *Journal of Speech and Hearing Research*, **12**, 462–496.

Darley, F.L., Aronson, A.E. and Brown, J.R. (1975) *Motor Speech Disorders*, W.B. Saunders, Philadelphia.

De La Torre, R., Mier, M. and Boshes, B. (1960) Studies in Parkinsonism: IX. Evaluation of respiratory function: preliminary observations. *Quarterly Bulletin of the Northwestern University Medical School*, **34**, 232–236.

DeLong, M.R. (1990) Primate models of movement disorders of basal ganglia origin. *Trends in Neurosciences*, **13**, 281–285.

Deuschl, G., Mischke, G. and Schenck, E. (1990) Symptomatic and essential rhythmic palatal myoclonus. *Brain*, **113**, 1645–1672.

Drummond, S. and Fitzpatrick, A. (2004) Speech and swallowing performances in tardive dyskinesia: a case study. *Journal of Medical Speech Language Pathology*, **12**, 9–19.

Drummond, S. (2008) Tardive dyskinesia, in *Clinical Management of Sensorimotor Speech Disorders*, 2nd edn (ed. M.R. McNeil), Thieme, New York, pp. 396–397.

Drysdale, A.J., Ansell, J. and Adeley, J. (1993) Palatopharyngo-laryngeal myoclonus: an unusual cause of dysphagia and dysarthria. *Journal of Laryngology & Otology*, **107**, 746–747.

Duffy, J. (1995) *Motor Speech Disorders: Substrates, Diagnosis and Management*, Mosby, St Louis.

Eidelberg, D. (1992) Positron emission tomography studies in Parkinsonism. *Neurology Clinics*, **10**, 421.

Enderby, P. (1986) Relationships between dysarthric groups. *British Journal of Disorders of Communication*, **21**, 180–197.

Enderby, P. (2008) Huntington's disease, in *Clinical Management of Sensorimotor Speech Disorders*, 2nd edn (ed. M.R. McNeil), Thieme, New York, pp. 331–333.

Evidente, V.G.H. (2000) Understanding essential tremor: differential diagnosis and options for treatment. *Postgraduate Medicine*, **108** (5), 138–139.

Faheem, A.D., Brightwell, D.R., Burton, G.C. and Struss, A. (1982) Respiratory dyskinesia and dysarthria from prolonged neuroleptic use: tardive dyskinesia? *American Journal of Psychiatry*, **139**, 517–518.

Ferguson, A. (1992) Speech control in persistent tardive dyskinesia: a case study. *European Journal of Disorders of Communication*, **27**, 89–93.

Feve, A., Angelard, B. and Lacau St Guily, J. (1995) Laryngeal tardive dyskinesia. *Journal of Neurology*, **242**, 455–499.

Filion, M. and Tremblay, L. (1991) Abnormal spontaneous activity of globus pallidus neurons in monkeys with MPTP-induced Parkinsonism. *Brain Research*, **547**, 142.

Filion, M., Tremblay, L. and Bedard, P.J. (1988) Abnormal influences of passive limb movement on the activity of globus pallidus neurons in Parkinsonian monkeys. *Brain Research*, **444**, 165.

Flint, A.J., Black, S.E. and Campbell-Taylor, I. (1992) Acoustic analysis in the differentiation of Parkinson's disease and major depression. *Journal of Psycholinguistic Research*, **21**, 383–399.

Folstein, S.E. (1989) Huntington's disease: a disorder of families, in *The Johns Hopkins Series in Contemporary Medicine and Public Health*, Johns Hopkins University Press, Baltimore, p. 251.

Forrest, K. and Weismer, G. (1995) Dynamic aspects of lower lip movement in Parkinsonian and neurologically normal geriatric speakers' production of stress. *Journal of Speech and Hearing Research*, **38**, 260–272.

Freed, D. (2000) *Motor Speech Disorders: Diagnosis and Treatment*, Singular-Thompson Learning, San Diego.

Friedhoff, A. (1982) Gilles de la Tourette syndrome, *Advances in Neurology*, **35**, 335–339.

Gamboa, J., Jimenez-Jimenez, F.L., Nieto, A. et al. (1997) Acoustic voice analysis in patients with Parkinson's disease treated with dopaminergic drugs. *Journal of Voice*, **11**, 314–320.

Gerratt, B.R. (1983) Formant frequency fluctuation as an index of motor steadiness in the vocal tract. *Journal of Speech and Hearing Research*, **26**, 297–304.

Gerratt, B.R., Goetz, C.G. and Fisher, H.B. (1984) Speech abnormalities in tardive dyskinesia. *Archives of Neurology*, **41**, 273–276.

Gerratt, B.R., Hanson, D.G. and Berke, G.S. (1987) Glottographic measures of laryngeal function in individuals with abnormal motor control, in *Laryngeal Function in Phonation and Respiration* (eds T. Baer, C. Sasaki and K. Harris), College Hill Press, Boston, pp. 521–531.

Goldenberg, J., Ferraz, M.B., Fonseca, A. *et al.* (1992) Sydenham chorea: clinical and laboratory findings. Analysis of 187 cases. *Revista Paulista de Medicina*, **110**, 152–157.

Golper, L., Nutt, J., Rau, M. and Coleman, R. (1983) Focal cranial dystonia. *Journal of Speech and Hearing Disorders*, **48**, 128–134.

Gracco, L.C., Marek, K.L. and Gracco, V.L. (1993) Laryngeal manifestations of early Parkinson's disease: imaging and acoustic data. *Neurology*, **43** (Suppl. 2), A285.

Guttman, M., Kish, S.J., and Furukawa, Y. (2003) Current concepts in the diagnosis and management of Parkinson's disease. *Canadian Medical Association Journal*, **168**, 293–301.

Hammen, V.L., Yorkston, K.M. and Beukelman, D.R. (1989) Pausal and speech duration characteristics as a function of speaking rate in normal and Parkinsonian dysarthric individuals, in *Recent Advances in Clinical Dysarthria* (eds K.M. Yorkston and D.R. Beukelman), College Hill Press, Boston, pp. 213–223.

Hanson, D.G. (1991) Neuromuscular disorders of the larynx. *Otolaryngologic Clinics of North America*, **24**, 1035–1051.

Hanson, D.G., Gerratt, B.R. and Ward, P.H. (1983) Glottographic measurement of vocal dysfunction: a preliminary report. *Annals of Otology, Rhinology and Laryngology*, **92**, 413–420.

Hanson, W.R. and Metter, E.J. (1980) DAF as instrumental treatment for dysarthria in progressive supranuclear palsy: a case report. *Journal of Speech and Hearing Disorders*, **45**, 268–275.

Hartelius, L., Carlstedt, A., Ytterberg, M. *et al.* (2003) Speech disorders in mild and moderate Huntington disease: results of dysarthria assessment of 19 individuals. *Journal of Medical Speech Language Pathology*, **11**, 1–14.

Hedreen, J.C. and Folstein, S.E. (1995) Early loss of neostriatal striosome neurons in Huntington's disease. *Journal of Neuropathology and Experimental Neurology*, **54**, 105–120.

Hirose, H. (1986) Pathophysiology of motor speech disorders (dysarthria). *Folia Phoniatrica et Logopaedica*, **38**, 61–88.

Hirose, H., Kiritani, S. and Sawashima, M. (1982) Patterns of dysarthric movement in patients with amyotrophic lateral sclerosis and pseudobulbar palsy. *Folia Phoniatrica et Logopaedica*, **34**, 106–112.

Hirose, H., Kiritani, S., Ushijima, Y. *et al.* (1981) Patterns of dysarthric movements in patients with Parkinsonism. *Folia Phoniatrica et Logopaedica*, **33**, 204–215.

Hirose, H., Sawashima, M. and Niimi, S. (1985) Laryngeal dynamics in dysarthric speech. Paper presented at the Thirteenth World Congress of Otorhinolaryngology, Miami Beach.

Ho, A.K., Bradshaw, J.L. and Iansek, R. (2000) Volume perception in Parkinsonian speech. *Movement Disorders*, **15**, 1125–1131.

Hoehn, M.M. and Yahr, M.D. (1967) Parkinsonism: onset, progression, and mortality. *Neurology*, **17**, 427–442.

Hoodin, R.B. and Gilbert, H.R. (1989a) Nasal airflows in Parkinsonian speakers. *Journal of Communication Disorders*, **22**, 169–180.

Hoodin, R.B. and Gilbert, H.R. (1989b) Parkinsonian dysarthria: an aerodynamic and perceptual description of velopharyngeal closure for speech. *Folia Phoniatrica et Logopaedica*, **41**, 249–258.

Hovestadt, A., Bogaard, J.D., Meerwaldt, J.D. *et al.* (1989) Pulmonary function in Parkinson's disease. *Journal of Neurology, Neurosurgery and Psychiatry*, **42**, 329–333.

Hunker, C., Abbs, J.H. and Barlow, S. (1982) The relationship between Parkinsonian rigidity and hypokinesia in the orofacial system: a quantitative analysis. *Neurology*, **32**, 755–761.

Jankovic, J. (1988) Cranial-cervical dysarthrias: an overview, in *Advances in Neurology: Facial Dyskinesias*, vol. 49 (eds J. Jankovic and E. Tolosa), Raven Press, New York, pp. 289–306.

Jankovic, J. (1995) Tardive syndromes and other drug-induced movement disorders. *Clinical Neuropharmacology*, **18**, 197–214.

Jankovic, J. (2006a) Huntington's disease, in *Neurological Therapeutics: Principles and Practice*, 2nd edn (ed. J.H. Noseworthy), Informa Healthcare, London, pp. 2869–2881.

Jankovic, J. (2006b) Treatment of dystonia. *Lancet Neurology*, **5**, 864–872.

Jeste, D.V. and Wyatt, R.J. (1982) *Understanding and Treating Tardive Dyskinesia*, Guilford Press, New York.

Johnson, J.A. and Pring, T.R. (1990) Speech therapy in Parkinson's disease: a review and further data. *British Journal of Disorders of Communication*, **25**, 183–194.

Kent, R.D. and Netsell, R. (1978) Articulatory abnormalities in the athetoid cerebral palsy. *Journal of Speech and Hearing Disorders*, **43**, 353–373.

Kent, R.D. and Rosenbek, J.C. (1982) Prosodic disturbance and neurological lesion. *Brain and Language*, **15**, 259–291.

Khan, R., Jampala, V.C., Dong, K. and Vedak, C.S. (1994) Speech abnormalities in tardive dyskinesia. *American Journal of Psychiatry*, **151**, 760–762.

King, J.B., Ramig, L.O., Lemke, J.H. and Harii, Y. (1994) Parkinson's disease: longitudinal changes in acoustic parameters of phonation. *Journal of Medical Speech Language Pathology*, **2**, 29–42.

Kluin, K.J., Gilman, S., Berent, S. and Gilman, S. (1993) Perceptual analysis of speech disorders in progressive supranuclear palsy. *Neurology*, **43**, 563–566.

Kulkarni, M. and Anees, S. (1996) Sydenham's chorea. *Indian Pediatrics*, **33**, 112–115.

Lance, J.W. and Adams, R.D. (1963) The syndrome of intention or action myoclonus as a sequel to anoxic encephalopathy. *Brain*, **87**, 111–133.

Langeveld, T.P.M., Drost, H.A., Frijns, J.H.M. *et al.* (2000) Perceptual characteristics of adductor spasmodic dysphonia. *Annals of Otology, Rhinology and Laryngology*, **109**, 741–748.

LaPointe, L., Case, J. and Duane, D. (1993) Perceptual-acoustic speech and voice characteristics of subjects with spastic torticollis, in *Motor Speech Disorders: Assessment and Treatment* (eds J. Till, K. Yorkston and D. Beukelman), Paul H. Brookes, Baltimore, pp. 40–45.

La Porta, M., Archambault, D., Ross-Chouinard, A. and Chouinard, G. (1990) Articulatory impairment associated with tardive dyskinesia. *Journal of Nervous and Mental Disease*, **178**, 660–662.

Laszewski, Z. (1956) Role of the Department of Rehabilitation in preoperative evaluation of Parkinsonian patients. *Journal of the American Geriatric Society*, **4**, 1280–1284.

Leenders, K.L. (1997) Pathophysiology of movement disorders studied using PET. *Journal of Neural Transmission* (Suppl. 50), 39.

Lethlean, J.B., Chenery, H.J. and Murdoch, B.E. (1990) Disturbed respiratory and prosodic function in Parkinson's disease: a perceptual and instrumental analysis. *Australian Journal of Human Communication Disorders*, **18**, 83–98.

Logemann, J.A. and Fisher, H.B. (1981) Vocal tract control in Parkinson's disease: phonetic feature analysis of misarticulations. *Journal of Speech and Hearing Disorders*, **46**, 348–352.

Logemann, J.A., Fisher, H.B., Boshes, B. and Blonsky, E.R. (1978) Frequency co-occurrence of vocal tract dysfunctions in the speech of a large sample of Parkinson's patients. *Journal of Speech and Hearing Disorders*, **43**, 47–57.

Ludlow, C.L. and Bassich, C.J. (1983) The results of acoustic and perceptual assessment of two types of dysarthria, in *Clinical Dysarthria* (ed. W.R. Berry), College Hill Press, San Diego, pp. 121–147.

Ludlow, C.L. and Bassich, C.J. (1984) Relationship between perceptual ratings and acoustic measures of hypokinetic speech, in *The Dysarthrias: Physiology, Acoustics, Perception, Management* (eds M.R. McNeil, J.C. Rosenbek and A.E. Aronson), College Hill Press, San Diego, pp. 163–195.

Martilla, J.R. and Rinne, U.K. (1991) Progression and survival in Parkinson's disease. *Acta Neurologica Scandinavia*, **84** (Suppl. 136), 24–28.

Martin, J.B. and Gusella, J.F. (1986) Huntington's disease: pathogenesis and management. *New England Journal of Medicine*, **315** (20), 1267–1276.

Matthews, W.B. and Glaser, G.H. (1984) *Recent Advances in Clinical Neurology*, Churchill Livingstone, Edinburgh.

Metter, E.J. and Hanson, W.R. (1986) Clinical and acoustical variability in hypokinetic dysarthria. *Journal of Communication Disorders*, **19**, 347–366.

Miller, W.C. and DeLong, M.R. (1987) Altered tonic activity of neurons in the globus pallidus and subthalamic nucleus in the primate MPTP model of parkinsonism, in *The Basal Ganglia II* (eds M.B. Carpenter and A. Jayaraman), Plenum, New York, p. 415.

Miller, L.G. and Jankovic, J. (1990) Drug-induced dyskinesias, in *Current Neurology*, vol. 10 (ed. S.H. Appel), Mosby-Yearbook, Chicago, pp. 127–136.

Mink, J.W. (2007) Functional organisation of the basal ganglia, in *Parkinson's Disease and Movement Disorders* (eds J. Jankovic and E. Tolosa), Lippincott Williams & Wilkins, Philadelphia, pp. 1–6.

Moore, C.A. and Scudder, R.H. (1989) Co-ordination of jaw muscle activity in Parkinsonian movement: description and response to traditional treatment, in *Recent Advances in Clinical Dysarthria* (eds K.M. Yorkston and D.R. Beukelman), College Hill Press, Boston.

Morris, J.G., Grattan-Smith, P., Jankelowitz, S.K. *et al.* (2002) Athetosis II: the syndrome of mild athetoid cerebral palsy. *Movement Disorders*, **17**, 1281–1287.

Mueller, P.B. (1971) Parkinson's disease: motor speech behaviour in a selected group of patients. *Folia Phoniatrica et Logopaedica*, **23**, 333–346.

Muenter, M.D., Daube, J.R. and Caviness, J.N. (1991) Treatment of essential tremor with methazolamide. *Mayo Clinic Proceedings*, **66** (10), 991–997.

Murdoch, B.E. (1990) *Acquired Speech and Language Disorders: a Neuroanatomical and Functional Neurological Approach*, Chapman & Hall, London.

Murdoch, B.E., Chenery, H.J., Bowler, S. and Ingram, J.C.L. (1989) Respiratory function in Parkinson's subjects exhibiting a perceptible speech deficit: a kinematic and spirometric analysis. *Journal of Speech and Hearing Disorders*, **54**, 610–626.

Murdoch, B.E., Manning, C.Y., Theodoros, D.G. and Thompson, E.C. (1995) Laryngeal function in hypokinetic dysarthria. Paper presented at the *23rd World Congress of the International Association of Logopedics and Phoniatrics*, Cairo, August 6–10.

Nausieda, P., Grossman, B., Koller, W. *et al.* (1980) Sydenham chorea: an update. *Neurology*, **30**, 331–334.

Obeso, J.A., Guridi, J. and DeLong, M.R. (1997) Surgery for Parkinson's disease. *Journal of Neurology, Neurosurgery and Psychiatry*, **62** (1), 2–8.

Platt, L., Andrews, G. and Howie, P. (1980) Dysarthria of adult cerebral palsy II. Phonemic analyses of articulation errors. *Journal of Speech and Hearing Research*, **23**, 41–45.

Ramig, L.A. (1986) Acoustic analyses of phonation in patients with Huntington's disease. *Annals of Otology, Rhinology and Laryngology*, **95**, 288–293.

Ramig, L.A., Scherer, R.C., Titze, I.R. and Ringel, S.P. (1988) Acoustic analysis of voices of patients with neurologic disease: rationale and preliminary data. *Annals of Otology, Rhinology and Laryngology*, **97**, 164–172.

Robbins, J.A., Logemann, J.A. and Kirshner, H.S. (1986) Swallowing and speech production in Parkinson's disease. *Annals of Neurology*, **19**, 283–287.

Sapienza, C.M., Walton, S. and Murry, T. (1999) Acoustic variations in adductor spasmodic dysphonia as a function of speech task. *Journal of Speech, Language and Hearing Research*, **42**, 127–140.

Sapienza, C.M., Walton, S. and Murry, T. (2000) Adductor spasmodic dysphonia and muscle tension dysphonia: acoustic analysis of sustained phonation and reading. *Journal of Voice*, **14**, 502–520.

Schapira, A.H.V. (2005) Present and future drug treatment for Parkinson's disease. *Journal of Neurology, Neurosurgery and Psychiatry*, **76**, 1472–1478.

Schonecker, M. (1957) Ein eigentümliches Syndrome im oralen Bereich bei Megaphenapplikation. *Nervenarzt*, **28**, 35.

Schuurman, P.R., Bosch, D.A. and Bossuyt, P.M. (2000) A comparison of continuous thalamic stimulation and thalamotomy for suppression of severe tremor. *New England Journal of Medicine*, **342** (7), 461–468.

Scott, S., Caird, F.I. and Williams, G.O. (1985) *Communication in Parkinson's Disease*, Croom Helm, London.

Serra-Mestres, J., Robertson, M.M. and Shetty, T. (1998) Palicoprolalia: an unusual variant of palilalia in Gilles de la Tourette's syndrome. *Journal of Neuropsychiatry and Clinical Neuroscience*, **10**, 117–118.

Simon, R., Arminoff, M. and Greenberg, D. (1999) *Clinical Neurology*, 4th edn, Appleton and Lange, Stamford.

Solomon, N.P. and Hixon, T.J. (1993) Speech breathing in Parkinson's disease. *Journal of Speech and Hearing Research*, **36**, 294–310.

Starr, P.A., Rau, S. and Davis, V. (2005) Spontaneous neuronal activity in human dystonia: comparison with Parkinson's disease and normal macaque. *Journal of Neurophysiology*, **93**, 3165–3176.

Steele, J.C., Richardson, J.C. and Olszewski, J. (1964) Progressive supra-nuclear palsy. *Archives of Neurology*, **10**, 333.

Strick, P.L., Dunn, R.P. and Picard, N. (1995) Macro-organization of the circuits connecting the basal ganglia with the cortical motor areas, in *Models of Information Processing in the Basal Ganglia* (eds J.C. Houk, J.L. Davis and D.G. Beiser), MIT Press, Cambridge, MA, pp. 117–130.

Svensson, P., Henningson, C. and Karlsson, S. (1993) Speech motor control in Parkinson's disease: a comparison between a clinical assessment protocol and a quantitative analysis of mandibular movements. *Folio Phoniatrica et Logopaaedica*, **45**, 157–164.

Swedo, S., Leonard, H., Schapiro, M. *et al.* (1993) Sydenham's chorea: physical and psychological symptoms of St Vitus dance. *Pediatrics*, **91**, 706–713.

Theodoros, D.G., Murdoch, B.E. and Thompson, E.C. (1995) Hypernasality in Parkinson's disease: a perceptual and physiological analysis. *Journal of Medical Speech Language Pathology*, **3**, 73–84.

Uitti, R.J. and Calne, D.B. (1993) Pathogenesis of idiopathic Parkinsonism. *European Neurology*, **33** (Suppl. 1), 6–23.

Valls-Sole, J. (2007) Neurophysiology of motor control and movement disorders, in *Parkinson's Disease and Movement Disorders* (eds J. Jankovic and

E. Tolosa), Lippincott Williams & Wilkins, Philadelphia, pp. 7–22.

Vernon, G.M. (1991) Drug-induced and tardive movement disorders. *Journal of Neuroscience Nursing*, **23**, 183–187.

Wasielewski, P.G., Burns, J.M. and Koller, W.C. (1998) Pharmacologic treatment of tremor. *Movement Disorders*, **13** (Suppl. 3), 90–100.

Weiner, W.J., Goetz, C.G., Nausieda, P. and Klawans, H.L. (1978) Respiratory dyskinesias: extrapyramidal dysfunction and dyspnea. *Annals of Internal Medicine*, **88**, 327–331.

Weismer, G. (1984) Acoustic descriptions of dysarthric speech: perceptual correlates and physiological inferences. *Seminars in Speech and Language*, **5**, 293–313.

Wichmann, T. and DeLong, M.R. (1998) Models of basal ganglia function and pathophysiology of movement disorders. *Neurosurgery Clinics of North America*, **9** (2), 223–236.

Wilcox, P.G., Bassett, A., Jones, B. and Fleetham, J.A. (1994) Respiratory dysrhythmias in patients with tardive dyskinesia. *Chest*, **105**, 203–207.

Wilson, S.K.A. (1912) Progressive lenticular degeneration: familial nervous disease associated with cirrhosis of the liver. *Brain*, **34**, 295.

Yoshida, K., Kaji, R., Shibasaki, H. and Iizuka, T. (2002) Factors influencing the therapeutic effect of muscle afferent block for oromandibular dystonia and dyskinesia and implications for their distinct pathophysiology. *International Journal of Oral and Maxillofacial Surgery*, **31**, 499–505.

Yoshida, K. and Iizuki, T. (2003) Jaw deviation dystonia evaluated by movement-related cortical potentials and treated with muscle afferent block. *Cranio – The Journal of Craniomandibular Practice*, **21**, 295–300.

Zraick, R., LaPointe, L., Case, J. and Duane, D. (1993) Acoustic correlates of vocal quality in spasmodic torticollis. *Journal of Medical Speech Language Pathology*, **1**, 261–269.

Zwirner, P. and Barnes, G.J. (1992) Vocal tract steadiness: a measure of phonatory and upper airway motor control during phonation in dysarthria. *Journal of Speech and Hearing Research*, **35**, 761–768.

Zwirner, P., Murry, T. and Woodson, G. (1991) Phonatory function of neurologically impaired patients. *Journal of Communication Disorders*, **24**, 287–300.

Dysarthrias associated with lesions in other motor systems

11

Ataxic dysarthria

The cerebellum is responsible for the coordination of muscular activity throughout the body. Although it does not itself initiate any muscle contractions, the cerebellum monitors those areas of the brain that do in order to coordinate the action of muscle groups and time their contractions so that movements involving the skeletal muscles are performed smoothly and accurately. Damage to the cerebellum or its connections leads to a condition called 'ataxia' in which movements become uncoordinated. Although even simple movements are affected by cerebellar damage, the movements most disrupted by cerebellar disorders are the more complex, multicomponent sequential movements, such as those involved in speech production. Following damage to the cerebellum, complex movements tend to be broken down or decomposed into their individual sequential components, each of which may be executed with errors of force, amplitude and timing, leading to uncoordinated movements. If the ataxia affects the muscles of the speech mechanism, the production of speech may become abnormal, leading to a cluster of deviant speech dimensions collectively referred to as 'ataxic dysarthria'.

To understand why the disturbed speech features characteristic of ataxic dysarthria following damage to the cerebellum occur, a knowledge of the basic neuroanatomy and functional neurology of the cerebellum is essential.

Neuroanatomy of the cerebellum

Gross anatomy of the cerebellum

Located posterior to the brainstem, the cerebellum occupies most of the posterior cranial fossa and is separated from the occipital and temporal lobes of the cerebrum by the tentorium cerebelli.

The cerebellum comprises two large cerebellar hemispheres which are connected by a mid-portion called the vermis (worm-like) (Figure 11.1). The cerebellar surface or cerebellar cortex consists of complexly folded ridges of grey matter, while the central core of the cerebellum consists of white matter in which are located several nuclear grey masses called the deep (cerebellar) nuclei.

A series of deep and distinct fissures divide the cerebellum into a number of lobes. Although different authors have classified the cerebellar lobes in different ways, most neurologists recognize

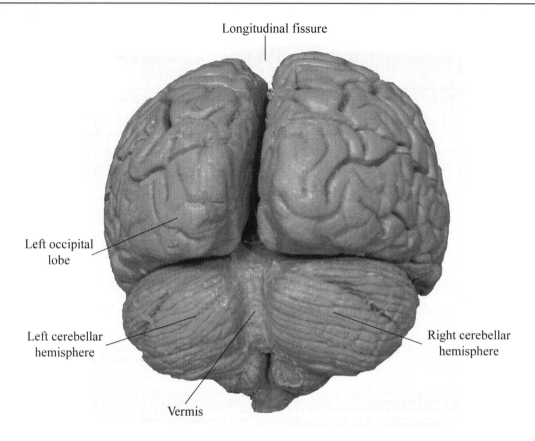

Longitudinal fissure

Left occipital lobe

Left cerebellar hemisphere

Right cerebellar hemisphere

Vermis

Figure 11.1 Posterior view of the brain showing the two cerebellar hemispheres located below the occipital lobes.

three different cerebellar lobes: the anterior lobe, the posterior lobe and the flocculonodular lobe (which includes the paired flocculi and the nodulus) (Figures 11.2 and 11.3). The anterior lobe, which can be seen from a superior view of the cerebellum, is that portion of the cerebellum that lies anterior to the primary fissure. It roughly corresponds to that part of the cerebellum called the paleocerebellum. The anterior lobe has a significant role in the regulation of muscle tone and receives its primary input from proprioceptors and exteroceptors in the head and body, including some from the vestibular system.

The largest portion of the cerebellum is the posterior lobe, also referred to as the neocerebellum. It is located between the other two lobes and is phylogenetically the newest portion of the cerebellum, being best developed in those animals, such as primates, that have a well-developed cerebral cortex. It functions in close association

with the cerebral cortex and is most concerned with the regulation of voluntary movements. In particular, it plays an essential role in the coordination of phasic movements and is the most important part of the cerebellum for the coordination of speech movements. The flocculonodular lobe comprises the nodulus and the paired flocculi and occupies the inferior rostal region of the cerebellum. The nodulus represents the rostral portion of the inferior vermis, while the flocculi are two small, irregular-shaped appendages attached to the inferior region of the cerebellum. Phylogenetically the flocculonodular lobe represents the oldest portion of the cerebellum and is also known as the archicerebellum. It functions in close association with the vestibular system and is therefore important in maintaining equilibrium and keeping the individual oriented in space.

The cerebellum is made up of both grey and white matter. As in the cerebral hemispheres,

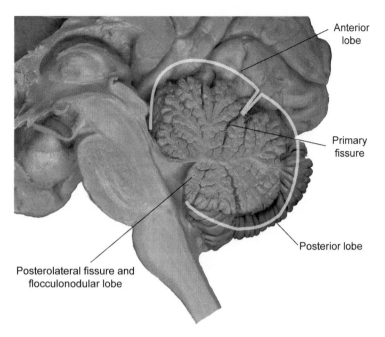

Figure 11.2 Mid-sagittal section through the brainstem and cerebellum showing the three cerebellar lobes.

most of the grey matter is found covering the surface of the cerebellum as cortex. The cerebellar cortex is highly folded into thin transverse folds, or folia. As a consequence of this extensive folding, in the region of 85% of the cerebellar cortex is concealed and its surface area is much larger than might be expected (about three-quarters of that of the cerebrum). Unlike the cerebral cortex, the cerebellar cortex is uniform throughout its structure.

The cerebellar, or deep nuclei

The central core of the cerebellum is made up of white matter in which are embedded four grey masses on either side of the midline. These grey masses are referred to as the cerebellar, or deep, nuclei (Figure 11.4). The largest and most medially placed of these nuclei is the dentate nucleus. Medial to the dentate nucleus are two smaller nuclei, the globose and emboliform nuclei (taken together called the interpositus), and most medial of all the deep nuclei is the fastigial nucleus. Most of the Purkinje cell axons, which carry impulses away from the cerebellar cortex, terminate in these nuclei. Some fibres from the cortex of the

flocculonodular lobe, however, bypass the deep nuclei and proceed to the brainstem.

The cerebellar peduncles

The cerebellum is attached to the brainstem on either side by three structures called the cerebellar peduncles (Figure 11.5). These peduncles consist of bundles of nerve fibres which convey impulses either to or from the cerebellum.

The largest of the cerebellar peduncles is the middle peduncle, or brachium pontis, which passes between the cerebellum and the pons. It is formed by the transverse fibres of the pons, which arise from the pontine nuclei. These fibres cross the midline to pass through the middle peduncle on the side opposite to their nucleus of origin to reach the cortex of the neocerebellum of the contralateral cerebellar hemisphere. The middle peduncle comprises afferent fibres belonging to the cortico-pontine-cerebellar pathway, which conveys information from the frontal and temporal lobes of the cerebrum to the cerebellum via the pons.

Fibres running between the medulla oblongata and the cerebellum comprise the inferior

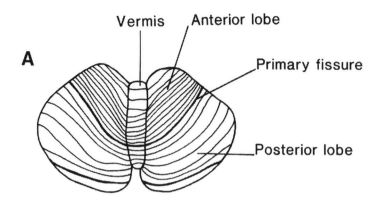

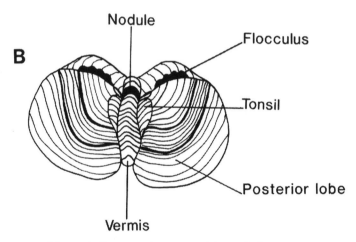

Figure 11.3   (A) Superior view of the cerebellum. (B) Inferior view of the cerebellum.

cerebellar peduncle, or restiform body. This peduncle is made up largely of afferent fibres, which pass to the cerebellum and include the posterior spinocerebellar tracts, the cuneocerebellar tracts, the olivocerebellar tract, the reticulocerebellar tract and vestibulocerebellar tract.

The superior cerebellar peduncle, or brachium conjunctivum, is connected to the midbrain at it junction with the pons. It carries most of the fibres that leave the cerebellum. These fibres originate in the dentate, globose and emboliform nuclei and pass to structures such as the contralateral red nucleus and the ventrolateral nucleus of the thalamus. Although the majority of the superior peduncle comprises efferent fibres, a small portion of it carries afferent fibres which include the

anterior spinocerebellar tract, the rubrocerebellar tract and the tectocerebellar tract.

Afferent and efferent connections

In order to coordinate muscular contractions, the cerebellum is linked to a large number of other parts of the nervous system by an extensive system of afferent and efferent fibres. Damage to these pathways can cause cerebellar dysfunction and possibly ataxic dysarthria, the same as damage to the cerebellum itself. All the afferent fibres to the cerebellum (i.e. those fibres conveying impulses to the cerebellum) terminate in the cerebellar cortex, giving off collateral fibres to the cerebellar nuclei on their way. The principal

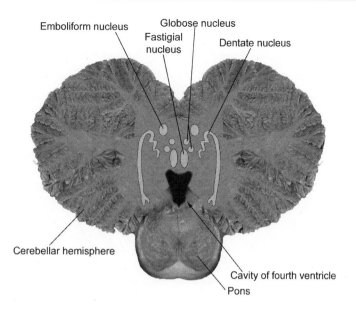

Figure 11.4 Location of the intracerebellar (deep) nuclei.

afferent projections to the cerebellum are listed in Table 11.1.

The afferent fibres originate from three major sources: the cerebrum and brainstem, the vestibular nuclei and the spinal cord. All of the afferent pathways arising from the cerebrum and many of those originating in the spinal cord undergo synaptic interruption in the brainstem, so that secondary fibres are relayed to the cerebellum from brainstem centres, which receive primary descending fibres from the cerebral cortex and ascending fibres from the spinal cord. The ma-

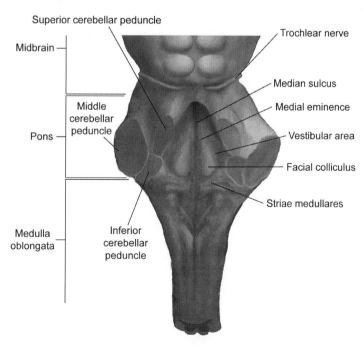

Figure 11.5 Posterior surface of the brainstem showing the cerebellar peduncles. (Note: the cerebellum has been removed.)

Table 11.1 Principal afferent projections to the cerebellum.

Origin in central nervous system	Pathway	Specific site of origin	Peduncle	Termination in cerebellum
Cerebral cortex	Cerebro-pontine-cerebellar	Primarily the motor cortex of the frontal lobe. Secondary fibres project from the pontine nuclei	Middle	Posterior lobe
Brainstem	Olivocerebellar	Inferior olivary nuclear complex	Inferior	All lobes and deep nuclei
	Rubrocerebellar	Red nucleus in midbrain	Superior	Posterior lobe and deep nuclei
	Reticulocerebellar	Reticular formation in brainstem	Inferior and middle	All lobes and deep nuclei
	Tectocerebellar	Midbrain quadrigeminal bodies	Superior	Anterior and posterior lobe
	Cuneocerebellar	Cuneate nuclei	Inferior	Primarily anterior lobe
	Vestibulocerebellar	Vestibular nuclei	Inferior	Flocculonodular lobe
	Trigeminocerebellar	Trigeminal nucleus	Superior	Anterior lobe
Spinal cord	Spinocerebellar	Various peripheral receptors such as muscle spindles and Golgi tendon organs	Inferior and superior	Anterior lobe

jor afferent pathway originating from the cerebral cortex is the cortico-ponto-cerebellar pathway (Figure 11.6). Although virtually all areas of the cerebral cortex contribute fibres to this pathway, it originates primarily in the motor cortex and projects to the ipsilateral pontine nuclei. From here, secondary fibres project primarily to the cortex of the neocerebellum in the contralateral cerebellar hemisphere. It is via the cortico-ponto-cerebellar tract that the cerebellum receives information regarding volitional movements that are in progress or are about to take place.

Afferent pathways to the cerebellum, which also project from the brainstem, arise in structures such as the olive (olivocerebellar tract), the red nucleus (rubrocerebellar tract), the reticular formation (reticulocerebellar tract), the midbrain (tectocerebellar tract) and the cuneate nucleus (cuneocerebellar tract). The inferior olivary nucleus in the medulla oblongata receives major input from the cerebral cortex, caudate nucleus, globus pallidus, red nucleus, brainstem reticular formation and spinal cord and projects mainly crossed fibres to the neocerebellum. The cuneate

nuclei receive input from the spinal cord and project to the ipsilateral paleo- and neocerebellum. Fibres from the vestibular nuclei project ipsilaterally to the flocculonodular lobe.

Cutaneous and proprioceptive information from the entire body also reaches the cerebellum. That from the face reaches the cerebellum either directly or via the trigeminal nucleus (trigeminocerebellar tract), while that from the remainder of the body is carried in the spinocerebellar tracts to the anterior lobe of the cerebellum (Figure 11.7). The signals transmitted in these tracts originate in various receptors such as muscle spindles, Golgi tendon organs, joint receptors and skin receptors. They inform the cerebellum of the momentary status of muscle contraction, the degree of tension on the muscle tendons, the positions of parts of the body and the forces acting on the surfaces of the body.

All of the efferent tracts from the cerebellum arise in the deep nuclei. None arises directly from the cerebellar cortex, which transmits its output signals only through the deep nuclei. Efferent signals are transmitted to many portions of the

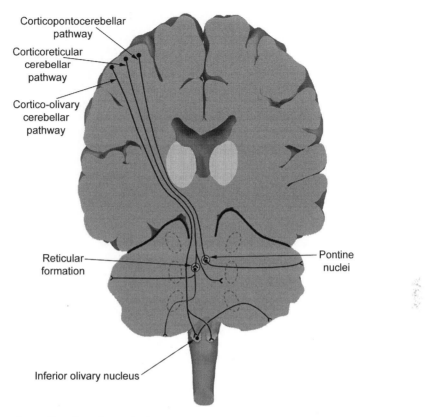

Corticopontocerebellar pathway

Corticoreticular cerebellar pathway

Cortico-olivary cerebellar pathway

Reticular formation

Pontine nuclei

Inferior olivary nucleus

Figure 11.6 Cerebellar afferent fibres from the cerebral cortex.

central nervous system, including the motor cortex via the thalamus, the basal ganglia, the red nucleus, the reticular formation of the brainstem and the vestibular nuclei. The principal cerebellar efferent fibres are summarized in Table 11.2.

A diagrammatic representation of the cerebellar efferent fibres is shown in Figure 11.8.

Most fibres from the dentate nucleus project to the thalamus with some fibres also passing to the red nucleus, the olive and the reticular formation. The globose and emboliform nuclei project mainly to the red nucleus, the olive and brainstem reticular formation. The major projection of the fastigial nucleus is to the vestibular nuclei and, to a lesser extent, to the reticular formation.

Efferent fibres from the dentate nuclei and interpositus nuclei project to the contralateral ventrolateral (and ventroanterior nucleus) of the thalamus. These thalamic nuclei, in turn, project fibres to the motor areas of the frontal lobe. By way of this pathway, the cerebellum can influ-

ence the functioning of the motor cortex. Important fibres passing from the interpositus nuclei and dentate nucleus also project to the contralateral red nucleus, where they influence the activity of the rubrospinal tract. In the midbrain, the rubrospinal tract decussates to the opposite side and passes through the brainstem to the lateral funiculus of the spinal cord. Each cerebellar hemisphere is thus linked principally with the same side of the body by means of a double decussation in the midbrain. Other fibres from the red nucleus project to the thalamus and thus may connect the cerebellum to the basal ganglia and cerebral cortex. The fastigial nucleus sends fibres to the vestibular nuclei in the brainstem to modify the activity of the vestibulospinal tracts and thereby influence muscle tone important for maintaining body posture and equilibrium. Projections from the cerebellar nuclei also travel to the reticular formation, where they enable cerebellar modification of the activity of the reticulospinal tracts.

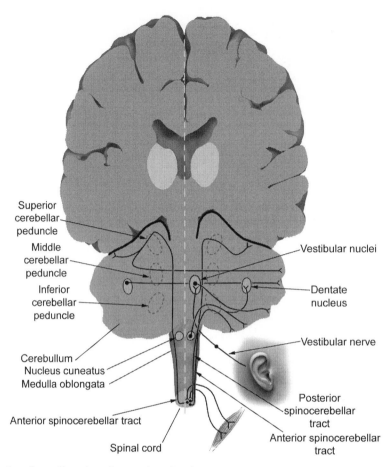

Figure 11.7 Cerebellar afferent fibres from the spinal cord and inner ear.

Table 11.2 Principal efferent projections from the cerebellum.

Pathway	Deep nuclei of origin	Destination	Peduncle
Cerebellothalamic	Dentate nucleus and interpositus nucleus	Contralateral thalamus (ventrolateral and ventroanterior nuclei). Secondary fibres project from here to the motor cortex of the frontal lobe	Superior and inferior
Cerebellorubral	Interpositus nucleus and dentate nucleus	Contralateral red nucleus	Superior
Cerebelloreticular	Fastigial nucleus, dentate nucleus and interpositus nucleus	Ipsilateral and contralateral reticular nuclei	Superior and inferior
Cerebellovestibular	Fastigial nucleus	Ipsilateral and contralateral vestibular nuclei	Inferior

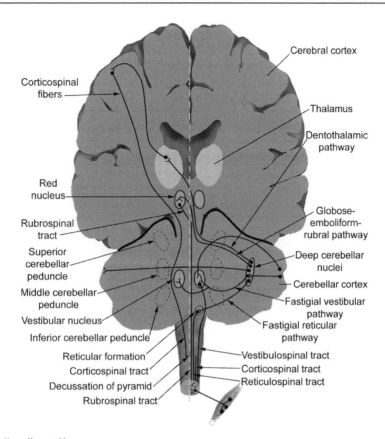

Figure 11.8 Cerebellar efferent fibres.

Overall, the extensive afferent and efferent connections of the cerebellum form a feedback loop by which the cerebellum can both monitor and modify motor activities taking place in various parts of the body to produce a smooth, coordinated motor action. Through its afferent supply, the cerebellum receives input from a number of different regions of the nervous system regarding motor activities either already in progress or about to occur. Further, by means of its efferent connections, the cerebellum is able to modify motor actions initiated elsewhere in the central nervous system.

Function of the cerebellum in voluntary motor activities

The cerebellum does not, itself, initiate any muscular activities. Rather, it functions only to coordinate those motor activities initiated elsewhere in the central nervous system. Voluntary move-ments can take place in its absence, but such movements are clumsy and disorganized. Although the role of the cerebellum in motor activities is not known with certainty, a variety of functions have been proposed by different authors. Some researchers have suggested that the function of the cerebellum is to exercise revisory control over the motor commands issued by the motor cortex (Ito, 1970; Eccles, 1973). Figure 11.9 illustrates the basic cerebellar pathways that may be utilized by the cerebellum to coordinate voluntary movements.

Briefly, it is proposed that, when motor impulses are transmitted from the motor cortex to the lower motor neurones via the pyramidal and extrapyramidal pathways (see Chapter 9), collateral impulses are also transmitted simultaneously to the cerebellum primarily via the pontocerebellar tract and, to a lesser extent, by way of the olivocerebellar tract. Consequently, for every voluntary motor movement performed, not only do

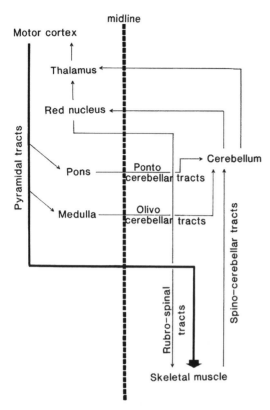

Figure 11.9 Pathways for cerebellar control of voluntary movements.

here via the superior peduncle to the ventrolateral nucleus of the thalamus. The thalamus in turn relays the cerebellar output back to the motor cortex where the stimulus first originated to modify the activity of the corticospinal and corticobulbar tracts. Thus, it can be readily recognized that the circuit described represents a complicated feedback loop beginning in the motor cortex and returning to the motor cortex. Eccles (1973) suggested that the commands from the motor cortex are imprecise and provisional, requiring for their refinement the continuous action of the cerebellar feedback loop. In this way, the motor cortex may depend on the cerebellum and its connections to modify its grossly formed neural instructions to the muscles.

The cerebellum acts as a servo-mechanism to damp muscle movements and stop them at their point of intention. It appears to compare the intentions of the motor cortex with the actual performances by the various muscles, and if the body parts are not moving in accordance with the intentions of the motor cortex, the 'error' between these two is calculated by the cerebellum so that appropriate and immediate corrections can be made. Ordinarily, the motor cortex transmits a greater volley of impulses than needed to perform each intended movement. Consequently, the cerebellum must act to inhibit the motor cortex at the appropriate time after the muscle has begun to move. The rate of movement is automatically assessed by the cerebellum and the length of time required for the body part to reach the point of intention is calculated. Appropriate inhibitory impulses are then transmitted by the cerebellum to the motor cortex to inhibit the agonist muscle (the muscle responsible for producing the movement) and to excite the antagonist muscle (the muscle that opposes or has the opposite action to the agonist muscle). In this way, the cerebellum is able to apply a 'braking', or damping, mechanism to stop the movement at the precise point of intention. If the cerebellum is damaged, the damping action is impaired and overshooting of the point of intention occurs. The conscious centres at the cerebrum recognize that this overshooting has occurred and initiate movement in the opposite direction. However, overshooting may then occur in the opposite direction and thus the body part

the muscles receive activating signals but also the cerebellum receives the same signals at the same time.

Once the muscles respond to the motor impulses by contracting, various proprioceptive receptors, such as muscle spindles, Golgi tendon organs and joint receptors, transmit information back to the cerebellum by way of the spinocerebellar and trigeminocerebellar tracts. It has been suggested that one function of the cerebellum may be to regulate the sensitivity of the muscle spindles so that optimum feedback regarding the state of muscle contraction can be supplied to the higher centres as a movement is performed (Gilman, 1969). The cerebellum interprets the afferent proprioceptive information and integrates it with the information received from the motor cortex (Konorski, 1967). Subsequently, impulses are transmitted from the cerebellar cortex, where the integration takes place, to the deep nuclei, particularly the dentate nucleus, and from involved in the movement may oscillate back and forth past the intended point for several cycles. This effect is called 'intention tremor'.

In addition to being able to initiate damping actions, the cerebellum is also able to predict the future positions of moving parts of the body. Cerebellar damage leads to a disturbance in this ability, and consequently the patient may be unable to gauge the distance and speed of body movements, an inability referred to as 'dysmetria'. Dysmetria, in combination with the inability to apply appropriate damping mechanisms, leads to the decomposition of body movements in patients with cerebellar disorders, especially those movements that require the coordinated action of a number of individual muscles. In complex motor acts, contraction of the individual muscles must be timed in such a way that one movement leads to the next in a smooth and orderly fashion. When the cerebellum becomes dysfunctional, the patient is unable to correctly time the beginning of the individual sequential movements that comprise the overall motor act. As a result, sequential movements may begin too early or too late and the overall movement pattern breaks down. Speech is an extremely complex motor act, requiring the coordinated contraction of a large number of individual muscles. It is not surprising, therefore, that speech production may be seriously affected in patients with disorders affecting the cerebellum or its connections.

Involuntary or postural movements controlled by the extrapyramidal system are also modified by the cerebellum in a similar manner to voluntary movements. Even reflex actions mediated through the spinal cord or brainstem are affected by the cerebellum. The major difference in the cerebellum's role in coordinating involuntary, as opposed to voluntary, motor activities is that different pathways are used. Motor impulses that originate in the basal ganglia and reticular formation and pass to the lower motor neurones via the extrapyramidal system are conveyed to the cerebellum via the olivocerebellar tract. Corrective signals from the cerebellum are passed to the muscles via the major descending pathways of the extrapyramidal system, namely the reticulospinal, rubrospinal and vestibulospinal tracts (see Chapter 9) rather than via the corticospinal

and corticobulbar pathway, as in the case of voluntary movements.

Clinical signs of damage to the cerebellum

Disorders of the cerebellum and/or the fibres leading to and from the cerebellum are accompanied by a number of characteristic signs which include disorders of movement, posture and muscle tone. Clinical signs usually appear on the same side of the body as the cerebellar lesion. Different symptoms result from cerebellar damage depending on the part of the cerebellum involved. Broadly, cerebellar disorders can be divided into those that affect the vestibulocerebellum (flocculonodular lobe) and those affecting the main mass of the cerebellum (the corpus cerebelli, which includes both the anterior and posterior lobes). Obviously, in many disorders both the corpus cerebelli and the flocculonodular lobe are involved.

Isolated damage to the flocculonodular lobe is most commonly associated with the presence of a tumour, usually a medulloblastoma and is associated with a disturbance in equilibrium called 'archicerebellar syndrome'. Patients are unsteady and have a tendency to fall backwards, forwards or to one side when standing on a narrow base with their eyes open. Some patients, in fact, are unable to maintain an upright position. Their gait is staggering and they tend to walk on a wide base. Other signs may also be present if the tumour later invades other parts of the cerebellum.

Damage to the corpus cerebelli or its connections is associated with a group of symptoms commonly collectively called 'neocerebellar syndrome', although the paleocerebellum is also usually involved. Destruction of small portions of the corpus cerebelli causes no detectable abnormality in motor function. It appears that the remaining areas of the cerebellum can compensate for the damaged part. More severe and enduring dysfunction of the cerebellum, however, occurs if either the deep nuclei or superior cerebellar peduncle are involved. When the lesion involves the cerebellum unilaterally, as is usually the case, the motor disturbance occurs on the same side as the lesion.

Box 11.1 Clinical Signs of Neocerebellar Syndrome

- Ataxia
- Dysmetria
- Decomposition of movement
- Dysdiadochokinesia
- Hypotonia
- Asthenia
- Tremor
- Rebound phenomenon
- Disturbance of posture and gait
- Nystagmus
- Dysarthria

The characteristic signs of neocerebellar syndrome are listed in Box 11.1.

As indicated above, complex movements, such as those required for speech production or the movement of an entire limb to a new position, depend on the proper sequencing of composite simple movements (composition). Further, they are also dependent on the contraction of synergistic muscles to provide postural fixation of certain joints to allow for the precise movement of other joints (synergia: cooperative action of muscles). Cerebellar dysfunction causes errors in both of these parameters, leading to slowing, dysmetria, dyssynergia and decomposition of movement. In the case of alternating movements, dysdiadochokinesia also results. The resulting uncoordinated, clumsy and disorganized muscular activity is termed 'ataxia'. Ataxia is the principal sign of cerebellar dysfunction.

The presence of dysmetria is evidenced by the patient's inability to stop a movement at the desired point. For example, when reaching for an object, the patient's hand may either overshoot the intended point or stop short of the intended point. Dyssynergia is reflected in the separation of a series of voluntary movements that normally flow smoothly and in sequence into a succession of mechanical or puppet-like movements (decomposition of movement). It may also be manifest as movement abnormalities, such as the delayed starting and stopping of movements. 'Dysdiadochokinesia' refers to an inability to perform rapid

alternating movements, such as rapidly moving the tongue from one side of the mouth to the other and back several times. To be performed rapidly such movements require considerable coordination by the cerebellum and are, therefore, severely disturbed in patients with cerebellar disorders.

A decrease in muscle tone (hypotonia) is also usually evident in cerebellar disorders (as can be ascertained by palpation of the muscles), and muscles affected by cerebellar lesions tend to be weaker and tire more easily than normal muscles (asthenia). The reduction in muscle tone may result from reduced muscle spindle sensitivity possibly because of an inadequate alpha motor neurone discharge as a result of the cerebellar damage. Tremor is another feature of cerebellar disease. It usually takes the form of an intention tremor and is seen during movement but is absent at rest. Disturbances of posture and gait may be very pronounced, the patient possibly being unable to maintain an upright posture and walking in a staggering fashion with a broad base of support.

The presence of rebound phenomenon can be demonstrated by asking patients to flex their elbow against resistance offered by the observer when their hand is only a small distance from their face and then suddenly releasing the forearm. Normally the movement of the forearm in the direction of flexion (i.e. towards the face) is quickly arrested by contraction of the extensor muscle (triceps). Cerebellar damage, however, delays this contraction with the result that patients may strike themselves in the face. Nystagmus may also be present, especially if the lesion encroaches upon the vermis.

Finally, as a result of dyssynergia and decomposition of the movement of the muscles of the speech mechanism during speech production, ataxic dysarthria may be present in association with some cerebellar lesions. The characteristics of ataxic dysarthria are discussed in detail below.

Diseases of the cerebellum associated with ataxic dysarthria

The cerebellum can be affected by a variety of different pathological conditions (Table 11.3), all

Table 11.3 Diseases of the cerebellum associated with ataxic dysarthria.

Diseases	Example	General features
Congenital anomalies	Cerebellar agenesis	Partial to almost total non-development of the cerebellum. May in some cases not be associated with any clinical evidence of cerebellar dysfunction. In other cases, however, a gait disturbance may be evident in addition to limb ataxia (especially involving the lower limbs) and dysarthria
Chromosomal disorders	Trisomy	Diffuse hypotrophy (underdevelopment) of the cerebellum may be present, which may be associated with either no clinical symptoms of cerebellar dysfunction through to marked limb ataxia
Trauma	Penetrating head wounds (e.g. bullet wounds)	May be associated with either mild slowly developing cerebellar dysfunction or rapid, severe cerebellar dysfunction
Vascular disease	Occlusion of anterior inferior cerebellar artery	Hypotonia and ipsilateral limb ataxia
	Occlusion of posterior inferior cerebellar artery	Dysarthria, nystagmus, ipsilateral limb ataxia and disordered gait and station
	Occlusion of superior cerebellar artery	Disordered gait and station. Ipsilateral hypotonia, ipsilateral limb ataxia and intention tremor. Occasionally dysarthria
Infections	Cerebellar abscess	Most frequently caused by purulent bacteria but can also occur with fungi. Cerebellar abscesses most frequently arise by direct extension from adjacent infected areas such as the mastoid process or from otologic disease
Tumours	Medulloblastomas, astrocytomas and ependymomas	Primary tumours of the cerebellum occur more frequently in children than adults. Medulloblastomas occur most commonly in the midline of the cerebellum in children and usually have a rapid course with a poor prognosis. Astrocytomas are more benign than medulloblastomas and generally occur in children of an older age group than medulloblastomas. Ependymomas are relatively slow growing and again are more common in children than adults
Toxic metabolic and endocrine disorders	Exogenous toxins, for example industrial solvents, carbon tetrachloride, heavy metals and so on.	Signs of cerebellar involvement usually associated with symptoms of diffuse involvement of the central nervous system following these intoxications rather than appearing in isolation to other neurological deficits
	Enzyme deficiencies, for example pyruvate dehydrogenase deficiency	Ataxia most marked in the lower limbs
	Hypothyroidism	Cretins show poor development of the cerebellum. Ataxia present in 20–30% of myxoedema cases
Hereditary ataxias	Friedreich's ataxia	The most commonly encountered spinal form of hereditary ataxia. Pathological degeneration primarily involves the spinal cord with degeneration of neurones occurring in the spinocerebellar tracts. Some degeneration of neurones in the dentate nucleus and brachium conjunctivum may also occur. The first clinical sign of the disease is usually clumsiness of gait. Later limb ataxia (especially involving the lower extremities) also occurs. A large percentage of cases also exhibit dysarthria and nystagmus and cognitive deficits may also be present
Demyelinating disorders	Multiple sclerosis	Usually associated with demyelination in a number of regions of the central nervous system including the cerebellum. Consequently, the dysarthria, if present, usually takes the form of a mixed dysarthria rather than purely an ataxic dysarthria. Paroxysmal ataxic dysarthria may occur as an early sign of multiple sclerosis

of which may be associated with the occurrence of ataxic dysarthria.

In general the signs and symptoms of cerebellar dysfunction are the same, regardless of aetiology, with the exception that in those disorders in which the lesion is slowly progressive (e.g. tumour cases), symptoms of cerebellar deficiency are much less severe than where the lesion develops acutely (e.g. cerebrovascular accidents and head trauma). Further, considerable recovery from the effects of an acute lesion can usually be expected.

Clinical characteristics of ataxic dysarthria

Ataxic dysarthria results from damage to the cerebellum and/or its connections. Although it may occur in association with severe, acute cerebellar lesions, being most evident in the early stages of such disorders and then slowly subsiding, ataxic dysarthria most frequently occurs as a late sign of more slowly developing bilateral or generalized cerebellar damage. If ataxic dysarthria is a prominent and early sign of cerebellar damage, it has been suggested that this indicates that the lesion involves the mid-portion of the vermis, as this region is believed by some researchers to be the primary locus for the coordination of motor speech (Lothman and Ferrendelli, 1980).

The disrupted speech output exhibited by individuals with cerebellar lesions has often been termed 'scanning speech', a term probably first used by Charcot (1877). According to Charcot (1877), 'the words are as if measured or scanned: there is a pause after every syllable, and the syllables themselves are pronounced slowly' (p. 192). The most predominant features of ataxic dysarthria include a breakdown in the articulatory and prosodic aspects of speech. According to Brown, Darley and Aronson (1970), the 10 deviant speech dimensions most characteristic of ataxic dysarthria can be divided into three clusters: articulatory inaccuracy, characterized by imprecision of consonant production, irregular articulatory breakdowns and distorted vowels; prosodic excess, characterized by excess and equal stress, prolonged phonemes, prolonged

intervals and slow rate; and phonatory-prosodic insufficiency, characterized by harshness, monopitch and monoloudness. Brown, Darley and Aronson (1970) believed that the articulatory problems were the product of ataxia of the respiratory and lingual-facial-buccal musculature, and prosodic excess was thought by these authors to result from slow movements. The occurrence of phonatory-prosodic insufficiencies was attributed to the presence of hypotonia.

Respiratory function in ataxic dysarthria

Perceptual correlates of respiratory inadequacy have been noted in a number of perceptual studies of ataxic dysarthria (Kluin *et al.*, 1988; Chenery, Ingram and Murdoch, 1991). In a study of 16 subjects with ataxic dysarthria, Chenery, Ingram and Murdoch (1991) reported the presence of significantly reduced ratings of respiratory support for speech as well as a respiratory pattern characterized by sudden forced inspiratory and expiratory sighs. Kluin *et al.* (1988) documented subjective reports of audible inspiration in ataxic dysarthric speakers investigated in their laboratory.

Evidence is also available from physiological studies to suggest that speech breathing is disturbed in ataxic dysarthria. Murdoch *et al.* (1991) employed both spirometric and kinematic techniques to investigate the respiratory function of a group of 12 subjects with ataxic dysarthria associated with cerebellar disease. Their results showed that almost one-half of the ataxic cases had vital capacities below the normal limits of variation. In addition, the ataxic dysarthric speakers also demonstrated unusual patterns of chest wall two-part contribution to lung volume change, including the presence of abdominal and ribcage paradoxing, abrupt changes in movements of the ribcage and abdomen and a tendency to initiate utterances at lower than normal lung volume levels. Murdoch *et al.* suggested that these findings were an outcome of impaired coordination of the chest wall and speculated that such respiratory anomalies had the potential to underlie some of the prosodic abnormalities observed in ataxic dysarthria.

Laryngeal function in ataxic dysarthria

Phonatory disturbances are frequently listed among the most deviant or most frequently occurring perceptually deviant speech dimensions in ataxic dysarthria (Brown, Darley and Aronson, 1970; Darley, Aronson and Brown, 1975; Enderby, 1986; Chenery, Ingram and Murdoch, 1991). The perceptual features listed that can be attributed to laryngeal dysfunction in ataxic dysarthria include disorders of vocal quality (e.g. a harsh voice, strained/strangled phonation, pitch breaks, vocal tremor), impairment of pitch level (e.g. elevated or lower pitch) and deficits in variability of pitch and loudness (e.g. monopitch, monoloudness, excess loudness variation). It should be noted that, as indicated by Darley, Aronson and Brown (1975), although attributed to phonatory dysfunction, many of the above speech deviations could also result, at least partly, from dysfunction at other levels of the speech production mechanism (e.g. the respiratory system).

Unfortunately, only one study reported to date has used physiological instrumentation to investigate laryngeal activity in ataxic dysarthria. Grémy, Chevrie-Muller and Garde (1967) used electroglottography to identify increased variability of vocal fold vibrations in ataxic subjects.

Velopharyngeal function in ataxic dysarthria

The presence of hypernasal speech and nasal emission is not a commonly reported feature of ataxic dysarthria, suggesting that functioning of the velopharyngeal port may be normal in patients with cerebellar lesions. Duffy (1995) did report, however, that in some rare cases ataxic subjects may exhibit mild hyponasality, possibly as a consequence of improper timing of velar and articulatory gestures for nasal consonants. Oral examination of patients with cerebellar disorders most often reveals that elevation of the soft palate during phonation is normal.

Articulatory and prosodic function in ataxic dysarthria

The most prominent features of ataxic dysarthria involve a breakdown in articulatory and prosodic aspects of speech. The imprecise articulation leads to the improper formation and separation of individual syllables, leading to a reduction in intelligibility while the disturbance in prosody is associated with loss of texture, tone, stress and rhythm of individual syllables.

As indicated earlier, Brown, Darley and Aronson (1970) concluded that the 10 deviant speech dimensions perceived to be the most characteristic of ataxic dysarthria fell into three clusters: articulatory inaccuracy, prosodic excess and phonatory-prosodic insufficiency. Based on the performance of ataxic speakers on the Frenchay Dysarthria Assessment, Enderby (1986) also observed perceptual correlates of articulatory and prosodic inadequacy to be prominent among the 10 features she believed to be the most characteristic of ataxic dysarthria, including poor intonation, poor tongue movement in speech, poor alternating movement of the tongue in speech, reduced rate of speech, reduced lateral movement of the tongue, reduced elevation of the tongue, poor alternating movement of the lips and poor lip movements in speech.

In addition to the perceptual studies of ataxic dysarthria mentioned above, a number of researchers have used acoustic and/or physiological procedures to study the articulatory and prosodic aspects of ataxic dysarthria. Kent, Netsell and Abbs (1979) examined the acoustic features of five patients with ataxic dysarthria. They reported that the most marked and consistent abnormalities observed in the spectrograms of these speakers were alterations in the normal timing patterns and a tendency towards equalized syllable durations. These authors concluded that general timing is a major problem in ataxic dysarthria. Further, they speculated that ataxic speakers fail to decrease syllable duration when appropriate because such reductions require flexibility in sequencing complex motor instructions. The lack of flexibility may lead to a syllable-by-syllable motor control strategy with subsequent abnormal stress patterns.

Only a few studies reported to date have used physiological instrumentation to investigate the functioning of the articulators in ataxic dysarthria. In support of the concept that ataxic speakers are impaired in motor control,

McClean, Beukelman and Yorkston (1987) reported the case of an ataxic speaker who performed poorly on a non-speech visuomotor tracking task involving the lower lip and jaw. Netsell and Kent (1976) analysed articulatory position and movements in ataxic speakers using cineradiography. They observed a number of abnormal articulatory movements, including abnormally small adjustments of anterior posterior tongue movements during vowel production, which they thought might form the basis of the perception of vowel distortions. Although movements of the lips, tongue and jaw were generally coordinated, these authors reported that individual movements of these structures were often slow. In addition, they noted that articulatory contacts for consonant production were occasionally incomplete.

Hirose, Kiritani and Sawashima (1978) used an X-ray microbeam technique and electromyography to investigate articulatory dynamics in two dysarthric patients, one of whom had cerebellar degeneration. In particular, they examined the movement patterns in the jaw and lower lip. Their results showed that the ataxic speaker demonstrated inconsistency in articulatory movements, being characterized by inconsistency in both range and velocity of movement. Further, Hirose, Kiritani and Sawashima (1978) found that electromyography evidenced a breakdown of rhythmic patterns in articulatory muscles during syllable repetition. Overall, the findings of Hirose, Kiritani and Sawashima (1978) are consistent with the perception that ataxic speech contains irregular articulatory breakdowns.

In an examination of four ataxic speakers, McNeil *et al.* (1990) investigated isometric force and static position control of the upper and lower lip, tongue and jaw during non-speech tasks. They reported that the ataxic speakers had greater force and position instability than normal speakers, although impairment on one task did not necessarily predict impairment on other tasks.

Mixed dysarthria

A number of nervous system disorders affect more than one level of the motor system. Con-sequently, in addition to the more 'pure' forms of dysarthria discussed previously, speech pathologists in clinical practice often encounter patients who exhibit what are called 'mixed dysarthrias'. Dysarthria of this latter type may occur in patients with cerebrovascular accidents, head trauma, brain tumours, inflammatory diseases and degenerative conditions. The three neurological diseases that account for most cases of mixed dysarthria are amyotrophic lateral sclerosis, Wilson's disease and multiple sclerosis. Of the neurological diagnoses associated with mixed dysarthria, degenerative diseases including amyotrophic lateral sclerosis and Wilson's disease account for 63% of cases with mixed dysarthria, while demyelinating conditions such as multiple sclerosis are responsible for 6% of these patients (Duffy, 1995). The type of dysarthria associated with each of these conditions together with their epidemiology, prognosis and neurological symptoms is discussed below.

Amyotrophic lateral sclerosis

Amyotrophic lateral sclerosis is a form of motor neurone disease characterized by selective and progressive degeneration in the corticospinal and corticobulbar pathways and in the motor neurones associated with the cranial nerves and anterior horn cells of the spinal cord. The intellectual abilities of the patient remain intact. Because it involves the progressive degeneration of both upper and lower motor neurones, the condition is associated with a speech disorder with characteristics of both a pseudobulbar and bulbar palsy, that is a spastic-flaccid dysarthria. Indeed, according to Duffy (1995), amyotrophic lateral sclerosis has been identified as the predominant cause of spastic-flaccid dysarthria, with 88% of cases attributed to this condition.

The incidence rate of amyotrophic lateral sclerosis is 0.5–2.4 per 100 000 population (Kurtzke, 1991). Despite numerous clinical investigations, little is known regarding the aetiology of amyotrophic lateral sclerosis. Bannister (1985) has suggested that the cause may be a variety of hereditary, traumatic, toxic or viral influences that bring about motor neurone degeneration in susceptible subjects. Hypothyroidism, lead poisoning and autoimmune disease have been reported to produce an amyotrophic lateral sclerosis-like condition, with the exception that the symptoms are reversible. Some authors have suggested that the presence of a persistent polio virus may be the cause of the disease. Several different inherited forms of the disorder have been reported (Patten, 1987), including a sex-linked and autosomal dominant form. A predominance of males are affected by amyotrophic lateral sclerosis, with an average male-to-female ratio of approximately 1.5 : 1.0 (Gubbay *et al.*, 1985). Definitive diagnosis requires the presence of upper and lower motor neurone signs in the bulbar region and at least two other spinal regions (cervical, thoracic or lumbosacral), or in three spinal regions.

Amyotrophic lateral sclerosis is a fatal disorder that develops primarily between the ages of 50 and 70 years with a median age at onset of 66 years. The median duration of the disease is about three years from onset to death (most commonly from pulmonary infections), with longer durations occurring in patients who experience onset of symptoms before 50 years of age (Tandan, 1994). The mode of onset is usually insidious and the relative prominence of symptoms depends upon which motor neurones are most affected. In general, patients with bulbar involvement have a poorer prognosis than those in whom dysfunction is limited to the extremities.

Degeneration of both upper and lower motor neurones produces signs of both upper and lower motor neurone lesions, although the signs of one may predominate at any one time. Spastic paralysis is present unless degeneration of the lower motor neurones is far advanced. Upper motor neurone signs such as hyperactive muscle stretch reflexes, spasticity, a positive Babinski sign and a positive sucking reflex may be present in addition to signs of lower motor neurone involvement, such as muscle atrophy and fasciculations. The most important feature of the disorder as far as speech is concerned is an all-pervading weakness of the bulbar musculature. Damage to the bulbar musculature inevitably produces problems in swallowing, aspiration, saliva control and speech (Hillel and Miller, 1987).

No effective treatments for amyotrophic lateral sclerosis are currently available. Administration of riluzole may reduce mortality and slow progression of the condition possibly by blocking glutamatergic transmission in the central nervous system. Despite prolonging disease duration by approximately 10%, riluzole does not produce any noticeable improvement in patient strength or well-being. Adverse effects include fatigue, dizziness, gastrointestinal disorders, reduced pulmonary function and a rise in liver enzymes. Symptomatic treatments such as the use of anticholinergic drugs (e.g. glycopyrrolate, amitriptyline, etc.) to reduce drooling of saliva may provide improvements in patient comfort and safety. A semi-liquid diet or feeding via a nasogastric tube may be required for severe dysphagia.

Dysarthria in amyotrophic lateral sclerosis

The presence of a severe speech disorder is a common finding in amyotrophic lateral sclerosis. Carrow *et al.* (1974) reported that 97% of their sample of 79 subjects exhibited one or more deviant speech symptoms. Because the disorder is progressive in nature, the characteristics of the speech disorder tend to change over time. Initially, the dysarthria may present as either flaccid or spastic with a predominance of either type as the disease progresses. In those cases where upper motor neurone involvement predominates, the dysarthric speech disturbance is associated with spasticity of the tongue, the presence of primitive reflexes and emotional lability, consistent with pseudobulbar palsy (Gallagher, 1989). Bulbar dysfunction resulting in dysarthria and/or dysphagia has been found to occur in most individuals with amyotrophic lateral sclerosis (Dworkin and Hartman, 1979). The clinical signs of the dysarthria resulting from predominantly lower motor neurone involvement (bulbar palsy) consist of fasciculations, weakness, atrophy and reduced mobility of the tongue, and lip and jaw muscle dysfunction (Tandan, 1994). The most deviant speech characteristics seen in association with this condition therefore represent a mixture of those deviant speech dimensions which occur in bulbar (phonatory and resonatory incompetence) and pseudobulbar palsy (prosodic excess and insufficiency, articulatory and resonatory incompetence and phonatory stenosis) (Darley, Aronson and Brown, 1975).

Perceptual features of dysarthria in amyotrophic lateral sclerosis. Based on a perceptual analysis of the speech abilities of 30 patients with amyotrophic lateral sclerosis, Darley, Aronson and Brown (1975) found that the 10 most dominant speech deviations were imprecise consonants, hypernasality, harsh voice quality, slow rate, monopitch, short phrases, distorted vowels, low pitch, monoloudness and excess and equal stress. In fact, characteristics such as distortion of vowels, slow rate, shortness of phrases and imprecision of consonants are more deviant in this condition than in any other neurological disorder. Further, they reported the presence of three prosodic alterations in amyotrophic lateral sclerosis that do not appear in either bulbar or pseudobulbar palsy: prolongation of intervals, prolongation of phonemes and inappropriate silences.

A larger study by Carrow *et al.* (1974) involving 79 patients with motor neurone disease (the majority of whom exhibited amyotrophic lateral sclerosis) revealed a predominance of abnormal phonatory and resonatory features in the speech of these subjects. Eighty (80%) of the amyotrophic lateral sclerosis patients exhibited harshness, 65% were breathy, 63% demonstrated vocal tremor, while 60% of the patients were perceived to exhibit a strained/strangled vocal quality. Hypernasality was perceived to be the most prevalent abnormal resonatory feature, occurring in 75% of these patients. Imprecision of consonants and impaired intelligibility were evident in 57 and 47% of the subjects, respectively, with a strong association apparent between the presence of tongue atrophy and dysphagia and poor intelligibility (Carrow *et al.*, 1974).

Kent and colleagues conducted several studies to determine the contribution of articulatory errors made by subjects with amyotrophic lateral sclerosis to their reduced speech intelligibility. Kent *et al.* (1990), using a phonetic feature analysis (Kent *et al.*, 1989), identified a number of phonetic errors in the speech of 25 male patients with amyotrophic lateral sclerosis. These included frequent phonatory (initial /h/ vs vowel; voicing contrast for syllable-initial consonants),

velopharyngeal (stop vs nasal consonant) and articulatory (stop vs affricate articulation; palatal vs alveolar fricatives; high vs low vowel; presence or absence of syllable-final consonant) errors. The five most affected phonetic features – initial voicing contrast, palatal vs alveolar place of articulation, fricative vs affricative manner of articulation, stop vs nasal consonant and initial /h/ vs vowel – were found to be highly correlated with the subjects' level of speech intelligibility ranging from 41 to 99%. Examination of individual cases of amyotrophic lateral sclerosis also revealed that speech motor functions failed to decline at a uniform rate with disease progression and that a common phonetic error pattern was not related to overall intelligibility deficits in these subjects (Kent *et al.*, 1990). Furthermore, phonetic contrast analysis of the speech output of patients with amyotrophic lateral sclerosis has revealed gender differences with respect to laryngeal function. Kent *et al.* (1994) suggested that the segmental functions of the larynx (e.g. voicing control) were particularly vulnerable to amyotrophic lateral sclerosis in male patients, while female subjects failed to exhibit high proportions of phonetic contrast errors indicative of impaired voicing control. Speech intelligibility appeared to be less affected by laryngeal dysfunction in women than in their male counterparts (Kent *et al.*, 1992). The most severely affected phonetic contrasts for the female subjects included those related mainly to articulation and resonance. These contrasts were highly correlated with the subjects' levels of intelligibility.

The link between intelligibility and specific articulatory deficits in amyotrophic lateral sclerosis was investigated by Riddell *et al.* (1995). They assessed 29 highly intelligible male and female subjects with amyotrophic lateral sclerosis, using the phonetically based intelligibility test (Kent *et al.*, 1989) and the Frenchay Dysarthria Assessment (Enderby, 1983), to ascertain the type of phonetic errors that may occur with early speech changes, as well as associated subsystem deficits. Although only a relatively small number of phonetic errors were elicited compared to previous studies (Kent *et al.*, 1990, 1992), two of the seven most frequently occurring phonetic errors involved voicing (final voicing, initial voicing contrasts), and were suggestive of laryngeal involvement at an early stage of the disease and consistent with previous findings of impaired laryngeal control in subjects with amyotrophic lateral sclerosis (Ramig *et al.*, 1990). In addition, the frequent contrast errors relating to vowels (high vs low vowel, vowel duration) demonstrated by the amyotrophic lateral sclerosis subjects were consistent with perceptual reports of high incidences of vowel distortion and physiological evidence of impaired tongue function (Darley, Aronson and Brown, 1975; DePaul and Brooks, 1993; Langmore and Lehman, 1994).

As would be expected, given the progressive nature of amyotrophic lateral sclerosis, speech intelligibility has been reported to decline over time in this condition. Kent *et al.* (1991) reported that the speech intelligibility of a 53-year-old woman with amyotrophic lateral sclerosis declined from 98 to 48% over a two-year period, with phonetic features such as voicing contrast, place and manner of articulation, stop vs nasal contrast and a number of features related to syllable shape being the most affected by progressive deterioration in speech.

Acoustic features of dysarthria in amyotrophic lateral sclerosis. A number of abnormal acoustic features have been identified in the speech of patients with amyotrophic lateral sclerosis. Compared to control subjects, these characteristics include abnormal fundamental frequency (Fo), which is either too high or too low (Kent *et al.*, 1992, 1994), reduced Fo range (Rosenfield *et al.*, 1991), equivocal abnormalities of jitter, shimmer and harmonic-to-noise ratio, increased stop-gap and syllabic vowel durations, reduced maximum vowel duration, a decrease in the number of syllables per phrase, poorly defined voice onset time distinctions for initial voiced and voiceless stops, and multiple amplitude and frequency modulations of various frequencies and magnitudes associated with rapid voice tremor, or 'flutter', (Caruso and Burton, 1987; Ramig *et al.*, 1990; Aronson *et al.*, 1992; Kent *et al.*, 1992, 1994; Turner and Weismer, 1993). These acoustic findings, in part, serve to quantify previous perceptual observations in that they reflect articulatory and laryngeal dysfunction involving slow, weak and unstable movements of the articulators and

the laryngeal musculature during speech (Duffy, 1995).

Physiological features of dysarthria in amyotrophic lateral sclerosis. In addition to the findings of studies based on perceptual and acoustic analysis, further light has been shed on the nature of the speech disturbance in amyotrophic lateral sclerosis by physiological investigations. In particular, tongue strength and mobility have been reported to be severely reduced in patients with this condition. Dworkin and Hartman (1979) used a combination of a pressure transducer and the measurement of lingual alternate motion rates to follow the progression of amyotrophic lateral sclerosis in a 49-year-old man. They found that tongue strength was less than 25% of that found in normal men and that the alternate motion rate of the tongue was nearly a third of the rate usually found in normal adult men. A pressure gauge was also used by Dworkin (1980) to measure tongue strength in patients with this condition. He found that both the anterior and lateral tongue strength was reduced in amyotrophic lateral sclerosis. Further, Dworkin, Aronson and Mulder (1980) found that there was a high negative correlation between tongue force and severity of articulation defect and between syllable rate and severity of articulation defect. The findings of Dworkin and co-workers were supported by those of DePaul *et al.* (1988). Using custom-designed force transducers, they found that the tongue muscles are more severely affected in amyotrophic lateral sclerosis than the facial muscles and muscles of mastication.

A greater impairment in tongue strength compared to the jaw and lower lip has since been identified in subsequent studies of patients with amyotrophic lateral sclerosis (DePaul and Brooks, 1993; Langmore and Lehmen, 1994). In a study utilizing measures of maximum voluntary contraction and rate of change of force, DePaul and Brooks (1993) found that the tongue was more impaired than the lip and jaw in a group of 10 mildly impaired males with amyotrophic lateral sclerosis, irrespective of time post-onset and the site of the initial symptoms. Jaw strength and rate of change of force were not found to be significantly reduced overall, although four subjects demonstrated substantial reductions in the rate of change of force of the jaw. While tongue and lower lip rate of change of force and tongue weakness were found to be related to the degree of speech severity, none of these measures was correlated with speech intelligibility. DePaul and Brooks (1993) suggested that the lack of correlation between these measures and speech intelligibility was due to the fact that only low levels of lip and tongue force were required to produce speech and that multiple orofacial muscle groups could compensate for each other so that speech intelligibility was maintained.

Similar findings were obtained by Langmore and Lehman (1994), who examined physiological deficits in the orofacial system in individuals with amyotrophic lateral sclerosis. Maximum strength and maximum rate of repeated contraction of the tongue tip, lower lip and jaw were measured with strain gauge force transducers. As a group, the 10 patients with bulbar and corticobulbar forms of amyotrophic lateral sclerosis demonstrated significantly reduced strength and speed of movement in the orofacial structures compared to a control group, with the tongue generally more affected than the lip and jaw. Tongue strength and speed were both consistently impaired, with tongue strength showing a larger decrement in relation to normal subjects. In general, however, rate measures were found to be more highly correlated with the perceived severity of dysarthria in these subjects, than were measures of muscle strength, indicating the slower rate was a more sensitive indicator of increasing severity of dysarthria than decreasing strength. Langmore and Lehman (1994) suggested this relationship was due to the fact that only a small percentage (10%) of maximum articulatory muscle strength is generated during speech and that, because speech is usually produced at close to maximal rate (Kent, Kent and Rosenbek, 1987), a slight reduction in rate will be perceived as abnormal.

The impairment to the lingual musculature that the above findings indicate supports the suggestion of DePaul *et al.* (1988) that the hypoglossal nucleus is affected more early and more severely than the motor trigeminal and facial nuclei in amyotrophic lateral sclerosis. The acoustic results of Caruso and Burton (1987) also support

the finding that tongue strength (Dworkin, Aronson and Mulder, 1980) and speed of articulatory movements (Hirose, Kiritani and Sawashima, 1982) are impaired in patients with amyotrophic lateral sclerosis.

Few physiological studies of velopharyngeal function in individuals with amyotrophic lateral sclerosis have been reported. Hirose, Kiritani and Sawashima (1982) identified abnormal velopharyngeal function in a case with amyotrophic lateral sclerosis using an X-ray microbeam pellet tracking system. During the repetitive production of the syllable /ka/, it was noted that the velum failed to maintain normal elevation for each vowel following the consonant. On a maximum rate repetition task, involving the syllable /ten/, the subject with amyotrophic lateral sclerosis performed at a slower rate compared to the normal subject and the degree of velum elevation for /t/ was noted to gradually reduce during the repetition series. These findings were considered to reflect fatigue of the velopharyngeal musculature (Hirose, Kiritani and Sawashima, 1982).

Impaired respiratory function is widely regarded as one of the major debilitating features of amyotrophic lateral sclerosis. Consequently, impaired respiratory support could be expected to impact speech production in this population. Both spirometric and kinematic investigations of speech breathing in patients with amyotrophic lateral sclerosis have been conducted to determine the lung capacities and patterns of chest wall movement in these individuals. Studies have identified reduced lung capacities and aberrant chest wall movements in patients with amyotrophic lateral sclerosis (Putnam and Hixon, 1984). Putnam and Hixon (1984) suggested that reduced vital capacities in this population were related to fatigue and/or weakness of any components of the chest wall. Abnormal chest wall movements observed in these cases included sudden and frequent slope changes and paradoxical movements of the ribcage and abdomen. It was proposed by Putnam and Hixon (1984) that the abrupt slope changes observed in their subjects were a result of ribcage/abdominal 'groping' due to a reduction in the afferent feedback for fine-motor control of chest wall coordination associated with the disease process or a manifestation of the efforts of the ribcage and abdomen to counteract fatigue during speech.

Multiple sclerosis (disseminated sclerosis)

Multiple sclerosis is the most common primary demyelinating disease and is a major cause of neurological disability in young adults in most Western countries. In general, the disease occurs with a different incidence and prevalence in different geographic regions, being most common in the temperate areas of the world and rare in the tropics. In about two-thirds of cases, the condition is characterized by periods of exacerbation and remission so that the course of the disease is variable. In the remaining one-third, the course of the disorder is progressive without remissions. Death may occur at 3–6 months post-onset in some cases while other multiple sclerosis patients may still be active up to 40 years post-onset. The period between exacerbation may be as short as a few weeks or as long as 20–30 years. The average number of fresh exacerbations is about 0.4 per patient per year. The prognosis in multiple sclerosis varies from case to case. Approximately 20% of patients have only minor symptoms. About 10–15% eventually become bedridden or wheelchair-bound. The majority of multiple sclerosis patients, however, have a significant disabling problem but never become bedridden or wheelchair-bound.

Multiple sclerosis principally attacks young adults, with the peak onset occurring between 20 and 40 years of age. Most studies show the mean onset between 31 and 33 years of age. Although cases with onset < 10 years or > 60 years of age have been documented, they are exceedingly rare. In addition, women are slightly more affected than are men. The cause of the disease is unknown. About 10% of cases are familial and there is some evidence of metabolic, immunological, inflammatory and viral factors having an influence on the disease. The most popular aetiological theory centres around a 'slow virus' being activated by an unknown event. Precipitating factors have been found to include influenza, upper respiratory tract infections, fevers, pregnancy and so on.

The most important clinical and pathophysiological lesions in multiple sclerosis occur in the white matter of the central nervous system. Demyelination causes scarring (sclerosis) of the brain tissue which is evidenced at autopsy as irregular grey islands called 'plaques' in the white matter. The plaques may vary in size from microscopic to large lesions visible to the naked eye and represent areas of myelin loss with relative preservation of axons and neurone cell bodies. The significance of the plaques is that they interfere with nerve impulse conduction. As the plaques may affect a number of different parts of the central nervous system, including the white matter of the cerebral hemispheres, brainstem, cerebellum, spinal cord and optic pathways, the neurological signs and symptoms of multiple sclerosis vary widely.

The signs and symptoms exhibited by patients with multiple sclerosis are dependent upon which part of the central nervous system is affected. Optic neuritis is often one of the first symptoms to be manifest and may in some cases precede other manifestations by years. Motor difficulties in the form of weakness, clumsiness and/or ataxia of gait are also commonly found and are often among the early signs of the disease. Visual complaints are also quite common and may involve acute or progressive loss of vision. Diplopia is also common and sensory symptoms including paraesthesias of the extremities, dysesthesias and loss or impairment of sensation are also frequent. Symptoms of autonomic dysfunction including evidence of incontinence and increased anal reflex may also occur. Bulbar signs are frequent and consequently dysarthria and dysphagia are common features and may progress to a level that makes speech unintelligible and swallowing food virtually impossible. Other less frequently seen symptoms include vertigo, tinnitus, hearing loss, seizures, trigeminal neuralgia and involuntary facial motor activity. Patients with multiple sclerosis may also exhibit symptoms related to mood, behaviour, memory or other higher cognitive functions. If present, symptoms related to memory defect and mild to moderate blunting of higher cortical functions usually occur late and in patients with rather extensive disease. (For a full description of the neuropathophysiology, aetiology, clinical features and medical treatment of multiple sclerosis see Chapter 7.)

Dysarthria in multiple sclerosis

Dysarthria is the most common communication disorder affecting individuals with multiple sclerosis. Reports vary as to the proportion of multiple sclerosis patients who present with dysarthria. Less than half of a series of 168 patients with multiple sclerosis examined by Darley, Brown and Goldstein (1972) exhibited significant speech deviations. Figures of between 20 and 47% have been suggested by other workers (Enderby and Phillip, 1986; Hartelius, Svensson and Bubach, 1993). Surveys of multiple sclerosis populations, conducted by Beukelman, Kraft and Freal (1985) and Hartelius and Svensson (1994), have reported incidences of speech disturbances in 23 and 44% of respondents, respectively. The severity of dysarthria in individuals with multiple sclerosis would appear to be mild initially, with an increase in speech impairment corresponding to an increase in the overall severity of the disease, the number of neurological systems involved and the general deterioration in functioning of the individual (Darley, Brown and Goldstein, 1972; Beukelman, Kraft and Freal, 1985). Indeed, the dysarthria associated with multiple sclerosis can be severe enough to warrant augmentative communication (Beukelman, Kraft and Freal, 1985).

Given the potential of diffuse central nervous system involvement in multiple sclerosis, it is generally accepted that the dysarthria associated with multiple sclerosis is predominantly mixed, although specific types of dysarthria may present in some individuals at various stages of the disease. The type of dysarthria exhibited by the individual will be dependent, therefore, upon the sites of demyelination. Duffy (1995) concluded that, based on perceptual evidence and knowledge of neurological involvement (Farmakides and Boone, 1960; Darley, Brown and Goldstein, 1972), ataxic and spastic dysarthria and a mixed ataxic-spastic dysarthria were the most frequently observed forms of dysarthria demonstrated by individuals with multiple sclerosis, although any

other types or combinations of dysarthria may present in association with this disease. Despite the fact that dysarthria is a recognized clinical symptom of multiple sclerosis, research has been sadly lacking in this area. While a few studies examining the perceptual and acoustic features of the dysarthric speech disturbance in multiple sclerosis have been conducted, the physiological bases of the speech disorder have not yet been addressed, apart from some preliminary investigations of respiratory and articulatory function.

Perceptual features of dysarthria in multiple sclerosis. The earliest description of the dysarthric speech disturbance evident in multiple sclerosis was provided by Charcot (1877), who described the speech disorder as slow and drawling with the words measured, or 'scanned', such that a pause occurred after every syllable. Although the presence of scanning speech has been referred to or identified in other groups of patients with multiple sclerosis (Farmakides and Boone, 1960; FitzGerald, Murdoch and Chenery, 1987), Darley, Brown and Goldstein (1972) found that only 14% of their subjects demonstrated scanning speech patterns, that is excess and equal stress on syllables. Duffy (1995) concluded that scanning speech was not the predominant perceptual feature of the dysarthria associated with multiple sclerosis.

Of the perceptual studies reported in the literature, the majority have identified impairments in the respiration, phonation, resonance and articulation of persons with multiple sclerosis. Farmakides and Boone (1960), in a study of 82 subjects with multiple sclerosis, observed the presence of excessive nasality, weak phonation, impaired respiratory control, a reduced rate of speech and difficulties with pitch variability and voiced/voiceless distinctions. In the most extensive perceptual study of the speech of 168 individuals with multiple sclerosis, Darley, Brown and Goldstein (1972) found that impaired loudness control and harshness were the most frequently perceived deviant speech dimensions, occurring in 77 and 72% of cases, respectively. Abnormal articulation was evident in approximately half of the subjects, while restricted use of vocal variations for emphasis, impaired pitch control, hypernasality, inappropriate pitch level and breathiness were perceived to be present in 20–40% of the subjects. Similar abnormal speech features and frequencies of occurrence were identified by Hartelius, Svensson and Bubach (1993) in all but two subjects within a group of 30 subjects with multiple sclerosis, using a clinical dysarthria assessment tool. Comparison of results between the two studies, however, should be viewed with caution, because of methodological differences. In a group of subjects severely affected by multiple sclerosis, FitzGerald, Murdoch and Chenery (1987) identified a higher frequency of the occurrence of deviant speech features compared to the Darley, Brown and Goldstein (1972) study. All of the subjects were perceived to demonstrate impaired respiratory support for speech while 91% of cases exhibited impaired pitch variation and steadiness, prolonged intervals and a harsh vocal quality. Prosodic deficits (reduced phrase length, excess and equal stress, reduced rate), imprecision of consonants, hoarseness and impaired loudness variation were perceived to be present in the speech of 78–87% of the subjects with multiple sclerosis. In general, the observed deviant speech features were mild. The abnormal articulation of consonants noted in these subjects was found to contribute the most to variations in overall intelligibility, while impaired respiratory support for speech was found to be highly associated with deviations in vocal quality, volume control and articulation (FitzGerald, Murdoch and Chenery, 1987).

Acoustic features of dysarthria in multiple sclerosis. As yet, the acoustic features of the dysarthric speech disturbance associated with multiple sclerosis have received limited attention in the research literature. The earliest attempt to investigate these characteristics was undertaken by Scripture (1916), who used a primitive phonautograph method to record the production of sustained vowels in 20 subjects with a diagnosis of disseminated sclerosis. Small, irregular waves were identified in the recordings and attributed to laryngeal ataxia, a result of sudden changes in laryngeal muscle tension. Using more sophisticated speech waveform measurements, Haggard (1969) confirmed the presence of a significant, but not consistent, tendency for patients with dissem-

inated sclerosis to demonstrate irregular phonatory onset.

Hartelius, Nord and Buder (1995) examined the durational, articulatory and phonatory acoustic features of five subjects with multiple sclerosis compared to the speech of two normal speakers. Durational measurements indicated that three of the five subjects with multiple sclerosis demonstrated a slower speaking rate involving more frequent pausing than normal speakers, longer vowel and word durations and a tendency towards equalization of syllable length in these words. The latter finding was consistent with the perceptual feature of excess and equal stress. Articulatory acoustic features identified in the subjects with multiple sclerosis included inadequate closure of stops characterized by continuous frication or spirantization, continuous voicing, presence of nasal formants during stop production, continuous frication superimposed on the formant patterns of vocalic segments, instability of voicing onset following stop release, reduced rate of second formant (F_2) transition and flatter F_2 transitions extending over 50% of the total vowel duration. Acoustic analysis of the phonation of subjects with multiple sclerosis failed to reveal any remarkable differences compared to the normal subjects in relation to fundamental frequency and range during a text reading task. Spectrum analysis of the Fo of sustained vowels, however, identified the presence of tremor in the voices of subjects with multiple sclerosis, with predominant instabilities occurring between 1 and 4 Hz. Interestingly, one of the subjects with multiple sclerosis with no perceptual speech disturbance demonstrated a slight tremor at around 4 Hz, suggestive of a subclinical manifestation of multiple sclerosis. The preliminary acoustic findings of Hartelius, Nord and Buder (1995) appeared to correlate with the underlying neuromotor dysfunction of each speaker with multiple sclerosis and, therefore, lend themselves to further investigation in larger groups of dysarthric subjects with multiple sclerosis to further define the acoustic features of the dysarthric speech disturbance in this population.

Physiological features of dysarthria in multiple sclerosis. Despite the relatively high incidence of dysarthria in multiple sclerosis, there is a paucity of research regarding the physiological nature of motor speech impairment associated with this condition. In one of the few reported physiological studies of articulatory function in multiple sclerosis, Murdoch *et al.* (1998) used lip and tongue transducer systems to assess articulatory function in 16 individuals with multiple sclerosis. They reported that individuals with multiple sclerosis exhibited significantly impaired tongue performance on tasks of strength, endurance and rate measures compared to normal controls. In particular, the subjects with dysarthria associated with multiple sclerosis demonstrated reduced maximum tongue strength, decreased endurance and a reduction in repetitive tongue movements. Further, Murdoch *et al.* (1998) reported the presence of lingual dysfunction in the absence of lip dysfunction. The pattern of differential impairment of the tongue and lips observed in relation to maintenance of strength is consistent with studies of other neurological conditions such as amyotrophic lateral sclerosis (DePaul and Brooks, 1993) and Parkinson's disease (Barlow and Abbs, 1983).

Subsequently, Murdoch, Gardiner and Theodoros (2000a) used electropalatography to document the location and timing of tongue-to-palate contacts during speech production in a 52-year-old male with dysarthria associated with slow, progressive multiple sclerosis. They reported that the subject with multiple sclerosis demonstrated only limited disruption to tongue-to-palate spatial configurations for the initial consonants assessed, with tongue placement for each phoneme being, in general, anatomically correct. However, the presence of articulatory 'overshooting' in some contact patterns was suggestive of a mild impairment in their subject's lingual motor control. Duffy (1995) stated that articulatory overshooting may occur owing to incoordination in force, accuracy, speed and range of tongue movements.

Velopharyngeal function has been reported to be intact in multiple sclerosis (Murdoch, Theodoros and Ward, 2000b). Using an accelerometric technique, Murdoch, Theodoros and Ward (2000b) reported that their group of 16 subjects with multiple sclerosis showed no significant difference in nasality compared to a group of normal controls, a finding consistent with other documented objective evaluations of velopharyngeal function in multiple sclerosis. Using oral manometry, Darley, Brown and Goldstein (1972) reported the presence of velopharyngeal dysfunction in only three of their 155 (2%) subjects with multiple sclerosis. As in the case of velopharyngeal function, other researchers have failed to identify laryngeal dysfunction in persons with multiple sclerosis based on electroglottographic and aerodynamic measures (Theodoros, Murdoch and Ward, 2000).

In contrast, impaired respiratory function has been reported in multiple sclerosis. Darley, Brown and Goldstein (1972) reported decreased vital capacities in their speakers with multiple sclerosis, with 11% of the subjects with multiple sclerosis demonstrating abnormally rapid respiration rates. While there have been no other studies of respiratory function specifically targeting the multiple sclerosis population, Murdoch *et al.* (1991), in a study of the respiratory kinematics of speakers with cerebellar disease, included nine subjects with multiple sclerosis in their cohort of 12. Abnormal coordination of the ribcage and abdomen during speech breathing, together with irregular chest wall movements, were identified in the majority of the subject group (Murdoch *et al.*, 1991).

Research into the perceptual, acoustic and physiological characteristics of multiple sclerosis remains limited. Extensive investigations of the dysarthric speech disorder evident in this population, in particular the physiological features of each subsystem of the speech production mechanism, are urgently required to ensure that appropriate treatment procedures can be instigated for the significant proportion of individuals with multiple sclerosis who exhibit dysarthria.

Wilson's disease (hepatolenticular degeneration)

Wilson's disease, or hepatolenticular degeneration, is a rare, inborn metabolic disorder caused by the body's inability to process dietary copper. As a result, copper accumulates in the tissues of the body, especially in the brain, liver and cornea of the eye. The most severely affected parts of the brain are the basal ganglia, although lesser degrees of copper deposition may also occur in the cerebellum, brainstem and other parts of the cerebrum. Of the basal ganglia, the corpus striatum is most involved with damage usually more marked in the putamen than in the caudate nucleus. Cirrhosis of the liver is also present and the deposition of copper in the eye gives a greenish-brown colour to the cornea (Kayser–Fleisher rings).

The condition is inherited in an autosomal recessive manner (Bearn, 1960) occurring in approximately one in every 30 000 of the population (Stremmel *et al.*, 1991). The clinical presentation of Wilson's disease includes neurological, hepatic, haematological and, in some cases, psychiatric symptoms (Adams and Victor, 1991; Oder *et al.*, 1991; Stremmel *et al.*, 1991). Although a distinctive sign of the disease is the presence of golden, brown (Kayser–Fleischer) rings around the cornea of the eyes, consistent with copper deposits, the initial symptoms are often non-specific and may result in delays in diagnosis (approximately 1.7 to 2 years) and subsequent treatment (Oder *et al.*, 1991; Stremmel *et al.*, 1991). The most common clinical signs and symptoms of the disease identified by investigators have included mainly Parkinsonian and hyperkinetic neurological behaviours. Stremmel *et al.* (1991) in a group of 51 subjects with Wilson's disease included dysarthria, tremor, writing difficulties, ataxic gait, hepatomegaly, splenomegaly and thrombocytopenia, while other investigators have reported the presence of dysdiadochokinesia, dystonia, rigidity, facial masking, wing-beating tremor, bradykinesia, dysphagia, drooling and gait and postural abnormalities (Adams and Victor, 1991; Oder *et al.*, 1991).

Many of the neurological signs and symptoms identified in patients with Wilson's disease have been partially supported by radiological data derived from computerized tomography (CT), magnetic resonance imaging (MRI) and positron emission tomography (PET). Most cerebral lesions were identified in the caudate, putamen, pallidum, subcortical white matter, midbrain and pons with evidence of generalized cerebral atrophy (Prayer *et al.*, 1990). The possible pathophysiological basis of the movement disorders observed in patients with Wilson's disease has been investigated using PET. As a result of a reduced uptake of fluorodopa, Snow *et al.* (1991) suggested that the nigrostriatal dopaminergic pathway was involved in patients with Wilson's disease who demonstrated neurological impairment. MRI findings are characterized by reduced T_1-weighted and increased T_2-weighted images of the putamen, pars compacta of the substantia nigra, periaqueductal grey matter, pontine tegmentum and thalamus (Keller *et al.*, 1999). In combination with basal ganglia hyperdensity, ventricular dilation and atrophy of the cerebral cortex, brainstem and cerebellum on CT, these findings are suggestive of widespread atrophy from the oxidative action of the copper toxicity. Abnormal dopamine, noradrenaline and serotonin neurotransmitter metabolism has also been reported in Wilson's disease (Portala *et al.*, 2001). The severity of neurological symptoms has been shown to be correlated with reduced PET-demonstrated glucose metabolism in the corpus striatum, thalamus, cerebral cortex and cerebellum (Lauterbach, 2002).

Although patients with Wilson's disease are a heterogeneous group, Oder *et al.* (1993) have identified three subgroups of persons with Wilson's disease, based on clinical findings and MRI data. The first subgroup consisted of subjects who exhibited bradykinesia, rigidity, cognitive impairment and an organic mood syndrome while demonstrating dilatation of the third ventricle. Focal thalamic lesions were evident in subjects exhibiting ataxia, tremor and reduced functional capacity, while a third subgroup with focal lesions in the putamen and pallidum exhibited dyskinesia, dysarthria and an organic personality syndrome.

Although Wilson's disease results in progressive neurological and hepatic degeneration, the condition has been shown to be amenable to treatment if diagnosed before excessive accumulation of copper and permanent damage occurs in body organs. Treatment regimens include a low copper diet, potassium sulfide to reduce copper absorption and a copper-chelating agent, D-penicillamine, which facilitates copper excretion (Duffy, 1995). In cases of adverse reactions or poor responses to D-penicillamine, other copper-depleting agents, such as trientine, zinc and tetrathiomolybdate, have been used in the treatment of Wilson's disease (Scheinberg, Jaffe and Sternlieb, 1987).

Dysarthria in Wilson's disease

A mixed ataxic-hypokinetic-spastic dysarthria is a prominent feature of Wilson's disease and is often one of the earliest neurological symptoms of the condition. In fact, dysarthria is considered a characteristic feature of the disease and has been reported to occur in 51 to 81% of patients (Martin, 1968; Starosta-Rubinstein *et al.*, 1987; Oder *et al.*, 1991; Stremmel *et al.*, 1991). The disordered speech takes the form of a mixed dysarthria consisting of mainly spastic, ataxic and hypokinetic components (Duffy, 1995). Starosta-Rubinstein *et al.* (1987) identified a predominance of spastic dysarthric components in the mixed dysarthria exhibited by their subjects, occurring in 76%, while features of ataxic dysarthria and hypokinetic dysarthria were evident in 69 and 59%, respectively. Slow hyperkinetic dystonia has also been observed in these patients to varying degrees (Starosta-Rubinstein *et al.*, 1987). The combination of dysarthria types and the level of severity varies widely amongst individuals with the disease (Berry *et al.*, 1974).

To date, there have been very few investigations of the dysarthric speech disturbance evident in patients with Wilson's disease. While the perceptual characteristics of the disturbed speech have been addressed to some extent (Berry *et al.*, 1974), no studies have endeavoured to define the physiological and acoustic features of the dysarthric speech disturbance in this population.

Perceptual features of dysarthria in Wilson's disease. Berry *et al.* (1974) found positive neurological signs of ataxia, rigidity or spasticity in their 20 patients with Wilson's disease. They noted that the most prominent speech characteristics of the dysarthria exhibited by their subjects were similar to the most prominent deviant speech dimensions exhibited by patients with Parkinson's disease. Reduced stress, monopitch, monoloudness and imprecise consonants were the four most highly ranked features in the Wilson's disease patients. The same four deviant speech dimen-

sions were also reported by Darley, Aronson and Brown (1969a,b) to be the most highly ranked speech abnormalities in Parkinson's patients. Further, subjects with Wilson's disease were reported by Berry *et al.* (1974) to share the deviant speech dimensions of irregular articulatory breakdown with cerebellar disorders, hypernasality with pseudobulbar palsy and inappropriate silences with Parkinson's disease. Overall, Berry *et al.* (1974) determined that the speech deviations seen in their patients with Wilson's disease fell into four clusters: prosodic insufficiency (monopitch, monoloudness, reduced stress), as seen in hypokinetic and spastic dysarthria; phonatory stenosis (low pitch, strained voice, harsh voice), as reported in spastic dysarthria; prosodic excess (slow rate, prolonged phonemes, prolonged intervals, excess and equal stress), as observed in ataxic dysarthria; and articulatory/resonatory inadequacy (hypernasality, imprecise consonants), as seen in spastic dysarthria and dysarthria associated with amyotrophic lateral sclerosis and chorea.

Pharmacological (D-penicillamine) and dietary treatment of Wilson's disease has been reported to improve the speech of patients with this condition, provided that treatment is commenced prior to permanent neurological or hepatic damage occurring (Berry *et al.*, 1974; Darley, Aronson and Brown, 1975). Day and Parnell (1987) described a case of Wilson's disease in which a severe dysarthria persisted, however, despite drug and dietary control.

Summary

Damage to the cerebellum or its connections results in ataxia, a condition in which muscular activity and movements become uncoordinated. If the muscles of the speech production mechanism are involved, the production of speech is disturbed leading to a cluster of speech impairments collectively referred to as 'ataxic dysarthria'. The condition can be associated with a wide range of neurological disorders that involve the cerebellum, including cerebrovascular accidents, brain tumours and so on. The most prominent features of ataxic dysarthria include a breakdown in the articulatory and prosodic aspects of speech.

Many neurological disorders cause disruption to more than one level of the motor system, leading to production of what are called 'mixed dysarthrias'. The clinical features of mixed dysarthrias are dependent on the levels of the motor system affected. For example, if both the upper and lower motor neurones are involved, the resulting mixed dysarthria would be expected to exhibit features of both a spastic and flaccid dysarthria (spastic-flaccid dysarthria), whereas if the upper motor neurones and the cerebellum were involved, the resulting dysarthria would be spastic-ataxic dysarthria. The three neurological diseases that account for the majority of cases of mixed dysarthria are amyotrophic lateral sclerosis, Wilson's disease and multiple sclerosis. Amyotrophic lateral sclerosis is associated with a progressive spastic-flaccid dysarthria, while Wilson's disease causes a mixed ataxic-hypokinetic-spastic dysarthria. The type of dysarthria exhibited by persons with multiple sclerosis is dependent on the site of demyelination but frequently manifests as a mixed ataxic-spastic dysarthria. However, other types or combinations of dysarthria may also manifest in multiple sclerosis.

References

Adams, R.D. and Victor, M. (1991) *Principles of Neurology*, McGraw-Hill, New York.

Aronson, A.E., Ramig, L.O., Winholtz, W.S. and Silber, S.R. (1992) Rapid voice tremor, or 'flutter', in amyotrophic lateral sclerosis. *Annals of Otology, Rhinology and Laryngology*, **101**, 511–518.

Bannister, R. (1985) *Brain's Clinical Neurology*, Oxford University Press, Edinburgh.

Barlow, S.M. and Abbs, J.H. (1983) Force transducers of the evaluation of labial, lingual and mandibular motor impairments. *Journal of Speech and Hearing Research*, **26**, 616–621.

Bearn, A.G. (1960) A genetic analysis of thirty families with Wilson's disease (hepatolenticular degeneration). *Annals of Human Genetics*, **24**, 33–43.

Berry, W.R., Darley, F.L., Aronson, A.E. and Goldstein, N.P. (1974) Dysarthria in Wilson's disease. *Journal of Speech and Hearing Research*, **17**, 169–183.

Beukelman, D.R., Kraft, G.H. and Freal, J. (1985) Expressive communication disorders in persons with multiple sclerosis: a survey. *Archives of Physical Medicine and Rehabilitation*, **66**, 675–677.

Brown, J.R., Darley, F.L. and Aronson, A.E. (1970) Ataxic dysarthria. *International Journal of Neurology*, **7**, 302–318.

Caruso, A.J. and Burton, E.S. (1987) Temporal acoustic measures of dysarthria associated with amyotrophic lateral sclerosis. *Journal of Speech and Hearing Research*, **30**, 80–87.

Carrow, E., Rivera, V., Mauldin, M. and Shamblin, L. (1974) Deviant speech characteristics in motor neuron disease. *Archives of Otolaryngology*, **100**, 212–218.

Charcot, J.M. (1877) *Lectures on the Diseases of the Nervous System*, New Sydenham Society, London.

Chenery, H.J., Ingram, J.C.L. and Murdoch, B.E. (1991) Perceptual analysis of speech in ataxic dysarthria. *Australian Journal of Human Communication Disorders*, **18**, 19–28.

Darley, F.L., Aronson, A.E. and Brown, J.R. (1969a) Differential diagnostic patterns of dysarthria. *Journal of Speech and Hearing Research*, **12**, 246–269.

Darley, F.L., Aronson, A.E. and Brown, J.R. (1969b) Clusters of deviant speech dimensions in the dysarthrias. *Journal of Speech and Hearing Research*, **12**, 462–496.

Darley, F.L., Aronson, A.E. and Brown, J.R. (1975) *Motor Speech Disorders*, W.B. Saunders, Philadelphia.

Darley, F.L., Brown, J.R. and Goldstein, N.P. (1972) Dysarthria in multiple sclerosis. *Journal of Speech and Hearing Research*, **15**, 229–245.

Day, L.S. and Parnell, M.M. (1987) Ten year study of a Wilson's disease dysarthria. *Journal of Communication Disorders*, **20**, 207–218.

DePaul, R., Abbs, J.H., Caligiuri, M. *et al.* (1988) Hypoglossal, trigeminal, and facial motoneuron involvement in amyotrophic lateral sclerosis. *Neurology*, **38**, 281–283.

DePaul, R. and Brooks, B.R. (1993) Multiple orofacial indices in amyotrophic lateral sclerosis. *Journal of Speech and Hearing Research*, **36**, 1158–1167.

Duffy, J.R. (1995) *Motor Speech Disorders: Substrates, Differential Diagnosis, and Management*, Mosby-Year Inc., Baltimore.

Dworkin, J.P. (1980) Tongue strength measurement in patients with amyotrophic lateral sclerosis:

qualitative and quantitative procedures. *Archives of Physical Medicine and Rehabilitation*, **61**, 422–424.

Dworkin, J.P., Aronson, A.E. and Mulder, D.W. (1980) Tongue force in normals and in dysarthric patients and amyotrophic lateral sclerosis. *Journal of Speech and Hearing Research*, **23**, 828–837.

Dworkin, J.P. and Hartman, D.E. (1979) Progressive speech deterioration and dysphagia in amyotrophic lateral sclerosis: case report. *Archives of Physical Medicine and Rehabilitation*, **60**, 423–425.

Eccles, J.A. (1973) A re-evaluation of cerebellar function in man, in *New Developments in Electromyography and Clinical Neurophysiology*, vol. 3 (ed. J. Desmedt), Karger, Basel, pp. 451–469.

Enderby, P.M. (1983) *Frenchay Dysarthria Assessment*, College Hill Press, San Diego.

Enderby, P. (1986) Relationships between dysarthric groups. *British Journal of Disorders of Communication*, **21**, 180–197.

Enderby, P. and Phillip, R. (1986) Speech and language handicap: towards knowing the size of the problem. *British Journal of Disorders of Communication*, **21**, 151–165.

Farmakides, M.N. and Boone, D.R. (1960) Speech problems in patients with multiple sclerosis. *Journal of Speech and Hearing Disorders*, **25**, 385–390.

FitzGerald, F., Murdoch, B.E. and Chenery, H.J. (1987) Multiple sclerosis: associated speech and language disorders. *Australian Journal of Human Communication Disorders*, **15**, 15–33.

Gallagher, J.P. (1989) Pathologic laughter and crying in ALS: a search for their origin. *Acta Neurologica Scandinavica*, **80**, 114–117.

Gilman, S. (1969) The mechanism of cerebellar hypotonia. *Brain*, **92**, 621–638.

Grémy, F., Chevrie-Muller, C. and Garde, E. (1967) Etude phoniatrique clinique et instrumentale des dysarthries. *Revue Neurologique*, **116**, 401–426.

Gubbay, S.S., Kahana, E., Zilber, N. *et al.* (1985) Amyotrophic lateral sclerosis: a study of its presentation and prognosis. *Journal of Neurology*, **232**, 295–300.

Haggard, M.P. (1969) Speech waveform measurements in multiple sclerosis. *Folia Phoniatrica et Logopaedica*, **21**, 307–312.

Hartelius, L., Nord, L. and Buder, E.H. (1995) Acoustic analysis of dysarthria associated with multiple sclerosis. *Clinical Linguistics and Phonetics*, **9**, 95–120.

Hartelius, L. and Svensson, P. (1994) Speech and swallowing symptoms associated with Parkinson's disease and multiple sclerosis: a survey. *Folia Phoniatrica et Logopaedica*, **46**, 9–17.

Hartelius, L., Svensson, P. and Bubach, A. (1993) Clinical assessment of dysarthria: performance on a dysarthria test by normal adult subjects, and by individuals with Parkinson's disease or with multiple sclerosis. *Scandinavian Journal of Logopedics and Phoniatrics*, **18**, 131–141.

Hillel, A.D. and Miller, R.N. (1987) Management of bulbar symptoms in amyotrophic lateral sclerosis, in *Advances in Experimental Medicine and Biology: Amyotrophic Lateral Sclerosis, Therapeutic, Psychological and Research Aspects*, vol. **29** (eds V. Cosi, A.C. Kato, P. Parlette and M. Poloni), Plenum Press, New York, pp. 275–302.

Hirose, H., Kiritani, S. and Sawashima, M. (1982) Patterns of dysarthric movement in patients with amyotrophic lateral sclerosis and pseudobulbar palsy. *Folia Phoniatrica et Logopaedica*, **34**, 106–112.

Hirose, H., Kiritani, S., Ushijima, T. and Sawashima, M. (1978) Analysis of abnormal articulatory dynamics in two dysarthric patients. *Journal of Speech and Hearing Disorders*, **43**, 96–105.

Ito, M. (1970) Neurophysiological aspects of cerebellar motor control system. *International Journal of Neurology*, **7**, 162–176.

Keller, R., Torta, R., Lagget, M. *et al.* (1999) Psychiatric symptoms of late onset of Wilson's disease: neuroradiological findings, clinical features and treatment. *Italian Journal of Neurological Sciences*, **20**, 49–54.

Kent, J.F., Kent, R.D., Rosenbek, J.C. *et al.* (1992) Quantitative description of the dysarthria in women with amyotrophic lateral sclerosis. *Journal of Speech and Hearing Disorders*, **35**, 723–733.

Kent, R.D., Kent, J.F. and Rosenbek, J.C. (1987) Maximum performance tests of speech production. *Journal of Speech and Hearing Disorders*, **52**, 367–387.

Kent, R.D., Kent, J.F., Weismer, G. *et al.* (1989) Relationships between speech intelligibility and the slope of the second-formant transitions in dysarthric subjects. *Clinical Linguistics and Phonetics*, **3**, 347–358.

Kent, R.D., Kent, J.F., Weismer, G. *et al.* (1990) Impairment of speech intelligibility in men with amyotrophic lateral sclerosis. *Journal of Speech and Hearing Disorders*, **55**, 721–728.

Kent, R.D., Kim, H.H., Weismer, G. *et al.* (1994) Laryngeal dysfunction in neurological disease: amyotrophic lateral sclerosis, Parkinson disease, and stroke. *Journal of Medical Speech-Language Pathology*, **2**, 157–175.

Kent, R.D., Netsell, R. and Abbs, J.H. (1979) Acoustic characteristics of dysarthria associated with cerebellar disease. *Journal of Speech and Hearing Research*, **22**, 627–648.

Kent, R.D., Sufit, R.L., Rosenbek, J.C. *et al.* (1991) Speech deterioration in amyotrophic lateral sclerosis: a case study. *Journal of Speech and Hearing Research*, **34**, 1269–1275.

Kluin, K.J., Gilman, S., Markel, D.S. *et al.* (1988) Speech disorders in olivopontocerebellar atrophy correlate with positron emission tomography findings. *Annals of Neurology*, **23**, 547–554.

Konorski, J. (1967) *Integrative Activity of the Brain*, University of Chicago Press, Chicago.

Kurtzke, J.F. (1991) Risk factors in amyotrophic lateral sclerosis. *Advances in Neurology*, **56**, 245–270.

Langmore, S.E. and Lehman, M.E. (1994) Physiologic deficits in the orofacial system underlying dysarthria in amyotrophic lateral sclerosis. *Journal of Speech and Hearing Research*, **37**, 28–37.

Lauterbach, E. (2002) Wilson's disease. *Psychiatric Annals*, **32**, 114–120.

Lothman, E.W. and Ferrendelli, J.A. (1980) Disorders and diseases of the cerebellum, in *Neurology*, vol. 5 (ed. R.N. Rosenberg), Grune & Stratton, New York, pp. 435–470.

Martin, J.P. (1968) Wilson's disease, in *Handbook of Clinical Neurology*, vol. 6 (eds P.J. Vinken and G.W. Bruyn), North-Holland Publishing Company, Amsterdam, pp. 267–278.

McClean, M.D., Beukelman, D.R. and Yorkston, K.M. (1987) Speech-muscle visuomotor tracking in dysarthric and nonimpaired speakers. *Journal of Speech and Hearing Research*, **30**, 276–282.

McNeil, M.R., Weismer, G., Adams, S. and Mulligan, M. (1990) Oral structure nonspeech motor control in normal, dysarthric, aphasic, and apraxic speakers: isometric force and static position. *Journal of Speech and Hearing Research*, **33**, 255–268.

Murdoch, B.E., Chenery, H.J., Stokes, P.D. and Hardcastle, W.J. (1991) Respiratory kinematics in speakers with cerebellar disease. *Journal of Speech and Hearing Research*, **34**, 768–780.

Murdoch, B.E., Gardiner, F. and Theodoros, D.G. (2000a) Electropalatographic assessment of articulatory dysfunction in multiple sclerosis: a case study. *Journal of Medical Speech-Language Pathology*, **8**, 359–364.

Murdoch, B.E., Spencer, T.J., Theodoros, D.G. and Thompson, E.C. (1998) Lip and tongue dysfunction in multiple sclerosis: a physiological analysis. *Motor Control*, **2**, 148–160.

Murdoch, B.E., Theodoros, D.G. and Ward, E.C. (2000b) Articulatory and velopharyngeal dysfunction in multiple sclerosis, in *Speech and Language Disorders in Multiple Sclerosis* (eds B.E. Murdoch and D.G. Theodoros), Whurr, London, pp. 47–63.

Netsell, R. and Kent, R. (1976) Paroxysmal ataxic dysarthria. *Journal of Speech and Hearing Disorders*, **41**, 93–109.

Oder, W., Grimm, G., Kollegger, H. *et al.* (1991) Neurological and neuropsychiatric spectrum of Wilson's disease: a prospective study of 45 cases. *Journal of Neurology*, **238**, 281–287.

Oder, W., Prayer, L., Grimm, G. *et al.* (1993) Wilson's disease: evidence of subgroups derived from clinical findings and brain lesions. *Neurology*, **43**, 120–124.

Patten, B.M. (1987) The syndromic nature of amyotrophic lateral sclerosis, in *Advances in Experimental Medicine and Biology: Amyotrophic Lateral Sclerosis, Therapeutic, Psychological and Research Aspects*, vol. **209** (eds V. Costi, A.C. Kato, P. Parlette and M. Poloni), Plenum Press, New York, pp. 303–319.

Portala, K., Levander, S., Westermark, K. *et al.* (2001) Pattern of neuropsychological deficits in patients with treated Wilson's disease. *European Archives of Psychiatry and Clinical Neuroscience*, **251**, 262–268.

Prayer, L., Wimberger, D., Kramer, J. *et al.* (1990) Cranial MRI in Wilson's disease. *Neuroradiology*, **32**, 211–214.

Putnam, A.H. and Hixon, T.J. (1984) Respiratory kinematics in speakers with motor neuron disease, in *The Dysarthrias: Physiology, Acoustics, Perception, Management* (eds M.R. McNeil, J.C. Rosenbek and A.E. Aronson), College Hill Press, San Diego, pp. 37–67.

Ramig, L.O., Scherer, R.C., Klasner, E.R. *et al.* (1990) Acoustic analysis of voice in amyotrophic lateral sclerosis. *Journal of Speech and Hearing Disorders*, **55**, 2–14.

Riddell, J., McCauley, R.J., Mulligan, M. and Tandan, R. (1995) Intelligibility and phonetic contrast errors in highly intelligible speakers with amyotrophic lateral sclerosis. *Journal of Speech and Hearing Research*, **38**, 304–314.

Rosenfield, D.B., Viswanath, N., Herbrich, K.E. and Nudelman, H.B. (1991) Evaluation of the speech motor control system in amyotrophic lateral sclerosis. *Journal of Voice*, 5, 224–230.

Scheinberg, I.H., Jaffe, M.E. and Sternlieb, I. (1987) The use of trientine in preventing the effects of interrupting penicillamine therapy in Wilson's disease. *New England Journal of Medicine*, 317, 209–213.

Scripture, B.W. (1916) Records of speech in disseminated sclerosis. *Brain*, 39, 445–477.

Snow, B.J., Bhatt, M., Martin, W.R.W. *et al.* (1991) The nigrostriatal dopaminergic pathway in Wilson's disease studied with positron emission tomography. *Journal of Neurology, Neurosurgery, and Psychiatry*, 54, 12–17.

Starosta-Rubinstein, S., Young, A.B., Kluin, K. *et al.* (1987) Clinical assessment of 31 patients with Wilson's disease. *Archives of Neurology*, 44, 365–370.

Stremmel, W., Meyerrose, K., Niederau, C. *et al.* (1991) Wilson disease: clinical presentation, treatment, and survival. *Annals of Internal Medicine*, 115, 720–726.

Tandan, R. (1994) Clinical features and differential diagnosis of classical motor neuron disease, in *Motor Neuron Disease* (ed. A.C. Williams), Chapman & Hall, London, pp. 3–27.

Theodoros, D.G., Murdoch, B.E. and Ward, E.C. (2000) Laryngeal and respiratory dysfunction in multiple sclerosis, in *Speech and Language Disorders in Multiple Sclerosis* (eds B.E. Murdoch and D.G. Theodoros), Whurr, London, pp. 64–79.

Turner, G.S. and Weismer, G. (1993) Characteristics of speaking rate in dysarthria associated with amyotrophic lateral sclerosis. *Journal of Speech and Hearing Research*, 36, 1134–1144.

Acquired childhood speech-language disorders

12

Introduction

Childhood speech-language disorders can be divided into developmental disorders and acquired disorders (Ludlow, 1980). Developmental disorders of speech and language are those which onset prior to the emergence of language (i.e. between birth and one year of age). Consequently, children with developmental speech-language disorders have never developed speech-language abilities normally. Although it is usually presumed that primary developmental speech-language disorders are caused by the dysfunctioning of the central nervous system, in most cases they have an idiopathic origin (i.e. the cause is unknown). Developmental speech-language disorders can, however, occur secondary to conditions such as peripheral hearing loss, mental retardation, cerebral palsy, child autism, birth trauma and environmental deprivation.

Acquired speech-language disorders, on the other hand, are disturbances in speech-language function that result from some form of cerebral insult after language acquisition has already commenced (Hecaen, 1976). The cerebral insult, in turn, can result from a variety of aetiologies, including head trauma, brain tumours, cerebrovascular accidents, infections, convulsive disorders (intractable epilepsy) and electroencephalographic abnormalities (Miller *et al.*, 1984). Typically, these children have commenced learning language normally and were acquiring developmental milestones at an appropriate rate prior to injury.

Of the two types of childhood speech-language disorders, the acquired variety most closely resembles the acquired adult communicative disorders discussed in earlier chapters. Despite this, the application of adult criteria and classifications to acquired speech-language disorders in children is problematic. It is important to remember that children, depending on age, are either beginning to develop or still developing speech and language concurrent with damage to the central nervous system. Consequently, interactions between the acquired and developmental mechanisms of motor speech-language disorders in children may complicate the use and application of adult classifications in the paediatric population (Murdoch and Hudson-Tennent, 1994a). Currently, the impact of a congenital or acquired central nervous system lesion on the developmental continuum of speech and language is unknown.

The difference in potential for the central nervous system to recover from, or compensate for, brain injury exhibited by children and adults is also a significant factor that limits the application of adult criteria to childhood speech-language disorders. Specifically, the potential of the central nervous system to recover from brain trauma sustained at a young age has often been reported as favourable relative to the recovery expected following brain damage in adults. It is also possible that the relationship between site of lesion and type of speech and/or language impairment determined in adults will not be readily applicable to the developing central nervous system.

Although for many decades attempts were made to categorize acquired childhood aphasia using adult aphasia classification systems (e.g. Goodglass and Kaplan, 1972), these attempts largely failed. The mere intention to compare language impairment in children to that exhibited by adults violates the nature of the developing brain and does not take into account the most essential variables and features that determine the latter. The developing brain displays progressive and regressive events during which axons, dendrites, synapses and neurones show exuberant growth and major loss leading to a remodelling of neural circuitry (wiring). This period of remodelling is hypothesized to be a time during which environmental factors can have a major impact on cortical organization. Different neural systems and associated capabilities are affected by environmental input at highly variable periods, supporting the idea that they develop along distinct time courses (Maurer and Lewis, 1998). Hence, differences in the rate of differentiation and degree of specialization are apparent within language as well. For example, aspects of semantic and grammatical processing differ markedly in the degree to which they depend on language input. Specifically, grammatical processing appears more vulnerable to delays in language experience compared to semantics (Neville and Bavelier, 2000). However, it is not only developmental plasticity that distinguishes an infant's brain but also the form of plasticity these brains exhibit in response to brain damage in the course of recovery that is significantly higher in the paediatric population.

In particular, there appear to be two major differences between acquired aphasia in children and aphasia in adults. First, the recovery process is described as being more rapid and complete in children (Lenneberg, 1967). Second, in the majority of cases, acquired childhood aphasia is predominantly non-fluent, its major features being mutism and lack of spontaneity of speech (Alajouanine and Lhermitte, 1965; Hecaen, 1976; Fletcher and Taylor, 1984). Further, with some rare exceptions, the acquired aphasia in children does not appear to fall into clear-cut syndromes evocative of the well-known aphasia subtypes described in adults (see Chapter 2).

The most commonly used system for the classification of the dysarthrias, at least with respect to adult disorders, has been that devised by Darley, Aronson and Brown (1975). Their system, also known as the Mayo Clinic classification system identifies six different types of dysarthria (flaccid, spastic, hypokinetic, hyperkinetic, ataxic, mixed dysarthria) which presumably reflect underlying pathophysiology (i.e. spasticity, weakness, etc.) and correlates with the site of the lesion in the nervous system. Whether this same system can be used for the developing central nervous system, however, is still debateable. Some studies have reported an inconclusive relationship between the site and features of paediatric dysarthria (Bak, van Dongen and Arts, 1983). Investigations that have attempted to compare the features of paediatric dysarthria following damage to the cerebellum and brainstem with those of adult dysarthric speakers with damage to the same areas have also been equivocal. Comparisons between the deviant speech characteristics identified for adults and children with acquired dysarthrias have revealed some overlap, but differences have also been evident that require further investigation (Murdoch and Hudson-Tennent, 1994a). Unfortunately, currently there is a paucity of literature available that provides a clear description of the nature and course of specific forms of childhood dysarthria. Consequently, until such time as empirical speech data are available to enable derivation of a classification system specific to childhood dysarthria, it would seem appropriate that a system of classification, such as the Mayo Clinic system, be used to define dysarthria in children in the same way it is used to define the equivalent speech disorders in adults.

Many texts on speech-language disorders published previously have paid only scant attention to acquired speech-language disorders in childhood. This chapter will review acquired childhood speech-language disorders in terms of their aetiology and clinical features.

Acquired childhood aphasia

More than a century after the first descriptions of acquired aphasia in children was reported in the late 1800s (Cotard, 1868, cited in Guttmann, 1942; Bernhardt, 1885; Freud, 1897), little conclusive information is available to help clinicians in the management of the cases they may find in their caseloads. Little also is understood about the linguistic pathology from which to derive the most effective and efficient treatment strategies. From the limited number of studies reported in the literature, a traditional description of childhood acquired aphasia has emerged. In the past, it has often been stated that acquired childhood aphasia is rare; however, when it does occur it is characterized by an initial period of mutism followed by a non-fluent, motor type of language impairment with no accompanying comprehension deficit or other features of a fluent type of aphasia (e.g. jargon, logorrhea, paraphasia). In addition, acquired childhood aphasia was usually regarded as being transitory in nature, with affected individuals making a good recovery.

In recent years, many of these earlier held views of acquired childhood aphasia have been challenged. For instance, although acquired childhood aphasia appears to be predominantly that of a non-fluent aphasia, this pattern of language disturbance is by no means invariant and fluent aphasia does occur in some cases. Further, acquired childhood aphasia is not as rare as previously thought and, despite the rapid recovery seen in some cases, 25–50% of children who develop acquired aphasia still have aphasic symptoms in the longer term. It is to these children we will now turn our attention.

Clinical features of acquired childhood aphasia

Although there is some variation between reports in the literature, the symptoms most reported in the classical studies to be characteristic of acquired childhood aphasia include: initial mutism (suppression of spontaneous speech), followed by a period of reduced speech initiative; a non-fluent speech output; simplified syntax (telegraphic expression); impaired auditory comprehension abilities (particularly in the early stages post onset) and impairment in naming; dysarthria; and disturbances in reading and writing (primarily in the acute stage post onset). Most authors suggest that fluent aphasia and receptive disorders of oral speech such as literal and verbal paraphasic errors, logorrhea and perseverations are only rarely found in children with acquired aphasia. There is, however, evidence to suggest that the age of the child has a role to play in determining whether these symptoms occur in a particular case. Some authors are of the opinion that the primarily non-fluent pattern of aphasia is only prevalent in children who are less than 10 years of age at the onset of the aphasia (Poetzl, 1926; Guttmann, 1942; Alajouanine and Lhermitte, 1965). For example, Alajouanine and Lhermitte (1965) found that the predominant features of the acquired aphasia demonstrated by children at <10 years of age included: decreased auditory comprehension; severe writing deficit and no logorrhea, paraphasias or perseveration. These same authors, however, reported that the acquired aphasia demonstrated by children >10 years of age is a more fluent form of aphasia, with paraphasia present, less frequent articulatory and phonetic disintegration and disturbed written language. Other authors, however, are of the opinion that the non-fluent type of aphasia is the pattern present in older children as well as the younger ones (Basser, 1962; Benson, 1972; Assal and Campiche, 1973; Hecaen, 1976). In recent years, the classic descriptions of acquired childhood aphasia have been questioned by the findings of studies that have shown that a fluent aphasia with paraphasias may be exhibited by children in the early stages post onset. In this chapter, the features of acquired childhood aphasias as described in the classic studies will be outlined first and the findings of more recent studies discussed later.

Classic descriptions of acquired childhood aphasia

Since the first reports of acquired childhood aphasia (Bernhardt, 1885; Freud, 1897), the condition has largely been regarded as being characterized by aphasia of the non-fluent type. Indeed, most contemporary authors describe non-fluency as the most prevailing clinical feature of acquired aphasia in children (Satz and Bullard-Bates, 1981; Carrow-Woolfolk and Lynch, 1982). Even those children with focal lesions involving the posterior language centre exhibit fluent aphasia less frequently than adults with similar lesions do.

A reduction in all expressive activities, including oral, written and gestural, has been reported to occur in children with acquired aphasia (Alajouanine and Lhermitte, 1965). Certainly, mutism is a frequently reported early symptom of acquired childhood aphasia. When present, the period of suppressed spontaneous speech may last from a few days to months. Hecaen (1983) carried out a retrospective study involving 56 acquired aphasia children ranging from 3.5 to 15 years of age, with brain lesions resulting from a variety of aetiologies, including trauma, tumour and haematoma. Hecaen found mutism to be the predominant clinical symptom in the initial stage post onset, occurring in 47% of his acquired child aphasics. When analysed according to lesion type, however, Hecaen found that only 20% of cases with progressive brain lesions (e.g. tumours) exhibited an initial mutism, while 85% of acute head trauma patients demonstrated this symptom in the early stages post onset. Further, the findings of Hecaen's study showed that mutism was exhibited more frequently by children with frontal rolandic lesions (63%) than children with temporal lesions (10%).

Following the period of mutism when speech returns, there is often a period during which the aphasic child is unwilling to speak (Guttmann, 1942; Alajouanine and Lhermitte, 1965). This period has also been described as representing a loss or reduction of 'speech initiative' (Hecaen, 1976, 1983). Increased incentives and encouragements are required in this period to get the child to produce even the few words they are capable of producing.

Alajouanine and Lhermitte (1965) offered a purely psychological reason for the presence of mutism in children with acquired aphasia. They proposed that the suppression of spontaneous speech might be the result of a psychological reaction experienced by the children in response to their inability to communicate. Alajouanine and Lhermitte (1965) noted that children tend to isolation, refusal and silence in response to conflict or difficulties. Further, these authors also observed that the unwillingness of aphasic children to speak after speech returns is similar to the behaviour of normal children when faced with a difficult problem they cannot solve and wish to put aside.

Although a number of authors have reported that children with acquired aphasia exhibit telegraphic expression or simplified syntax (Bernhardt, 1885; Guttmann, 1942; Alajouanine and Lhermitte, 1965), few have described the spoken syntax of these children in detail. Aram, Ekelman and Whitaker (1986) examined the spontaneous spoken syntax of 16 children with acquired cerebral lesions to either the left or the right hemisphere and compared it to that of a group of appropriately matched control subjects. These workers found that children with unilateral left hemisphere lesions performed less well on most measures of spoken syntax (including both simple and complex sentence structure) than the control subjects. Specifically, children with left cerebral lesions had a shorter mean length of utterance, lower developmental sentence scores, lower percentages of total sentences correct, a smaller number of main verbs and interrogative reversals, fewer sentences containing conjunctions or embedded clauses and produced a greater percentage of complex sentences in error compared to the children in the control group. On the other hand, the syntactic limitations of children with right cerebral lesions were limited primarily to errors on simple sentence measures and were far less pervasive than the syntactic errors observed in the children with left hemisphere lesions. They had a shorter mean length of utterance, produced more simple sentences in error and produced developmentally earlier negatives than the control subjects did.

Although there is general agreement that expressive language problems are common in acquired childhood aphasia, there has been considerable debate over the years concerning the presence of deficits in auditory comprehension in this group of children. By far the majority of early researchers in this field considered impairments in auditory comprehension a rare occurrence in children with acquired aphasia (Bernhardt, 1885; Guttmann, 1942). Alajouanine and Lhermitte (1965) reported the presence of auditory comprehension deficits in about one-third of their acquired childhood aphasia cases. It has been suggested by Hecaen (1976, 1983) that, when present, disturbances in auditory comprehension occur almost exclusively in the early stages post onset of aphasia and disappear rapidly and virtually completely. Consequently, as different authors may have examined children with acquired aphasia at different stages post onset, this may account for the variability relating to the presence of impaired auditory comprehension abilities in childhood acquired aphasics reported in the literature. Further confusion arises when patient age considerations are taken into account. In some studies, auditory comprehension problems have been reported to be rare in child acquired aphasics <10 years of age (Guttmann, 1942; Basser 1962; Assal and Campiche, 1973).

Diminished verbal stock or an impoverished lexicon is another commonly reported symptom of acquired childhood aphasia (Bernhardt, 1885; Alajouanine and Lhermitte, 1965; Collignon, Hecaen and Angerlerques, 1968). This was noted by Hecaen (1983) to occur in the late stages. He reported that 44% of his sample of acquired childhood aphasics had naming problems (not of a paraphasic type), which tended to persist. In fact, Hecaen observed that naming problems are commonly present when the child returns to school and consequently is often mentioned explicitly in their school reports.

Hesitations have also been noted in the speech of children with acquired aphasia by various authors (e.g. Bernhardt, 1885; Guttmann, 1942). It is possible that these either are the result of the dysarthria sometimes being reported as present in these children (Guttmann, 1942: Hecaen, 1976, 1983) or, alternatively, reflect the word-finding problems also reported to occur in this population. Hecaen (1983) listed dysarthria as a common finding in association with acquired childhood aphasia, 52% of his 56 subjects exhibiting a dysarthric disturbance. According to Hecaen, the factor having the greatest influence in determining the occurrence of dysarthria is the localization of the underlying lesion. Hecaen reported that 81% of children with anterior lesions exhibited a dysarthria as part of their aphasic disturbance, while only 20% of cases with temporal lesions exhibited a dysarthria. Alajouanine and Lhermitte (1965) found dysarthria with paralytic and dystonic features (see Chapter 10) in 22 out of their total of 32 cases.

A disorder vaguely referred to as a 'reading problem' is often included by authors in the list of symptoms they regard as characteristic of acquired childhood aphasia. Alajouanine and Lhermitte (1965), for instance, reported the presence of a 'reading problem' in 18 out of the 32 children with acquired aphasia in their study. Unfortunately, however, in the majority of studies reported in the literature there has been no attempt made to define the nature of the observed reading disturbance in any further detail other than to merely document its presence. Most authors, for instance, give no indication as to the relative effects of the condition on the children's ability to read aloud versus their ability to read for comprehension. It is possible that the general lack of differentiation in most descriptions of the reading abilities of children with acquired aphasia may be due to the fact that reading disorders, although common in the acute stage post onset, in most cases disappear rapidly and completely (Hecaen, 1976, 1983).

A writing deficit is also a commonly reported feature of acquired childhood aphasia (Branco-LeFèvre, 1950; Alajouanine and Lhermitte, 1965; Hecaen, 1976, 1983). Alajouanine and Lhermitte (1965) noted that the written language of all 32 of their child subjects with acquired aphasia was disturbed, there being a severe disorder in spontaneous writing, writing to dictation and copying in over half their subjects. In 25% of their cases, copied writing only was possible. Dysorthographia (the misspellings often being based on phonetic disturbances) was also observed in the spontaneous writing and writing to dictation of a number (five out of 32) of their acquired aphasic cases. Hecaen (1976) described the writing disorder observed in his subjects as one of the most frequent, most persistent and most variable of all the symptoms of acquired childhood aphasia.

Contemporary descriptions of acquired childhood aphasia

Although, based on descriptions contained in 'landmark' studies such as those conducted by Bernhardt (1885), Guttmann (1942); Alajouanine and Lhermitte (1965), Gloning and Hift (1970) and Hecaen (1976), acquired childhood aphasia, has over past years been generally regarded as being of a non-fluent type, a number of later publications have documented the occurrence of an initial fluent aphasia in children with neurological impairment (Visch-Brink and van de Sandt-Koenderman, 1984; van Dongen, Loonen and van Dongen, 1985; Van Hout, Evrard and Lyon, 1985; Van Hout and Lyon, 1986). In addition, although the majority of 'landmark' studies also stressed the absence or rarity of receptive speech disorders such as paraphasias, logorrhea and perseveration, especially in children under 10 years of age, more recent reports in the literature have documented the occurrence of these features in the spontaneous speech and test responses of children with acquired aphasia. Consequently, although the rarity of paraphasic errors and logorrhea was once thought to illustrate the unique character of acquired childhood aphasia compared to adult aphasia, the findings of recent studies suggest a need to reappraise the traditional concept of the clinical features of acquired aphasia in children.

As pointed out by Visch-Brink and van de Sandt-Koenderman (1984), the term 'rarity' when used to describe the presence of paraphasias in cases of acquired childhood aphasia appears to be used somewhat loosely in the literature.

Alajouanine and Lhermitte (1965), who stressed the 'rarity' of paraphasias, actually observed paraphasic errors in the spontaneous speech of seven out of the 32 children with acquired aphasia in their study. Likewise, Gloning and Hift (1970) observed paraphasias in the spontaneous speech of four out of eight of their acquired aphasic children. Included among Guttmann's (1942) subjects were four cases described extensively, two cases of whom produced paraphasias (one child for at least a year post-onset).

Visch-Brink and van de Sandt-Koenderman (1984) found that, of the 14 children with acquired aphasia they studied, the spontaneous speech of eight was marked by the occurrence of paraphasias: four of these children were reported in detail, with their aphasia classified according to type (fluent/non-fluent/mixed) and their paraphasic errors categorized as literal, verbal and neologism. They concluded that in no sense of the word could paraphasias be regarded as rare in their sample of children with acquired aphasia since over half of the children produced paraphasias in their spontaneous speech and a single child could produce many paraphasias. Moreover, paraphasias occurred in all forms of aphasia including fluent, non-fluent and mixed aphasias.

Van Hout, Evrard and Lyon (1985) examined from onset of aphasia or emergence from coma 16 children with acquired aphasia, 11 of whom (ranging in age from four to 10.8 years) presented with 'non-classic' symptoms. These authors also found paraphasias in the language output of the children once speech reappeared after a period of initial mutism. Indeed, Van Hout, Evrard and Lyon (1985) suggested that paraphasias are the rule rather than the exception in acquired childhood aphasia. Furthermore, in half of the cases they studied, paraphasic errors were not limited only to the acute stage post onset. They divided their subjects into three groups according to the evolution of paraphasias over time. In one group the paraphasic errors resolved within a few days, in the second group paraphasia resolved in a few months and in the third group paraphasia was still present at greater than one year post-onset.

A fluent aphasia was reported by van Dongen, Loonen and van Dongen (1985) in three of the 27 acquired aphasic children referred to their clinic over a four-year period. Their findings demonstrated that an adult-like fluent aphasia can occur in children <10 years of age, and consequently they challenged the view that acquired aphasia is always non-fluent and devoid of paraphasias. Although all three subjects with fluent aphasia had posterior lesions, van Dongen, Loonen and van Dongen (1985) emphasized that posterior lesions do not invariably result in fluent aphasia in children.

A case of Wernicke's aphasia in a 10-year-old boy resulting from herpes simplex encephalitis was described by Van Hout and Lyon (1986). The symptoms exhibited by this case were similar to those associated with Wernicke's aphasia in adults and included a severe comprehension deficit, jargon output, logorrhea and anosognosia. The recovery pattern exhibited by this case resembled the pattern described for a sensory aphasia by Buckingham and Kertesz (1974). His rapid recovery of writing skills was atypical of that usually reported for cases of acquired childhood aphasias. Thus, the case as described by Van Hout and Lyon (1986) differs considerably from the usual case of acquired childhood aphasia, where logorrhea and anosognosia are rare and writing disorders are one of the more persistent language deficits. Van Hout and Lyon (1986) attributed the Wernicke's aphasia observed in their subject to the nature of the lesion itself and not to the age of the subject. In herpes simplex encephalitis, the lesions are profoundly destructive (Barringer, 1978) and consequently this condition causes more severe lesions in the temporal lobes than are seen in other varieties of lesions which affect the brain in childhood.

Although it is not immediately clear why the clinical features of acquired childhood aphasia reported by earlier researchers (e.g. Alajouanine and Lhermitte, 1965) differ from those of subsequent workers (e.g. van Dongen, Loonen and van Dongen, 1985), several explanations have been proposed. One possible reason for the disparity could be the difference in the time post onset that the subjects were examined in the different studies. For instance, Visch-Brink and van de Sandt-Koenderman (1984) suggested that it is possible that the presence or absence of neologisms in the spontaneous speech output of children with ac-

quired aphasia might be related to the time post onset that the subjects were examined. In their study, the subjects were examined within a few days post-onset of aphasia and neologisms were recorded. On the other hand, Alajouanine and Lhermitte (1965) made their observations a number of months post-onset and did not report the presence of neologisms in the spontaneous speech of their acquired aphasic children. It is possible therefore, that by the time that Alajouanine and Lhermitte (1965) examined their subjects, a number of symptoms, including the presence of neologism, may have disappeared. Van Hout, Evrard and Lyon (1985) also suggested that the time post onset may be a factor underlying the disparity between the earlier and more recent studied in terms of whether so-called positive signs such as paraphasias, perseveration, sterotypics and so on were recorded or not. Since they observed that some positive signs persisted long after the acute stage in half of the cases they studied, Van Hout, Evrard and Lyon (1985) believed that the time post onset of the language examination does not wholly account for the difference in clinical signs described in the earlier versus more recent studies of acquired childhood aphasia.

Another possible reason for the variation in clinical features of acquired childhood aphasia reported in earlier versus more recent studies lies in the nature of the criteria used to select the aphasic subjects. In many earlier studies, subjects were only included if they had a concomitant hemiparesis or hemiplegia, as this was taken as being indicative of the presence of brain damage and hence served to delineate acquired aphasia from developmental language disorders. As pointed out by Woods and Teuber (1978), however, such a selection criterion could result in a bias towards children with anterior lesions and hence a motor-type of aphasia. It is possible, therefore, that this could explain the lack of paraphasias, logorrhea and so on reported in may earlier studies of acquired childhood aphasia.

Van Dongen, Loonen and van Dongen (1985) suggested that differences in aetiology may provide another reason for the discrepancy between reports. They believed that when the aetiology is head trauma recovery may be observed within a short time, so that the fluent characteristics of the aphasia may be either not recognized or not recorded.

Van Hout, Evrard and Lyon (1985) proposed that variations in methodology could best account for the differences between their findings and the descriptions of acquired childhood aphasia in earlier studies. As in the majority of other reports, their subjects were also reluctant to speak. If Van Hout, Evrard and Lyon (1985) had limited their study simply to a clinical examination of spontaneous speech, as many of the earlier researchers had done, they believed that positive signs such as paraphasias, logorrhea and so on would have been 'masked' by the children's lack of spontaneity or mutism. They suggested that it was the testing itself and the encouragement they provided that enabled the acquired aphasic children in their sample to overcome their unwillingness to speak and thereby produce the observed positive signs.

In summary, clinically the aphasia pattern observed in cases of acquired childhood aphasia appears in most cases to resemble that of a non-fluent aphasia. Often, there is an initial mutism followed by a period of reduced speech initiative together with a diminished lexicon, simplified syntax, hesitations and dysarthria. Disturbances in reading and writing are also common. Variations to this pattern of language disturbance, however, do exist and fluent aphasia does occur in some cases. According to Satz and Bullard-Bates (1981), it is unknown whether the variations in the manifestations of acquired childhood aphasia are related to either age/maturation mechanisms or age-independent factors such as lesion site, lesion size, aetiology, type of lesion or time post onset of assessment.

Recovery from acquired childhood aphasia

The consequences of cerebral lesions incurred in childhood are generally regarded as less serious than those incurred in adult life (Basser, 1962; Teuber, 1975). Consequently, it is generally agreed that the prognosis for recovery in acquired childhood aphasia is much better than that expected in adult aphasia (Guttmann, 1942;

Basser, 1962; Alajouanine and Lhermitte, 1965; Lenneberg, 1967). The often described complete or near-complete recovery of language function following lesions of the left cerebral hemisphere in childhood is frequently cited as being indicative of the 'plasticity' of the immature brain, whereby the non-damaged areas of the brain are capable of assuming language function. Although the mechanisms underlying compensation are not fully understood, the good recovery from acquired childhood aphasia has been attributed to processes which include the transfer of language function to the undamaged portions of the left cerebral hemisphere and/or the intact right cerebral hemisphere. Some authors (e.g. Satz and Bullard-Bates, 1981), however, suggest that the speed of recovery sometimes witnessed in children with acquired aphasia is incompatible with a transfer of language to and a learning of language by the right hemisphere.

Another proposed explanation for the often good recovery exhibited by children with acquired aphasia is that both hemispheres contain mechanisms for language and that language therefore need not be relearned in the minor hemisphere. Under normal circumstances, in the majority of children, the language mechanisms in the right hemisphere are inhibited by those in the left such that only the left hemisphere develops complex language function. According to this proposal, damage to the left hemisphere in children causes a 'release from inhibition' in the right hemisphere allowing it to assume a greater role in language function.

Although for some time it has been generally believed that the prognosis of acquired aphasia in children is good, the findings of several studies reported in the literature suggest that the recovery is not as complete as stated. In fact, there are a variety of opinions expressed in the literature concerning the prognosis of acquired aphasia in children, ranging from favourable declarations of complete recovery to more guarded predictions of only partial recovery. In describing the recovery of language function in acquired childhood aphasia, many authors make reference only to 'clinical recovery'. A number of researchers, however, have emphasized that despite apparent clinical recovery subtle but persistent language deficits may persist, even in those cases where the left hemisphere injury was acquired as early as during intrauterine life (Alajouanine and Lhermitte, 1965; Woods and Carey, 1979; Rankin, Aram and Horwitz, 1981; Vargha-Khadem, Gorman and Watters, 1985).

Satz and Bullard-Bates (1981) reviewed the literature relating to the prognosis of acquired childhood aphasia and concluded that although spontaneous recovery occurs in the majority of children with this disorder it by no means occurs in all cases. Of the cases included in the studies they reviewed, 25–50% remained unremitted by one year post-onset. Alajouanine and Lhermitte (1965) reported that 75% of their acquired aphasic subjects attained normal or near-normal language by one year post-onset. Of the eight children who had an unfavourable course in their study, six had massive lesions, one showed mental deterioration and one died. One-third of the children with acquired aphasia studied by Hecaen (1976) attained complete recovery within a period of six weeks to two years post-onset. Carrow-Woolfolk and Lynch (1982) suggested that the recovery period in cases of acquired childhood aphasia may extend up to five years. Even in those cases where recovery from aphasia occurs, however, there are often serious cognitive and academic problems which remain (Satz and Bullard-Bates, 1981). For instance, the majority of children with acquired aphasia appear to have difficulty following a normal progression through school (Hecaen, 1976; Chadwick, 1985). None of the 32 children with acquired aphasia studied by Alajouanine and Lhermitte (1965) showed normal progress in the long term. According to these authors, school subjects requiring the use of language (first language study, foreign languages, history, geography, etc.) are more difficult for these children than subjects such as mathematics.

Factors influencing recovery from acquired childhood aphasia

A number of different factors which may influence the recovery of language in acquired childhood aphasia have been identified by various authors. These factors include: the site of the lesion, the size and side of the lesion, the aetiology, the associated neurological disturbances, the age at onset, the type and severity of the aphasia and the presence of electroencephalographic abnormalities. As pointed out by van Dongen and Loonen (1977), however, the wide diversity of aetiologies, the severities of aphasia and the length of follow-up reported in the various studies of acquired childhood aphasia make it difficult to work out which of the factors are the most important in determining the final outcome of the aphasia. According to Satz and Bullard-Bates (1981), our current knowledge is inadequate for determining which factors assist and which factors impede recovery.

Influence of age at onset. The prognostic factor that has perhaps received the greatest attention in the literature is the age at onset. Lenneberg (1967) stated that the prognosis of acquired aphasia in children is directly related to the age at onset of aphasia and that any aphasia incurred after the age of puberty does not remit entirely. Various authors agree that there are considerable differences in prognosis with age. Penfield (1965) claimed that in children aged <10 years with acquired aphasia, there is a good chance of the reacquisition of lost verbal skills within one year, although such recovery may occur at the expense of other non-verbal skills. In support of this claim, Carrow-Woolfolk and Lynch (1982) suggested that children younger than three years of age with cerebral lesions follow normal language acquisition after an initial pause of all language development. Vargha-Khadem, Gorman and Watters (1985) found that as the age of aphasia onset increases (at least in children > five years old), the language impairment becomes progressively worse. Ten years of age is considered by many authors the upper limit for complete language recovery (Oelschlaeger and Scarborough, 1976), cerebral lesions incurred after this time causing a persistent language deficit. There is an unconfirmed premise that cerebral plasticity is lost by the age of 10 years as a result of the development of cerebral dominance or laterized specialization of language function.

Despite the support provided by the above studies that age at onset is an important prognostic determinant in acquired childhood aphasia, not all authors have been able to find a relationship between the age at aphasia onset and recovery. Further, a number of reports in the literature actually contradict the information provided by the more supportive studies outlined above. For instance, Hecaen (1976) described three cases of children with acquired aphasia with onset at 14 years of age who showed excellent recovery patterns. Although Alajouanine and Lhermitte (1965) reported a difference in the symptomatology between children with acquired aphasia <10 years and aphasic children >10 years of age, they found no significant difference in the speed of recovery between these two age groups. Likewise, Van Hout, Evrard and Lyon (1985) found no direct relationship between the age at onset and the rate of disappearance of paraphasias in children with acquired aphasia. With such conflicting empirical data, it is obvious that as yet the relationship between age at onset and recovery in acquired childhood aphasia is uncertain.

Influence of type and severity of aphasia. With regard to the type of aphasia, Guttmann (1942) emphasized the good prognosis of a purely motor aphasia, especially in young children. Van Dongen and Loonen (1977) also found the type of aphasia exhibited in the acute stage post onset to be of prognostic significance. They reported that five out of the six children with an initial amnestic aphasia recovered from aphasia, but only one of the seven children with mixed aphasia showed recovery. The findings of van Dongen and Loonen (1977) lend support to an earlier claim by Assal and Campiche (1973) that mixed aphasia has a poor prognosis. Van Dongen and Loonen (1977) also found a significant relationship between the severity of the comprehension deficit at the onset of acquired childhood aphasia and a poor recovery from aphasia.

Influence of aetiology. No systematic studies relating aetiology to recovery from acquired childhood aphasia have been reported in the literature. Guttmann (1942), however, reported that children with head trauma improve more than those with vascular disease. Likewise, van Dongen and Loonen (1977) also found that most children with traumatic aphasia recovered completely. Infection (e.g. encephalitis) was found to

be more frequent in children with the most severe aphasia and persistent paraphasias by Van Hout, Evrard and Lyon (1985). A number of authors, including Mantovani and Landau (1980) have suggested that the prognosis for recovery from acquired aphasia associated with convulsive disorder is much worse than for other acquired childhood aphasias.

Influence of extent and side of lesion. The findings of a number of studies have suggested a link between the extent of the cerebral lesion and the persistence of aphasic symptoms in children with acquired aphasia (Alajouanine and Lhermitte, 1965; Hecaen, 1976, 1983). As mentioned previously, six of the eight aphasic children with unfavourable language outcomes in the study conducted by Alajouanine and Lhermitte (1965) had extensive cerebral lesions, suggesting that the larger the cerebral lesion the poorer the prognosis for recovery. Hecaen (1983) found bilateral lesions frequently linked with persistent aphasic symptoms. Van Hout, Evrard and Lyon (1985) also concluded that bilateral lesions may negatively influence the outcome of the language disturbance in acquired childhood aphasia based on their findings that the aphasic children with the most persistent paraphasias and who exhibited the most severe aphasic disorder in their sample all had bilateral brain lesions. Other authors, including Collignon, Hecaen and Angerlerques (1968) and Gloning and Hift (1970) have also stressed that severe bilateral lesions are indicative of a poor prognosis for recovery in acquired childhood aphasia.

Based primarily on the findings of studies published prior to the 1940s, it was for many years considered that there was a higher incidence of aphasia following right cerebral lesions in children than in adults. This belief led to the formulation of the 'equipotentiality' hypothesis, which states that at birth each cerebral hemisphere has the same potential to develop language function and that the lateralization of language and the development of cerebral dominance occurs as the child matures (Lenneberg, 1967). Subsequent studies, however, have shown that the frequency of aphasia from right cerebral hemisphere lesions in right-handed children is similar to that in right-handed adults (Satz and Bullard-Bates, 1981; Carter, Hohenegger and Satz, 1982). Satz and Bullard-Bates (1981) stated that, after infancy, the risk of aphasia is significantly greater following left-brain damage than right-brain injury regardless of the age of the individual. Furthermore, crossed aphasia (i.e. aphasia occurring after right hemisphere damage in right-handed individuals) is rare in both adults and children, particularly after 3–5 years of age and perhaps earlier. Woods and Teuber (1978) suggested that in the studies carried out earlier than the 1940s, prior to the widespread use of antibiotics, there may have been biased estimations relating to the handedness distribution of subjects with acquired aphasia in that, in the cases observed, there may have been undetected bilateral brain damage caused by infections.

In addition to the extent and side of lesion, it has also been suggested by several authors that the localization of the cerebral lesion influences recovery from acquired childhood aphasia. Van Hout, Evrard and Lyon (1985) suggested that the localization of the lesion is a more important prognostic variable than the extent of the lesion. Alajouanine and Lhermitte (1965) also indicated that recovery from acquired aphasia in children is dependent upon the site as well as the extent and reversibility of the lesion. It should be noted, however, that although these latter authors suggested a link between lesion localization and recovery they did not provide any specific examples of how the site of the cerebral damage influences the prognosis for recovery. Although Hecaen (1983) found that all language symptoms, including auditory and written comprehension, were more disturbed following anterior than following temporal lesions in children, he did not list the site of lesion as a factor involved in the determination of the outcome of the aphasic disturbance.

Influence of the presence of encephalographic abnormalities. The relationship between changes in the electroencephalographic pattern and recovery in children with acquired aphasia is controversial. Some authors have reported that recovery correlates with a disappearance of abnormalities in the electroencephalographic trace, while others have been unable to find any link

between these two factors. Shoumaker *et al.* (1974) found that improved language abilities in children with acquired aphasia associated with convulsive disorder corresponded with an improvement in the electroencephalographic pattern. Likewise, van Dongen and Loonen (1977) found that recovery of language function in a group of children with acquired aphasia resulting from a variety of aetiologies (including convulsive disorder) was associated with a reduction in electroencephalographic abnormalities. Other authors, however, including Gascon *et al.* (1973) and McKinney and McGreal (1974), were unable to demonstrate a correlation between improved electroencephalographic patterns and improved language. Of the 24 children with acquired aphasia who were reported to have recovered in the study conducted by Alajouanine and Lhermitte (1965), 16 still suffered severe motor sequelae and electroencephalographic disturbances. Alajouanine and Lhermitte (1965) interpreted this finding as an indication that recovery does not result from the reversibility of the lesion.

Influence of concomitant neurological disturbances. Concomitant neurological disturbances represent another variable that has been implicated as a factor which influences recovery from acquired childhood aphasia. As in the case of the prognostic variables discussed above, however, the findings reported in the literature relating to the importance of associated neurological signs as a prognostic indicator in children with acquired aphasia tend to be contradictory. Lange-Cosack and Tepfner (1973) reported that there is minimal or no recovery in traumatic aphasic subjects who have suffered coma for more than seven days. On the other hand, Hecaen (1976) questioned the importance of coma as a prognostic indicator in cases of acquired childhood aphasia, he being unable to demonstrate a clear relationship between the occurrence and duration of coma and the severity and persistence of the language deficit.

In summary, although a number of different factors have been suggested as having prognostic significance in acquired childhood aphasia, currently there is an insufficient amount of information available to determine which of these factors are unequivocally favourable or unfavourable for recovery.

Acquired childhood aphasia of different aetiologies

The general clinical features of acquired childhood aphasia described previously are largely based on the findings of studies which have included aphasic children with a variety of underlying aetiologies, including trauma, vascular lesions, tumours, infections and convulsive disorder. As well as influencing the prognosis for recovery of language function in cases of acquired childhood aphasia, there is some evidence that the aetiology also has an important influence on the type of aphasia that is exhibited. It is no longer possible to assume that the effects of slow-onset lesions (e.g. tumours) on language are the same as those of rapid-onset lesions (e.g. cerebrovascular accidents and head trauma). Further, children who have suffered traumatic head injuries characteristically exhibit expressive language deficits and typically show good recovery. In cases of acquired childhood aphasia following vascular lesions, the prognosis for recovery is poorer and the aphasic symptoms more variable and more persistent (Guttmann, 1942; van Dongen and Loonen, 1977). In addition, although acquired childhood aphasia can be caused by a similar range of disorders of the nervous system as adult aphasia, the relative importance of each of the different causes to the occurrence of language disturbances in children differs from the situation seen in adults. For instance, although in peacetime cerebrovascular accidents are the most common cause of aphasia in adults, the most common cause of acquired childhood aphasia is traumatic brain injury. Consequently, instead of describing the linguistic skills of groups of children with acquired aphasia resulting from different causes, as has occurred in the past, there is a need to examine the clinical features of the acquired childhood aphasia associated with each aetiology separately.

Acquired childhood aphasia following vascular disorders

Cerebrovascular disorders constitute a much smaller proportion of the neurological diseases of childhood than they do of adulthood. However, they occur more frequently than generally thought and are a significant cause of morbidity and mortality in the childhood population. The incidence of cerebrovascular accidents in children has been estimated as 2.6 per 100 000 of the population.

Virtually all the diseases of blood vessels which affect adults may at some time also occur in children (Bickerstaff, 1972; Salam-Adams and Adams, 1988). Despite this, the causes of vascular diseases of the brain in children differ from those in adults. For instance, degenerative disorders such as atherosclerosis affect primarily the middle-aged and elderly and are rare in childhood (Moosy, 1959). Some vascular diseases of the brain, such as embolism arising from subacute or acute bacterial endocardial valvular disease, occur at all ages, while others, such as vascular disorders associated with congenital heart disease, are peculiar to childhood.

'Acute hemiplegia of childhood' is a term used by many paediatricians and neurologists to describe the sudden onset of hemiplegia in children. A wide variety of vascular diseases of the brain, including both occlusive and haemorrhagic disorders, have been described under this heading.

Idiopathic childhood hemiplegia. The most commonly reported and dramatic syndrome resulting from an ischaemic stroke in childhood is idiopathic childhood hemiplegia. This syndrome involves the sudden onset of hemiplegia as a result of a unilateral brain infarct of unknown origin and can affect children from a few months of age up to 12 years of age (Bickerstaff, 1972). According to Bickerstaff (1972), females are affected more than males in a ratio of about 3 : 2.

The cause of idiopathic childhood hemiplegia has been argued for many years and a variety of possible causes have been proposed, including: polioencephalitis (Strumpell, 1884), encephalitis (Adams, Cammermeyer and Denny-Brown, 1949; Bernheim, 1956; Brandt, 1962), venous thrombosis (Bernheim, 1956; Brandt, 1962; Norman, 1962), demyelination (Wyllie, 1948), epilepsy (Norman, 1962) and occlusion of the internal carotid artery (Duffy *et al.*, 1957; Goldstein and Burgess, 1958; Bickerstaff, 1964). Although there appears to be some agreement that arterial occlusion is the most common cause of idiopathic childhood hemiplegia, the reason for the occlusion is less certain. For reasons indicated above, atheroma cannot be implicated in childhood. Studies using carotid angiograms have demonstrated the presence of thrombosis of either the common or the internal carotid arteries in some cases of idiopathic childhood hemiplegia (Salam-Adams and Adams, 1988). Bickerstaff (1964) suggested that roughening of the wall of the internal carotid artery as a result of arteritis secondary to throat, tonsillar or cervical gland infection might be the causal factor in some instances. Further, in some reported cases neither angiography nor post-mortem examination was able to demonstrate the presence of vascular lesions, suggesting that in these cases an embolus may have temporarily blocked a cerebral artery and then later broken up before the angiogram was taken or the post-mortem performed (Salam-Adams and Adams, 1988).

Other vascular occlusive disorders in childhood. A number of other vascular occlusive disorders peculiar to childhood can also cause ischaemic strokes in children. These disorders include: vascular disease associated with congenital heart disease, arteritis (inflammation of an artery) of various types, sickle cell anaemia, vascular occlusion associated with irradiation of the base of the brain, moyamoya and strokes associated with homocystinuria and Fabry's angiokeratosis.

Ischaemic strokes associated with congenital heart disease occur most frequently in the first two years of life, corresponding to the stage when congenital heart disease has its greatest frequency (six per 1000 live births) (Salam-Adams and Adams, 1988). Banker (1961) reported that of the childhood cerebrovascular accident cases examined by him, 28% were associated with congenital heart disease, making it the single most common cause of cerebrovascular accidents in his study.

Various type of arteritis, including that associated with lupus erythematosus and occurring secondary to infections in the tonsillar fossa and lymph glands in the neck, have been reported to cause ischaemic stroke in children (Bickerstaff, 1964; Davie and Cox, 1967; Salam-Adams and Adams, 1988). Lupus erythematosus is a diffuse inflammatory disease that involves the kidneys, skin, haematological system, the central nervous system and occasionally the liver. It is more common in females than males with a ratio of about 10 : 1. Although the average onset is around 30 years of age, symptoms can occur in the first decade of life (Bell and Lastimosa, 1980). Neurological complications have been reported to occur in up to 75% of patients (Tindall, 1980), with seizures being the most common single neurological symptom. Hemiplegia secondary to cerebral arteritis, which is either transitory or permanent, occurs in approximately 5% of patients with lupus erythematosus. If permanent neurological loss occurs, it is correlated with obstruction of one of the major extracranial or intracranial blood vessels. A case of lymphadenitis (inflammation of the lymph nodes) in the region of the carotid bifurcation and extending to involve the artery was described by Schnüriger (1966, cited in Bickerstaff, 1972). Bickerstaff (1972) reported damage to the carotid artery near its passage past the tonsillar fossa, possibly resulting from arteritis due to a throat infection.

Both arterial and venous occlusions leading to cerebral infarction have been observed in children with sickle cell disease, an inherited blood disorder occurring primarily in persons of African origin (Salam-Adams and Adams, 1988). Likewise, cerebral infarcts have been reported subsequent to cobalt radiation of the base of the brain for treatment of a variety of neoplastic disorders in children, including craniopharyngiomas and pituitary adenomas.

Another vascular disorder of childhood that may cause vascular occlusion of the internal carotid artery is moyamoya disease. Patients with this condition present with headache, seizures, stroke-like episodes, visual symptoms and mental retardation as well as, in some cases, a movement disorder, a gait disturbance and/or a speech deficit. Typically, the symptoms are bihemispheric. Moyamoya disease is characterized by the presence of a network of fine anastomotic blood vessels at the base of the brain called a rete mirabile. The aetiology of moyamoya disease is uncertain. There have been some suggestions that the condition is a congenital disorder involving retention of the embryonal rete mirabile. Alternatively, the network of anastomoses may be the consequence of an acquired disorder involving occlusion of the carotid arteries. It is possible, therefore, that several types of arterial disease in childhood may lead to moyamoya.

Complications of certain hereditary metabolic diseases may also occasionally cause occlusive vascular disease in children. Two such conditions where this may occur include homocystinuria and Fabry's disease. Both of these conditions result from enzyme deficiencies and both, amongst other effects, may cause structural damage to the blood vessels, leading to thrombosis. Homocystinuria, resulting from a lack of cystathionine-synthetase, manifests as mental retardation. Ischaemic strokes arising from either arterial or venous thrombosis may be experienced by persons with this disorder in late childhood, adolescence or adult life. Likewise, Fabry's disease, a sex-linked disorder affecting males and resulting from a deficiency in galactosyl hydrolase, may also cause structural changes in the blood vessels, leading to thrombosis and stroke (Adams and Lyon, 1982).

Brain haemorrhage in childhood. Spontaneous intracranial haemorrhage is much less common in children than in adults. Two major types of cerebral haemorrhage occur in childhood: one type occurring secondary to haematological diseases such as leukaemia, sickle cell disease, haemophilia and thrombocytopenic purpura, the second type occurring secondary to vascular abnormalities such as arteriovenous malformations. It is noteworthy that haemorrhage resulting from rupture of saccular (berry) aneurysms is rare in childhood (Bickerstaff, 1972). In addition, the majority of arteriovenous malformations manifest as brain haemorrhage or in some other way during the third decade of life. Only approximately 10% of arteriovenous malformations cause haemorrhage or other problems in childhood.

Few studies of acquired aphasia occurring secondary to vascular disorders in children have been reported in the literature. Those studies that have been published, however, suggest that the pattern of language symptoms is similar to that seen in cases of adult aphasia of vascular origin (Dennis, 1980; Aram *et al.*, 1983). Aram *et al.* (1983) documented the course of acquired apha-

sia following a vascular lesion in the putamen, anterior limb of the internal capsule and lateral portion of the head of the caudate nucleus in the left hemisphere of a right-handed seven-year-old girl. These workers reported that symptoms were similar to those listed for adult aphasics with equivalent subcortical lesions, the child exhibiting a right-sided hemiplegia, mutism, oral apraxia and a comprehension deficit but no dysarthria. At six months post-onset, the only persisting problems were a mild hemiparesis and minor spelling difficulties. Dennis (1980) noted a significant degree of both expressive and receptive aphasia in a nine-year-old girl following an infarct of vascular origin in the left temporal parietal region.

In addition to the two single case studies mentioned above, a number of cases of acquired childhood aphasia resulting from vascular lesions have also been described as a part of some studies which have included children with acquired aphasia resulting from a variety of aetiologies (e.g. Hecaen, 1983). Hecaen (1983) noted that all six children in his sample with a vascular aetiology exhibited aphasia. He reported that the most frequent language symptom exhibited by these children was a writing disorder. The next most frequent symptoms were mutism, articulatory disorders and naming disorders. Auditory comprehension deficits were present in half of these cases, while paraphasias and reading disorders were exhibited by only two out of the six children.

Overall, the lack of studies dealing specifically with acquired childhood aphasia following vascular disorder means that little is known about the prognosis for recovery from acquired aphasia in children with vascular origin. Guttmann (1942) and van Dongen and Loonen (1977), however, have reported that children with acquired aphasia of vascular origin recover language less well than those with aphasia resulting from traumatic head injuries do.

Acquired childhood aphasia following traumatic brain injury

Traumatic brain injury (TBI) is the leading cause of death and permanent disability in children and adolescents. Epidemiological studies indicate that the incidence of TBI in childhood is approximately 200 per 100 000 per year, with male children having a higher incidence of TBI than female children have in a ratio of around 1.8 : 1. Disabilities demonstrated by children who survive TBI range from persistent vegetative state through mental and physical disabilities, language disorders, academic difficulties and dysarthria. TBI is the major cause of acquired childhood aphasia.

The prognosis for recovery shown by children who have suffered mild head injuries has been reported to be excellent. Although the prognosis for recovery from severe head injuries is less certain, it is reported to be better than for adults. This difference may be the outcome of two factors. First, it may be due to the different nature of the impacts causing TBI in children versus adults and, second, it may be related to differences in the basic mechanisms of brain damage following TBI in the two groups, which in turn are related to differences in the physical characteristics of children's heads and adults' heads. The majority of instances of childhood TBI result from falls (this is particularly the case for infants and toddlers) or low-speed (30–60 km/h) pedestrian or bicycle accidents that involve a motor vehicle. Consequently, many paediatric head injuries are associated with a lesser degree of injury resulting from rotational acceleration. Adults on the other hand are more likely to sustain TBI as a result of high-speed motor vehicle accidents, which by their nature are more likely to yield greater diffuse brain injury. Road traffic accidents are considered the most common cause of long-term morbidity following TBI in childhood. Evidence is available that indicates that the type of brain injury resulting from severe head trauma depends on the physical properties of the individual's brain and skull. These physical properties are known to differ in a number of ways between children and adults, thereby contributing to different patterns of brain injury following head trauma in each group. First, an infant's brain weight is 15% of body weight progressing through to only 3% of body weight in adults. Second, the existence of unfused sutures and open fontanelles makes the skull of an infant and young child pliable, allowing a greater degree of deformation and possibly a greater ability to absorb the energy of physical

impact. (The biomechanics of TBI are discussed in Chapter 4.)

Performance on formal language tests. Contrary to the traditional view that children make a rapid and full recovery from TBI, a number of later studies have documented the existence of persistent language deficits subsequent to severe TBI in children. Gilchrist and Wilkinson (1979) reported that almost two-thirds of young people with severe TBI exhibit aphasic-type disorders. Areas of language function reported to be deficient in children following TBI include: verbal fluency (Chadwick *et al.*, 1981a,b; Slater and Bassett, 1988; Jordan, Ozanne and Murdoch, 1990), object naming (Levin and Eisenberg, 1979a,b; Jordan, Ozanne and Murdoch, 1988, 1990), word and sentence repetition (Levin and Eisenberg, 1979a,b) and written output (Ewing-Cobbs *et al.*, 1985, 1987). Unfortunately, the specific methodological approaches employed by different researchers to document the language abilities of children with TBI vary widely from study to study, making it difficult to determine the pattern of language impairment in this population. For instance, in some studies children with TBI have been included in larger groups of children with language difficulties arising from other neurological conditions (e.g. cerebrovascular accident, brain tumour, etc.), making the identification of specific areas of language impairment associated with TBI difficult (e.g. Alajouanine and Lhermitte, 1965; Hecaen, 1976). In addition whereas some earlier researchers utilized aphasia batteries (e.g. Levin and Eisenberg, 1979a,b; Ewing-Cobbs *et al.*, 1985, 1987) to assess the language abilities of children with TBI, other, later, researchers have used tests more appropriate for paediatric subjects (e.g. Jordan, Ozanne and Murdoch, 1988). The present chapter will provide a historical overview of research into the effects of childhood TBI on language abilities in an attempt to establish the status of our understanding of the nature of language impairments in this population.

The language abilities of a group of 32 children with acquired aphasia associated with a variety of aetiologies, including TBI, cerebrovascular malformation, aneurysm and occlusion of the middle cerebral artery among others, was evaluated by Alajouanine and Lhermitte (1965). They reported that the most obvious feature of the language disorder exhibited by the children in their group was a reduction in 'expressive activities', with each child demonstrating a reduction in oral and written language and a reduction in the use of gestures.

Hecaen (1976) reported the language features of a group of 26 cases of acquired childhood aphasia of mixed aetiology which included 16 cases of head trauma. The associated aphasia was described by Hecaen as being characterized by a period of mutism followed by the recovery of language, marked by decreased initiation of speech, naming disorders, dyscalculia and dysgraphia. Although less frequent, receptive language disorders were observed in one-third of the children with aphasia examined by Hecaen (1976). Owing to the wide range of aetiologies included in the subject groups examined by Alajouanine and Lhermitte (1965) and Hecaen (1976), however, any attempt to attribute the language features to any one aetiological group such as TBI must of necessity be guarded.

Performance on standard aphasia tests. The early investigations of language in groups comprising only children with TBI used standardized instruments such as aphasia batteries and tests of specific language behaviours to determine the profile of language impairment. For example, the Neurosensory Center Comprehensive Examination for Aphasia (NCCEA) (Spreen and Benton, 1969) was used by Levin and Eisenberg (1979a) to examine the language abilities of a group of children and adolescents with closed head injury. Deficits in auditory comprehension were identified in 11% of the group and verbal repetition was impaired in only 4%. Dysnomia for objects presented visually or tactually to the left hand were identified in about 12% of the group studied.

Ewing-Cobbs *et al.* (1985) also examined the language abilities of a group of children and adolescents with TBI using the NCCEA. Their findings showed that during the early stages of recovery (less than six months post-trauma) a significant proportion of their subjects demonstrated linguistic impairments. In particular, naming disorders, dysgraphia and reduced verbal

productivity were prominent. These authors concluded that the language disorder identified was evidence of a 'subclinical aphasia' rather than a frank aphasia disturbance. Ewing-Cobbs *et al.* (1985) speculated that, from a developmental perspective, the type of speech-language impairment incurred from a TBI is related to the language skills that are in primary ascendancy at the time of the injury. Further, comparison of recovery related to the severity of injury indicated that children with moderate/severe TBI were more likely to demonstrate poorer performance on the naming and graphic subtests when compared to their mildly head-injured counterparts. In a further study of 23 children and 33 adolescents with TBI, Ewing-Cobbs *et al.* (1987) identified 'clinically significant language impairment' in a large proportion of their subjects, with expressive and graphic functions most affected.

Performance on paediatric language tests. The most comprehensive series of studies to have documented the language abilities of children with TBI using tests developed for paediatric application is that reported by Jordan and colleagues (Jordan, Ozanne and Murdoch, 1988; Jordan, Cannon and Murdoch, 1992; Jordan and Murdoch, 1990a, 1993, 1994). Jordan, Ozanne and Murdoch (1988) assessed the language abilities of a group of 20 TBI children, aged between eight and 16 years of age, at least 12 months post-injury using the Test of Language Development series and the NCCEA. They found the TBI group to be mildly language-impaired when compared to the language abilities of a group of age- and sex-matched, non-neurologically impaired controls. In particular, these investigators identified the presence of a specific deficit in naming in the TBI group. The linguistic impairment exhibited by the TBI children studied by Jordan, Ozanne and Murdoch (1988), however, did not conform to any recognized developmental language disorder. Rather, it was noted by these researchers that the observed language disturbance was similar to that reported to occur following TBI in adults in that their children with TBI also presented with a 'subclinical aphasia' characterized by dysnomia. Jordan, Ozanne and Murdoch (1988) concluded that, in contrast to the traditional view that the immature brain makes a rapid and full recovery following traumatic injury, TBI in children can produce long-term and persistent language deficits. In a follow-up study of the same group of children with TBI 12 months later, Jordan and Murdoch (1990a) observed that the naming deficit had persisted while at the same time verbal fluency abilities had deteriorated.

The high level language functioning of a group of 11 children with severe TBI was assessed by Jordan, Cremona-Meteyard and King (1996). Their findings indicated that the children with severe TBI had a lesser ability to create sentences with reference to social stimuli and a reduced ability to interpret ambiguous or figurative expressions than a group of matched controls. In contrast, Jordan, Cremona-Meteyard and King noted that the children with severe TBI were similar to the control children in their ability to make inferences. Jordan, Cannon and Murdoch (1992) investigated the linguistic performance of a group of mildly head-injured children in adulthood but failed to identify any persistent linguistic deficits for this group, even in the very long term. In contrast, however, Jordan and Murdoch (1994) were able to identify late linguistic sequelae from 10 to 34 years following severe TBI sustained during childhood. Although overall scores achieved by these subjects fell within the average range on standardized tests of adolescent language development, scores were lower for the severely traumatically brain injured individuals than for controls on measures of lexical recognition and retrieval as well as auditory comprehension of grammatically complex commands. Interestingly, a generalized reduction in linguistic skills across all areas of language competence assessed (syntax, semantics, pragmatics) was noted, suggesting a lack of specificity of linguistic impairment in their sample. It would appear, therefore, that children with mild TBI may be relatively spared in terms of persistent linguistic deficits when compared to their severely traumatically brain injured counterparts, although marked variability in linguistic outcomes is evident within the severe TBI group.

In summary, contrary to the long-held view that children make a rapid and full recovery from TBI, a number of studies have documented the existence of persistent language deficits subsequent to severe TBI in childhood. In particular, studies of language function after paediatric TBI have shown that expressive oral language skills, including verbal fluency and naming to confrontation, are most consistently compromised, whereas receptive language is less impaired and tends to recover earlier after injury. The observed language impairment is often characterized initially by reduced verbal output or, in its most severe form, mutism, which is followed in the longer term by subtle high-level language deficits. Subclinical language disturbance, as reflected in impoverished verbal fluency, dysnomia and decreased word-finding ability is consistently reported in the literature. Frank aphasia, however, occurs in only a very small proportion of children suffering from TBI, if at all. The pattern of language impairment reported subsequent to childhood TBI is, therefore, similar in many ways to that reported in the literature relating to adult TBI (see Chapter 4).

Discourse abilities. As indicated above, traditional studies of the linguistic abilities of children who have suffered a TBI have focused primarily on the use of standard language assessment procedures to document the characteristics of the language impairment exhibited by this population. In particular, many studies have utilized aphasia batteries to describe the linguistic skills of children with TBI. Unfortunately, many authors agree that traditional language measures may not adequately identify the range of language difficulties manifest in persons with TBI (Chapman *et al.*, 1992; Jordan, Cannon and Murdoch, 1992; McDonald, 1992, 1993). In many instances, despite the existence of subtle, high level linguistic deficits, people with TBI tend to score within normal limits on traditional aphasia tests (Levin, Benton and Grossman, 1982; Jordan and Murdoch, 1990a; Chapman *et al.*, 1992; Jordan, Cannon and Murdoch, 1992; McDonald, 1993). Further, despite the apparent recovery of language function as identified by structured language measures, both children and adults have been shown to have persistent deficits at the discourse level of language following TBI (Mentis and Prutting, 1987; Dennis and Barnes, 1990; McDonald, 1992, 1993; Chapman *et al.*, 1998).

Consequently in an attempt to better define the scope of communicative impairment in children with TBI, many researchers have recently advocated the use of discourse measures to identify those aspects of the language disorder that have proven elusive to traditional language batteries (Ewing-Cobbs *et al.*, 1985; Jordan, Ozanne and Murdoch, 1988; Dennis and Barnes, 1990; Dennis and Lovett, 1990).

According to Dennis and Lovett (1990), 'discourse' refers to the use of communicative language in context. Discourse reflects the complex interaction between cognition, linguistic and information-processing abilities (Chapman, Levin and Lawyer, 1999). Given that children with severe TBI exhibit deficits in a variety of cognitive functions, including attention, memory, visuospatial function and psychosocial function among others in addition to linguistic impairments, discourse analysis may provide a better indication of communicative ability following childhood TBI than structured linguistic measures does. Although a variety of different discourse types are recognized, including descriptive, conversational, narrative, procedural and expository discourse, by far the majority of studies that have investigated the discourse abilities of children with TBI have used narrative discourse (Campbell and Dollaghan, 1990; Jordan, Murdoch and Buttsworth, 1991; Chapman *et al.*, 1992, 1998; Dennis, Jacennik and Barnes, 1994; Chapman, 1995).

Performance on narrative discourse tasks. Narrative tasks provide the opportunity to examine 'complex language, sequencing of events, children's ability to make information explicit for the listener, and the knowledge of story structure' (Olley, 1989, p. 44). In addition, Liles *et al.* (1989) suggested that story-generation tasks are useful in rendering characterizations of language use in high-level TBI subjects. Consequently, the inclusion of narrative tasks in a test battery for children with TBI has been seen by several research groups as having the potential to provide valuable information for documenting further the linguistic characteristics of the TBI population. To that end Jordan, Murdoch and Buttsworth (1991) used a story-generation task to examine

the story grammar skills and intersentential cohesion abilities of a group of 20 children with TBI aged 8–16 years and 1–4 years post-injury. Performance of the children with TBI was compared to that of a group of non-neurologically impaired accident victims matched for age, sex and socioeconomic status. No significant differences were found between the narrative skills of the children with TBI and the matched controls on any of the story grammar measures or use of cohesive devices. Jordan, Murdoch and Buttsworth (1991) inferred that the story-generation task used in their study might not have yielded optimal narrative performance. In contrast, based on narratives collected during a storytelling task, Chapman *et al.* (1992) reported deficits in the story grammar skills of 20 children and adolescents with TBI when tested at least one year post-injury. In particular their findings indicated that the discourse of children with severe TBI differed from that of normal controls on both language and information structures, the severe TBI cases producing less language and less information than the normal children in retelling a story. Further, the subjects with severe TBI differed from those with mild/moderate TBI on information structure measures of narratives. The disruption in story structure was reported by Chapman *et al.* (1992) to be characterized primarily by the omission of critical setting and action information.

Chapman *et al.* (1998) used a storytelling task to investigate the effects of severe TBI on discourse in children who were 6–8 years of age at the time of testing. In order to consider age-at-injury effects, these workers compared the narratives of children who sustained a TBI before the age of five years to those children aged greater than five years at the time of injury. The results indicated that severe TBI has a deleterious effect on discourse in young children. In particular, Chapman *et al.* (1998) reported that their TBI cases exhibited marked reductions in the overall amount of information (propositions), in the structural completeness and in the expression of the central semantic meaning (gist) of the story. In contrast, measures of sentential length and complexity did not differ between the severe TBI and control subjects. Consistent with the findings of Jordan, Murdoch and Buttsworth (1991), the ability of the children with severe TBI to manipulate certain cohesive devices (e.g. use of reference and connectors) was comparable to those of the control subjects. Although no significant differences were found by Chapman *et al.* (1998) according to age at injury, these researchers suggested that there was a consistent pattern of generally poorer discourse for the early-injured group (i.e. less than five years of age at the time of injury).

Ewing-Cobbs *et al.* (1998) examined linguistic structure, cohesion and thematic recall of the narrative discourse of two groups of children with TBI selected on the basis of the presence or absence of acute language disturbance. A sibling comparison group was also included. Based on a storytelling task, the language-impaired TBI group produced fewer words and utterances than the sibling group, their stories being characterized by fewer complete referential and lexical ties and more referential errors, which Ewing-Cobbs *et al.* (1998) suggested were indicative of difficulty conjoining meaning across sentences. In addition, the language-impaired TBI group was reported to recall only one-third of the propositions needed to maintain the story theme and made more errors sequencing the propositions than the other two groups did. The language-impaired TBI group, however, did not differ from the other two groups on measures of the rate and fluency of speech production, number or length of mazes, use of conjunctives or naming errors. Overall, the majority of the findings reported by Ewing-Cobbs *et al.* (1998) are consistent with those of Chapman *et al.* (1992) who, as noted earlier, reported a reduction in the number of words, number of sentences and amount of core information retained in the narratives of children and adolescents with severe TBI in conjunction with preservation of syntactic complexity and fluency.

Performance on conversational discourse tasks. To date, only two studies of the conversational discourse abilities of children with TBI have been reported (Campbell and Dollaghan, 1990; Jordan and Murdoch, 1990b). Campbell and Dollaghan (1990) collected a series of spontaneous conversation samples from nine children and adolescents with TBI over a period of approximately 13 months. At the time of initial assessment 2–16

weeks post-injury, significant differences in all measures of expressive language were identified when compared to a normal control group. Significant improvement occurred, however, in the TBI group over the 13 months between the initial and final assessment. Although at the final follow-up the TBI group was reported to produce fewer utterances than the controls produced, their performance on other measures – including total number of words, total number of different words, mean length of utterances in morphemes, percentage of complex utterances and percentage of utterances within mazes – was the same as the controls. Campbell and Dollaghan (1990) did note, however, that the patterns of deficit and recovery in the TBI group were heterogeneous with five of the nine TBI cases continuing to exhibit marked deficits. Jordan and Murdoch (1990b) elicited conversations from a group of 20 children with TBI and examined the conversational skills using the Clinical Discourse Analysis (Damico, 1985). No significant differences were found between the performance of the TBI children and a group of matched controls on this measure of conversational competency. Jordan and Murdoch (1990b) cautioned, however, that the children with TBI in their study were all between one and five years post-injury at the time of testing. They highlighted the need for further research of a prospective nature examining the performance of children with TBI throughout the course of recovery on measures of conversational competency to clarify the relationship between time post injury and the occurrence of conversational error behaviours.

In summary, evidence is available to suggest that the discourse abilities of children with TBI are impaired in a number of ways compared to normals. As yet, however, the relationship between factors such as age at injury, lesion site and size, severity of injury, and so on and the occurrence of deficits in discourse skills is unknown.

Acquired childhood aphasia associated with brain tumours

Intracerebral tumours are a recognized cause of acquired aphasia in children (Alajouanine and Lhermitte, 1965; Hecaen, 1976;

Carrow-Woolfolk and Lynch, 1982; Brown, 1985; van Dongen, Loonen and van Dongen, 1985; Rekate *et al.*, 1985; Hudson, Murdoch and Ozanne, 1989). Neoplasms of the posterior cranial fossa (i.e. those involving the cerebellum, pons, fourth ventricle and cisterna magna) occur more frequently in children than supratentorial tumours do (Matson, 1956; Gjerris, 1978; Segall *et al.*, 1985). Cerebellar astrocytoma is the most common type of posterior fossa tumour in childhood, occurring most frequently in children between five and nine years of age (Cuneo and Rand, 1952; Matson, 1969). Fortunately, cerebellar astrocytomas are also highly curable and have an excellent prognosis following surgical removal. Next to cerebellar astrocytoma, medulloblastoma is the most frequent tumour type involving structures within the posterior cranial fossa in children. Generally, these latter tumours involve children at a younger age than do cerebellar astrocytomas, their maximum incidence being with the age range of 3–7 years (Delong and Adams, 1975). Although initially cerebellar astrocytoma and medulloblastoma may present in a similar manner, the prognosis of these two tumours types is quite different. While astrocytoma has a very favourable prognosis, medulloblastoma has a poor prognosis for recovery. The third most frequently encountered tumour of the posterior cranial fossa is the ependymoma. This neoplasm grows from the floor of the fourth ventricle and affects children who are at a similar age to those affected by the medulloblastoma and, like the medulloblastoma, ependymoma has a poor prognosis with a high proportion of tumours recurring after surgical removal.

Considering their location in the central nervous system, it would not be expected that posterior fossa tumours would cause language problems. A number of secondary effects, however, are associated with these tumours, which can, in some cases, lead to language deficits. Many posterior fossa tumours either originate from or invade the fourth ventricle of the brain. As a result, hydrocephalus may occur following obstruction of the flow of cerebrospinal fluid. Subsequent compression of the cerebral cortex could lead to dysfunction in the central speech-language centres. In addition, radiotherapy administered after sur-

gical removal of posterior fossa tumours, in order to prevent tumour spread or recurrence, has been reported to cause aphasia in some adults and intellectual deficits in some children (Broadbent, Barnes and Wheeler, 1981; Meadows *et al.*, 1981; Duffner, Cohen and Thomas, 1983; Burns and Boyle, 1984). Further, the negative effects of radiotherapy have been reported to appear as delayed reaction, so that any associated language deficit may only appear in the long term (Hodges and Smith, 1983).

Given that tumours located in the posterior cranial fossa represent the most common form of brain tumours in children, research conducted in the area of linguistic deficits resulting from treatment and/or surgery following childhood tumour has had its focus particularly on those located in that region of the brain (Hudson, Murdoch and Ozanne, 1989; Hudson and Murdoch, 1992a,b; Murdoch and Hudson-Tennent, 1994b). In fact, the most extensive investigations of the language abilities of children treated for posterior fossa tumours to date have been carried out by Murdoch and colleagues. The aforementioned researchers found that these children performed significantly below their peers on both receptive and expressive language tasks. Results of these studies (e.g. Hudson and Murdoch, 1992b) indicated that these children might not be competent language users when compared to their matched controls. Areas of impairment included auditory comprehension, oral expression and in particular reduced higher-level language abilities, with deficiencies in understanding and manipulating complex, abstract language structures (Hudson and Murdoch, 1992a).

Hudson, Murdoch and Ozanne (1989) investigated the speech-language abilities of a group of children who had undergone surgery to remove a posterior fossa tumour. They reported that although dysarthria and language impairment were not the inevitable outcome of such surgery, in some cases speech and/or language deficits did occur. Four of the six cases they assessed exhibited a language impairment. In particular, they observed that those children who had undergone radiotherapy post surgery appeared to have a greater chance of long-term impairment than those who did not. Although they recognized that radiotherapy may be vital for the long-term survival of children who have undergone surgery to remove brain tumours, Hudson, Murdoch and Ozanne (1989) emphasized the need for the medical team (including speech-language pathologists) to be aware of the possible long-term effects that radiotherapy may have on language abilities.

Rekate *et al.* (1985) studied six children who had experienced acute bilateral damage to large areas of both cerebellar hemispheres as a result of the presence of tumours. Their sample included four children with medulloblastoma, one with astrocytoma and one with ependymoma. All six children were described as being mute for 1–3 months post-surgery, the muteness in most cases resolving to a mild residual cerebellar (ataxic) dysarthria. One subject was described by Rekate *et al.* as having normal speech six months post-onset. Volcan, Cole and Johnson (1986) reported the case of an eight-year-old girl who had a right hemiparesis, truncal ataxia, signs of cerebellar dysfunction and muteness subsequent to the removal of a medulloblastoma from her fourth ventricle. Within two weeks post-surgery, she had regained monosyllabic speech but was described as having a monotone and dysarthria.

Acquired childhood aphasia following infection

Infectious disorders of the central nervous system are recognized as a significant cause of acquired childhood aphasia. Van Dongen, Loonen and van Dongen (1985) reported that of 27 children with acquired aphasia referred to their clinic over a four-year period, 15% had a history of infectious disease. Similarly, Van Hout, Evrard and Lyon (1985) noted that 38% of their child cases with acquired aphasia had an infectious disorder.

Although the brain and its membranous coverings can be infected by the same range of microorganisms as other organs of the body, in the majority of cases of acquired childhood aphasia with infectious disease reported in the literature, the infectious disorder involved has been herpes simplex encephalitis. Two antigenic types of herpes simplex virus (HSV) are now recognized, type 1 (HSV-1) and type 2 (HSV-2). HSV-1 is responsible for almost all cases of sporadic encephalitis in children and adults. HSV-2,

which causes congenital herpes, produces aseptic meningitis in the adult and encephalitis in the neonate.

HSV appears to involve primarily the basomedial portion of the frontal and temporal lobes and may present as an intracranial space-occupying lesion. As a result of the destructive nature of the lesions associated with infectious disorders, and in particular herpes simplex encephalitis, the language disorder associated with this disease tends to be more severe than in acquired aphasia resulting from other causes. Van Hout and Lyon (1986) reported a case of Wernicke's aphasia in a 10-year-old boy subsequent to herpes simplex encephalitis. Their subject exhibited a number of features atypical of the usual descriptions of acquired childhood aphasia in that he exhibited symptoms such as a severe comprehension deficit, neologistic jargon, logorrhea and anosognosia, the latter two features in particular usually being described as lacking in aphasic children. Van Hout and Lyon attributed the severe language disorder evidenced by their subject to the destructive bilateral damage to the temporal lobes caused by herpes simplex encephalitis.

Acquired childhood aphasia associated with convulsive disorder

Landau and Kleffner (1957) reported the first cases of acquired childhood aphasia with convulsive disorder. Landau–Kleffner syndrome, also known as 'acquired epileptic aphasia' or 'acquired verbal agnosia', appears to result from a heterogeneous group of conditions with variable aetiologies (Deonna *et al.*, 1977). Onset has been reported to occur between the ages of two and 13 years with the majority of children experiencing their first loss of language function somewhere between three and seven years of age. Most authors agree that males are affected twice as often as females (Cooper and Ferry, 1978; Msall *et al.*, 1986).

Acquired epileptic aphasia is characterized by an initial deterioration of language comprehension followed by disruption of the child's expressive abilities. In some cases, the onset of language deterioration is abrupt, while in others the language disturbance develops gradually.

Comprehension may be totally lost or reduced to understanding only short phrases and simple instructions (Worster-Drought, 1971). These receptive deficits have been interpreted in various ways. Some authors consider them a specific deficit in phonological decoding. In numerous cases of Landau–Kleffner syndrome, however, the inability to identify auditory information, which extends to non-verbal stimuli, has been classified as an auditory agnosia involving language as well as environmental sounds. Often owing to a reduced comprehension ability, the presence of a hearing loss is suspected in the early stages of the disorder and many of the subjects are initially thought to be deaf. However, in the majority of cases, their audiogram is within normal limits (Cooper and Ferry, 1978; Van Harskamp, van Dongen and Loonen, 1978; Van de Sandt-Koenderman *et al.*, 1984). In association with the reduction in comprehension, the spontaneous speech of the child also changes.

In most reported cases, expressive language impairments succeed the onset of auditory comprehension deficits, with either a progressive loss of vocabulary and/or phonological disturbances. Expressively the child may become 'mute, use jargon or produce odd sounds, exhibit misarticulations, inappropriate substitution of words and anomia, or resort to gestures and grunts' (Cooper and Ferry, 1978, p. 177). Unlike acquired childhood aphasia following focal unilateral lesions, in Landau–Kleffner syndrome jargon aphasia with paraphasia and neologisms is often observed before the complete loss of language function that may last several months or even years. Over the course of the condition, the degree of language impairment often fluctuates, with periods of transient recovery after the introduction or change of an antiepileptic drug.

Preceding, co-occurring with, or following the language deterioration there may be a series of convulsive seizures (Van de Sandt-Koenderman *et al.*, 1984). Although seizures do occur often, they are not the defining feature of the syndrome. Miller *et al.* (1984) reported that of those cases that exhibit seizures 43% experience the seizures before the language regression, 16% display co-occurrence of seizures and language regression and 41% experience seizures sometime after the

language regression. Regardless of whether there are clinically observable seizures, however, all patients with the syndrome exhibit epileptiform discharges in their electroencephalograms (Deonna, Fletcher and Voumard, 1982). The electroencephalographic abnormalities usually take the form of bilateral synchronous disturbances, frequently with a temporal predominance (Gascon *et al.*, 1973; Deonna, Fletcher and Voumard, 1982). Other clinical measures, such as X-ray, arteriography, computerized tomography and cerebrospinal fluid examination, usually yield completely normal results.

In addition to the language disorder, a number of other associated problems may also occur in acquired epileptic aphasia. Emotional problems have been reported in a number of cases (Miller *et al.*, 1984) and behavioural problems such as aggressiveness, temper outbursts, refusing to respond, inattention, withdrawal and hyperactivity occur frequently (Gascon *et al.*, 1973; Deonna *et al.*, 1977; Campbell and Heaton, 1978). One surprising feature of this syndrome is that the child's non-verbal intelligence usually remains unimpaired (Miller *et al.*, 1984).

As previously mentioned, the cause of acquired epileptic aphasia is unknown. Miller *et al.* (1984) pointed out that speculation regarding the neurological basis of this syndrome is likely to continue until a non-invasive assessment of cortical structure and function is better developed. Despite this, however, several hypotheses as to the pathogenesis of aphasia with convulsive disorder have been proposed. Landau and Kleffner (1957) together with Sato and Dreifuss (1973) postulated that the speech-language regression may be the result of functional ablation of the primary cortical language areas by persistent electrical discharges. Gascon *et al.* (1973), however, suggested that the electrical discharges displayed by these children occur secondary to a lower level subcortical de-afferenting process and that the discharges are not directly responsible for the aphasia.

As for the actual cause of the convulsive disorder, the data on which several hypotheses are based were obtained from pathoanatomical studies (Miller *et al.*, 1984). One hypothesis proposes that there exists a pathogenetic mechanism related in an unknown way to the convulsive disorder (Gascon *et al.*, 1973). For instance, there may be an unusual genetic pattern of cerebral organization that makes a child particularly sensitive to brain damage or seizure activity as far as language is concerned (Deonna *et al.*, 1977). Another hypothesis suggests that the convulsive disorder and language loss is caused by an active low-grade selective encephalitis that affects the temporal lobes (Worster-Drought, 1971; McKinney and McGreal, 1974). It has also been suggested that acquired epileptic aphasia may be caused by vascular disorders. A diminished vascular supply in the territory of the left middle cerebral artery was found in one subject with this disorder examined by Rapin *et al.* (1977).

The prognosis of aphasia with convulsive disorder is unclear. Van de Sandt-Koenderman *et al.* (1984) caution that many reports concentrate on the medical aspects of the syndrome, whilst the aphasia is poorly described. Consequently, the many contradictory statements about the prognosis may be due to the variation in the particular aspect of the disorder being described as recovering. A medical examination of children may declare them 'completely recovered' when there may be still demonstrable aphasic characteristics evidenced if sufficiently sensitive testing is carried out. Often the language recovery in acquired epileptic aphasia is very limited. Miller *et al.* (1984) stated that over 80% of cases reported in the literature have receptive and expressive deficits that persist for longer than six months. In general, it appears that the prognosis for recovery is poor if there has been no progress one year post-onset. As indicated above, some children with this disorder go through periods of exacerbations and remissions. Mantovani and Landau (1980) found that children who exhibit this latter type of course have a relatively good prognosis.

Summary

Although for a long time it has been believed that acquired aphasia in children is primarily of the non-fluent type, in recent years this belief has been challenged by studies which have demonstrated that fluent aphasias can be observed in children if language examination is carried out in the early

stages post-onset. In addition, there is now evidence to suggest that the type of aphasia resulting from brain damage in children varies according to the underlying aetiology. Clearly, there is a need for more research to further elucidate the specific clinical features of each of the speech-language deficits associated with the various neurological disorders which may cause acquired childhood aphasia.

Acquired childhood dysarthria

As outlined in Chapter 1, contraction of the muscles of the speech mechanism is regulated by nerve impulses originating in the motor cortex that are conveyed to the muscles by way of the descending motor pathways. Components of the neuromuscular system that can be disrupted by lesions to cause dysarthria include motor areas of the cerebral cortex, cerebellum, basal ganglia system, brainstem, peripheral nervous system, neuromuscular junction as well as the muscles of the speech mechanism themselves.

Acquired childhood dysarthria of different aetiologies

The major aetiologies of acquired childhood dysarthria include traumatic brain injury, intracerebral tumours and cerebrovascular accidents. In addition, genetic disorders are also sometimes the cause of childhood dysarthria, including Duchenne muscular dystrophy and Huntington's disease (see Chapter 10).

Acquired childhood dysarthria following traumatic brain injury

Persistent dysarthria is a commonly reported sequela of severe TBI in children. Despite this, few studies have investigated the incidence and nature of dysarthria following TBI acquired in childhood. The majority of studies that do exist tend to report only the presence or frequency of dysarthria but do not go on to provide an analysis of the speech disorder. The small number of the studies that have attempted to further define the nature of dysarthria subsequent to TBI in children have been case studies (Murdoch and Horton, 1998; Murdoch *et al.*, 1999; Cahill, Murdoch and Theodoros, 2000) or have examined only one aspect of the speech production mechanism (Stierwalt *et al.*, 1996). Murdoch *et al.*(1999), in a study of the effects of real-time continuous visual biofeedback in the treatment of speech breathing disorders, examined the motor speech function of one child with severe dysarthria subsequent to TBI using perceptual and instrumental measures and observed impairments in all of the speech subsystems. Similarly, Murdoch and Horton (1998) identified a range of impairments across the speech production mechanism, using both perceptual and instrumental assessments, in single case studies of children with dysarthria subsequent to TBI. In the most comprehensive series of studies completed to date, Cahill, Murdoch and Theodoros (2002, 2003, 2005) examined 24 children who had acquired a TBI, using both perceptual and instrumental measures and found that each child presented with a differing profile of speech subsystem deficits, ranging from no dysarthria through to moderate/severe dysarthria.

These findings are not unexpected given that the diffuse, non-specific nature of TBI can lead to damage in many areas of the central nervous system, resulting in impairment in one or more of the motor speech subsystems. More specifically, the perceptual and instrumental analysis of speech function in the group of children with TBI examined by Cahill and colleagues identified substantial impairments in prosody, velopharyngeal and articulatory function, as well as reduced lung capacity and impaired respiratory/phonatory control for speech but little impairment in laryngeal function.

Acquired childhood dysarthria associated with brain tumours

Dysarthria has been reported to occur subsequent to the diagnosis and treatment of posterior fossa tumours, with the presentation of the speech impairment ranging from transient mutism, to mild dysarthria, through to a persistent developmental

speech disorder. The literature, to date, predominantly documents the presence of transient cerebellar mutism subsequent to surgery for a posterior fossa tumour and that resolution to normal speech involves a period of dysarthria. There is some evidence, however, that in some individuals treated for posterior fossa tumours speech does not return to pre-morbid levels, implying the presence of a persistent dysarthria. The majority of reports, however, are not only based on small numbers of children but are also restricted to descriptions of the speech impairment based on perceptual speech analyses. A number of studies have labelled the speech disorder evident as cerebellar or ataxic dysarthria utilizing the Mayo Clinic classification. Unfortunately, in many of these studies the actual clinical features of the speech disorder were not elaborated, using the overall term of 'ataxic dysarthria' only as a descriptor.

In a recent published series of studies based on perceptual, acoustic and physiological assessments, Cornwell, Murdoch and Ward (2003; Cornwell *et al.*, 2004; Cornwell, Murdoch and Ward, 2005) determined that, although not all children treated for posterior fossa tumours exhibit a persistent dysarthria, in those cases where it does occur the nature of the deviant perceptual features usually reflects those associated with dysarthria in adults with cerebellar or lower motor neurone damage, dependent on tumour location within the posterior cranial fossa. In particular, where the tumour is primarily cerebellar in location the child usually exhibits a predominance of phonatory, articulatory and prosodic disturbances. Examination of the individual components of the speech musculature revealed that there was impairment to lip, tongue and laryngeal function both at rest and during the performance of non-speech and speech tasks, along with more minor deficits in palatal and respiratory function.

Acquired childhood dysarthria following cerebrovascular accident

Despite being a recognized sequela of cerebrovascular disorders, very few detailed descriptions of dysarthria resulting from cerebrovascular disorders in children have been reported. Horton *et al.* (1997) have provided the only detailed description of a child with dysarthria associated with basilar artery stroke based on a comprehensive assessment using both perceptual and physiological techniques. The physiological assessments indicated the most severe motor speech deficits to be in the respiratory and velopharyngeal subsystems with significant deficits also being apparent in the articulatory subsystem, collectively resulting in severely reduced intelligibility. Bak, van Dongen and Arts (1983) also described the perceptual features of the speech disorder exhibited by a child with a brainstem infarct following occlusion of the basilar artery. Specifically, the dysarthria in their case was characterized by imprecise consonants, distorted vowels, hypernasality and a breathy voice.

Acquired childhood dysarthria in relation to site of damage

As outlined in Chapter 9, components of the neuromuscular system that when damaged can lead to dysarthria include the lower motor neurones, upper motor neurones, extrapyramidal system (e.g. basal ganglia), cerebellum, neuromuscular junction as well as the muscles of the speech mechanism themselves.

On the basis of acoustic-perceptual judgements of speech and neuroanatomical data, Darley, Aronson and Brown (1969a,b) identified six different types of dysarthria in adults: flaccid, spastic, hypokinetic, hyperkinetic, ataxic and mixed (e.g. spastic-ataxic dysarthria). In that the same components of the neuromuscular system can be affected by neurological disorders in children as in adults, as pointed out above, it would seem appropriate that the dysarthria classification system devised by Darley, Aronson and Brown (1969a,b) be used to describe acquired dysarthrias in children in the same way as it is used to describe the equivalent speech disorders in adults. (For a full description of the neuropathophysiological basis and clinical features of the six different classifications of dysarthria see Chapters 9, 10 and 11.)

Flaccid dysarthria (lower motor neurone dysarthria)

Damage to the motor cranial nerves and spinal nerves represents lower motor neurone lesions. These lesions interrupt the conduction of nerve impulses from the central nervous system to the skeletal muscles. Where either the bulbar cranial nerves (V, VII, IX, X, XI, XII) and/or the spinal nerves that supply the muscles of respiration are involved, changes in speech collectively referred to as 'flaccid dysarthria' may result. In the case of the bulbar cranial nerves, the damage may involve the nerves either in their peripheral course or in their nuclei in the brainstem.

Symptoms of lower motor neurone lesions include a loss of muscle tone, muscle weakness, a loss or reduction of muscle reflexes, atrophy of the muscles involved and fasciculations. The actual name, flaccid dysarthria, is derived from the major symptom of lower motor neurone damage, flaccid paralysis. The characteristics of the speech deficit exhibited by patients with flaccid dysarthria vary from case to case depending upon which particular nerves are affected.

In addition to lesions in the lower motor neurones themselves, flaccid dysarthria can also result from either impaired nerve impulse transmission across the neuromuscular junction (such as occurs in myasthenia gravis) or disorders which involve the muscles of the speech mechanism themselves (e.g. muscular dystrophy).

The lower motor neurones that innervate the muscles involved in speech production can be damaged by a variety of neurological diseases, including viral infections (e.g. poliomyelitis), tumours, cerebrovascular accidents (e.g. embolization resulting from congenital heart disease), degenerative disorders and traumatic head injury. The general name applied to flaccid paralysis of the muscles supplied by nerves arising from the bulbar regions of the brainstem (which, with the exception of the respiratory muscles, include the muscles of the speech mechanism) is 'bulbar palsy'. Bulbar palsy can be caused by pathological conditions which affect either the cell body of the lower motor neurones in the cranial nerve nuclei or the axon of the lower motor neurone as it courses through the peripheral nerve. In particular, damage to cranial nerves V (trigeminal), VII (facial), X (vagus) and XII (hypoglossal) in their peripheral course can lead to flaccid dysarthria.

Trigeminal nerve disorders. The trigeminal nerves supply the muscles of mastication (temporalis, masseter, pterygoid), which in turn regulate the movement of the mandible. In children with unilateral trigeminal lesions, the mandible deviates towards the paralysed side when they are asked to open their mouth widely. This deviation is brought about by the unopposed contraction of the pterygoid muscles on the active side (i.e. the side opposite to the lesion). In addition, children will show a loss or reduction of muscle tone and atrophy in the muscles of mastication on the side of the lesion. Only minor alterations in speech occur, however, as a result of unilateral trigeminal lesions, in that movements of the mandible are impaired to only a small extent. A much more devastating effect on speech occurs following bilateral trigeminal lesions, the muscles responsible for the elevation of the mandible being too weak in many cases to approximate the mandible and maxilla. This inability, in turn, may prevent the tongue and lips from making the necessary contacts with oral structures for the production of labial and lingual consonants and vowels. Unilateral trigeminal lesions in children may result from traumatic head injury and brainstem tumours involving the pons. Bilateral flaccid paralysis of the masticatory muscles, on the other hand, may be seen in bulbar poliomyelitis.

Facial nerve disorders. The muscles of facial expression (e.g. orbicularis oris, buccinators, etc.) are supplied by the facial nerves. Unilateral facial nerve lesions cause flaccid paralysis of the muscles of facial expression on the same side as the lesion. Consequently, children with such lesions present with drooping of the mouth on the affected side and saliva may constantly dribble from the corner. In addition, as a result of the loss of muscle tone in the orbicularis oculi muscle, the lower eyelid may also droop. During smiling, the mouth is retracted on the active side but not on the child's affected side. Likewise, during frowning, the frontalis muscle on the side contralateral to the lesion will corrugate the forehead; however, on the side ipsilateral to the lesion no corrugation will occur. In cases of bilateral facial nerve paralysis, saliva may drool from both corners of the mouth and the lips may be slightly parted at rest.

Both unilateral and bilateral facial nerve lesions affect speech production. Children with facial nerve lesions are unable to seal their lips tightly and during speech air escapes between their lips during the build-up of intraoral pressure. Consequently, unilateral facial nerve lesions cause distortion of bilabial and labiodental consonants. Speech impairments associated with bilateral facial nerve lesions range from distortion to complete obliteration of bilabial and labiodental consonants.

A number of different acquired disorders can cause malfunctioning of the facial nerves in children. In some cases, the facial palsy may have an idiopathic origin, such as in Bell's palsy. Bell's palsy usually causes unilateral facial paralysis. Prognostically, in the region of 80% of Bell's palsy cases recover in a few days or weeks. Unilateral facial paralysis can also result from closed head injuries, damage to one or other facial nerve during the course of forceps delivery, compression of the facial nerve by tumour (e.g. acoustic neuroma) and damage to the facial nucleus by brainstem tumours (e.g. glioma).

Bilateral facial paralysis may occur in idiopathic polyneuritis (Guillain–Barré syndrome). In addition, sarcoidosis, bulbar poliomyelitis and some forms of basal meningitis may also cause facial diplegia, as can some congenital disorders such as congenital hypoplasia of the nuclei of the VIIth and VIth cranial nerves (Möbius syndrome).

Vagus nerve disorders. Among other structures, the vagus nerves supply the muscles of the larynx and the levator muscles of the soft palate. Lesions of the vagus nerves, therefore, can affect either the phonatory or resonatory aspects of speech production, or both, depending upon the location of the lesion along the nerve pathway. Lesions which involve the nucleus ambiguus in the medulla (as occurs in lateral medullary syndrome following occlusion of the posterior inferior cerebellar artery) or the vagus nerve near to the brainstem (e.g. in the region of the jugular foramen) cause paralysis of all the skeletal muscles supplied via the vagus. Children with this type of lesion present with a flaccid dysphonia characterized by moderate breathiness, harshness and reduced volume. Other voice problems that may be also present include diplophonia, short phrases and inhalatory stridor. These voice abnormalities result from paralysis of the vocal cord on the side of the lesion which tends to lie in a slightly abducted position. In addition to the voice problem, these children also present with hypernasality due to paralysis of the soft palate on the affected side.

Lesions of the vagus which involve the nerve at a point distal to the exit of the pharyngeal nerve (which supplies the levator of the soft palate) but proximal to the exit of the superior laryngeal nerve have the same effect on phonation as brainstem lesions. These lesions, however, do not cause hypernasality since the functioning of the levator veli palatini is not compromised. In those cases where the recurrent laryngeal nerve is involved, dysphonia in the absence of hypernasality is also present. In these latter cases, however, the cricothyroid muscles (the principal tensor muscles of the vocal cords) are not affected and the vocal cords are paralysed closer to the midline (the paramedian position). Consequently, although the voice is likely to be harsh and reduced in loudness, there is likely to be a lesser degree of the breathiness than is seen in those children with brainstem lesions involving the nucleus ambiguus. The recurrent laryngeal nerve can be injured during surgery to the neck (e.g. thyroidectomy) or occasionally during chest surgery, especially on the left side where the nerve loops around the aortic arch. Bilateral damage to the recurrent laryngeal nerves is rare.

Hypoglossal nerve disorders. With the exception of palatoglossus, all the extrinsic and all the intrinsic muscles of the tongue are controlled by the hypoglossal nerves. Unilateral hypoglossal nerve damage therefore, as might occur in either brainstem conditions such as medial medullary syndrome or peripheral nerve lesions such as submaxillary tumours, which compress one or other hypoglossal nerves, is associated with flaccid paralysis, atrophy and fasciculations in the ipsilateral side of the tongue. On protrusion the tongue deviates to the affected side.

In bilateral hypoglossal involvement, both sides of the tongue may be atrophied and show fasciculations. Although in this case protrusion occurs in the midline, the degree of protrusion may be severely limited. In addition, elevation of the tip and body to contact the alveolar ridge or hard palate may be difficult or impossible.

Although both phonation and resonation remain normal, lesions of the hypoglossal nerves therefore cause disturbances in articulation by interfering with normal tongue movement. The articulatory imprecision occurs especially during production of linguodental and linguopalatal consonants. In the case of unilateral lesions, any articulatory imprecision may be temporary in that most patients learn to compensate for unilateral tongue weakness within a few days. More serious articulatory impairments, however, are associated with bilateral hypoglossal nerve lesions. As indicated above, tongue movement in such cases may be severely restricted and speech sounds such as high front vowels and consonants that require elevation of the tongue tip to contact the upper alveolar ridge or hard palate (e.g. /t/, /d/, /l/, etc.) may be grossly distorted.

Hypoglossal nerve lesions are rare in children and more commonly result from damage to the hypoglossal nucleus in the brainstem than from damage to the peripheral nerve itself. Some isolated cases of damage to the hypoglossal nerve are seen as the result of the child falling with something (usually a pencil) in their mouth.

Multiple cranial nerve disorders. In addition to individual damage to each of the bulbar cranial nerves, flaccid dysarthria can also result from simultaneous damage to a number of cranial nerves. For example, lesions in the region of the jugular foramen (the exit point of IXth, Xth and XIth nerves) can cause the concurrent dysfunctioning of the pharynx, soft palate and larynx. The nerves passing through the jugular foramen can be affected by disorders such as tumours within the jugular foramen (i.e. glomus jugulare tumours), metastases involving the base of the skull and sarcoidosis.

Spastic dysarthria (upper motor neurone dysarthria)

Persistent spastic dysarthria is caused by bilateral disruption of the upper motor neurone supply to the bulbar cranial nerve nuclei. Lesions of upper motor neurones that can cause dysarthria may be located in the cerebral cortex, the internal capsule, the cerebral peduncles or the brainstem. Clinical signs of upper motor neurone lesions include: spastic paralysis or paresis of the involved muscles, little or no muscle atrophy, hyperactive muscle stretch reflexes (e.g. hyperactive jaw-jerk) and the presence of pathological reflexes (e.g. positive Babinski sign, positive rooting reflex, etc.).

In that the majority of the cranial nerve nuclei receive a bilateral upper motor neurone innervation, in general bilateral corticobulbar lesions are required to produce a permanent and severe spastic dysarthria. Usually only a transient impairment in articulation occurs subsequent to unilateral corticobulbar lesions. Such lesions cause a spastic paralysis or weakness in the contralateral lower half of the face, but not the upper part of the face, which may be associated with a mild, transient dysarthria due to weakness of the orbicularis oris. There is, however, no weakness of the forehead, muscles of mastication, soft palate (therefore no hypernasality), pharynx (therefore no swallowing problems) or larynx (therefore no dysphonia). In addition to the lower facial weakness, however, unilateral upper motor neurone lesions may produce a mild weakness of the tongue on the side opposite to the lesion.

The general name given to spastic paralysis of the bulbar musculature as a result of bilateral upper motor neurone lesions is 'pseudobulbar palsy' (supranuclear palsy). Pseudobulbar palsy, which takes its name from its clinical resemblance to bulbar palsy, may be associated with a variety of neurological disorders which bilaterally affect the upper motor neurones anywhere from their cell bodies, located in the motor cortex, through to their synapses with the appropriate lower motor neurones. Bilateral cerebrovascular accidents, multiple sclerosis, motor neurone disease, extensive neoplasms, congenital disorders, encephalitis and severe brain trauma are all possible causes of this syndrome. All aspects of speech production, including phonation, resonation, articulation and respiration, are affected in pseudobulbar palsy, but to varying degrees. Overall, pseudobulbar palsy is characterized by features such as

bilateral facial paralysis, dysphagia, hypophonia, bilateral hemiparesis, incontinence and bradykinesia.

Hypoxic ischaemic encephalopathy is the most common cause of spastic dysarthria in childhood. In most cases, this is associated with intrapartum asphyxia, although severe anoxic brain damage at any stage can cause the same disorder. Brainstem ischaemia with infarction resulting from embolization in association with congenital heart disease can also cause pseudobulbar palsy in children (as it can bulbar palsy). Spastic dysarthria may also be seen in children who have suffered head injuries with elevated intracranial pressure and a midbrain or upper brainstem shearing injury (as a result of a deceleration/acceleration type of injury). Although a common cause of pseudobulbar palsy in adolescents and young adults, disseminated sclerosis is not a common cause of spastic dysarthria in pre-pubertal children. Degenerative disorders, such as metachromatic leukodystrophy can also cause childhood pseudobulbar palsy.

Dysarthria associated with extrapyramidal syndromes

Diseases which selectively involve the extrapyramidal system without affecting the pyramidal pathways are referred to as 'extrapyramidal syndromes'. Movement disorders are the primary features of extrapyramidal syndromes and, where the muscles of the speech mechanism are involved, disorders of speech may occur. The major pathological changes associated with extrapyramidal disorders are located in the basal ganglia and their related nuclei (e.g. the substantia nigra).

Extrapyramidal syndromes share a number of related symptoms, which include: (1) hypokinesia (akinesia) – slowness and poverty of spontaneous movement; (2) hyperkinesia – abnormal involuntary movements; (3) rigidity of muscles; and (4) loss of normal postural reactions.

Hypokinetic dysarthria. The term 'hypokinetic dysarthria' was first used by Darley, Aronson and Brown (1969a,b) to describe the resultant complex pattern of perceptual speech characteristics associated with Parkinson's disease. Parkinsonism occurs most commonly in persons in their fifties and sixties. However, a syndrome which, like idiopathic Parkinson's disease in adults, is associated with either a reduced level of dopamine in the substantia nigra or blockage of the dopamine receptors in the basal ganglia, also occurs in childhood. This syndrome is referred to as 'hypokinetic dyskinesia'. In addition, a number of other conditions also predispose to the occurrence of Parkinson's disease in childhood. Drug-induced Parkinsonism, for instance, can occur at all ages and subacute meningitis, such as that seen in association with measles, may also present with a parkinsonian-like picture. Further, in past years, post-encephalitic Parkinsonism secondary to epidemic encephalitis was common in children.

The clinical picture of Parkinson's disease consists of four major groups of symptoms: tremor, rigidity of the muscles, akinesia and loss of normal postural fixing reflexes. According to Darley, Aronson and Brown (1975), features of the speech disorder seen in adult Parkinson's patients include: difficulty in initiating speech, once speech is started the speech becomes faster (festinant speech), reduced loudness, variable speech rate between subjects, some patients speaking at a slower than normal rate and others speaking at a slightly faster than normal rate and disturbed prosody (e.g. monopitch, reduced stress, monoloudness).

Hyperkinetic dysarthria. A variety of extrapyramidal disorders may cause hyperkinetic dysarthria. Each of these disorders is characterized by the presence of abnormal involuntary muscle contractions of the limbs, trunk, neck, face and so on which disturb the rhythm and rate of normal, motor activities, including those involved in speech production. The major extrapyramidal disorders that cause hyperkinetic dysarthria include myoclonic jerks, tics, chorea, athetosis, dyskinesia and dystonia.

According to the nature of the abnormal involuntary movements, hyperkinetic disorders are divided into quick hyperkinesias (e.g. myoclonic jerks, tics, chorea) and slow hyperkinesias (e.g. athetosis, dyskinesia, dystonia). In quick hyperkinesias, the abnormal involuntary movements are rapid and either unsustained or sustained only very briefly and occur at random in terms of the body part affected. In contrast, the abnormal involuntary movements seen in slow hyperkinesias build up to a peak slowly and are sustained for at least one second or longer. Muscle tone waxes and wanes, producing a variety of distorted postures.

Myoclonic jerks. These are abrupt, sudden, unsustained muscle contractions that occur irregularly. The muscles of the limbs as well as those of the speech mechanism can be affected. The muscles of the face, soft palate, larynx, diaphragm and so on may be involved either individually or in combination (e.g. palatopharyngolaryngeal myoclonus). Myoclonic jerks may be seen in children in association with diffuse metabolic, infectious or toxic disorders of the central nervous system such as diffuse encephalitis and toxic encephalopathies. In addition, they are also associated with convulsive disorders (epilepsy).

Tics. Tics are recurrent, but brief, unsustained compulsive movements that involve a relatively small part of the body. One distinctive childhood disease characterized by the progressive development of tics involving the face, neck, upper limbs and eventually the entire body is Tourette's disorder. In this condition, which usually has an onset between two and 15 years of age, uncontrolled vocalizations (e.g. grunting, coughing, barking, hissing, snorting) occur often as a result of involuntary contractions of the muscles of the speech mechanism. In addition, stuttering-like repetitions, unintelligible sounds and echolalia are also present in some cases. The cause of the condition is unknown, although it has been suggested that the pathophysiological basis of the disease is increased dopamine activity.

Chorea. Slower than myoclonic jerks, choreic contractions involve a single, unsustained, isolated muscle action that produces a short, rapid, uncoordinated jerk of part of the body, such as the trunk, limb, face, tongue and so on. These contractions are random in their distribution and their timing is irregular and unpredictable. When superimposed on the normal movements of the speech mechanism during speech production, choreic movements can cause momentary disturbances to the course of contextual speech. In fact, all aspects of speech can be disrupted in patients with chorea and the hyperkinetic dysarthria of chorea is characterized by a highly variable pattern of interference with articulation, phonation, resonation and respiration.

There are two major diseases in which choreic movements are present: Sydenham's chorea and Huntington's disease. The onset of Sydenham's chorea usually occurs between five and 10 years of age, females being affected more than males. In many instances, Sydenham's chorea appears to be associated with either streptococcal infections (strep-throat) or rheumatic heart disease. Huntington's disease is an inherited disorder which, although it can manifest in childhood, usually has its onset in adult life.

Athetosis. Athetoid movements are characterized by a continuous, arrhythmic, slow, writhing-type of muscle movement. These movements are always the same in the same patient and cease only during sleep. Although athetoid movements primarily involve the limbs, the muscles of the speech mechanism, including the muscles of the face, tongue and so on may also be affected, causing facial grimacing, protrusion and writhing of the tongue and difficulty in speaking and swallowing. Athetoid movements disrupt these functions by interfering with the normal contraction of the muscles involved. In most cases, athetosis forms part of a complex of neurological signs, including those of cerebral palsy, that result from a disordered development of the brain, birth injury or other aetiological factors. The condition is usually associated with pathological changes in the corpus striatum and cerebral cortex.

Dyskinesia (lingual-facial-buccal dyskinesia). Miller and Keane (1978) defined dyskinesia as an 'impairment of the power of voluntary movements'. Although, according to this definition, all involuntary movements could be described as 'dyskinetic', only two dyskinetic disorders are described under this heading: tardive dyskinesia and levodopa-induced dyskinesia. Tardive dyskinesia is a well-recognized side effect of long-term neuroleptic treatment (treatment with a pharmacological agent having an antipsychotic action),

while levodopa-induced dyskinesia results from the use of levodopa in the treatment of Parkinson's disease. In that the muscles of the tongue, face and oral cavity are often most affected, these two disorders are also termed lingual-facial-buccal dyskinesias. In both conditions, the basic pattern of abnormal involuntary movement is one of repetitive, slow writhing, twisting, flexing and extending movements, often with a mixture of tremor.

Dystonia. Dystonia tends to involve large parts of the body. The abnormal involuntary movements are slow and sustained for prolonged periods and may produce grotesque posturing and bizarre writhing movements. Although these involuntary movements mostly involve the trunk, neck and proximal parts of the limbs, the muscles of the speech mechanism can also be affected. A variety of conditions lead to dystonia, including encephalitis, head trauma, vascular diseases and drug toxicity (especially the more potent tranquilizers).

Ataxic dysarthria

Ataxic dysarthria is a motor speech disorder associated with damage to the cerebellum or its connections, in which a breakdown in the articulatory and prosodic aspects of speech are the predominant features. Although the cerebellum itself does not initiate any muscle contractions, it acts to coordinate muscle actions initiated by other parts of the brain (e.g. the motor cortex and basal ganglia) so that those movements are performed smoothly and accurately.

Damage to the cerebellum or its connections leads to a condition called 'ataxia' in which movements performed by skeletal muscles become uncoordinated. If the muscles of the speech mechanism are involved, speech production may become abnormal, leading to a cluster of deviant speech dimensions collectively called 'ataxic dysarthria'. Clinically, the signs of damage to the cerebellum include ataxia, dysmetria, decomposition of movement, dysdiadochokinesia, hypotonia, asthenia, tremor, rebound phenomena, disturbance of posture and gait, nystagmus and dysarthria.

As indicated above, breakdown in the articulatory and prosodic aspects of speech are the predominant features of ataxic dysarthria. The imprecise articulation results in the improper formation and separation of individual syllables, leading to a reduction in intelligibility, while the disturbance in prosody is associated with the loss of texture, tone, stress and rhythm of individual syllables. The dysprosody results in slow, monotonous and improperly measured speech, often termed 'scanning speech'.

There are a number of different causes of acquired ataxia in childhood, including: posterior fossa tumours (e.g. medulloblastomas, cerebellar astrocytomas, etc.), traumatic head injury, infections (e.g. cerebellar abscess), degenerative disorders (e.g. metachromatic leukodystrophy) and toxic, metabolic and endocrine disorders (e.g. heavy metal poisoning).

Mixed dysarthria

Some disorders of the nervous system affect more than one level of the neuromuscular system. Consequently, in addition to the more 'pure' forms of dysarthria outlined above, clinicians may also be confronted by patients who exhibit 'mixed dysarthrias'. These may be caused by a variety of conditions, including cerebrovascular accidents, head trauma, brain tumours, inflammatory diseases and degenerative conditions. A mixed ataxic-hypokinetic-spastic dysarthria may be seen in children with Wilson's disease (see Chapter 11).

Summary

Acquired childhood speech-language disorders are defined as disturbances in speech-language function that result from some form of cerebral insult after language acquisition has already commenced. A variety of aetiologies may cause acquired speech-language disorders in children, including head trauma, brain tumours, cerebrovascular accidents, infections, convulsive disorders and electroencephalographic abnormalities. Based on early studies, for many years acquired childhood aphasia was considered primarily a non-fluent, motor type of language impairment, its major features being initial mutism and lack of spontaneity of speech with no accompanying comprehension deficit or other features of a fluent type of aphasia (e.g. jargon, logorrhea and paraphasia). Further, it was usually regarded as being transitory in nature, affected individuals making a good recovery. In recent years, however, this earlier held view of acquired childhood aphasia has been challenged in that it is now known that the non-fluent pattern is by no means invariant, with fluent aphasia with paraphasic errors occurring in some cases, especially in the early stages post-onset. Further, despite rapid recovery occurring in some cases, in the region of 25–50% of children who experience acquired aphasia still show aphasic symptoms in the longer term.

To date, a well-researched system for the classification of acquired speech disorders in children has not been developed. Consequently, acquired childhood dysarthria tends to be classified the same way as equivalent speech disorders in adults according to the Mayo Clinic classification system. The major aetiologies of acquired childhood dysarthria include traumatic brain injury, intracerebral tumours (particularly those involving the posterior cranial fossa) and cerebrovascular accidents. Persistent dysarthria has been reported to occur in children in association with each of these neurological disorders.

References

Adams, R.D., Cammermeyer, J. and Denny-Brown, D. (1949) Acute necrotizing hemorrhagic encephalopathy. *Journal of Neuropathy and Experimental Neurology*, 8, 1–29.

Adams, R.D. and Lyon, G. (1982) *Neurology of Hereditary Metabolic Diseases of Children*, McGraw-Hill, New York.

Alajouanine, T. and Lhermitte, F. (1965) Acquired aphasia in children. *Brain*, 88, 553–662.

Aram, D.M., Ekelman, B.L. and Whitaker, H.A. (1986) Spoken syntax in children with acquired unilateral hemisphere lesions. *Brain and Language*, 27, 75–100.

Aram, D.M., Rose, D.F., Rekate, H.L. and Whitaker, H.A. (1983) Acquired capsular/striatal aphasia in childhood. *Archives of Neurology*, **40**, 614–617.

Assal, G. and Campiche, R. (1973) Aphasie et troubles du langage chez l'enfant après contusion cérébrale. *Neurochirurgie*, **19**, 399–406.

Bak, E., van Dongen, H.R. and Arts, W.F.M. (1983) The analysis of acquired dysarthria in childhood. *Developmental Medicine and Child Neurology*, **25**, 81–94.

Banker, B.Q. (1961) Cerebral vascular disease in infancy and childhood. *Neuropathology and Experimental Neurology*, **20**, 127–140.

Barringer, J.R. (1978) Herpes simplex infections of the nervous system, in *Handbook of Clinical Neurology*, vol. **34** (eds D. Vinken and G. Bruyn), North-Holland Publishing Company/Elsevier, Amsterdam, pp. 346–368.

Basser, L.S. (1962) Hemiplegia of early onset and the faculty of speech with special reference to the effects of hemispherectomy. *Brain*, **85**, 427–460.

Bell, R.D. and Lastimosa, A.C.B. (1980) Metabolic encephalopathies, in *Neurology*, vol. 5 (ed. R.N. Rosenberg), Grune & Stratton, New York, pp. 115–164.

Benson, D.F. (1972) Language disturbances of childhood. *Clinical Proceedings Children's Hospital of Washington*, **28**, 93–100.

Bernhardt, M. (1885) Ueber die spastiche cerebralparalyse im kindersatter (hemiplegia spastica infantalis), nebst einem excurse uber: aphasie bei kindern. *Archiv für Pathologische Anatomie und Physiologic und für Klinische Medecin*, **102**, 26–80.

Bernheim, M. (1956) Thrombophlebitis cerebrales. *Annals of Paediatrics (Basel)*, **187**, 153–160.

Bickerstaff, E.R. (1964) Aetiology of acute hemiplegia in childhood. *British Medical Journal*, **2**, 82–87.

Bickerstaff, E.R. (1972) Cerebrovascular disease in infancy and childhood, in *Handbook of Clinical Neurology: Vascular Diseases of the Nervous System Part II* (eds P.J. Vinken and G.W. Bruyn), North-Holland Publishing Company, Amsterdam, pp. 412–441.

Branco-LeFèvre, A.F. (1950) Contribuicao para o estu do da psicopatologia da afasia en criancas. *Archivos Neuro-Psyquiatrica (San Paulo)*, **8**, 345–393.

Brandt, S. (1962) Causes and pathogenic mechanisms of acute hemiplegia in childhood. *Little Club Clinics in Developmental Medicine*, **6**, 7–11.

Broadbent, V.A., Barnes, N.D. and Wheeler, T.K. (1981) Medulloblastoma in childhood: long-term results of treatment. *Cancer*, **48**, 26–30.

Brown, J.K. (1985) Dysarthria in children: neurologic perspective, in *Speech and Language Evaluation in Neurology: Childhood Disorders* (ed. J.K. Darby), Grune & Stratton, New York, pp. 252–273.

Buckingham, H. and Kertesz, A. (1974) A linguistic analysis of fluent aphasia. *Brain and Language*, **1**, 43–61.

Burns, M.S. and Boyle, M. (1984) Aphasia after successful radiation treatment: a report of two cases. *Journal of Speech and Hearing Disorders*, **19**, 107–111.

Cahill, L.M., Murdoch, B.E. and Theodoros, D.G. (2000) Variability in speech outcome following severe childhood traumatic brain injury: a report of three cases. *Journal of Medical Speech-Language Pathology*, **8**, 347–352.

Cahill, L.M., Murdoch, B.E. and Theodoros, D.G. (2002) Perceptual analysis of speech following traumatic brain injury in childhood. *Brain Injury*, **16**, 415–446.

Cahill, L.M., Murdoch, B.E. and Theodoros, D.G. (2003) Perceptual and instrumental analysis of laryngeal function following traumatic brain injury in childhood. *Journal of Head Trauma Rehabilitation*, **18**, 268–283.

Cahill, L.M., Murdoch, B.E. and Theodoros, D.G. (2005) Articulatory function following traumatic brain injury in childhood: a perceptual and instrumental approach. *Brain Injury*, **19**, 41–58.

Campbell, T.F. and Dollaghan, C.A. (1990) Expressive language recovery in severely brain-injured children and adolescents. *Journal of Speech and Hearing Disorders*, **55**, 567–581.

Campbell, T.F. and Heaton, E.M. (1978) An expressive speech program for a child with acquired aphasia: a case study. *Human Communication (Summer)*, **89**, 102.

Carrow-Woolfolk, E. and Lynch, J. (1982) *An Integrative Approach to Language Disorders in Children*, Grune & Stratton, Orlando, FL.

Carter, R.L., Hohenegger, M.K. and Satz, P. (1982) Aphasia and speech organization in children. *Science*, **218**, 797–799.

Chadwick, O. (1985) Psychological sequelae of head injury in children. *Developmental Medicine and Child Neurology*, **27**, 72–75.

Chadwick, O., Rutter, M., Brown, G. *et al.* (1981a) A prospective study of children with head injuries:

II cognitive sequelae. *Psychological Medicine*, **11**, 49–61.

Chadwick, O., Rutter, M., Shaffer, D. and Shrout, P.E. (1981b) A prospective study of children with head injuries: IV specific cognitive deficits. *Journal of Clinical Neuropsychology*, **8**, 101–120.

Chapman, S.B. (1995) Discourse as an outcome measure in pediatric head-injured populations, in *Traumatic Brain Injury in Children* (eds S.H. Broman and M.E. Michel), Oxford University Press, New York, pp. 95–116.

Chapman, S.B., Culhane, K.A., Levin, H.S. *et al.* (1992) Narrative discourse after closed head injury in children and adolescents. *Brain and Language*, **43**, 42–65.

Chapman, S.B., Levin, H.S. and Lawyer, S.L. (1999) Communication problems resulting from brain injury in children: special issues of assessment and management, in *Communication Disorders Following Traumatic Brain Injury* (eds S. McDonald, L. Togher and C. Code), Psychology Press, Hove, pp. 235–269.

Chapman, S.B., Levin, H.S., Wanek, A. *et al.* (1998) Discourse after closed head injury in young children: relation of age to outcome. *Brain and Language*, **61**, 420–449.

Collignon, R., Hecaen, H. and Angerlerques, G. (1968) A propos de 12 cas d'aphasie acquis chez l'enfant. *Acta Neurologica et Psychiatrica Belgica*, **68**, 245–277.

Cooper, J.A. and Ferry, P.C. (1978) Acquired auditory verbal agnosia and seizures in childhood. *Journal of Speech and Hearing Disorders*, **43**, 176–184.

Cornwell, P.L., Murdoch, B.E. and Ward, E.C. (2003) Perceptual evaluation of motor speech following treatment for childhood cerebellar tumour. *Clinical Linguistics and Phonetics*, **17**, 597–615.

Cornwell, P.L., Murdoch, B.E. and Ward, E.C. (2005) Differential motor speech outcomes in children treated for midline cerebellar tumour. *Brain Injury*, **19**, 119–134.

Cornwell, P.L., Murdoch, B.E., Ward, E.C. and Kellie, S. (2004) Acoustic investigation of vocal fold quality following treatment of childhood cerebellar tumour. *Folia Phoniatrica et Logopaedica*, **56**, 93–107.

Cuneo, H.N. and Rand, C.W. (1952) *Brain Tumors of Childhood*, Charles C. Thomas, Springfield, IL.

Damico, J. (1985) Clinical discourse analysis: a functional approach to language assessment, in *Communication Skills and Classroom Success* (ed. C.S. Simon), Taylor & Francis, London, pp. 165–203.

Darley, F.L., Aronson, A.E. and Brown, J.R. (1969a) Differential diagnostic patterns of dysarthria. *Journal of Speech and Hearing Research*, **12**, 246–269.

Darley, F.L., Aronson, A.E. and Brown, J.R. (1969b) Clusters of deviant speech dimensions in dysarthrias. *Journal of Speech and Hearing Research*, **12**, 462–496.

Darley, F.L., Aronson, A.E. and Brown, J.R. (1975) *Motor Speech Disorders*, W.B. Saunders, Philadelphia.

Davie, J.C. and Cox, W. (1967) Occlusive disease of the carotid artery in children. *Archives of Neurology*, **17**, 313–323.

Delong, G.R. and Adams, R.D. (1975) Clinical aspects of tumours of the posterior fossa in childhood, in *Handbook of Clinical Neurology: Tumours of the Brain and Skull* (eds P.J. Vinken and G.W. Bruyn), North-Holland Publishing Company, Amsterdam, pp. 375–397.

Dennis, M. (1980) Strokes in childhood. 1. Communicative intent, expression and comprehension after left hemisphere arteriopathy in a right-handed nine-year-old, in *Language Development and Aphasia in Children* (ed. R.W. Reiber), Academic Press, New York, pp. 79–103.

Dennis, M. and Barnes, M.A. (1990) Knowing the meaning, getting the point, bridging the gap, and carrying the message: aspects of discourse following closed head injury in childhood and adolescence. *Brain and Language*, **39**, 428–446.

Dennis, M., Jacennik, B. and Barnes, M.A. (1994) The content of narrative discourse in children and adolescents after early-onset hydrocephalus and in normally developing age peers. *Brain and Language*, **46**, 129–165.

Dennis, M. and Lovett, M.W. (1990) Discourse ability in children after brain-damage, in *Discourse Ability and Brain Damage: Theoretical and Empirical Perspectives* (eds Y. Joanette and H.H. Brownell), Springer-Verlag, New York, pp. 199–223.

Deonna, T., Beaumanoir, A., Gaillard, F. and Assal, G. (1977) Acquired aphasia in childhood with seizure disorder: a heterogeneous syndrome. *Neuropadiatrie*, **8**, 263–273.

Deonna, T., Fletcher, P. and Voumard, C. (1982) Temporary regression during language acquisition: a linguistic analysis of a $2\frac{1}{2}$ year old child with epileptic aphasia. *Developmental Medicine and Child Neurology*, **24**, 156–163.

van Dongen, H.R. and Loonen, M.C.B. (1977) Factors related to prognosis of acquired aphasia in children. *Cortex*, **13**, 131–136.

van Dongen, H.R., Loonen, M.C.B. and van Dongen, K.J. (1985) Anatomical basis for acquired fluent aphasia in children. *Annals of Neurology*, **17**, 306–309.

Duffner, P.K., Cohen, M.E. and Thomas, P.R.M. (1983) Late effects of treatment on the intelligence of children with posterior fossa tumours. *Cancer*, **51**, 233–237.

Duffy, P.E., Portney, B., Mauro, J. and Wehrle, P.E. (1957) Acute infantile hemiplegia secondary to spontaneous carotid thrombosis. *Neurology*, 7, 664–666.

Ewing-Cobbs, L., Brookshire, B., Scott, M.A. and Fletcher, J.M. (1998) Children's narratives following traumatic brain injury: linguistic structure, cohesion and thematic recall. *Brain and Language*, **61**, 395–419.

Ewing-Cobbs, L., Fletcher, J.M., Levin, H.S. and Landry, S.H. (1985) Language disorders after pediatric head injury, in *Speech and Language Evaluation in Neurology: Childhood Disorders* (ed. J.K. Darby), Grune & Stratton, Orlando, FL, pp. 97–112.

Ewing Cobbs, L., Levin, H.S., Eisenberg, H.M. and Fletcher, J.M. (1987) Language functions following closed head injury in children and adolescents. *Journal of Clinical and Experimental Neuropsychology*, **9**, 575–592.

Fletcher, J.M. and Taylor, H. (1984) Neuropsychological approaches to children: towards a developmental neuropsychology. *Journal of Neuropsychology*, **6**, 39–57.

Freud, S. (1897) *Infantile Cerebral Paralysis*, University of Miami Press, Coral Gables, FL.

Gascon, G., Victor, D., Lombroso, C.T. and Goodglass, H. (1973) Language disorder, convulsive disorder and electroencephalographic abnormalities. *Archives of Neurology*, **28**, 156–162.

Gilchrist, E. and Wilkinson, M. (1979) Some factors determining prognosis in young people with severe head injuries. *Archives of Neurology*, **36**, 355–359.

Gjerris, F. (1978) Clinical aspects and long-term prognosis of infratentorial intracranial tumours in infancy and childhood. *Acta Neurologica Scandinavica*, **57**, 31–52.

Gloning, K. and Hift, E. (1970) Aphasie im vorschulalter. *Zeitschrift Nervenheilkunde*, **28**, 20–28.

Goldstein, S.L. and Burgess, J.P. (1958) Spontaneous thrombosis of the internal carotid artery in a seven year old child. *American Journal of Disorders of Childhood*, **95**, 538–540.

Goodglass, H. and Kaplan, E. (1972) *The Assessment of Aphasia and Related Disorders*, Lea and Febiger, Philadelphia.

Guttmann, E. (1942) Aphasia in children. *Brain*, **65**, 205–219.

Hecaen, H. (1976) Acquired aphasia in children and the ontogenesis of hemispheric functional specialization. *Brain and Language*, **3**, 114–134.

Hecaen, H. (1983) Acquired aphasia in children: revisited. *Neuropsychologia*, **21**, 581–587.

Hodges, S. and Smith, R.W. (1983) Intracranial calcification and childhood medulloblastoma. *Archives of Disease in Childhood*, **58**, 663–664.

Horton, S.K., Murdoch, B.E., Theodoros, D.G. and Thompson, E.C. (1997) Motor speech impairment in a case of childhood basilar artery stroke: treatment directions derived from physiological and perceptual assessment. *Pediatric Rehabilitation*, **1**, 163–177.

Hudson, L.J. and Murdoch, B.E. (1992a) Chronic language deficits in children treated for posterior fossa tumour. *Aphasiology*, **6**, 135–150.

Hudson, L.J. and Murdoch, B.E. (1992b) Language recovery following surgery and CNS prophylaxis for the treatment of childhood medulloblastoma: a prospective study of three cases. *Aphasiology*, **6**, 17–28.

Hudson, L.J., Murdoch, B.E. and Ozanne, A.E. (1989) Posterior fossa tumours in childhood: associated speech and language disorders post surgery. *Aphasiology*, **3**, 1–18.

Jordan, F.M., Cannon, A. and Murdoch, B.E. (1992) Language abilities of mildly closed head injured children 10 post-injury. *Brain Injury*, **6**, 39–44.

Jordan, F.M., Cremona-Meteyard, S. and King, A. (1996) High-level linguistic disturbances subsequent to childhood closed head injury. *Brain Injury*, **10**, 729–738.

Jordan, F.M. and Murdoch, B.E. (1990a) Linguistic status following closed head injury: a follow-up study. *Brain Injury*, **4**, 147–154.

Jordan, F.M. and Murdoch, B.E. (1990b) A comparison of the conversational skills of closed head injured children and normal children. *Australian Journal of Human Communication Disorders*, **18**, 69–82.

Jordan, F.M. and Murdoch, B.E. (1993) A prospective study of the linguistic skills of children with closed head injuries. *Aphasiology*, **7**, 503–512.

Jordan, F.M. and Murdoch, B.E. (1994) Severe closed head injury in childhood: linguistic outcomes into adulthood. *Brain Injury*, 8, 501–508.

Jordan, F.M., Murdoch, B.E. and Buttsworth, D.L. (1991) Closed head injured children's performance on narrative tasks. *Journal of Speech and Hearing Research*, 34, 572–582.

Jordan, F.M., Ozanne, A.E. and Murdoch, B.E. (1988) Long-term speech and language disorders subsequent to closed head injury in children. *Brain Injury*, 2, 179–185.

Jordan, F.M., Ozanne, A.E. and Murdoch, B.E. (1990) Performance of closed head injured children on a naming task. *Brain Injury*, 4, 27–32.

Landau, W.M. and Kleffner, F.R. (1957) Syndrome of acquired aphasia with convulsive disorder in children. *Neurology*, 10, 915–921.

Lange-Cosack, H. and Tepfner, G. (1973) *Das Hirntrauma im Kinder und Jugendalter*, Springer-Verlag, Berlin.

Lenneberg, E. (1967) *Biological Foundations of Language*, John Wiley & Sons, Inc., New York.

Levin, H.S., Benton, A.L. and Grossman, R.G. (1982) *Neurobehavioural Consequences of Closed Head Injury*, Oxford University Press, New York.

Levin, H.S. and Eisenberg, G.M. (1979a) Neuropsychological impairment after closed head injury in children and adolescents. *Journal of Pediatric Psychology*, 4, 389–402.

Levin, H.S. and Eisenberg, G.M. (1979b) Neuropsychological outcome of closed head injury in children and adolescents. *Child's Brain*, 5, 281–292.

Liles, B.Z., Coelho, C.A., Duffy, R.J. and Zalagens, M.R. (1989) Effects of elicitation procedures on the narratives of normal and closed head injured adults. *Journal of Speech and Hearing Disorders*, 54, 356–366.

Ludlow, C. (1980) Children's language disorders: recent research advances. *Annals of Neurology*, 7, 497–507.

Mantovani, J.F. and Landau, W.M. (1980) Acquired aphasia with convulsive disorder: course and prognosis. *Neurology*, 30, 524–529.

Matson, D.D. (1956) Cerebellar astrocytoma in childhood. *Pediatrics*, 18, 150–158.

Matson, D.D. (1969) *Neurosurgery of Infancy and Childhood*, Charles C. Thomas, Springfield, IL.

Maurer, D. and Lewis, T.L. (1998) Overt orienting toward peripheral stimuli: normal development and underlying mechanisms, in *Cognitive Neuroscience of Attention: A Developmental Perspective* (ed. J.E. Richards), Lawrence Erlbaum, Hillsdale, NJ, pp. 51–102.

McDonald, S. (1992) Communication disorders following closed head injury: new approaches to assessment and rehabilitation. *Brain Injury*, 6, 283–292.

McDonald, S. (1993) Pragmatic language skills after closed head injury: ability to meet the informational needs of the listener. *Brain and Language*, 44, 28–46.

McKinney, W. and McGreal, D.A. (1974) An aphasic syndrome in children. *Canadian Medical Association Journal*, 110, 637–639.

Meadows, A.T., Massari, D.J., Fergusson, J. et al. (1981) Decline in IQ scores and cognitive dysfunction in children with acute lymphocytic leukaemia treated with cranial irradiation. *Lancet*, 2, 1015–1018.

Mentis, M. and Prutting, C.A. (1987) Cohesion in the discourse of normal and head injured adults. *Journal of Speech and Hearing Research*, 30, 88–98.

Miller, B.F. and Keane, C.B. (1978) *Encyclopedia and Dictionary of Medicine, Nursing and Allied Health*, W.B. Saunders, Philadelphia.

Miller, J.F., Campbell, T.F., Chapman, R.S. and Weismer, S.E. (1984) Language behaviour in acquired aphasia, in *Language Disorders in Children* (ed. A. Holland), College Hill Press, Baltimore, pp. 63–71.

Moosy, J. (1959) Development of cerebral arteriosclerosis in various age groups. *Neurology*, 9, 569–574.

Msall, M., Shapiro, B., Balfour, P.B. et al. (1986) Acquired epileptic aphasia: diagnostic aspects of progressive language loss in preschool children. *Neurology*, 25, 248–251.

Murdoch, B.E. and Horton, S.K. (1998) Acquired and developmental dysarthria in childhood, in *Dysarthria: A Physiological Approach to Assessment and Treatment* (ed. B.E. Murdoch), Stanley Thornes, Cheltenham, pp. 373–427.

Murdoch, B.E. and Hudson-Tennent, L.J. (1994a) Speech disorders in children treated for posterior fossa tumours: ataxic and developmental features. *European Journal of Disorders of Communication*, 29, 379–397.

Murdoch, B.E. and Hudson-Tennent, L.J. (1994b) Differential language outcomes in children treated for posterior fossa tumours. *Aphasiology*, 8, 507–534.

Murdoch, B.E., Pitt, G., Theodoros, D.G. and Ward, E.C. (1999) Real-time visual biofeedback in the treatment of speech breathing disorders following childhood traumatic brain injury: a report of one case. *Pediatric Rehabilitation*, 3, 5–20.

Neville, H.J. and Bavelier, D. (2000) Specificity and plasticity in neurocognitive development in humans, in *The New Cognitive Neurosciences* (ed. M.S. Gazzaniga), MIT Press, Cambridge, MA, pp. 83–98.

Norman, R.M. (1962) Neuropathological findings in acute hemiplegia in childhood. *Little Clubs Clinics in Developmental Medicine*, **6**, 37–48.

Oelschlaeger, M.L. and Scarborough, J. (1976) Traumatic aphasia in children: a case study. *Journal of Communication Disorders*, **9**, 281–288.

Olley, L. (1989) Oral narrative performance of normal and language impaired school aged children. *Australian Journal of Human Communication Disorders*, **17**, 43–65.

Penfield, W. (1965) Conditioning the uncommitted language cortex for language learning. *Brain*, **88**, 787–798.

Poetzl, T. (1926) Ueber sensorische aphasie in kindersalter. *Nasen-Ohrenklin*, **14**, 109–118.

Rankin, J.M., Aram, D.M. and Horwitz, S.J. (1981) Language ability in right and left hemiplegic children. *Brain and Language*, **14**, 292–306.

Rapin, I., Mattis, S., Rowan, J.A. and Golden, G.G. (1977) Verbal auditory agnosia in children. *Developmental Medicine and Child Neurology*, **119**, 192–207.

Rekate, H.L., Grubb, R.L., Aram, D.M. *et al.* (1985) Muteness of cerebellar origin. *Archives of Neurology*, **42**, 697–798.

Salam-Adams, M. and Adams, R.D. (1988) Cerebrovascular disease by age group, in *Handbook of Clinical Neurology: Vascular Diseases Part 1* (eds P.J. Vinken, G.W. Bruyn and H.L. Klawans), Elsevier Science Publishers, Amsterdam, pp. 197–221.

Sato, S. and Dreifuss, F.E. (1973) Electroencephalographic findings in a patient with developmental expressive aphasia. *Neurology*, **23**, 181–185.

Satz, P. and Bullard-Bates, C. (1981) Acquired aphasia in children, in *Acquired Aphasia* (ed. M.T. Sarno), Academic Press, New York, pp. 75–93.

Segall, H.D., Batnitzky, S., Zee, S. *et al.* (1985) Computed tomography in the diagnosis of intracarotid neoplasms in children. *Cancer*, **56**, 1748–1755.

Shoumaker, R., Bennett, D., Bray, P. and Curless, R. (1974) Clinical and EEG manifestations of an unusual aphasic syndrome in children. *Neurology*, **24**, 10–16.

Slater, E.J. and Bassett, S.S. (1988) Adolescents with closed head injuries. *American Journal of Diseases of Children*, **142**, 1048–1051.

Spreen, O. and Benton, A.L. (1969) *Neurosensory Centre Comprehensive Examination for Aphasia*, University of Victoria, Victoria, BC.

Stierwalt, J., Robin, D., Solomon, N. *et al.* (1996) Tongue strength and endurance: relation to speaking ability of children and adolescents following traumatic brain injury, in *Disorders of Motor Speech: Assessment, Treatment and Clinical Characteristics* (eds D. Robin, K. Yorkston and D. Beukelman), Paul H. Brooks, Baltimore, pp. 241–256.

Strumpell, A. (1884) Über die acute encephalitis die kinder. *Deutsch Medicine*, **57**, 212–215.

Teuber, H.L. (1975) Recovery of function after brain injury in man, in *Outcome of Severe Damage of the Central Nervous System* (eds R. Porter and D.W. Fitzsimons), CIBA Foundation symposium No. 34, Elsevier/Excerpta Medica, Amsterdam, pp. 146–163.

Tindall, R.S.A. (1980) Cerebrovascular disease, in *Neurology*, vol. 5 (ed. R.N. Rosenberg), Grune & Stratton, New York, pp. 41–77.

Van de Sandt-Koenderman, W.M.E., Smit, I.A.C., van Dongen, H.R. and van Hest, J.B.C. (1984) A case of acquired aphasia and convulsive disorder: some linguistic aspects of recovery and breakdown. *Brain and Language*, **21**, 174–183.

Van Harskamp, F., van Dongen, H.R. and Loonen, M.C.B. (1978) Acquired aphasia with convulsive disorders in children: a case study with a seven year follow up. *Brain and Language*, **6**, 141–148.

Van Hout, A., Evrard, P. and Lyon, G. (1985) On the positive semiology of acquired aphasia in children. *Developmental Medicine and Child Neurology*, **27**, 231–241.

Van Hout, A. and Lyon, G. (1986) Wernicke's aphasia in a 10 year old boy. *Brain and Language*, **29**, 268–285.

Vargha-Khadem, F., Gorman, A.M. and Watters, G.V. (1985) Aphasia and handedness in relation to hemispheric side, age, and injury and severity of cerebral lesion during childhood. *Brain*, **108**, 677–696.

Visch-Brink, E.G. and van de Sandt-Koenderman, M. (1984) The occurrence of paraphasias in the spontaneous speech of children with an acquired aphasia. *Brain and Language*, **23**, 258–271.

Volcan, I., Cole, G.P. and Johnson, K. (1986) A case of muteness of cerebellar origin. *Archives of Neurology*, **43**, 313–314.

Woods, B.T. and Carey, S. (1979) Language deficits after apparent clinical recovery from childhood aphasia. *Annals of Neurology*, **6**, 405–409.

Woods, B.T. and Teuber, H.L. (1978) Changing patterns of childhood aphasia. *Annals of Neurology*, **3**, 273–280.

Worster-Drought, C. (1971) An unusual form of acquired aphasia in children. *Developmental Medicine and Child Neurology*, **13**, 563–571.

Wyllie, W.G. (1948) Acute infantile hemiplegia. *Proceedings of the Royal Society of Medicine*, **41**, 459–466.

Index

Printed and bound by CPI Group (UK) Ltd, Croydon, CR0 4YY